Comprehensive Gynecology and Obstetrics

Series Editors

Ikuo Konishi
National Kyoto Medical Center
Kyoto
Japan

Hidetaka Katabuchi
Department of Obstetrics and Gynecology
Kumamoto University
Kumamoto
Japan

This series presents the current and future perspectives of medical science in gynecology and obstetrics. The authors fully describe the current understanding of a disease including clinical features, imaging, pathology, and molecular biology, and also include the historical aspects and theories for exploring the etiology of the disease. Also, recent developments in diagnostic strategy, medical treatment, surgery, radiotherapy, prevention, and better health-care methods are clearly shown. Thus, each volume in the series focuses on the scientific basis for the pathogenesis of a disease and provides clinical applications that make it possible to offer personalized treatment for each patient. Over the past 20 years, physicians have been working to develop a standard treatment and publish clinical guidelines for a disease based on epidemiological evidence, mainly through the use of randomized clinical trials and meta-analyses. Recently, however, comprehensive genomic and genetic analyses have revealed the differences and variations in biological characteristics even among patients with the same diagnosis and have been focusing on personalized therapy. Now all physicians and patients are entering a new world of "precision medicine" through the use of genomic evidence. We are confident that readers will greatly benefit from the contents of the series with its purview of the exciting and promising future of gynecology and obstetrics.

More information about this series at http://www.springer.com/series/13621

Mikio Mikami
Editor

Surgery for Gynecologic Cancer

Springer

Editor
Mikio Mikami
Department of Obstetrics and Gynecology
School of Medicine, Tokai University
Isehara
Japan

ISSN 2364-1932 ISSN 2364-219X (electronic)
Comprehensive Gynecology and Obstetrics
ISBN 978-981-13-1518-3 ISBN 978-981-13-1519-0 (eBook)
https://doi.org/10.1007/978-981-13-1519-0

This Springer imprint is published by the registered company Springer Nature Singapore Pte Ltd.
The registered company address is: 152 Beach Road, #21-01/04 Gateway East, Singapore 189721, Singapore

Preface

The field of gynecologic surgery has evolved in the last 2 decades—for example, the introduction of laparoscopic and robotic surgery and sentinel node biopsy. In Japan, that state of the art in gynecologic surgery was introduced slowly, carefully, and gradually because our history of gynecologic oncology has been based on gynecologic pathology, not surgery. However we also have the notable history of developing radical hysterectomy for cervical cancer. Minimally invasive surgery also started in the field of reproductive medicine, not gynecologic oncology, in 1970 in Japan. It has been prudent, therefore, for gynecologic oncologists in Japan to introduce minimally invasive surgery (MIS) in their field. Some gynecologic oncologists made a great effort to popularize MIS, so the Japanese national health insurance system eventually started to cover the surgery for endometrial cancer at an early stage and, in 2018, radical hysterectomy for early-stage cervical cancer as well. At the time of the annual meeting of the Society of Gynecologic Oncology in 2018 (SGO2018) in New Orleans, women undergoing radical hysterectomy for early cervical cancer had a significantly higher risk of disease recurrence and worse long-term survival with MIS, including robotic-assisted procedures, two separate studies showed. The prospective study showed that the number of disease recurrences after laparoscopic or robotic-assisted procedures was almost four times higher than the number of recurrences after open surgery, although the absolute numbers were small: 27 recurrences versus 7 in more than 600 patients. The difference translated into a hazard ratio for disease-free survival (DFS) of 3.74 (at 4.5 years) for MIS versus open surgery. A retrospective analysis, based on two national databases, also revealed a statistically significant trend toward declining survival as adoption of MIS increased. All audiences at SGO2018 including me were surprised to hear the result of both presentations, because they had believed that the outcome of MIS for early cervical cancer must be non-inferior to that of open surgery. What is one to think about these results? I recommend that gynecologic surgeons in Japan would have to make the evidence of the non-inferiority of MIS by creating a registry of MIS surgeries and show the benefits of unique Japanese ideas and procedures of MIS to outweigh those of open surgery. I believe Japanese surgeons perform meticulous, awe-inspiring surgeries, which bring great benefits to patients. I hope this book will be a lighthouse in the development of gynecologic surgery and will show clearly our belief that MIS is not inferior to open surgery.

This book presents the current principles and procedures of gynecologic surgeries. The authors have made great efforts to complete their own chapters of specific surgical methods, and I would like to express my sincere thanks to all of them for the successful contribution of their work. I am also grateful to Ms. Machi Sugimoto and Ms. Yoko Arai at Springer Japan for their kind co-operation with me in the publication of this book.

Kanagawa, Japan Mikio Mikami

Contents

Subspecialty Training of Gynecologic Surgery in Japan

1

Takuma Fujii

Abstract

Gynecologic oncologists are the surgeon and have wide range of knowledge regarding the methods of treating gynecologic cancers. It is critical to foster gynecologic oncologists in the society. The Japan society of gynecologic oncology has the fostering program for gynecologic oncologist as a specialist. As a surgeon, a requirement for specialist qualification is a minimum of 3 years of experience at designated training facilities. The trainees have experienced more than 150 patients with gynecologic cancer including surgery, radiotherapy, and chemotherapy. Gynecologic oncologists should also have knowledge regarding the diagnostic radiology, pathology, palliative care, clinical trials, and so on. In surgery, invasive cancer surgery should be performed in a minimum of 100 patients. It is stipulated that radical hysterectomy should be performed in a minimum of 15 patients. In contrast, the most critical issue that remains to be solved is a training for a laparoscopic surgery for malignancies. The popularity of the laparoscopic surgery in the training hospital in Japan was by far behind compared with the one in the USA. Additionally, there are fewer young physicians aspiring to become gynecologists. In general, the number of the gynecologic cancers will be increasing in an aging society. We are then afraid of the shortage of gynecologic oncologists in the future. In the university hospital, the instructor should find and foster medical students with aptitude in gynecologic oncology.

Keywords

Gynecologic cancer · Gynecologic oncologist · Education · Specialist

T. Fujii (✉)
Department of Obstetrics and Gynecology, School of Medicine, Fujita-Health University, Toyoake, Aichi, Japan
e-mail: fujiit44@fujita-hu.ac.jp

M. Mikami (ed.), *Surgery for Gynecologic Cancer*, Comprehensive Gynecology and Obstetrics, https://doi.org/10.1007/978-981-13-1519-0_1

1.1 The Position of Gynecologic Oncologists in the Environment Surrounding Medical Care in Japan

The characteristics of the Japanese medical health insurance system include the following: (1) the guarantee of public health insurance for all citizens, (2) free choice of the institution for medical care, (3) investment of public spending to maintain health insurance for all, and (4) provision of advanced medical services at a low medical fee. This system has helped maintain the highest medical standards and prolong the average life expectancy (Fig. 1.1). For cancer treatment, there are 250 general hospitals with more than 500 hospital beds, and approximately 100 university hospitals provide medical education and play a central role in the treatment of cancer patients [1]. Having institutions available where specialist medical care can be received nearby ensures the quality of medical care in Japan. Since many opinions indicated that the current concept of "specialist" was difficult to understand for the people of Japan, a new specialist system has been established in 2015 for doctors starting initial training [2]. For this specialist system reform, "the Japanese Board of Medical Specialties" was established. This specialty board certifies the specialist system for each basic medical field. If physicians undergo initial training for 2 years and subsequent basic specialty field

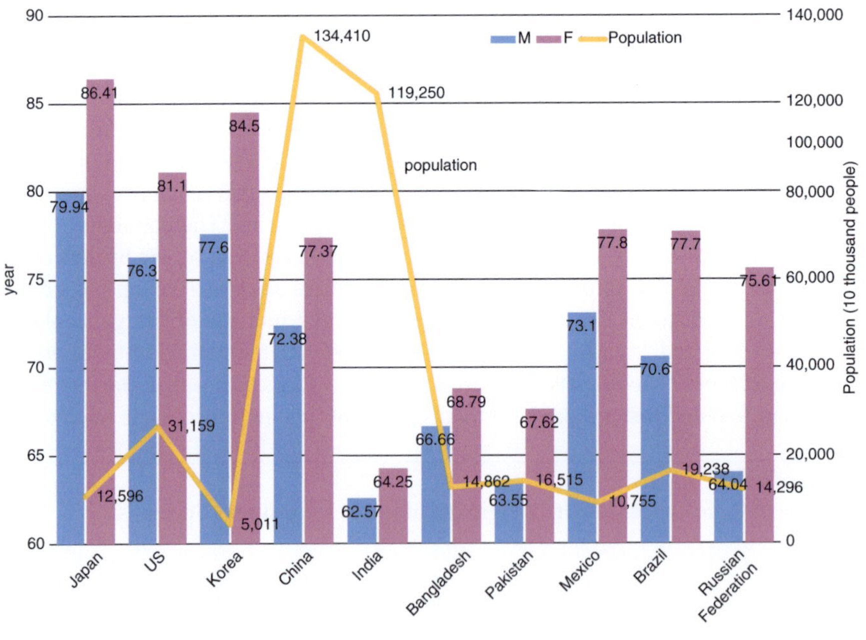

Fig. 1.1 Life expectancies at birth in selected countries [19]. *X*-axis, selected countries; left *Y*-axis, bar indicated average age of the lifetime in each country; and right *Y*-axis, estimated population in each country in 2011 but Japan in 2012. *M* male, *F* female

training for 3 years, new (specialty board) specialists will be certified starting in 2021. After that, there is a framework for acquiring subspecialties within each field, and gynecologic oncologists shall be designated as specialists who will receive a subspecialty rating. Although the Japan Society of Gynecologic Oncology (JSGO) specialist system was started in 2005, a time of profound reform for its educational program has been brought about by the new specialist system established by the Japanese Board of Medical Specialties. One of the characteristics of the board is to prevent the collapse of rural community-based health care. In Japan, a declining birthrate and an increasing aging population cause a remarkable fall in rural populations. The population is concentrated in metropolitan areas, whereas the rural population continues to decline, and this pace of rural depopulation is not expected to slow anytime in the near future. If the rural population decreases, the number of patients will also decrease. Specialists in rural areas will not be able to accumulate enough experience with the fewer number of patients. Although the educational system of the gynecologic oncologists in Japan had started following the American gynecologic oncologist model, this model may no longer suit future specialists under the Japanese Medical Specialty Board.

Additionally, there are fewer young physicians aspiring to become gynecologists. Furthermore, an increasing proportion of young physicians are women; as a result, there are concerns that there will be less active gynecologic oncologists. The qualification for gynecologic oncologists can be acquired after obtaining the qualification for obstetrics and gynecology. If the total number of obstetricians and gynecologists declines, then the number of gynecologic oncologists will spontaneously decline. The member of the Japanese Society of Obstetrics and Gynecology can obtain the certificate of the gynecological oncologists as well as specialists in perinatal care and reproductive medicine. Accordingly, young physicians who are qualified in obstetrics and gynecology subsequently choose one of these three fields. If the benchmark for being a gynecologic oncologist is too high, there was a risk of losing candidates who will choose this specialization.

In the Japanese public health-care insurance system, patients are provided advanced medical services at a low cost; however, as the government budget deficit is growing, there is a demand to reduce medical expenses. However, expensive methods in medical care, such as molecular targeting drugs and robot-assisted surgery, are gaining popularity. Therefore, if associated national health insurance points are considerably reduced and these new and expensive methods in medical care are introduced within insured health-care services, it will be detrimental to hospital management. To provide citizens with medical services considered truly effective for a reasonable fee, supporting evidence must be provided. One aim of JSGO is to foster a group of specialists to provide surgery-based multimodal cancer treatment, while they accumulate evidence through clinical trials of therapeutic outcomes to contribute to the development of future medical treatment [2].

1.2 Gynecological Cancers: Current State, Problems, and Associated Measures

1.2.1 Cervical Cancer

A requirement for specialist qualification is a minimum of 3 years of experience at designated training facilities, during which time candidates must have treated ≥150 patients with gynecologic cancer (surgery, radiotherapy, and chemotherapy) [2]. In surgery, invasive cancer surgery should be performed in a minimum of 100 patients, and it is stipulated that radical hysterectomy should be performed in a minimum of 15 patients [2]. In Japan, radical hysterectomy for early invasive cancer has been historically developed using the Okabayashi procedure, with a high popularization rate. This procedure is included in the requirements for becoming a certified gynecologic oncologist. The skills for this procedure are ideally passed from senior physicians to junior physicians. However, this surgery will be performed in less opportunity in the future. The popularization of concurrent radiation therapy has led to increased opportunity for performing radiotherapy as the first-line treatment, rather than surgery, depending on advanced stage of the disease [3–5]. Gynecologists and radiologists should discuss and determine which therapy is optimal in conference one by one. Laparoscopic surgery for early invasive cervical cancer is ready to be performed as advanced medical care. More laparoscopic surgery induces less open surgery cases, which is a problem for junior physicians to be trained in radical hysterectomy. In fact, there are three options such as open, laparoscopic, or robot-assisted surgery in a limited number of patients with cervical cancer. We should discuss how we teach three procedures for young doctors.

1.2.2 Uterine Cancer

The increase in obesity has led to a higher prevalence of uterine cancer than cervical cancer [6]. The figure presents the prevalence of uterine and ovarian cancer in the USA, Japan, and Korea [7] (Table 1.1). The lifetime risk of uterine cancer is 2% in

Table 1.1 Incidence of cancer among Japan, the USA, and Korea (2012)

	Organ	*N*	ASR	Cumulative risk
Japan	Cervix	9320	10.9	0.96
	Corpus	11,449	10.6	1.12
	Ovary	8921	8.4	0.84
USA	Cervix	12,966	6.6	0.61
	Corpus	49,645	19.5	2.39
	Ovary	20,874	8.0	0.90
Korea	Cervix	3299	9.5	0.95
	Corpus	2016	5.8	0.6
	Ovary	2349	6.8	0.69

N number of the patients with cancer, *ASR* age-standardized rates per 100,000 population
Cumulative risk (%): risk of the disease during 0–74 years of age

the USA, which is remarkably higher than in Japan and Korea. One reason for this is obesity, which is expected to gradually increase in Japan. In obese patients, open surgery carries a higher risk due to its invasiveness; therefore, laparoscopic surgery will be performed more often. At present, laparoscopic surgery for uterine cancer is covered by national health insurance and is no longer avoidable. The procedure is useful for early-stage uterine cancer. In recent years, robot-assisted laparoscopic surgery has drawn attention. To popularize robot-assisted surgery, the effectiveness of the procedure should be also examined.

1.2.3 Ovarian Cancer

The greater issue with ovarian cancer is the mortality rate rather than the prevalence [2]. As things currently stand, without any groundbreaking discoveries enabling the early detection of ovarian cancer, the number of mortalities is expected to rise. Early diagnoses of ovarian cancer are difficult, and it is unlikely that prognosis for the disease will improve in the near future. Currently, the only method associated with prolonged survival is treatment by a gynecologic oncologist. It has been reported that treatment by a gynecologic oncologist appears to extend the patient's life by approximately 6–9 months [8, 9]. In patients who undergo ovarian or tubal resection and are aged 20 years or younger, the risk of incomplete surgery is significantly lower if the operation is performed by a gynecologic oncologist [10]. Since complications also appear to occur significantly more frequently in patients who do not consult a gynecologic oncologist for surgery, some are of the opinion that skills related to surgery consulting should also be included in gynecologic oncologist training [11]. It would seem natural to consider that gynecologic oncologists would treat cases of ovarian cancer. However, no reports on the actual state of such treatment have been released in Japan. In the USA, approximately 40%–70% of patients with suspected ovarian cancer consult with a gynecologic oncologist. Reasons for such percentages are believed to be difficulty accessing such specialists as they tend to be concentrated at certain facilities and other factors such as the health insurance system [9, 12]. Furthermore, although it has also been reported that ovarian cancer should ideally be treated by gynecologic oncologists, it appears likely that nonspecialized physicians are conducting such treatment in actual clinical settings [13]. In the USA, the incidence of ovarian cancer is predicted to increase with the aging of society, with an increase of 19% forecast in the number of cases from 2010 to 2050 [6]. However, localization of gynecologic oncologists is a problem, and it is feared that the burden on physicians may increase in some areas [14]. Ovarian cancer may metastasize to the peritoneal cavity, and prognosis is reported to improve with combined resection of other organs within the peritoneal cavity, such as intestinal resection. Therefore, because there are considerable variations in surgical procedures depending on the extent of spread of the lesion or lesions, labor and surgery time also vary considerably. However, National Health Insurance points remain the same despite these differences. Given the lack of obstetrician/gynecologists, operating room nurses, and anesthesiologists in addition to factors such as the increase in sales tax putting pressure on hospital management, para-aortic lymph node dissection may have to be omitted when there are too few slots allocated for surgery at a particular hospital. Accordingly, ovarian cancer surgery, for which the time required is difficult to determine in advance, should be performed at "specialized cancer hospitals" at which there is a greater level of understanding regarding the disease.

1.3 Educational Issues for Gynecological Oncologists

1.3.1 Comprehensive Medical Care

Gynecologic oncologists must have extensive knowledge and medical ethics on a range of treatment methods for gynecologic cancers, and they must implement the latest surgery-based multimodal treatments for gynecologic cancers [2]. They provide medical care in collaboration with other departments and are required to have skills to perform the central role in medical care. Other specialist fields include various hospital departments for each cancer; specialists in pathology, diagnostic radiology, radiotherapy, and chemotherapy must interact with gynecologic oncologists. Gynecologic oncologists are also required to work with nurses and care managers involved in colostomy care, palliative care/end-of-life care, and home care. Knowledge on the social insurance system and long-term care insurance is required, and gynecologic oncologists should be familiar with the cost of medical care [15]. Cancer treatment is not limited to surgery, radiotherapy, or anti-cancer therapy. Half of the cancer cases are not early-stage cancers; thus, palliative care is another important aspect in cancer care. We believe that making young doctors understand palliative therapy is extremely important in their education.

1.3.2 Surgical Education

How are surgical skills acquired? In the past, young doctors were introduced to surgery as a senior's surgical assistant and learned different procedures by observation. However, changes in the social environment, such as ethical concerns, individual abilities, and the need to acquire a complex and high level of skill, have made it increasingly difficult to learn procedures using conventional techniques today. Therefore, it is becoming more important than ever to make an accurate assessment of the behaviors of highly performing individuals, i.e., their surgical competency and education assessment. Because surgical mentors have not learned the educational method, they faced to the great difficulty in teaching. Instructors at teaching hospitals, such as university hospitals, feel burdened by the troubles of teaching and experience many difficulties despite spending a lot of time in this obligatory task, and it is not unusual for them to move to private hospitals. Physicians in the USA specializing in laparoscopic surgery often move to private hospitals for this reason

[16]. The level of difficulty in teaching laparoscopic surgery is remarkably higher than that in teaching open surgery. In open surgery, a medical instructor can assume what trainees are thinking or attempting by seeing the movement of their manipulation with the scalpel, scissors, and forceps. The instructor can then help them develop the surgical field and assist with the procedure to effectively teach them. In laparoscopic surgery, the instructor might not understand what a trainee is performing until immediately before the maneuver as the movement of instruments is viewed on a monitor. The critical difference with open surgery is that the movement of the operator's hands cannot be seen in a widely developed surgical field. Furthermore, the visible surgical field differs depending on the placement of a camera, which largely depends on the skill in camera placement. In laparoscopic surgery, once a mistake is made, it can cause serious complications. Laparoscopic surgery is extremely difficult and involves arduous labor for the medical instructor. As a result, there is a severe shortage of medical instructors at teaching hospitals. Whether laparoscopic surgery, including robot-assisted surgery, will gain popularity in Japan may depend on instructions in the future. The Japanese Society for Gynecologic Oncology aims to popularize laparoscopic surgery; they are planning to hold nationwide seminars.

Trainees beginning laparoscopic surgery should start it gradually as there are multiple training methods other than performing it on an actual patient. It is important to thoroughly observe surgical procedures and understand the movement of the staff and the setup in the operating room. The surgical procedure and skills can be verified through surgical videos. In Japan, limited simulations using cadavers and animals are performed because of ethical reasons, anatomical differences, and the high cost involved. Nevertheless, these methods are indispensable experiences and should be required before performing the actual surgery.

For the concurrent resection of other organs, the person who performs these procedures greatly differs between Japan and the western countries. In Japan, there is no additional surgical remuneration for physicians, and the fee is determined based on national health insurance points according to the disease category, so there is no incentive for gynecologists to resect other organs such as the intestine, bowel, or spleen. Considering the risk of postoperative complications, intestinal resection is generally performed by a surgeon. At present, a very limited number of gynecologists perform intestinal resection.

1.3.3 Understanding Radiology and Pathology

Radiotherapy is a one of the fundamental treatments for cancer, and knowledge on this radiotherapy is required [2]. Gynecologic oncologists share clinical information with radiotherapists to set the optimal irradiation field, and they should be involved in determining the treatment plan. The latest 3D radiation therapy and IMRT have enabled more precise pinpoint irradiation; sharing accurate information has become all the more important.

The pathological diagnosis in gynecology is difficult in general. There is a high rate of complaints made in the USA related to gynecologic tumors [17], so this problem is not unique to Japan. Regular conferences should be held with pathologists for having detailed discussions on individual cases. The diagnostic criteria for ovarian cancer have recently changed, which has made the diagnosis increasingly difficult.

1.3.4 Understanding Clinical Trials

Clinical trials are conducted to develop "better methods of treatment" for patients, and the results are returned to patients as evidence [2]. There is no doubt that the results of clinical trials have altered conventional standard treatments and contributed to medical advances. The Gynecologic Oncology Group (GOG) 111 trial, which led to combined cisplatin and paclitaxel therapy becoming the standard treatment for ovarian cancer, had a very strong impact [18]. Because clinical trials require an appropriate number of patients to be registered, gathering patients at specific facilities is very effective for such trials. It is important that specialists have an understanding of clinical trials and are educated to proactively encourage medical practitioners and patients to participate in such trials.

1.4 Summary

Training at integrated institutions is important for improving skills, but training at hospitals with few patients is not advisable for physicians and patients. In the USA, there are approximately 100 institutions with gynecologic oncologists, which are unevenly distributed [11]. However, training facilities meet strict criteria and accumulate a considerable number of cases. Therefore, it is an ideal environment that facilitates clinical trials and makes it easy to accumulate evidence.

By contrast, hospitals are scattered throughout Japan. While hospitals are accessible nearby, institutions that meet standards similar to those of hospitals in the USA are extremely limited. Given the limited resources, we have no choice but to independently improve individual skills.

Unlike the situation in the USA, it is very difficult for physicians to be transferred due to differences in the working conditions unique to Japan. Nonetheless, specialized training should be conducted at an integrated institution if circumstances allow it. Fostering leaders in gynecologic oncology is an important mission, and it can be accomplished by returning to local communities after obtaining specialist qualifications to provide medical skills in gynecologic cancer and by teaching younger physicians. Among these activities, educating medical students at university hospitals with a medical department is of utmost importance. Unless students with aptitude in gynecologic oncology are discovered and fostered, future human resources will be depleted in this field. I would like to emphasize that physicians working at university hospitals should be given a special incentive in this mission to train the next generation.

Acknowledgments The author would like to thank Ms. Usui, a secretary at the Department of Obstetrics and Gynecology, Fujita Health University, for the expert help in the formatting and the preparation of the manuscript.

References

1. Yamaguchi K. Overview of cancer control programs in Japan. Jpn J Clin Oncol. 2002;32(Suppl):S22–31.
2. Fujii T. Changing state of gynecologic oncologist specialty in Japan. J Obstet Gynaecol Res. 2016;42(5):481–8. https://doi.org/10.1111/jog.12970.
3. Japan Society of Obstetrics and Gynecology. Gynecologic tumor committee report-2002. Acta Obstet Gynaecol Jpn. 2005;57(5):990–1046.
4. Japan Society of Obstetrics and Gynecology. Gynecologic tumor committee report-2008. Acta Obstet Gynaecol Jpn. 2010;62(3):827–910.
5. Japan Society of Obstetrics and Gynecology. Gynecologic tumor committee report-2012. Acta Obstet Gynaecol Jpn. 2014;66(3):995–1038.
6. Wallace AH, Havrilesky LJ, Valea FA, Barnett JC, Berchuck A, Myers ER. Projecting the need for gynecologic oncologists for the next 40 years. Obstet Gynecol. 2010;116(6):1366–72. https://doi.org/10.1097/AOG.0b013e3181fc3a22.
7. globocan. 2012. http://globocan.iarc.fr/Pages/online.aspx
8. Giede KC, Kieser K, Dodge J, Rosen B. Who should operate on patients with ovarian cancer? An evidence-based review. Gynecol Oncol. 2005;99(2):447–61. https://doi.org/10.1016/j.ygyno.2005.07.008.
9. Stewart SL, Rim SH, Richards TB. Gynecologic oncologists and ovarian cancer treatment: avenues for improved survival. J Womens Health (2002). 2011;20(9):1257–60. https://doi.org/10.1089/jwh.2011.3053.
10. Eskander RN, Bristow RE, Saenz NC, Saenz CC. A retrospective review of the effect of surgeon specialty on the management of 190 benign and malignant pediatric and adolescent adnexal masses. J Pediatr Adolesc Gynecol. 2011;24(5):282–5. https://doi.org/10.1016/j.jpag.2011.03.012.
11. Aviki EM, Rauh-Hain JA, Clark RM, Hall TR, Berkowitz LR, Boruta DM, et al. Gynecologic oncologist as surgical consultant: intraoperative consultations during general gynecologic surgery as an important focus of gynecologic oncology training. Gynecol Oncol. 2015;137(1):93–7. https://doi.org/10.1016/j.ygyno.2015.01.536.
12. Goff BA, Miller JW, Matthews B, Trivers KF, Andrilla CH, Lishner DM, et al. Involvement of gynecologic oncologists in the treatment of patients with a suspicious ovarian mass. Obstet Gynecol. 2011;118(4):854–62. https://doi.org/10.1097/AOG.0b013e31822dabc6.
13. Committee Opinion No. 477: the role of the obstetrician-gynecologist in the early detection of epithelial ovarian cancer. Obstet Gynecol. 2011;117(3):742–6. https://doi.org/10.1097/AOG.0b013e31821477db.
14. Shalowitz DI, Vinograd AM, Giuntoli RL, 2nd. Geographic access to gynecologic cancer care in the United States. Gynecol Oncol 2015;138(1):115–120. doi:https://doi.org/10.1016/j.ygyno.2015.04.025.
15. Hoffman MS, Bodurka DC. Surgical education and training program development for gynecologic oncology: American perspective. Gynecol Oncol. 2009;114(2 Suppl):S47–51. https://doi.org/10.1016/j.ygyno.2008.12.023.

16. Rogers RM. Chapter 6. Training the gynecologic surgeon. In: Rock JA, Jones HW, editors. Te Linde's operative gynecology. 10th ed. Philadelphia, PA: Lippincott Williams & Wilkins; 2011. p. 73–9.
17. Troxel DB. An insurer's perspective on error and loss in pathology. Arch Pathol Lab Med. 2005;129(10):1234–6. https://doi.org/10.1043/1543-2165(2005)129[1234:aipoea]2.0.co;2.
18. McGuire WP, Hoskins WJ, Brady MF, Kucera PR, Partridge EE, Look KY, et al. Cyclophosphamide and cisplatin compared with paclitaxel and cisplatin in patients with stage III and stage IV ovarian cancer. N Engl J Med. 1996;334(1):1–6. https://doi.org/10.1056/nejm199601043340101.
19. Life expectancies at birth in selected countries. In: Cancer statics in Japan '14. Foundation for Promotion of Cancer Research. 2014. http://ganjoho.jp/data/reg_stat/statistics/brochure/2014/cancer_statistics_2014.pdf.

Gynecologic Oncology Fellowship Training in the United States

2

Laurie L. Brunette, Barbara A. Goff, Lynda D. Roman, and Koji Matsuo

Abstract

Gynecologic oncology is a growing field composed of physicians who have completed subspecialty training in the comprehensive care of women with gynecologic malignancies including cancers of the uterine cervix, uterine corpus, fallopian tubes, ovaries, vagina, vulva, and other rare gynecologic tumors. They are proficient in performing surgery not just on pelvic organs, but in gastrointestinal, urologic, plastic and reconstructive, and other abdominal and pelvic surgical techniques through a variety of approaches in order to treat newly diagnosed and recurrent gynecologic malignancies. They are also knowledgeable in chemotherapeutic and targeted therapies, radiation therapy, critical care, and palliative care. Gynecologic oncologists understand and advance the field through research in risk factors, prevention, and treatment of these cancers that afflict over 100,000 US women annually. After completing a 4-year obstetrics and gynecology residency, an additional 3- or 4-year fellowship program is necessary to become a gynecologic oncologist. These fellowship programs are regulated and accredited by a central, national agency, the Accreditation Council for Graduate Medical Education (ACGME). Strict requirements are in place ensuring that graduating fellows are competent in patient care, surgery, medical knowledge, and research but are also professional and ethical physicians who efficiently function within and contribute to the greater medical community. In this chapter, we describe the

L. L. Brunette (✉) · L. D. Roman · K. Matsuo (✉)
Division of Gynecologic Oncology, Department of Obstetrics and Gynecology, University of Southern California, Los Angeles, CA, USA

Norris Comprehensive Cancer Center, University of Southern California, Los Angeles, CA, USA
e-mail: Laurie.Brunette@med.usc.edu; Koji.Matsuo@med.usc.edu

B. A. Goff
Division of Gynecologic Oncology, Department of Obstetrics and Gynecology, University of Washington, Seattle, WA, USA

M. Mikami (ed.), *Surgery for Gynecologic Cancer*, Comprehensive Gynecology and Obstetrics, https://doi.org/10.1007/978-981-13-1519-0_2

history, structure, and admissions process of gynecologic oncology fellowship in the United States and explore the current education and demographics of gynecologic oncology fellows and the role of gynecologic oncologists in the education of future specialists and treatment of US women afflicted with gynecologic cancers.

Keywords
Gynecologic oncology · Fellowship · Obstetrics and gynecology · Gynecologic surgery

2.1 The History of Gynecologic Oncology in the United States

Gynecologic oncology was first recognized in the United States as a unique medical and surgical subspecialty of obstetrics and gynecology in the late 1960s. Prior to this, obstetricians and gynecologists relied heavily on other surgical and medical services to provide adequate care to women with gynecologic malignancies. The Society of Gynecologic Oncologists (SGO) was founded in 1969 with the purpose of "identifying the principles, knowledge, and skills related to gynecologic malignancies; guide the development of a subspecialty devoted exclusively to this field; and promote research, education, and practice of the subspecialty [1]." In the 1970s, gynecologic oncologists began using chemotherapy and were first allowed to earn hospital privileges in gastrointestinal and urinary tract surgery. The field has continued to expand in number, and novel treatment modalities and diagnostic tools are continuously incorporated. Today, SGO has approximately 2000 members which includes primarily gynecologic oncologists, as well as medical oncologists, pathologists, radiation oncologists, hematologists, surgical oncologists, obstetrician/gynecologists, nurses, nurse practitioners, physician assistants, social workers, fellows-in-training, residents, and other allied healthcare professionals interested in the treatment and care of women's cancer.

In 1972 a gynecologic oncology subspecialty board was created, and accredited fellowship training programs began to be established [2]. There has been an increase in the number of fellowship programs and positions over time, and in 2018, there will be 50 accredited programs (Table 2.1). The gynecologic oncology fellowship programs were previously managed by the American Board of Obstetrics and Gynecology (ABOG). As of 2017, all accredited gynecologic oncology fellowships will be managed by the Accreditation Council for Graduate Medical Education (ACGME) (www.acgme.org).

ACGME defines a gynecologic oncologist as a subspecialist in obstetrics and gynecology who has advanced knowledge of the comprehensive management of patients with gynecologic malignancies. This includes familiarity with those diagnostic and therapeutic procedures necessary for the total care of a woman at risk for or diagnosed with gynecologic cancer or precursors and complications resulting

Table 2.1 Gynecologic oncology fellowships in the United States by length and location

Program	Location (City, State)
Three-year programs	
Brigham and Women's Hospital	Boston, MA
Case Western Reserve University/University Hospitals Cleveland Medical Center	Cleveland, OH
Cedars-Sinai Medical Center	Los Angeles, CA
Cleveland Clinic Foundation	Cleveland, OH
Duke University Hospital	Durham, NC
Icahn School of Medicine of Mount Sinai	New York, NY
Johns Hopkins University	Baltimore, MD
Massachusetts General Hospital	Boston, MA
Mayo Clinic College of Medicine and Science	Rochester, MN
McGaw Medical Center of Northwestern University	Chicago, IL
Medical College of Georgia	Augusta, GA
Montefiore Medical Center/Albert Einstein College of Medicine	Bronx, NY
New York Presbyterian Hospital (Columbia Campus)	New York, NY
New York University School of Medicine	New York, NY
Ohio State University/Mt Carmel Hospital Program	Columbus, OH
Stanford Health Care-Sponsored Stanford University	Stanford, CA
SUNY Health Science Center at Brooklyn	Brooklyn, NY
Temple University Hospital/Fox Chase Cancer Center	Philadelphia, PA
UCLA David Geffen School of Medicine/UCLA Medical Center	Los Angeles, CA
University of Alabama Medical Center	Birmingham, AL
University of California (Davis) Health System	Sacramento, CA
University of California (San Francisco)	San Francisco, CA
University of Chicago	Chicago, IL
University of Colorado	Aurora, CO
University of Iowa Hospitals and Clinics	Iowa City, IA
University of Kentucky College of Medicine	Lexington, KY
University of Michigan Hospitals and Health Centers	Ann Arbor, MI
University of Minnesota Medical School	Minneapolis, MN
University of North Carolina Hospitals	Chapel Hill, NC
University of Oklahoma Health Sciences Center	Oklahoma City, OK
University of Pennsylvania Health System	Philadelphia, PA
University of South Florida	Tampa, FL
University of Southern California/LAC+USC Medical Center	Los Angeles, CA
University of Tennessee	Germantown, TN
University of Virginia Medical Center	Charlottesville, VA
University of Wisconsin Hospitals and Clinics	Madison, WI
UPMC Medical Education/Magee Women's Hospital	Pittsburgh, PA
Yale-New Haven Medical Center	New Haven, CT
Four-year programs	
Brown University (Women and Infants Hospital of Rhode Island)	Providence, RI
Detroit Medical Center/Wayne State University	Detroit, MI
Jackson Memorial Hospital/University of Miami	Miami, FL
Memorial Sloan Kettering Cancer Center	New York, NY
National Capital Consortium/Walter Reed National Military Medical Center	Bethesda, MD
University of Buffalo/Roswell Park Cancer Institute	Buffalo, NY
University of California (Irvine)	Orange, CA

(continued)

Table 2.1 (continued)

Program	Location (City, State)
University of California (San Diego) Medical Center	La Jolla, CA
University of Texas M.D. Anderson Cancer Center	Houston, TX
University of Texas Southwestern Medical School	Dallas, TX
University of Washington	Seattle, WA
Washington University/BJH/SLCH Consortium (alternates between 3 and 4 years)	St. Louis, MO

Listed in alphabetic order

therefrom [3]. Gynecologic oncologists are a small group of highly skilled clinicians and surgeons who treat a relatively high proportion of malignancies affecting women. In the United States, 852,630 women are expected to be diagnosed with cancer in 2017 [4]. Of these, 107,470 women will be diagnosed with gynecologic malignancies including cancers of the uterine cervix, uterine corpus, fallopian tubes, ovaries, vulva, vagina, and other rare tumors. This results in 12.6% of all US female malignancies being treated by gynecologic oncologists. Most gynecologic oncologists provide comprehensive care to their patients from diagnosis to cure or end of life and incorporate surgical and medical management, critical care, and palliative care. Some gynecologic oncologists do not personally provide aspects of this treatment, but still function as the leader of a multidisciplinary team of medical oncologists, radiation oncologists, other surgical specialists, reproductive endocrinologists, geneticists, and palliative and critical care specialists to provide comprehensive care to their patients. This differs from most other oncologic specialties in which the surgeons are not responsible for the other aspects of the patient's cancer care. In order to gain the surgical, clinical, communication, and research skills that are essential to becoming a gynecologic oncologist, it is necessary to pursue fellowship training after completion of a 4-year obstetrics and gynecology residency.

2.2 Gynecologic Oncology Fellowship Structure and Education

As of 1996, all gynecologic oncology fellowships were required to be at least 36 months in length of training and must include at least 12 months of research and 24 months of clinical training [5]. As of 2017, 24% of programs are 48 months in length. These 4-year programs generally have more time dedicated to research than 3-year programs, but may provide additional time in clinical training as well.

In a 2016 study, applicants reported choosing a 3-year versus 4-year program based on surgical volume, patient population, faculty, and/or reputation 43% of the time, whereas 28% reported it was where they happened to match, but not what they preferred. Nineteen percent chose a program based on the amount of research time available, and 10% expressed a desire for a 3-year fellowship so they could enter the workforce and earn a higher income sooner [6]. There was no difference between the rates of acquiring an academic position afterward between those attending a

3-year and 4-year program (58 vs. 52%). Graduates of 4-year programs were more likely to hold advanced degrees (48 vs. 20%, $p < 0.001$) and have more than ten publications at the completion of fellowship (43 vs. 18%, $p < 0.001$). Forty percent of those fellows with advanced degrees received them during fellowship.

ACGME has outlined a list of six core competencies expected of graduating gynecologic oncology fellows: Patient Care and Procedural Skills, Medical Knowledge, Practice-Based Learning and Improvement, Interpersonal and Communication Skills, Professionalism, and Systems-Based Practice (Fig. 2.1) [3]. As part of the first core competency of *Patient Care and Procedural Skills* (Fig. 2.2), fellows must be able to competently manage gynecologic cancer and its complications. This includes radical operations performed on the female reproductive organs; dissection of inguinal, pelvic, and para-aortic lymph nodes; and adjunctive procedures such as cystoscopy, proctoscopy, sigmoidoscopy, paracentesis, thoracentesis, and placement of central venous catheters. They also must be competent at the administration of chemotherapeutic drugs and targeted therapeutics and the recognition of complications that may result from the use of such agents. While graduating fellows do not administer radiation, they usually make the decision of when it is

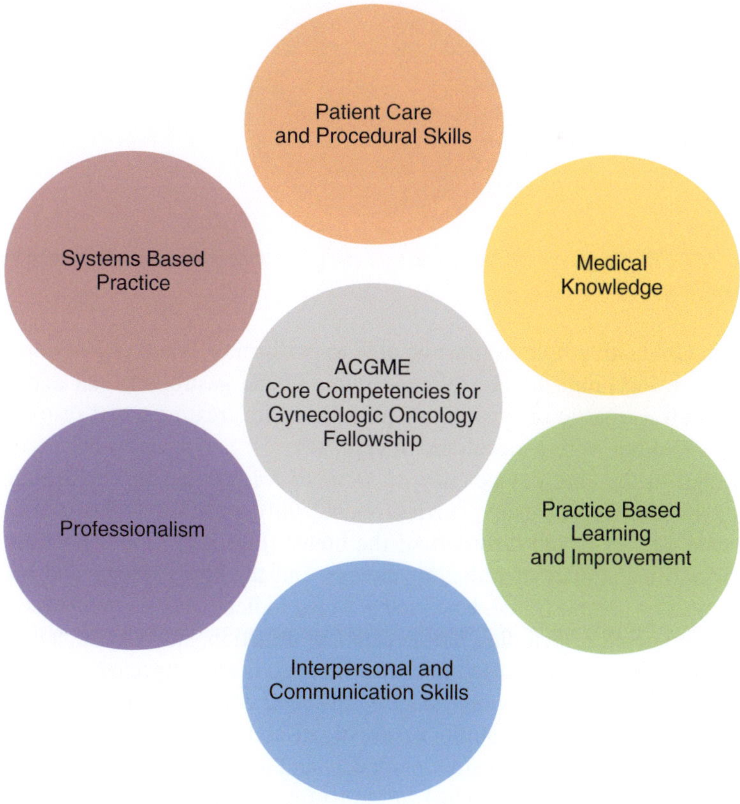

Fig. 2.1 ACGME core competencies for gynecologic oncology fellowship

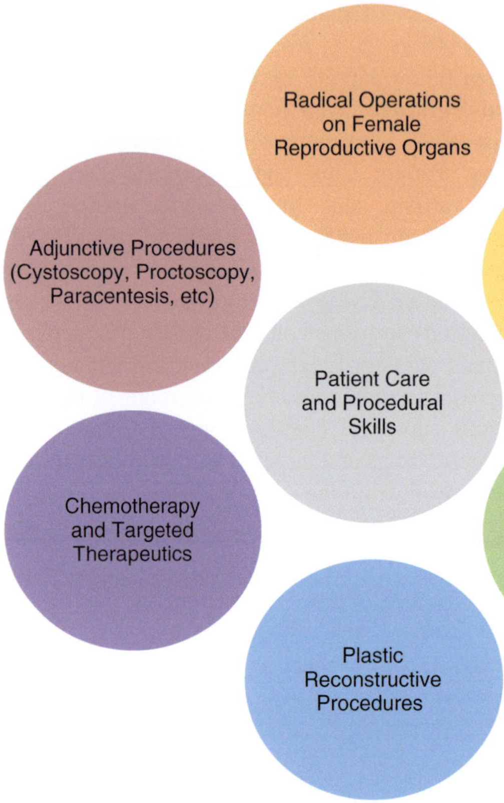

Fig. 2.2 ACGME components of the patient care and procedural skills core competency for gynecologic oncology fellows

indicated. Graduating fellows must be able to perform or, when appropriate, direct care teams to accomplish surgical procedures of the gastrointestinal and urinary tracts as well as plastic reconstructive procedures for treatment and restoration of function in women with gynecologic malignancy.

Essential to the core competency of *Medical Knowledge* are the principles of gynecologic pathology, cancer genetics, oncofertility, critical care, hospice and palliative care medicine, and disorders of the breast (Fig. 2.3). Understanding of the methods and techniques of radiation therapy and the radiobiology and radiation physics must be demonstrated. Knowledge of the indications for chemotherapy and targeted therapeutics, including the mechanism of action, side effects, advantages, and disadvantages of agents used in cancer therapy, is also expected.

The *Practice-Based Learning and Improvement* core competency dictates that fellows must demonstrate the ability to investigate and evaluate their care of patients, to appraise and assimilate scientific evidence, and to continuously improve patient care based on constant self-evaluation and lifelong learning. Fellows must also demonstrate *Interpersonal and Communication Skills* as part of the fourth core

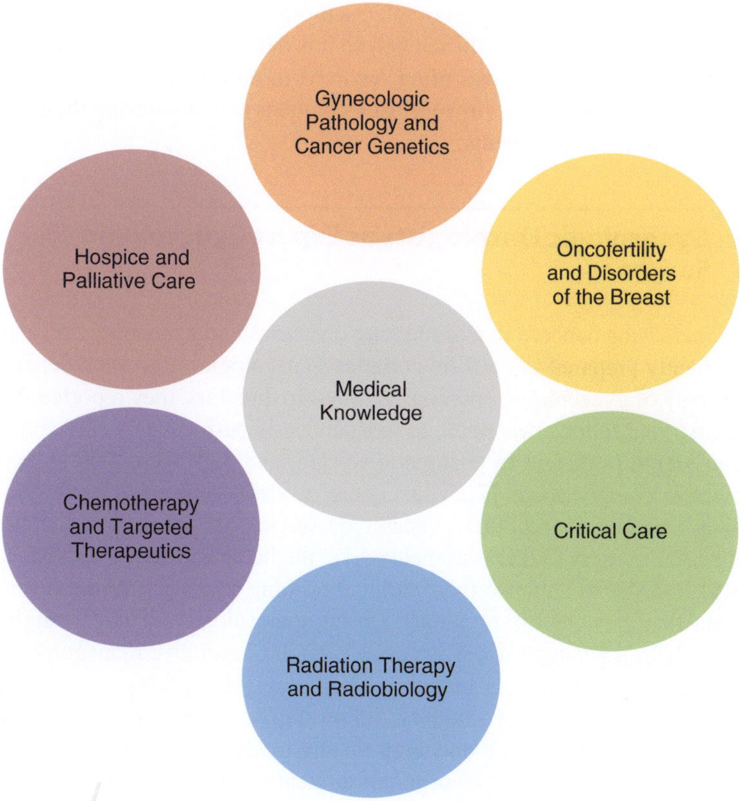

Fig. 2.3 ACGME components of medical knowledge core competency for gynecologic oncology fellows

competency. These skills should result in the effective exchange of information and collaboration with patients, their families, and health professionals.

As part of the two remaining core competencies (*Professionalism and Systems-Based Practice*), fellows must demonstrate a commitment to carrying out professional responsibilities and an adherence to ethical principles. They must also demonstrate an awareness of and responsiveness to the larger context and system of healthcare, as well as the ability to call effectively on other resources in the system to provide optimal healthcare.

Beyond the core competencies, fellows are expected to participate in a scholarly activity that will enhance his or her understanding of the latest scientific techniques and encourage interaction with other scientists. The minimum 12 months of dedicated research curriculum must include didactic instruction in research design, grant writing, research methodology, scientific writing, and presentation skills. Fellows should graduate prepared to pursue research funding and academic positions and be an independent investigator if they desire. They must be given the opportunity to present their academic contributions to the gynecologic oncology community, and each fellow must complete a thesis and defend it during fellowship. The thesis is required to be published before it is defended during the board certification process. Fellows are also often involved in enrolling patients into clinical trials to test novel therapeutics or surgical techniques and monitoring their response and reactions to these treatments.

2.3 Gynecologic Oncologists as Expert Gynecologic Surgeons

There is increasing concern that graduating obstetrics and gynecology residents are not sufficiently prepared to perform complex gynecologic surgeries independently. In one survey of gynecologic oncology fellowship directors, they reported that only 44% of first-year fellows were able to independently perform a hysterectomy, 63% were considered proficient in postoperative care, and 52% were able to recognize postoperative complications [7]. Thus, some residents seek additional training in gynecologic oncology and other gynecologic surgery subspecialties such as minimally invasive surgery (MIS) or female pelvic medicine and reconstructive surgery (FPMRS) in order to enhance their surgical training and increase the diversity of techniques that they can offer patients. During gynecologic oncology training, fellows hone their skills in preoperative evaluation, postoperative management, and a variety of surgical techniques including open, vaginal, laparoscopic, and robotic approaches to gynecologic procedures. Fellowship programs vary on whether they rely solely on the gynecologic oncology faculty to teach the fellows the necessary surgical skills or whether they incorporate surgical services such as urology, breast, colorectal, and hepatobiliary surgery. Many programs also incorporate surgical simulators, animal labs, cadaver labs, and instructional videos to achieve this end.

The field of gynecologic oncology has undergone a dramatic change after the introduction of robotic surgery, which first gained US Food and Drug Administration (FDA) approval for gynecologic surgery in 2005. In 2013, 31% of hysterectomies completed in the United States were performed robotically, resulting in a decrease in the use of open and vaginal techniques [8]. A survey of gynecologic oncology fellows and fellowship directors in 2010 showed that 95% of respondents reported having at least one robot at their institution, 95% utilize it, and 94% of fellows plan on performing robotic surgery after completing their fellowship training [9]. Structured training of gynecologic oncology fellows in robotic surgeries has also become increasingly important. Multiple institutions have published data on the success of their robotic training programs which may include didactic and hands-on training, instructional videos, assistance at the operating room table, and ultimately performance of segments of the procedure in tandem with the attending physician [10–13].

Owing to this additional training in surgical techniques and familiarity with difficult dissection and removal of malignant masses, gynecologic oncologists are generally considered the most skilled of the gynecologic surgeons. This has resulted in an increasing number of patients being referred to gynecologic oncologists for complex or challenging gynecologic surgeries, even if malignancy is not suspected. Many obstetricians and gynecologists also rely on gynecologic oncologists to assist with challenging obstetrics cases, such as those with abnormal placentation that may require hysterectomies at the time of cesarean delivery [14, 15].

2.4 Gynecologic Oncology Fellowship Application Process

All matriculating US fellows must have satisfactorily completed an accredited ACGME or Royal College of Physicians and Surgeons of Canada (RCPSC) obstetrics and gynecology residency. Candidates submit their application to a centralized agency, the Electronic Residency Application Service (ERAS®) (www.amc.org/services/eras/). Applications include demographic information, medical school transcripts, and scores from US Medical Licensing Exams (USMLE®) and/or Comprehensive Osteopathic Medical Licensing Examination of the United States (COMLEX-USA) and Council on Resident Education in Obstetrics and Gynecology (CREOG) exams. They also submit a curriculum vitae including details of their higher education, research publications and presentations, volunteer activities, work experience, and honors and awards. Letters of recommendation are required and are often from residency program directors, department chairs, gynecologic oncologists, and other research and clinical mentors. After reviewing the applications, programs offer a subset of applicants in-person interviews which usually occur in the spring and summer the year prior to the fellows' expected start date. After interviews are conducted, applicants and fellowship programs rank each other in order of desirability. These preferences are then entered into the National Resident Matching Program (NRMP®) (www.nrmp.org), also known as The Match®, which uses a computerized mathematical algorithm to match applicants to positions based on these preferences. Each fellowship program accepts one or two applicants per year. Rarely, programs may not participate in The Match® if they do not have a position available or if they offer the position to someone outside of The Match®. The number of programs participating in The Match® and the number of positions offered through The Match® over time are represented in Fig. 2.4.

Gynecologic oncology is considered one of the most competitive subspecialties of obstetrics and gynecology, demonstrated by match rates ranging from 52% to 74%, since 2004. The number of applicants participating in the NRMP Match® has been steadily increasing over time (Fig. 2.5). In 2017, there were 83 applicants who entered The Match®, and 54 (65%) of them matched. Various surveys of gynecologic oncology fellows have been conducted that demonstrate the characteristics of applicants to the specialty. In a survey of gynecologic oncology fellows in 2000, 80% had completed their residency at a university program, and 33% worked with gynecologic oncology fellows during their residency. Twenty-five percent took time off in between residency and fellowship to improve their application. Most fellows planned to go into academics (78%), and 20% planned to go into combined academic/private practice [2]. This was similar to rates found in a 2003 survey in which 78% of responding gynecologic oncology fellows planned to pursue academic

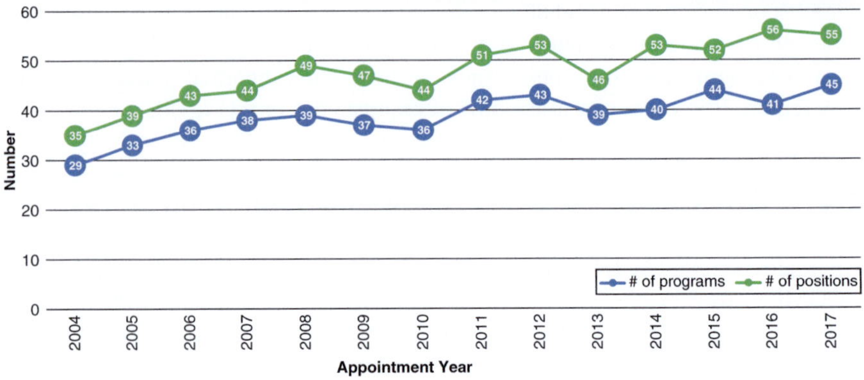

Fig. 2.4 Number of US gynecologic oncology fellowship programs and positions in the NRMP Match® from 2004 to 2017. National Resident Matching Program, Results and Data: Specialties Matching Service 2008–2017 Appointment Year. National Resident Matching Program, Washington, DC. 2008–2017. http://www.nrmp.org/match-data/fellowship-match-data

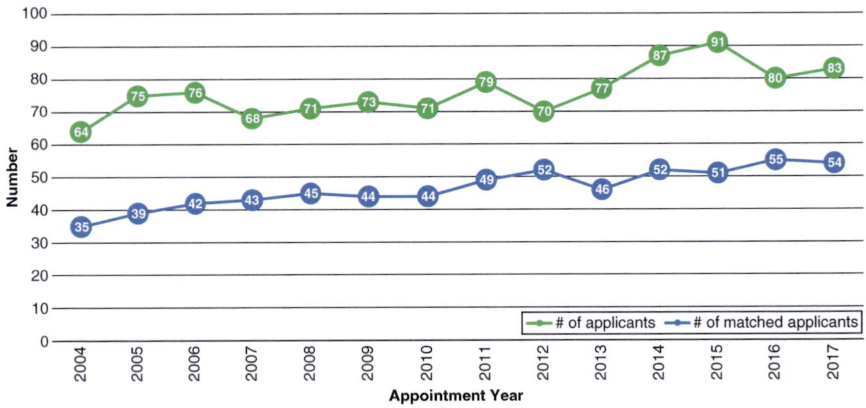

Fig. 2.5 Number of total and matched applicants to US gynecologic oncology programs participating in the NRMP Match® from 2004 to 2017. National Resident Matching Program, Results and Data: Specialties Matching Service 2008–2017 Appointment Year. National Resident Matching Program, Washington, DC. 2008-2017. http://www.nrmp.org/match-data/fellowship-match-data/

positions upon graduating [5]. A study in 2013 showed that applicants had ample prior research experience with 66% of those who matched having one to three published manuscripts and 16% having more than three [16]. Given the competitive nature and the focus on training academicians, there is even some concern that applicants to gynecologic oncology are including unverified publications and honors on their applications [17].

Most recently, in a survey of 58 applicants to gynecologic oncology fellowship, the highly qualified nature of matched applicants was demonstrated [16]. Seventy-one percent of respondents matched including 49% of applicants matching at the program they ranked first and 86% matching to one of the programs they ranked in their top four. Successful applicants applied to and interviewed at multiple programs. Seventy-six percent applied to at least 26 programs. Half of applicants who did not match interviewed at less than five programs, and only 4% of those who matched interviewed at less than five programs. Ninety-eight percent of applicants had attended an allopathic medical school, while only 2% graduated from an osteopathic medical school. A quarter of applicants were members of the Alpha Omega Alpha (AOA) Honor Medical Society. Applicants had extensive research experience including 77% who had done at least one poster presentation, 82% had at least one published manuscript, and 77 had given at least one oral presentation. Additionally, 82% had a letter of recommendation from a nationally known specialist, and 60% did a visiting elective.

Every year there are applicants who do not match into gynecologic oncology, and some elect to apply again in the future after committing years to improving their application. This may include performing additional clinical or basic science research, publishing manuscripts and presenting at national meetings, practicing as obstetrician and gynecologists and honing surgical skills, completing other fellowships (minimally invasive surgery, palliative care, surgical oncology, research fellowships, or others), or seeking mentorship from experts in the field of gynecologic oncology.

2.5 Gynecologic Oncology Fellow and Faculty Demographics

When practicing SGO members were surveyed; 52% held academic positions, 21% were in private practice, 20% had a combination of private practice and academic involvement, and 7% had other types of practices [6]. In a 2014 survey of gynecologic oncology applications, 75, 5, 14, and 5% were Caucasian, Black, Asian, and others, respectively [16]. SGO data show that overall women comprise 36% of gynecologic oncologists and 42% of academic gynecologic oncology faculty [18, 19]. Historically, obstetrics and gynecology and gynecologic oncology were male-dominated fields, and senior faculty and leadership roles remain dominated by men [18, 20, 21]. However, for over 20 years, more than half of obstetrics and gynecology residents are women [22]. The proportion of female obstetrics and gynecology faculty physicians increased from 30% in 1994 to 50% in 2008, and obstetrics and gynecology now have the largest proportion of women residents of any specialty (83%) [23, 24]. Similarly, gynecologic oncology fellows are now disproportionately female (74%) [19]. Gender disparities are seen among this subspecialty as well with only 21% of division directors being female, and among the gynecologic oncologists who are department chairs, 21% are women [18, 20].

A survey in 2015 of work-life balance among current gynecologic oncology fellows revealed that the median age was 32 years old (range 28–39 years old). Seventy-seven percent were married or partnered, and 41% had children. Time spent at work exceeded 60 h per week for 71% of fellows and exceeded 80 h per week for 44%. Only 22% were satisfied with work-life balance during fellowship [25]. However, 87% of fellows reported overall satisfaction with their fellowship [2]. Areas that could improve fellowship satisfaction were formal didactics and time for self-education.

In response to concerns about the number of hours residents and fellows were working, the ACGME instituted an 80-h work week limit on all trainees across all medical specialties in 2003. It has continued to revise policies on work hour restrictions to improve patient care and safety while optimizing resident and fellow education. These policies were most recently revised in July 2017 [26] and include guidelines regarding work hours and supervision of trainees as well as recommendations for how to improve the well-being of trainees with attention to preventing fatigue, burnout, and mental illness. These issues face physicians across all medical specialties, but gynecologic oncologists may be at particular risk for stress and burnout due to long hours, high patient volumes, busy surgical schedules, and the emotional stress of caring for oncologic patients and end of life care. Surveys of SGO members reveal that 30% of gynecologic oncologists scored high for emotional exhaustion, 30% screened positive for depression, 15% screened positive for alcohol abuse, 34% reported impaired quality of life, and only 19% were satisfied with work-life balance [27, 28]. Female gynecologic oncologists appear to be at higher risk for burnout, fatigue, and dissatisfaction with work-life balance than their male counterparts [27, 29], which is of major concern given the growing number of women in the field. Younger gynecologic oncologists are also at increased risk for burnout and work-related stress [27, 28]. These issues clearly impact personal physician well-being as well as patient care and have larger individual and societal implications, such as impacts on families, physician professional and academic productivity, and physician dropout rates which could lead to a shortage of gynecologic oncologists in the future [30–32]. The SGO assembled a wellness task force to address these issues and published specialty-specific data as well as recommendations for potential solutions [30]. They advocate for the integration of wellness education into the core curriculum of training programs to promote healthy lifestyles and burnout prevention strategies early in physicians' careers.

2.6 The Future of Gynecologic Oncology

Despite concerns about stress and burnout, 80–90% of gynecologic oncology fellows and faculty repeatedly report high levels of satisfaction with their subspecialty choice [25, 27, 29]. The number of gynecologic oncology applicants, fellows, and faculty continues to increase. As the population of the United States becomes generally more elderly, the need for specialists in the care of gynecologic malignancies is also rising. Research and development of novel therapeutics and surgical techniques continues to drive the field toward improved survival rates and quality of life for women with gynecologic malignancies. Gynecologic oncologists are trained to become lifelong learners and to adapt to these new technologies and needs of their patients. The majority of gynecologic oncologists are also involved in training future physicians, with 82% reporting that they are involved in resident training and 35% with gynecologic oncology fellows [6]. In order to provide comprehensive training to gynecologic fellows and produce competent subspecialists in women's cancer care, fellowships must also constantly tailor their curriculum to provide the most cutting-edge knowledge and technical training, as well as meet the needs of the changing demographics and work-life balance demands of their fellows.

Acknowledgements *Support*: Ensign Endowment for Gynecologic Cancer Research (K.M.). *Disclosure*: None declared.

References

1. Berchuck A. Society of Gynecologic Oncologists. J Oncol Pract. 2007;3(2):108–9.
2. Scribner DR, Baldwin J, Gold MA. Factors affecting fellowship satisfaction among gynecologic oncology fellows. Gynecol Oncol. 2001;80(1):74–8.
3. ACGME. Program requirements for graduate medical education in gynecologic oncology (subspecialty of obstetrics and gynecology). Chicago, IL: Accreditation Council for Graduate Medical Education; 2016.
4. Siegel RL, Miller KD, Jemal A. Cancer statistics, 2017. CA Cancer J Clin. 2017;67(1):7–30.
5. Ramondetta LM, et al. Mentorship and productivity among gynecologic oncology fellows. J Cancer Educ. 2003;18(1):15–9.
6. Kesterson JP, et al. Evaluation of association between gynecologic oncology fellowship length and a career in academic medicine. J Cancer Educ. 2018;33(1):141–6.
7. Guntupalli SR, et al. Preparedness of obstetrics and gynecology residents for fellowship training. Obstet Gynecol. 2015;126(3):559–68.
8. Lim PC, et al. Multicenter analysis comparing robotic, open, laparoscopic, and vaginal hysterectomies performed by high-volume surgeons for benign indications. Int J Gynaecol Obstet. 2016;133(3):359–64.
9. Sfakianos GP, et al. Robotic surgery in gynecologic oncology fellowship programs in the USA: a survey of fellows and fellowship directors. Int J Med Robot. 2010;6(4):405–12.
10. Lee PS, et al. Robotic-assisted laparoscopic gynecologic procedures in a fellowship training program. JSLS. 2009;13(4):467–72.
11. Hoekstra AV, et al. Robotic surgery in gynecologic oncology: impact on fellowship training. Gynecol Oncol. 2009;114(2):168–72.
12. Geller EJ, Schuler KM, Boggess JF. Robotic surgical training program in gynecology: how to train residents and fellows. J Minim Invasive Gynecol. 2011;18(2):224–9.
13. Soliman PT, et al. Successful incorporation of robotic surgery into gynecologic oncology fellowship training. Gynecol Oncol. 2013;131(3):730–3.
14. Silver RM, et al. Center of excellence for placenta accreta. Am J Obstet Gynecol. 2015;212(5):561–8.
15. Shamshirsaz AA, et al. Maternal morbidity in patients with morbidly adherent placenta treated with and without a standardized multidisciplinary approach. Am J Obstet Gynecol. 2015;212(2):218.e1–9.
16. Iqbal IJ, et al. Attributes of successfully matched versus unmatched obstetrics and gynecology fellowship applicants. Am J Obstet Gynecol. 2014;210(6):567.e1–8.
17. Frumovitz M, et al. Unverifiable accomplishments and publications on applications for gynecologic oncology fellowships. Obstet Gynecol. 2012;119(3):504–8.
18. Hill EK, et al. Gender differences in scholarly productivity within academic gynecologic oncology departments. Obstet Gynecol. 2015;126(6):1279–84.
19. Alvarez R. Society of gynecologic oncologists demographic data. Dallas, TX: American Board of Obstetrics & Gynecology; 2015.

20. Hofler L, et al. Subspecialty and gender of obstetrics and gynecology faculty in department-based leadership roles. Obstet Gynecol. 2015;125(2):471–6.
21. Hofler LG, et al. Comparison of women in department leadership in obstetrics and gynecology with those in other specialties. Obstet Gynecol. 2016;127(3):442–7.
22. Rayburn W. The obstetrician-gynecologist workforce in the United States: facts, figures, and implications 2011. Washington, DC: American Congress of Obstetricians and Gynecologists; 2011.
23. Rayburn WF, et al. Trends in the academic workforce of obstetrics and gynecology. Obstet Gynecol. 2010;115(1):141–6.
24. Colleges, A.o.A.M. 2014 physician specialty databook. Washington, DC: Association of American Medical Colleges; 2014.
25. Szender JB, et al. Evaluation of satisfaction with work-life balance among U.S. Gynecologic Oncology fellows: a cross-sectional study. Gynecol Oncol Rep. 2016;16:17–20.
26. ACGME. Common program requirements section VI with background and intent. Chicago, IL: Accreditation Council for Graduate Medical Education; 2017.
27. Rath KS, et al. Burnout and associated factors among members of the Society of Gynecologic Oncology. Am J Obstet Gynecol. 2015;213(6):824.e1–9.
28. Ramondetta LM, et al. Work related stress among gynecologic oncologists. Gynecol Oncol. 2011;123(2):365–9.
29. Szender JB, et al. Satisfaction with work-life balance among U.S. gynecologic oncologists, a cross-sectional study. Am J Clin Exp Obstet Gynecol. 2015;2(4):166–75.
30. Cass I, et al. Stress and burnout among gynecologic oncologists: a Society of Gynecologic Oncology Evidence-based Review and Recommendations. Gynecol Oncol. 2016;143(2):421–7.
31. Turner TB, et al. The impact of physician burnout on clinical and academic productivity of gynecologic oncologists: a decision analysis. Gynecol Oncol. 2017;146(3):642–6.
32. Gordinier ME, et al. Survey of female gynecologic oncologists and fellows: balancing professional and personal life. Gynecol Oncol. 2000;79(2):309–14.

Surgical Anatomy of Gynecologic Malignancies

3

Takuma Fujii

Abstract

Surgical anatomy is quite different from natural, textbook anatomy or systemic anatomy because the configuration of the organs becomes rearranged during the surgical process. It is important to know the original, precise topology of the organs and how the landscape changes during surgery, step by step. For example, knowledge of the uterine vessels is important for preservation of the uterus. Understanding the configuration of the nerves around the uterus, ureter, and bladder is important for preservation of bladder function. It is also crucial to know the configuration of vessels and nerves during lymphadenectomy or removal of recurrent tumors. When removing disseminated peritoneal tumors under the diaphragm, knowing the thickness of the diaphragm is useful. The anatomy described in this chapter is mainly based on cadaveric dissection. It must be noted that, in the dorsal field, organs such as vessels and nerves—the view of which is usually obscured during conventional surgery—may be exposed in a cadaver.

Keywords

Cadaver · Surgery · Radical hysterectomy · Anatomy

T. Fujii (✉)
Department of Obstetrics and Gynecology, School of Medicine, Fujita-Health University, Toyoake, Aichi, Japan
e-mail: fujiit44@fujita-hu.ac.jp

M. Mikami (ed.), *Surgery for Gynecologic Cancer*, Comprehensive Gynecology and Obstetrics, https://doi.org/10.1007/978-981-13-1519-0_3

3.1 Introduction

Surgical anatomy is quite different from natural, textbook anatomy. Once the scalpel makes the incision, the organs separate from each other, thereby altering the configuration from their original pattern. Views of the surgical field during radical hysterectomy and para-aorta lymphadenectomy are shown in this chapter. The locations of dorsal organs such as vessels and nerves, the view of which is usually obscured during conventional surgery, may be exposed in a cadaver. Understanding the precise surgical anatomy, however, is indispensable for performing surgery to remove gynecological malignancies.

3.2 Opening the Abdominal Cavity

It is important to know how to determine the appropriate incision line of the anterior lamina of the rectus abdominis muscle prior to opening the peritoneal cavity. The anterior lamina of the rectus sheath is exposed after incising the skin and fat tissue (Fig. 3.1a). The incision line of the sheath is set approximately

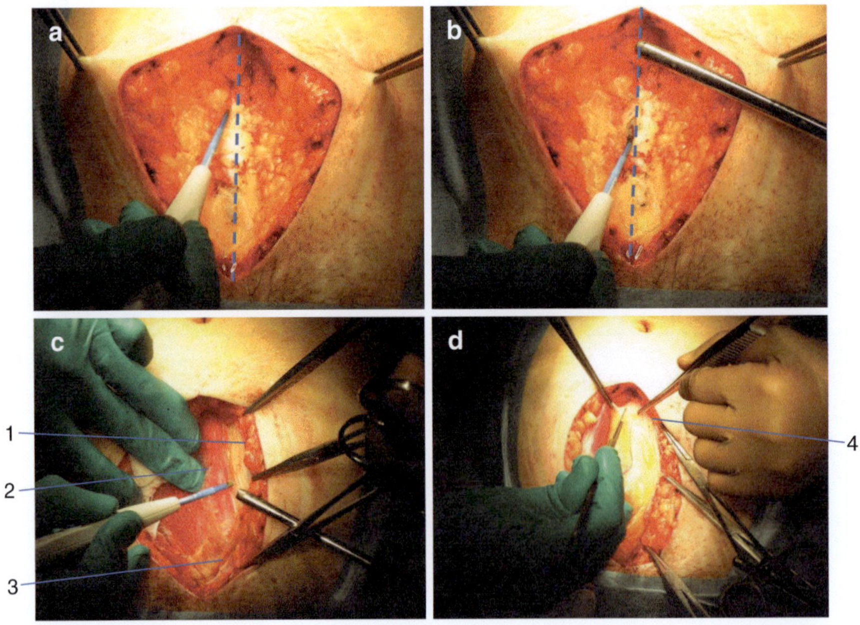

Fig. 3.1 Opening the abdominal cavity. (**a**) Dotted line indicates the midline of the body. (**b**) Incision line is set 2 mm from the right side of the midline. (**c, d**) 1, linea alba; 2, rectus abdominis muscle; 3, pyramidalis muscle; and 4, peritoneum

2 mm from the *right side* of the midline (Fig. 3.1b), and the linea alba is then easily found on the *left side*. The muscle is then detached from the linea alba (Fig. 3.1c). The next step is to incise the peritoneum (Fig. 3.1d). This technique is based on knowledge of the topology of the linea alba and anterior lamina of the rectus abdominis.

3.3 Inferior Epigastric Vessels in the Abdominal Wall

During trocar insertion into the side wall of the pelvic cavity for laparoscopic surgery (Fig. 3.2), it is important to avoid injuring the inferior epigastric vessel in the abdominal wall. The external iliac artery runs over the center of the inguinal ligament, and the external iliac vein runs medial to the artery. The inferior epigastric vessels branch off from the external iliac artery at the level of the inguinal ligament and run toward the cranial side parallel to the external iliac vessels until they reach under the rectus abdominis muscle.

3.4 Retroperitoneal Approach into the Pelvic Cavity from the Midline Incision of the Abdomen

Retroperitoneal cavity was developed from the midline incision of the abdomen. The configuration of the vessels, nerves and ureter was identified (Fig. 3.3).

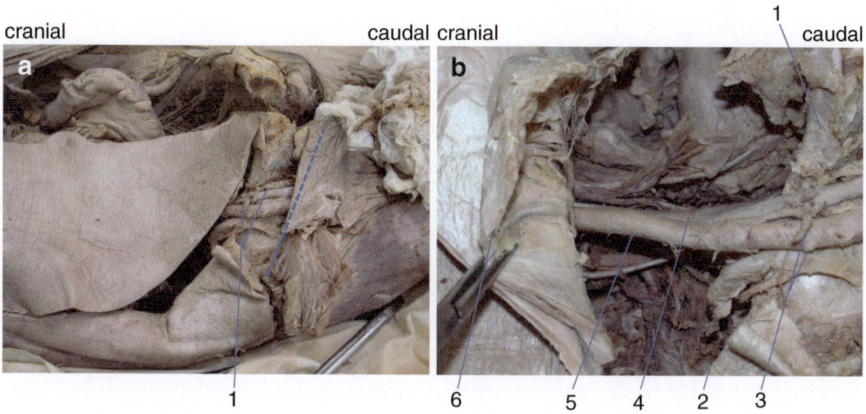

Fig. 3.2 (**a**) External artery and vein at the level of inguinal ligament. Dotted line indicates the right side of the inguinal ligament. 1. external iliac artery and vein. (**b**) Higher magnification of the site. 1, pubic tubercle; 2, right anterosuperior iliac spine; 3, stumps of the inferior epigastric vessels; 4, external iliac vein; 5, external iliac artery; and 6, stumps of the inferior epigastric vessels

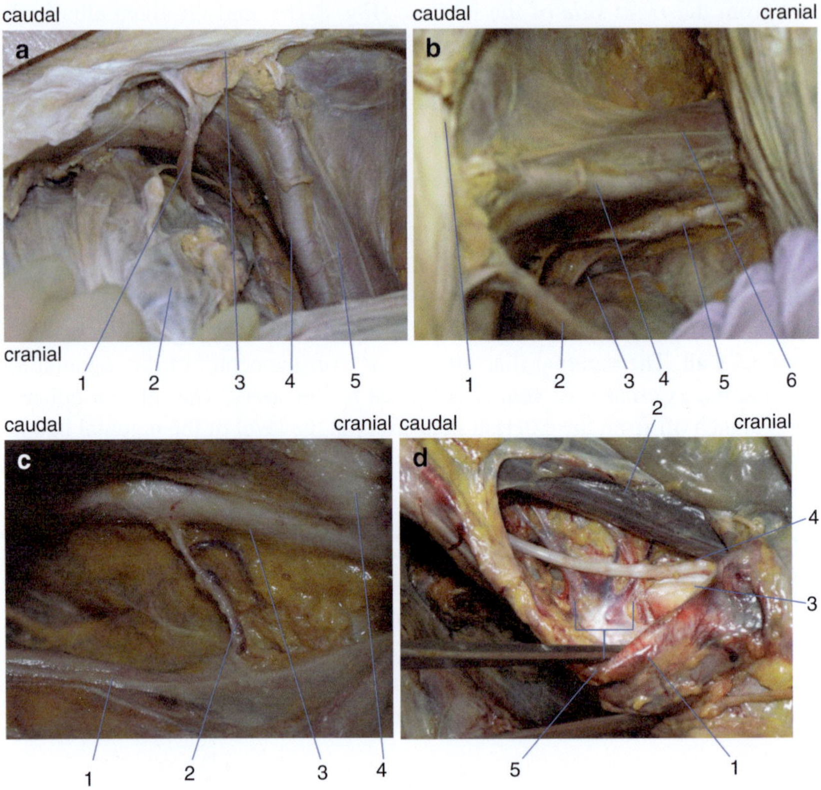

Fig. 3.3 (**a**) Vessels underneath the right round ligament run into the uterus. 1, right round ligament; 2, peritoneum; 3, inguinal ligament; 4, external iliac artery; and 5, iliopsoas muscle. (**b**) The uterine artery runs into the uterus. 1, inguinal ligament; 2, umbilical artery; 3, uterine artery; 4, external iliac artery; 5, internal iliac artery; and 6, iliopsoas muscle. (**c**) The nutrient vessel from the internal iliac artery runs into the ureter. 1, right ureter; 2, branch of the internal artery; 3, internal iliac artery; and 4, external iliac artery. (**d**) Vessels supplying the iliopsoas muscle run between the lumbosacral trunks and the obturator nerve. 1, right external iliac artery; 2, iliopsoas muscle; 3, lumbosacral trunk nerve; 4, obturator nerve; and 5, vessels from internal iliac vessels, which run toward the iliopsoas muscle

3.5 Anatomy of the Uterine Corpus and Cervix

Precise knowledge of the uterine cavity is necessary for trachelectomy. The histological and anatomical cervical appearances were not identical, as shown by the red lines (Fig. 3.4). After resecting the cervix, the remnant uterine cavity (measuring 4.5 cm long) met the minimum requirement for uterine preservation.

3.6 Anatomy of the Uterine Artery

The uterine artery branches into three major vessels in the cervix tissues (Fig. 3.5). The cervical connective tissues are dissected and the uterine artery is exposed. The corresponding veins are located underneath the uterine artery.

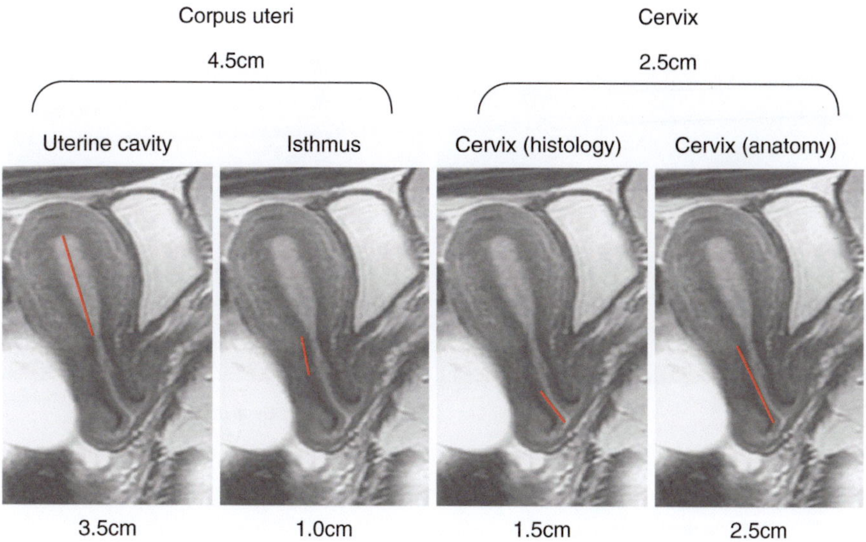

Fig. 3.4 These T2-weighted magnetic resonance images show the uterine cavity

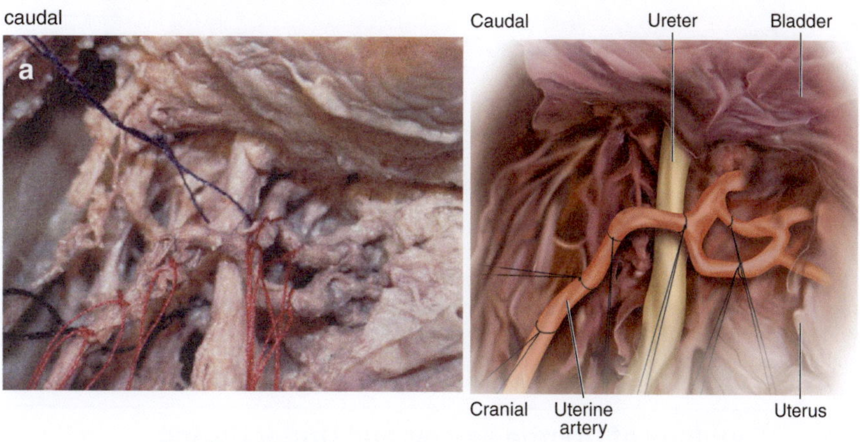

Fig. 3.5 The left uterine vessels were exposed from the connective tissues surrounding the uterus. (**a**) Left: The uterine artery branches into three major vessels (red strings). Blue string indicates the ureter. (**Right**) Drawing of the same area. (**b**) Left: Three symmetrical branches of the uterine veins (black strings) are located underneath the artery and across the ureter. (**Right**) Drawing of the same area

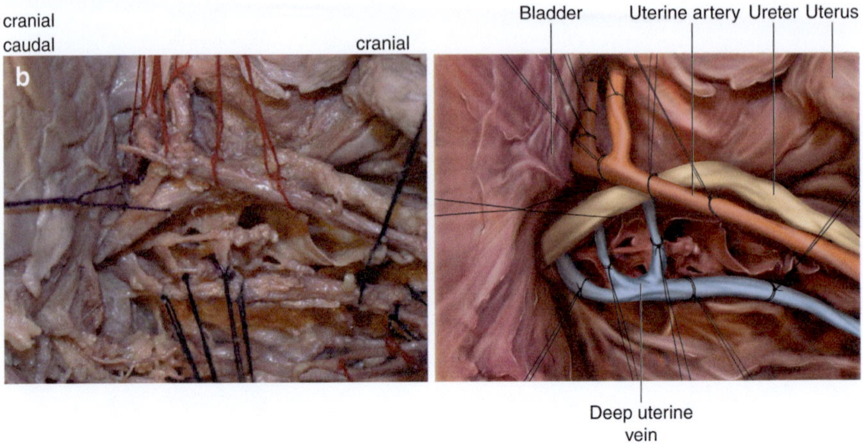

Fig. 3.5 (continued)

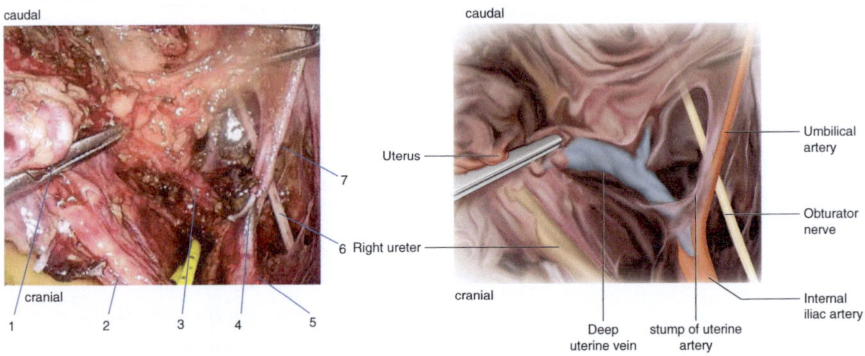

Fig. 3.6 Topology of the right side of uterine vessels and the ureter as seen during laparoscopic surgery. Ureter was displaced away (yellow vessel tape). 1, uterus; 2, right ureter; 3, deep uterine vein; 4, stump of uterine artery (white clip); 5, internal iliac artery; 6, obturator nerve; and 7, umbilical artery

3.7 Topology of Uterine Vessels and Ureter During Laparoscopic Surgery

The deep uterine vein runs parallel with the uterine artery. The origin of the uterine artery and emergence of the deep uterine vein were at the same level but across the ureter from each other. Hence, the site of origin of the uterine artery was the marker for the emergence of the deep uterine vein during laparoscopic surgery (Fig. 3.6).

3.8 Unroofing the Ureter Tunnel

The ureter tunnel is unroofed, as shown in Fig. 3.7. The anterior leaf of the ureter tunnel was dissected from the ureter and cervix (Fig. 3.7a). Of note, vessels in the posterior leaf of the ureter tunnel were observed clearly in the unfixed cadaver (Fig. 3.7b) while the nerves in the unfixed cadaver (Fig. 3.7c).

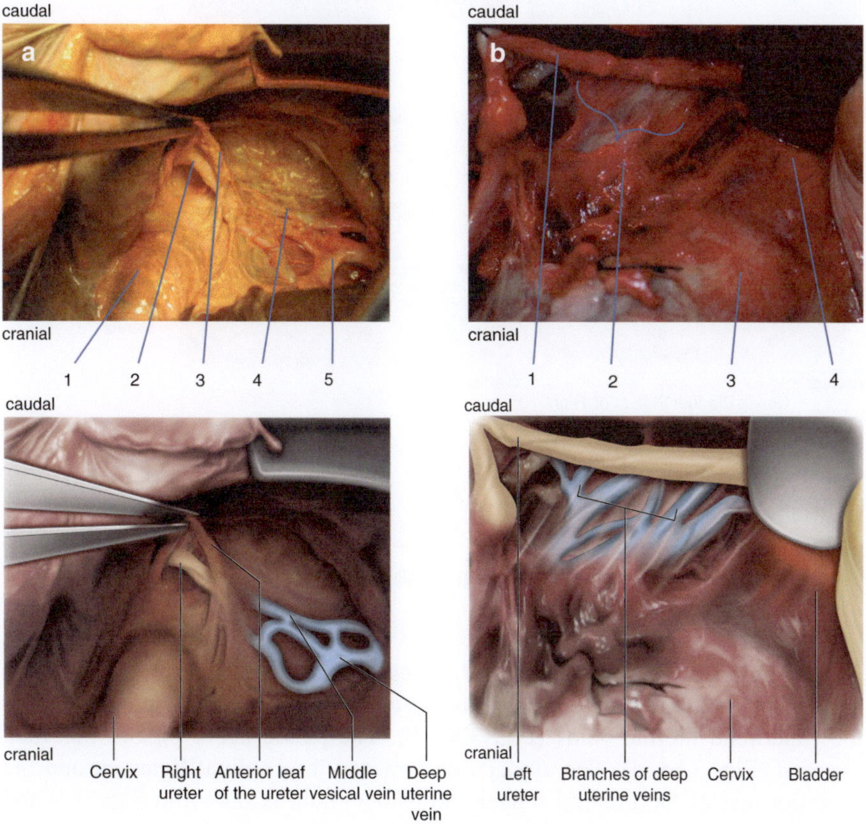

Fig. 3.7 Unroofing the anterior leaf of the ureter tunnel. (**a**) Anterior leaf of the right ureter tunnel was grasped by tweezer. 1, cervix; 2, right ureter; 3, anterior leaf of the ureter; 4, middle vesical vein; and 5, deep uterine vein. (**b**) Vessels of the left posterior leaf of the ureter tunnel were exposed in the unfixed cadaver. 1, left ureter; 2, branches of deep uterine veins; 3, cervix; and 4, bladder. (**c**) Nerves on the right side were recognized in the fixed cadaver. 1, cervix; 2, bladder; 3, plexus of nerves; and 4, right ureter. (**d**) 1, right ureter; 2, branch of the middle vesical vein; 3, deep uterine vein; 4, uterine artery; and 5, cervix

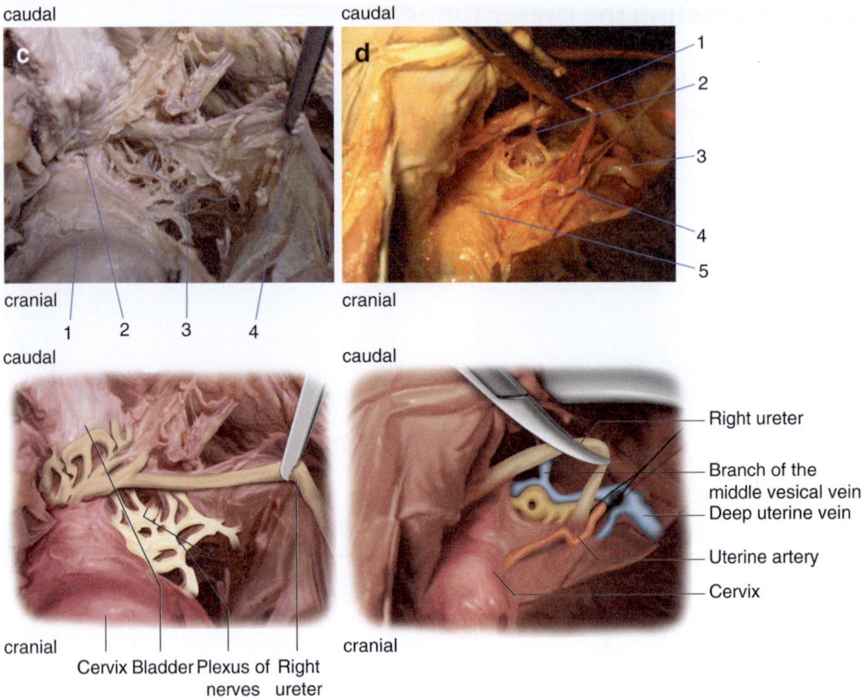

Fig. 3.7 (continued)

3.9 Configuration of the Cardinal Ligament (Paracervical Tissues)

The cardinal ligament was composed of vessels, nerves, and connective tissues. The right side of the deep uterine vein was exposed after incision and ligation of the superficial uterine veins (Fig. 3.8a, b). The pelvic nerve plexus was then exposed (Fig. 3.8c, d). The association between the cardinal ligament and the posterior leaf of the ureteral tunnel and paracolpium is shown in Figs. 3.9 and 3.10, respectively.

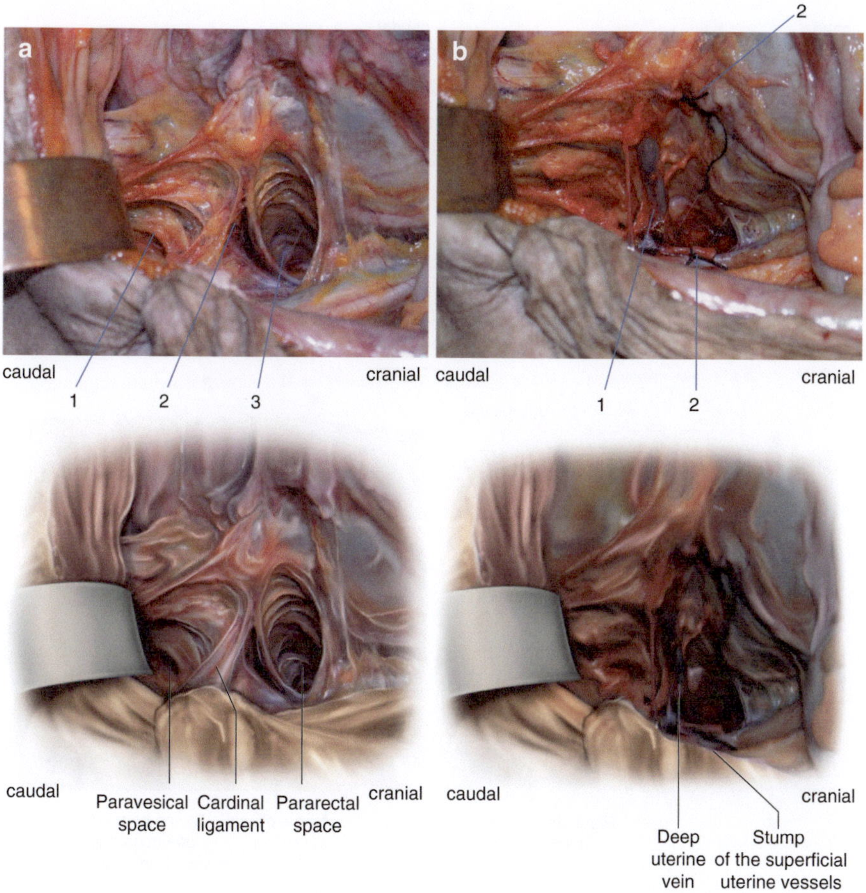

Fig. 3.8 Exposure of the deep uterine vein. (**a**) 1, right side of the paravesical space; 2, cardinal ligament; and 3, pararectal space. (**b**) 1, deep uterine vein; 2, stump of the superficial uterine vessels. (**c**) 1, right side of the deep uterine vessels; 2, vesical vein. (**d**) 1, nerve plexus; 2, stump of the deep uterine vein; and vesical vein, respectively

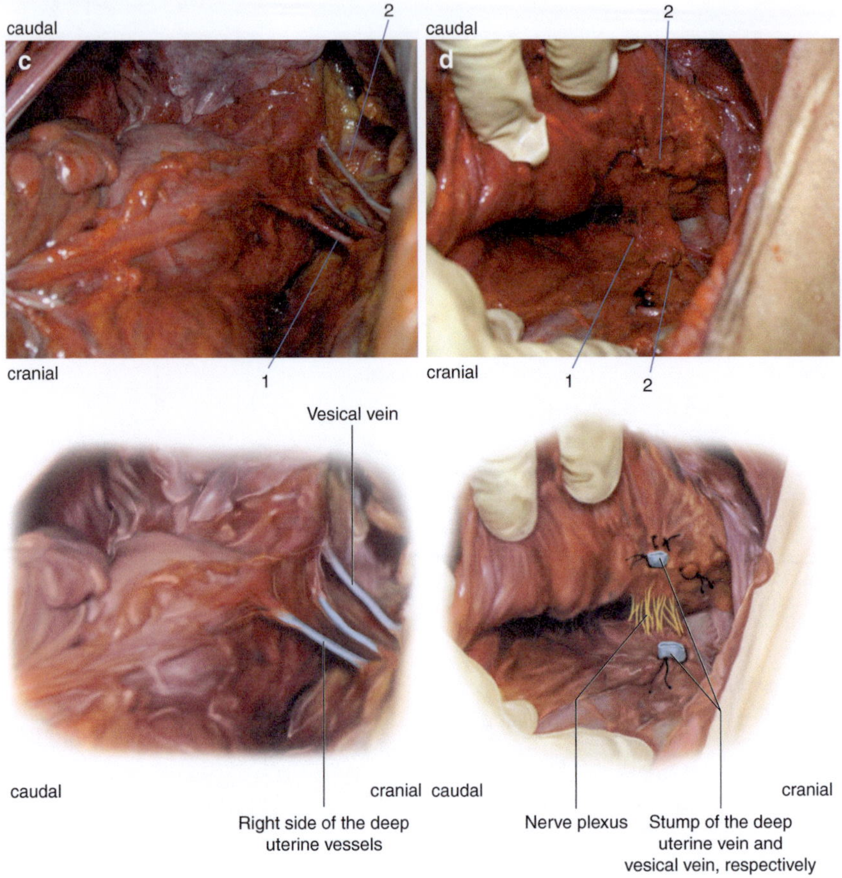

Fig. 3.8 (continued)

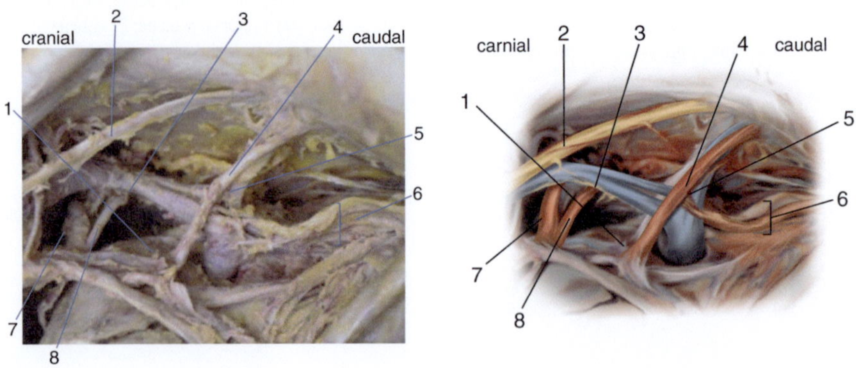

Fig. 3.9 To visualize the association between the left cardinal ligament and the posterior leaf of the ureteral tunnel, the connective tissues are partially removed at the cardinal ligament and posterior leaf of the ureteral tunnel. 1, left side of the connective tissue and nerves of the cardinal ligament; 2, obturator nerve; 3, deep uterine vein; 4, obturator artery; 5, obturator vein; 6, posterior leaf of the ureter tunnel; 7, inferior gluteal artery; 8, internal pudendal artery

3.10 Topology of the Cardinal Ligament, Posterior Leaf of the Ureteral Tunnel, and Paracolpium

The cardinal ligament, posterior leaf of the ureteral tunnel, and paracolpium are resected during radical hysterectomy (Fig. 3.10).

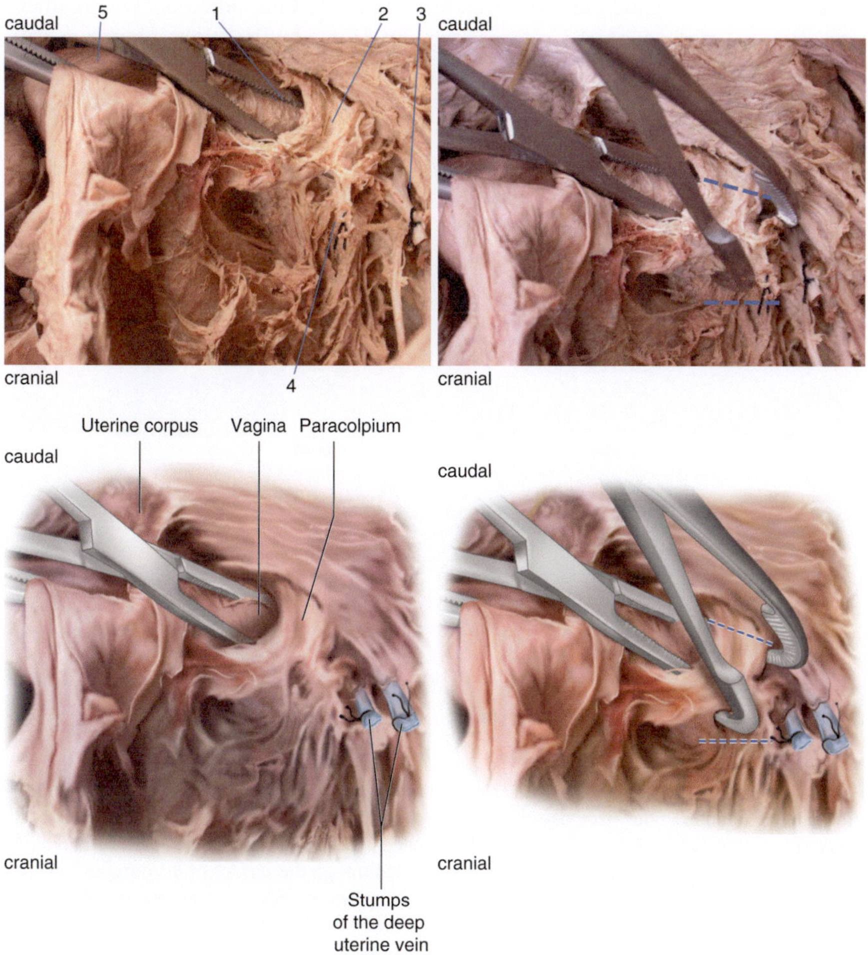

Fig. 3.10 (**Left**) Tissues of the right paracolpium were separated from the vaginal wall by the right forceps. The Kocher forceps seen in the left grasped the right side of the ligament of the ovary. 1, vagina; 2, paracolpium; 3 and 4, stumps of the deep uterine vein; and 5, uterine corpus. (**Right**) Dotted blue lines indicate the incision lines of the paracolpium and the cardinal ligament, respectively, for radical hysterectomy

3.11 Drainage from the Cervix to the Pelvic Cavity

If the vessel permeation in the cancer tissues was observed, the cancer cells might be spread through the vessels toward the other organs. It is a critical point why vessels should be resected in the radical hysterectomy. To visualize drainage from the cervix to the pelvic cavity, indigo carmine was injected into the cervix of the unfixed cadaver. Its course could then be traced through the left infundibulopelvic ligament (Fig. 3.11a), surface of the retroperitoneum (Fig. 3.11b), right obturator vein (Fig. 3.11c), right deep uterine vein (Fig. 3.11d), and right middle vesical vein (Fig. 3.11e).

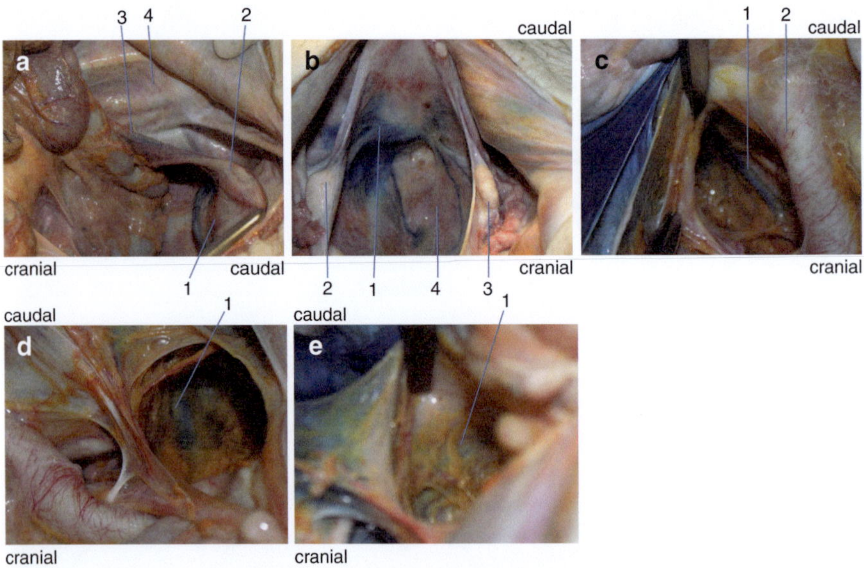

Fig. 3.11 Course of drainage from the cervix to the pelvic cavity. (**a**) Course through the infundibulopelvic ligament. View from the right side of the cadaver. Uterine body was not shown in this photo. It was located toward the left side of the photo. 1, cervix; 2, left ovary; 3, left infundibulopelvic ligament; and 4, external iliac artery. (**b**) Course through the surface of the retroperitoneum. 1, cervix; 2, left ovary; 3, right ovary; and 4, back surface of the retroperitoneum. (**c**) Course through the right obturator vein (1). 2, right external iliac artery. (**d**) Course through the right deep uterine vein (1). (**e**) Course through the right middle vesical vein (1)

3.12 Configurations of the Hypogastric Nerve, Deep Uterine Vein, and Middle Rectal Artery

The left deep uterine vein crosses over the hypogastric nerve, as shown in Figs. 3.12 and 3.13.

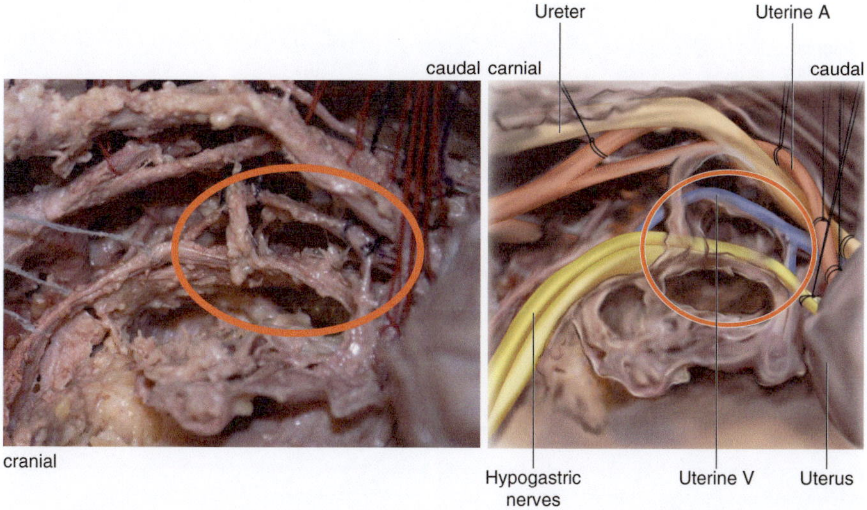

Fig. 3.12 (**Left**) Configuration of the hypogastric nerve (represented by sky blue strings) relative to the deep uterine vein (represented by black strings). (**Right**) Drawing of the same area. A, artery and V, vein

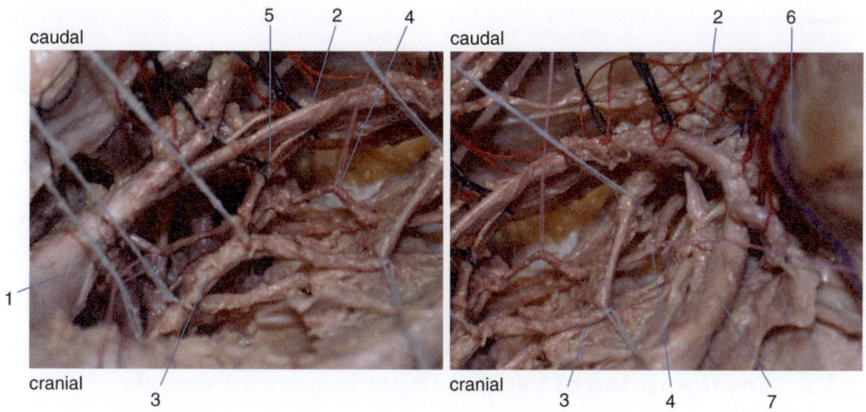

Fig. 3.13 (**Left**) Configuration of the hypogastric nerve relative to the middle rectal artery at the level of the initiation of the rectal artery. 1, internal iliac artery; 2, uterine artery (red strings); 3, hypogastric nerve (sky blue strings); 4, middle rectal artery (pink strings); 5, deep uterine vein (black); 6, uterine cervix; and 7, ureter. (**Right**) Configuration of the hypogastric nerve relative to the middle rectal artery at the level of the uterine artery

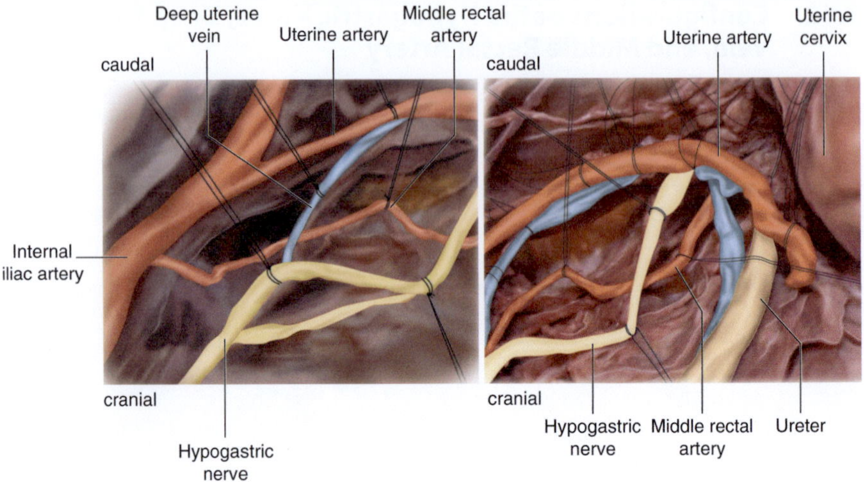

Fig. 3.13 (continued)

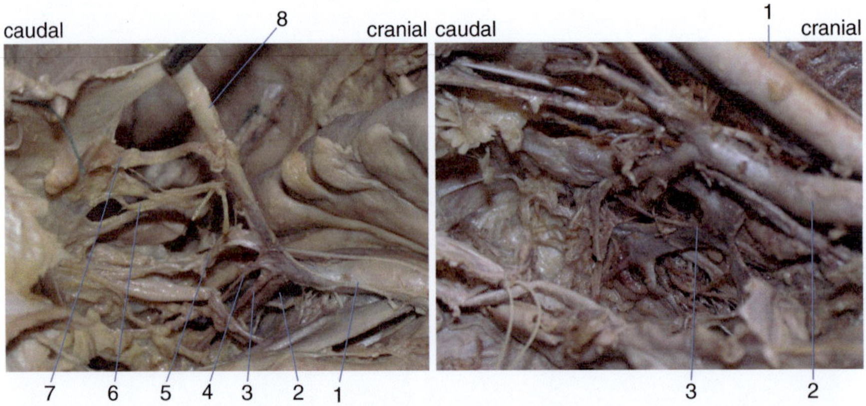

Fig. 3.14 Branches of the left internal iliac artery and vein (caudal side). (**Left**) 1, internal iliac artery; 2, inferior gluteal artery; 3, internal pudendal artery; 4, obturator artery; 5, uterine artery; 6, inferior vesical artery; 7, superior vesical artery; and 8, umbilical artery. (**Right**) Branches of the right internal iliac artery and vein (caudal side). 1, right external iliac artery; 2, internal iliac artery; and 3, trunk of internal iliac vein

3.13 Configuration of Various Other Important Vessels

The branches of the left internal iliac artery were configured in the plane. Once the artery was exposed, the bundle of arteries resembled strings of a harp (Fig. 3.14). Other important vessels are shown in Figs. 3.15, 3.16, 3.17, and 3.18.

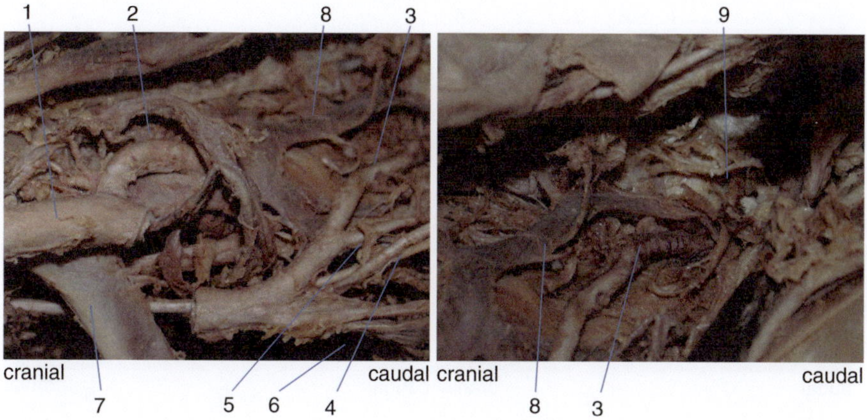

Fig. 3.15 Branches of the left internal iliac artery and vein (left: cranial site, right: caudal site). 1, left internal iliac artery; 2, inferior gluteal artery; 3, internal pudendal artery; 4, obturator artery; 5, middle rectal artery; 6, umbilical artery; 7, internal iliac vein; 8, pudendal vein; and 9, sacrospinous ligament

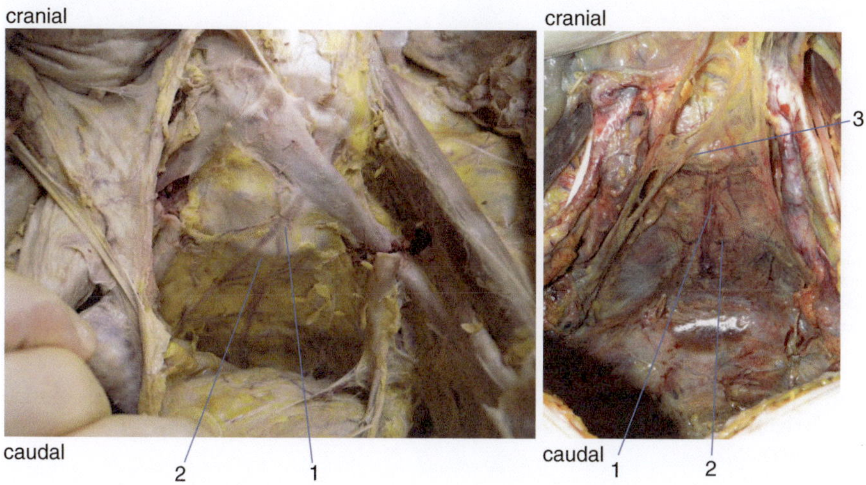

Fig. 3.16 Variant sacral vessels. (**Left**: fixed cadaver, **right**: unfixed cadaver).There are variant sacral vessels in the surface of the sacrum. 1, sacral vessels; 2, sacral promontory; and 3, superior hypogastric plexus

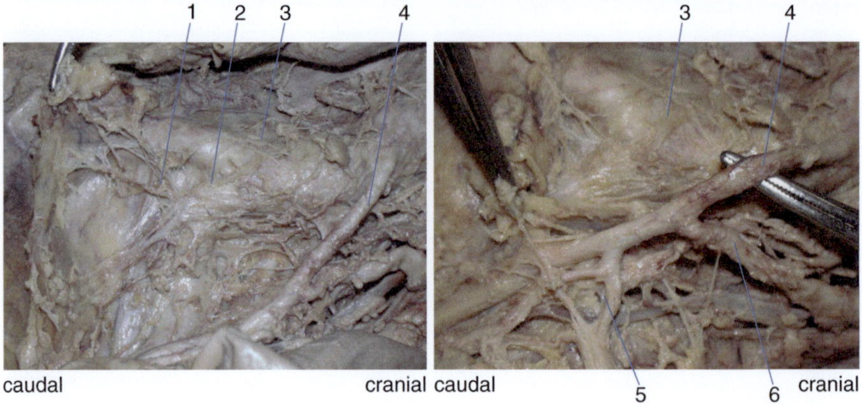

Fig. 3.17 Aorta and inferior mesenteric artery (**left**). 1, sacral promontory; 2, superior hypogastric plexus; 3, aorta; 4, inferior mesenteric artery; (**right**) magnification view of the inferior mesenteric artery 5, sigmoid artery; and 6, left colic artery

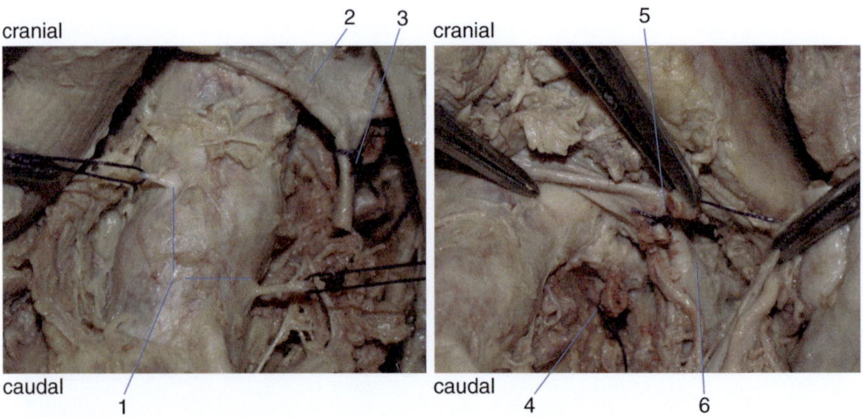

Fig. 3.18 Aorta and renal vessels. (**Left**)1, ovarian artery; 2, left renal vein; 3, left ovarian vein; (**right**) 4, stump of the second lumbar vein; 5, stump of the left renal vein; and 6, left renal artery

3.14 Diaphragm, Pleura, and Peritoneum

It is important to know the thickness of the diaphragm (Fig. 3.19) before removing disseminated peritoneal tumors from underneath it.

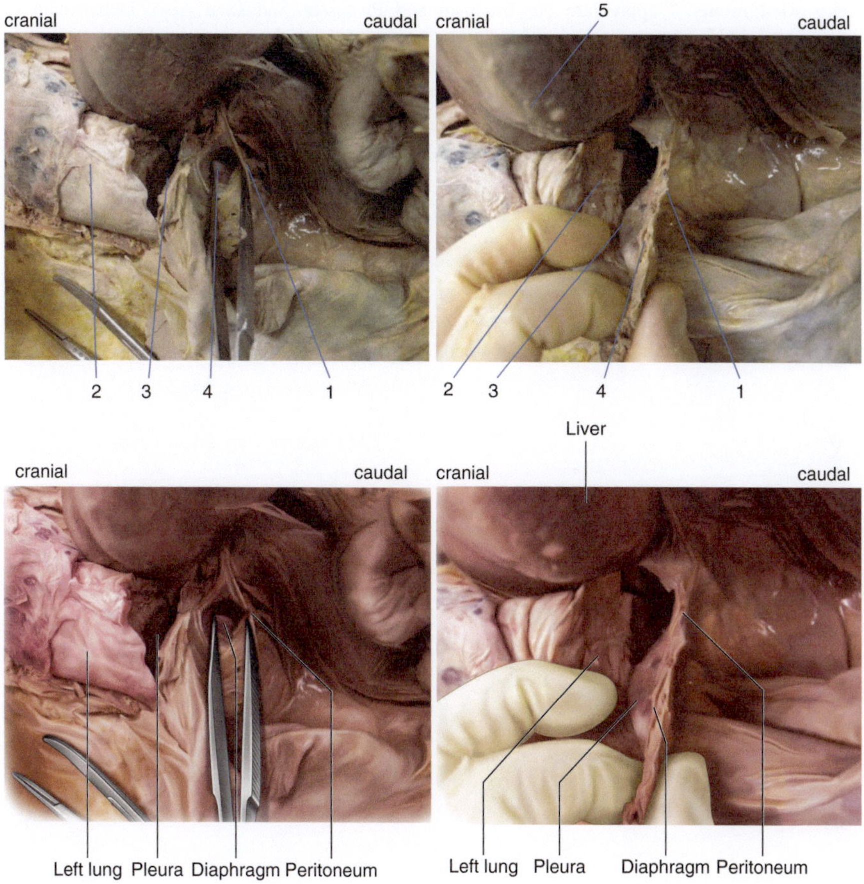

Fig. 3.19 Right side of the diaphragm, pleura, and peritoneum. 1, peritoneum. 2, right lung; 3, pleura; 4, diaphragm; and 5, liver

3.15 Summary

Views of the surgical field from various perspectives are shown in this chapter. Familiarity with the topology of the organs during surgery is critical for accomplishing high-quality surgery. Cadaveric studies such as DVD or contents [1, 2] are useful for deepening this knowledge. I strongly recommended the use of their information.

Notes This cadaveric study was performed at the Clinical Anatomy Laboratory, Department of Anatomy, Keio University, School of Medicine, Tokyo, Japan.

Acknowledgments I appreciate Dr. Imanishi and Professor Sadakazu Aiso, Department of Anatomy, Keio University, School of Medicine, for helping with the cadaveric study. I appreciate Dr. Torii, Department of Obstetrics and Gynecology, Fujita Health University, School of Medicine, and Professor Mikio Mikami, Tokai University, School of Medicine, for their critical comments.

References

1. Baggish MS, Karram MM. Atlas of pelvic anatomy and gynecologic surgery. 3rd ed. St. Louis, MO: Saunders; 2011.
2. Fujii T. Basic knowledge of robot-assisted laparoscopic surgical anatomy for the trainee of the gynecologic oncologists. Tokyo: META Corporation Japan Ltd.; 2016. http://kos.actioforma.net/products/contents/view_en/jp.co.metaco.MedicalKOS.12.298/2/

Conization

4

Yoichi Kobayashi

Abstract

Conization is the most important clinical procedure for patients with CIN3 and microinvasive carcinoma of the uterine cervix who need to preserve fertility. The main purposes of conization are confirmation of pathological diagnosis and treatment of CIN3 or early invasive cervical cancer. Preoperative evaluation should include cytology, colposcopy, and histology. Conization is performed with cold knife (CKC), laser, loop electrocautery (LEEP/LLETZ), and other devices. The treatment success of CKC, laser, and LEEP/LLETZ for CIN is reported to be about 90–98%, and there are no significant differences among these three procedures in treatment outcomes. The recurrence rate after conization has been reported to be approximately 5% regardless of surgical procedures, while age is a risk factor of recurrence. Human papilloma virus (HPV) testing is useful for detecting recurrence as well as cytology. Hemorrhage and cervical stenosis are the main complications after conization. Cone height is one of the risk factors for stenosis, while postmenopausal and postpuerperal amenorrheic women are also high risk for stenosis. Conization can also influence subsequent pregnancy. Treatment for CIN significantly increases the risk of preterm premature rupture of the membrane (pPROM) and preterm birth, and its risk is associated with cone height. CIN during pregnancy should be observed, and conization should be avoided except when invasive cancer cannot be excluded. Several trials have attempted to apply conization with pelvic lymphadenectomy for early invasive cervical cancer instead of radical trachelectomy. Further prospective studies should be conducted to establish these "less invasive" procedures to preserve fertility.

Y. Kobayashi (✉)
Department of Obstetrics and Gynecology, School of Medicine, Kyorin University, Mitaka-City, Tokyo, Japan
e-mail: yoichi@ks.kyorin-u.ac.jp

M. Mikami (ed.), *Surgery for Gynecologic Cancer*, Comprehensive Gynecology and Obstetrics, https://doi.org/10.1007/978-981-13-1519-0_4

Keywords
Cold knife · Laser · LEEP/LLETZ · Premature delivery · HPV · Bleeding Cervical

4.1 History

In the past, patients with cervical intraepithelial neoplasia 3 (CIN3) and microinvasive carcinoma of the uterine cervix had undergone hysterectomy. However, recently, conization has become the most important procedure for these patients especially when there is a need to preserve fertility. In Japan, among patients with carcinoma in situ (CIS), the proportions of those received hysterectomy and conization were 49.6% and 40.6%, respectively, in 1995, but the proportion of hysterectomy had decreased to 11.8% while that of conization had increased to 80.3% in 2013 [1, 2].

It is unclear when the first report of the "conization" procedure of the uterine cervix was published in the literature. A search for "cone biopsy and cervix" as keywords in PubMed shows a report from Crossen RJ to be the oldest publication on record; he described the history of conization in detail [3]. According to his manuscript, in 1815, Lisfranc reported the removal of a wedge-shaped block for presumed early cervical cancer, although later investigation demonstrated that these cases were not cancer but chronic inflammation [3]. Since then, many surgeons have attempted to improve the procedures and to reduce complications. In 1916, Sturmdorf devised his cold knife conization (CKC) technique with sutural coaptation of the vaginal cuff [3]. In 1935, Pendleton Tompkins compared trachelorrhaphy, amputation, and Sturmdorf operation, and he statistically demonstrated that the Sturmdorf operation was the most preferable in cure rate and had the lowest influence on subsequent pregnancies [3]. Thus, the Sturmdorf operation became the gold standard of conization performed by cold knife.

With the development of improved surgical devices, the cold knife has been replaced with other devices such as laser, electrical cautery (loop electrosurgical excisional procedure (LEEP)/large loop excision of the transformation zone (LLETZ)), and harmonic scalpel. Carbon dioxide (CO_2) laser for gynecology use was first described by Bellina [4]. Dorsey JH et al. reported on cone biopsy performed by CO_2 laser and demonstrated its advantages in both pathological diagnosis and low surgical complications [5]. But CO_2 laser technique is limited by the difficulties in setting instruments and its relatively longer surgical time for procedure. Kitsuki applied Nd:YAG laser for cervical conization and demonstrated satisfactory results compared to CO_2 laser [6]. Parallel to the development of laser, loop excisional technique was first introduced by Cartier et al. in the early 1980s, and then the LEEP technique was later developed. In 1992, another electrical cautery device, Shimodaira-Taniguchi cone biopsy probe, was developed to minimize the disadvantages of LEEP [7]. Konno et al. later reported conization using harmonic scalpel that could improve disadvantages of laser and LEEP [8]. As described, many new procedures and instruments have been established in accordance with technological development. Every procedure has its own characteristics, and the advantages and disadvantages of these methods are described below.

4.2 Principle and Indication

The main purposes of cervical conization are to confirm diagnosis and to treat the lesion. As a treatment modality, conization is able to preserve fertility and allow for subsequent pregnancy; thus, surgeons should make every effort to reduce reproductive and obstetrical complications. Indications for conization are shown in Table 4.1. Diagnostic conization should be performed if invasive cancer is suspected by cytology, but a histological diagnosis cannot demonstrate invasion. Conization can also be applied to evaluate depth of invasion and lymphovascular space invasion (LVSI) for the determination of subsequent surgical procedure in early invasive cancer (stage 1A).

Indications for treatment of CIN differ with various patient populations. According to the 2012 updated consensus guidelines for the management of abnormal cervical cancer screening and cancer precursors, therapeutic conization is unacceptable for CIN3 in pregnant women, and diagnostic excisional procedure is recommended only if invasion is suspected [9]. Special attention should be also paid to postpuerperal and postmenopausal women in performing conization since the incidence of cervical stenosis or occlusion after conization is considered higher in postpuerperal amenorrheic women; additionally, diagnosis of hematometra due to cervical occlusion could possibly be delayed in this subpopulation of patients [10]. In postmenopausal women, Hasegawa et al. reported that incidence of cervical stenosis is significantly higher compared to premenopausal women (59.1 vs. 8.3%) [11]. Based upon these findings, although conization is a less invasive procedure for CIN, conization should be only prudently offered to postmenopausal women. Hysterectomy might be a more preferable treatment for postmenopausal cases.

Table 4.1 Indication of conization of the uterine cervix

Therapeutic
1. Histologically diagnosed CIN3 or stage Ia1
2. Recurrent CIN2~3
3. Adenocarcinoma in situ (AIS)
Diagnostic
1. Suspected CIN3 or more lesion with unsatisfactory colposcopy (entire squamocolumnar junction cannot be visualized)
2. Diagnosis for AIS
3. Suspected (early) invasive cancer in cytology but no correspondence histology/colposcopic finding
4. To devaluate depth of invasion and LVSI for determination of following surgical procedure in early invasive cancer
5. Insufficient cytology or histology to warrant procedure

CIN cervical intraepithelial neoplasia, *LVSI* lymphovascular space invasion

4.3 Preoperative Evaluation

Before conization, preoperative evaluation is very important. When an abnormal Papanicolaou smear is confirmed, colposcopy followed by biopsy should be performed by an experienced colposcopist. Songveeratham et al. reported that 15% of high-grade squamous intraepithelial lesion (HSIL) cases are underdiagnosed by cytology [12]. Although the value of endocervical curettage (ECC) at colposcopy has been controversial, and while ECC has not been routinely performed, Fine et al. reported that preoperative ECC is associated with grade of dysplasia and suggest that routine ECC should be included as part of the preoperative assessment [13]. Pretorius et al. also concluded that ECC should be performed for the patients with abnormal cytology even when colposcopy is satisfactory [14].

4.4 Technique

In performing conization, historically cold knife has been used. Recently, in accordance with the development of new technologies and equipments, electrocautery (LEEP/LLETZ), laser, and harmonic scalpel have been applied for conization. A randomized prospective study comparing CKC, laser, and LEEP and their respective characteristics as reported by Mathevet et al. is summarized in Table 4.2 [15]. They concluded that laser conization is relatively costly and time-consuming and that laser and LEEP may induce artifact so that histological evaluation of the surgical margin is difficult. In a meta-analysis, LEEP/LLETZ is as effective as CKC with regard to recurrence rate, positive margin, residual disease as well as secondary hemorrhage and cervical stenosis [16]. As described, every procedure has its advantages and disadvantages; thus, the procedures should be selected by the surgeon according to the institutional settings, size and depth of the lesion, and/or economic status of the patients.

The scheme of our procedure for laser conization is shown in Fig. 4.1. Briefly, the patient is set in lithotomy position, and the speculum is inserted in the vagina. Acetic acid or Schiller's solution is used in order to determine the range of surgical resection. Hemostatic sutures using No. 2-0 Vicryl are placed at 3 and 9 o'clock positions. Local injection of vasoconstrictor is not routinely used in our institute. Four to eight sutures by No. 3-0 Vicryl are made just inside of the margin to retract

Table 4.2 Characteristics of cold knife, laser, and LEEP (modified ref. 15)

	Mean operative time	Mean blood loss	Mean cone volume	Difficulty of technique	Cost	Evaluation of margin
Cold knife	○	○	◎	○	◎	◎
Laser	○	○	○	○	X	○
LEEP	◎	◎	○	◎	○	X

LEEP loop electrosurgical excision procedure
◎: superior, ○: acceptable, X: inferior

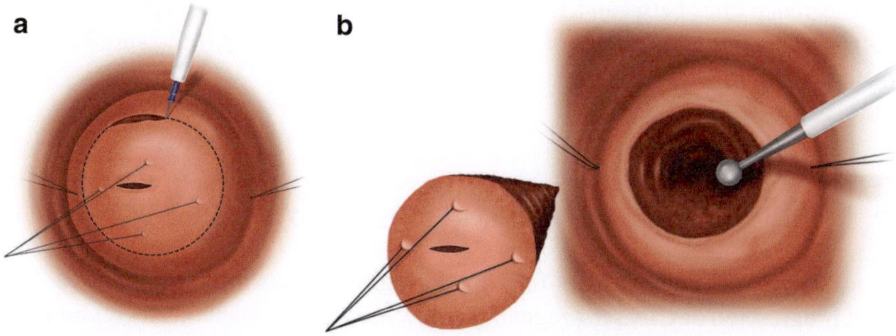

Fig. 4.1 Conization technique by laser. (**a**) After marking the line of incision 3–5 mm of outer margin with small spot by laser, cervix is cut by laser beam. (**b**) After removal of the specimen, hemostasis and vaporization are made by defocused laser spot or ball electrode

the lesion, and a knot is made on the thread at 12 o'clock to recognize orientation of the specimen [17]. Width and depth of conization could be determined individually according to the colposcopic findings. After marking the line of incision 3–5 mm of outer margin with small spots by laser, the cervix is cut by laser beam. During the procedure, if surgical mist or bleeding occurs, an aspirator is used during the procedure. After the desired depth is obtained, the upper margin is cut by scalpel so that the pathological diagnosis of the endocervical surgical margin is more readily possible. After removal of the specimen, hemostasis and vaporization are made by defocused laser spot or ball electrode. Additionally, the outer margin is vaporized to reduce recurrence of surgical margin-positive cases. We usually insert a 8 Fr Nelaton catheter into the uterine cavity to avoid stenosis; this will later be removed after about 1 week after conization, but insertion of catheter can be omitted. Absorbable hemostat such as oxidized cellulose is placed on the wound.

When using LEEP/LLETZ, excision in multiple fragments can complicate histopathological assessment, so surgeons should inform the pathologist on the precise orientation of the resected specimens. If CKC is performed, the surgeons should take care to minimize side effect such as hemorrhage and cervical stenosis [17].

Evidence to support use of antibiotics to reduce infectious complications after conization is insufficient, so routine use of antibiotics should be avoided [18].

4.5 Result and Outcome

According to a systematic review, the treatment success rates (no residual disease during follow-up) for CKC, laser conization, and LEEP/LLETZ for CIN are reported as 90–94%, 93–96%, and 91–98%, respectively, and there are no significant differences among these three procedures in treatment outcomes [19]. Even in unsatisfactory colposcopic examinations, there is no significant difference in the incidence of persistent or recurrent disease between LEEP and CKC for CIN [20]. For cervical adenocarcinoma in situ (AIS), there is no difference in residual and recurrence rates between LEEP and CKC. Conization is acceptable as a definitive treatment for Ia1 squamous cell carcinoma of the cervix if the surgical margin is negative [21, 22].

4.6 Influence of Conization for Pregnancy

The safety of delaying treatment for CIN during pregnancy has been reported. The risk of progression of CIN3 in pregnancy is low, and the spontaneous regression rate is high [23, 24]. For CIN1 to CIN3 in pregnant women, regression rates and persistence rates were reported 16.7–77.4% and 22.6–70.0%, respectively, while progression rates were 0–13.3% [25]. CIN3 in pregnancy is usually observed and should be re-evaluated at 6 weeks postpartum [9], and diagnostic conization during pregnancy is recommended only if invasion is suspected [9].

Adverse obstetrical outcomes after conization have been shown in number of studies. Sadler et al. reported that LEEP and laser conization were associated with significantly increased risk of preterm premature rupture of the membrane (pPROM), and if cone height is ≧1.7 cm, pPROM risk increased threefold compared with untreated women [26]. A systematic review and meta-analysis by Kyrgiou et al. showed that treatment for CIN significantly increased the risk of preterm birth. Relative risks (RRs) of preterm delivery according to the conization procedures are 2.70 (2.14–3.40) for CKC, 2.11 (1.26–3.54) for laser conization, and 1.56 (1.36–1.79) for LEEP/LLETZ, respectively. Cone depth is also associated with preterm delivery, and if cone depth is ≧20.0 mm, the RR increased to 4.91 (2.06–11.68). Chorioamnionitis and low birth weight are also significantly increased after conization [27].

For young women, the indication and application of conization should be sufficiently discussed. Chevreau et al. reviewed the age at LEEP on obstetrical outcome, and they found that age younger than 25 years at the time of LEEP is associated with extremely early preterm delivery (before 26 weeks) if cone depth is ≧15 mm [28]. It can perhaps be surmised that the cervix is a growing organ, and its length is significantly shorter in young women [29]. In these patients, vaporization might better be considered as a treatment option instead of conization. Mariya et al. reported there were no significant differences in cure rate, human papilloma virus (HPV) clearance rate, or recurrent rates between conization and vaporization groups, and no adverse pregnancy outcome was observed in the vaporization group [30]. In order to reduce the height of cone, Kim et al. reported "coin-shaped" conization. In their report, mean cone height was reduced from 14.0 mm to 12.8 mm, and it improved reduction rate of uterine cervical length over the subsequent pregnancy [31], but whether it could contribute to improve obstetrical outcome is still controversial. In order to minimize the incidence of adverse events as well as positive margin, Kawano et al. showed the cutoff value of cone length was 15 mm in single quadrant disease and 20 mm in two or more quadrant disease to avoid positive cone margin in women ≦40 years old [32].

4.7 Residual Disease/Recurrence

After treated for CIN, early detection of residual/recurrent disease is essential. Histology taken under colposcopy after conization has been reported to be highly negative, so colposcopy as the only postoperative test may not be suitable for follow-up after conization [33]. For follow-up after conization, cytology and screening of HPV can be useful for detecting recurrence. Nobbenhuis et al. reported sensitivity of HR-HPV test 6 months after treatment was higher than abnormal cervical cytology in posttreatment CIN2/CIN3 (90 vs. 62%) [34]. Additionally, co-testing with cytology and HPV testing at 12 and 24 months has been recommended as follow-up after conization [9].

The recurrence rate after conization has been reported to be approximately 5% regardless of surgical procedures [35]. Recognizing high-risk factors for recurrence after conization is important. It is well-known that a positive surgical margin is a risk factor for residual disease/recurrence after conization [36]. Age ≧50, parity ≧5, positive post-cone ECC, and multi-quadrant disease can also predict post-cone residual disease [37]. Tanaka et al. mentioned aged ≧46 was an independent risk factor for recurrent/persistent disease [35]. In multivariate analysis from Zhu et al., for patients with high-grade squamous intraepithelial lesion (HSIL) with positive margins after LEEP, age ≧35 was an independent risk factor [38]. Giannella et al. described HPV clearance after conization decreased with age; thus increasing age can be categorized as a risk for post-conization recurrence [39]. Park et al. reported positive margin and pre-cone HR-HPV load were the only significant factors predicting post-cone residual disease [36].

4.8 Complications

Several complications of conization have been reported. Intraoperative bleeding is a major complication but is rarely heavy and in most cases can be controlled by sutures and electrocoagulation. In our experience, most cases of bleeding can be controlled by ball electrode. Postoperative bleeding is a frequent complication. Usually, it takes 4–5 weeks for postoperative reepithelialization of the cervix. During this period, slight hemorrhage may occur, but in cases of massive hemorrhage, this will occur on the 8th to 12th day after conization because during this period the fibrino-leukocytic membrane covering the denuded cervix sloughs away [40]. Incidences of secondary hemorrhage of conization in LEEP, CKC, and laser were reported 5.3–10.1%, 0–9.4%, and 0.9–6.1%, respectively [15, 16, 41–45] (Table 4.3). Occasionally it requires hemostasis including suturing or packing and rarely requires blood transfusion, uterine artery embolization, or hysterectomy.

Table 4.3 Incidence of secondary hemorrhage and cervical stenosis after conization

	LEEP (%)	CKC (%)	Laser (%)
Secondary hemorrhage	5.3–10.1	0–9.4	0.9–6.1
Cervical stenosis	3.4–19	2.9–29	0–9

LEEP loop electrosurgical excision procedure, *CKC* cold knife conization

Cervical stenosis is another major problem after conization. Cone height is a risk of stenosis, but elderly age is another risk [35]. Incidences of postoperative cervical stenosis of CKC, LEEP, and laser conization were reported 3.4–19%, 2.9–29%, and 0–9%, respectively [15, 16, 41–45] (Table 4.3). As there is no standard definition of stenosis, these findings could not be simply compared. Special consideration for postmenopausal and postpuerperal amenorrheic women should be made because they are at high risk for cervical stenosis (see Chap. 4.2).

Although there is a possible risk of infection, major infection after conization in any procedures (CKC, LEEP, and laser) is approximately 0.1–2% [46, 47], but it will depend on the patients' status (history of pelvic inflammatory disease, etc.). Other uncommon complications of conization have been reported to include bladder perforation, peritonitis, intra-abdominal bleeding, pseudoaneurysm of uterine artery, and vaginal evisceration [45, 48–51].

4.9 Future Prospect

Although fertility-sparing surgery for International Federation of Gynecology and Obstetrics (FIGO) stage 1A1 with LVSI, 1A2, and small 1B1 cervical cancer patients is radical trachelectomy (RT) with pelvic lymphadenectomy, postoperative severe complications could occur as well as a high incidence of premature delivery in subsequent pregnancy. Thus, several trials have been performed to develop less invasive procedures for low-risk early-stage cervical cancer (histology; squamous cell carcinoma, adeno/adenosquamous cell carcinoma, tumor size <2 cm, stromal invasion <10 mm, no LVSI) [52]. Biliatis et al. performed loop biopsy with pelvic lymphadenectomy for 35 small-volume stage 1B1 cervical cancer patients, and there was no recurrence, and 7 full-term pregnancies have been achieved [53]. Fagotti et al. reported CKC and laparoscopic pelvic lymphadenectomy for early-stage cervical cancer. Four of 17 cases involved LVSI, and 2 patients received adjuvant chemotherapy, and no recurrence was observed after a median follow-up of 16 months. They concluded CKC and laparoscopic pelvic lymphadenectomy might be feasible as a fertility-sparing procedure instead of radical trachelectomy in selected and informed patients [54]. Literature review has demonstrated cone biopsy to be a feasible treatment of ≧stage 1A2 disease by Reade et al. including data from Fagotti et al. In this review, a total of 1163 cases received conization, and recurrence rate and death from disease were 2.0% and 0.7%, respectively [55]. Andikyan et al. reported cervical conization with sentinel lymph node (SLN) mapping could be acceptable for small-volume stage I cervical cancer [52]. Neoadjuvant chemotherapy followed by conization with lymphadenectomy for stage 1B2 disease case has also been attempted

[56]. In order to establish a less invasive procedure employing conization with warranted curative rate, further prospective studies should be conducted.

Acknowledgment The author much appreciates Ms. Mieko Kaneko for her skillful illustration and Dr. Atsushi Suzuki for his English support of manuscript.

References

1. Annual report of the committee on Gynecologic Oncology, the Japan Society of Obstetrics and Gynecology. Acta Obstet Gynaecol Jpn. 2000;52:855.
2. Annual report of the committee on Gynecologic Oncology, the Japan Society of Obstetrics and Gynecology. Acta Obstet Gynaecol Jpn. 2015;67:1885.
3. Crossen RJ. Wide conization of cervix; follow-up of 1,000 cases, 600 from 2 to 14 years. Am J Obstet Gynecol. 1949;57:187–206.
4. Bellina JH. Gynecology and laser. Cont Obstet Gynecol. 1974;4:24–74.
5. Dorsey JH, Diggs ES. Microsurgical conization of the cervix by carbon dioxide laser. Obstet Gynecol. 1979;54:565–70.
6. Kitsuki K. Studies on Nd:YAG laser therapy for cervical intraepithelial neoplasia. Nihon Gan Chiryo Gakkai Shi. 1990;25:2810–21, Japanese
7. Matsumura M, Ota T, Takeshima N, Takizawa K. Shimodaira-Taniguchi conization method: its utility and reliability. Int J Gynecol Cancer. 2010;20:1025–30.
8. Konno R, Akahira J, Igarashi T, Yamakawa H, Sato S, Yajima A. Conization of the cervix using harmonic scalpel. Tohoku J Exp Med. 1999;189:171–8.
9. Massad LS, Einstein MH, Huh WK, Katki HA, Kinney WK, Schiffman M, Solomon D, Wentzensen N, Lawson HW, 2012 ASCCP Consensus Guidelines Conference. 2012 updated consensus guidelines for the management of abnormal cervical cancer screening tests and cancer precursors. Obstet Gynecol. 2013;121:829–46.
10. Hirai K, Kanaoka Y, Sumi T, Yasui T, Nakai Y, Nishio J, Yamamasu S, Ishiko O. Occlusion of the external cervical os after conization in a postpuerperal amenorrheic woman. Arch Gynecol Obstet. 2004;270(1):64–6.
11. Hasegawa K, Torii Y, Kato R, Udagawa Y, Fukasawa I. The problems of cervical conization for postmenopausal patients. Eur J Gynaecol Oncol. 2016;37(3):327–31.
12. Songveeratham S, Kietpeerakool C, Khunamornpong S, Sribanditmongkol N, Srisomboon J. Preceding cervical cytology in women with high-grade squamous intraepithelial lesion. Arch Gynecol Obstet. 2011;283(6):1381–4.
13. Fine BA, Feinstein GI, Sabella V. The pre- and postoperative value of endocervical curettage in the detection of cervical intraepithelial neoplasia and invasive cervical cancer. Gynecol Oncol. 1998;71(1):46–9.
14. Pretorius RG, Zhang WH, Belinson JL, Huang MN, Wu LY, Zhang X, Qiao YL. Colposcopically directed biopsy, random cervical biopsy, and endocervical curettage in the diagnosis of cervical intraepithelial neoplasia II or worse. Am J Obstet Gynecol. 2004;191(2):430–4.
15. Mathevet P, Dargent D, Roy M, Beau G. A randomized prospective study comparing three techniques of conization: cold knife, laser, and LEEP. Gynecol Oncol. 1994;54(2):175–9.
16. Jiang YM, Chen CX, Li L. Meta-analysis of cold-knife conization versus loop electrosurgical excision procedure for cervical intraepithelial neoplasia. Onco Targets Ther. 2016;9:3907–15.
17. Jordan J, Martin-Hirsch P, Arbyn M, Schenck U, Baldauf JJ, Da Silva D, Anttila A, Nieminen P, Prendiville W. European guidelines for clinical management of abnormal cervical cytology, part 2. Cytopathology. 2009;20(1):5–16.
18. Kietpeerakool C, Chumworathayi B, Thinkhamrop J, Ussahgij B, Lumbiganon P. Antibiotics for infection prevention after excision of the cervical transformation zone. Cochrane Database Syst Rev. 2017;1:CD009957. https://doi.org/10.1002/14651858.CD009957.pub2.

19. Martin-Hirsch PP, Paraskevaidis E, Bryant A, Dickinson HO, Keep SL. Surgery for cervical intraepithelial neoplasia. Cochrane Database Syst Rev. 2010;6:CD001318. https://doi.org/10.1002/14651858.CD001318.pub2.
20. El-Nashar SA, Shazly SA, Hopkins MR, Bakkum-Gamez JN, Famuyide AO. Loop electrosurgical excision procedure instead of cold-knife conization for cervical intraepithelial neoplasia in women with unsatisfactory colposcopic examinations: a systematic review and meta-analysis. J Low Genit Tract Dis. 2017;21(2):129–36.
21. Sopracordevole F, Chiossi G, Barbero M, Cristoforoni P, Ghiringhello B, Frega A, Tortolani F, Boselli F, Clemente N, Ciavattini A, Italian Society of Colposcopy and Cervico-Vaginal Pathology. Surgical approach and long-term clinical outcome in women with microinvasive cervical cancer. Anticancer Res. 2014;34(8):4345–9.
22. Papakonstantinou K, Kyrgiou M, Lyons D, Soutter WP, Ghaem-Maghami S. Management of stage Ia1 squamous cervical cancer and the importance of excision margins: a retrospective study of long-term outcome after 25 years of follow-up. Am J Obstet Gynecol. 2014;211(6):625.e1–6.
23. Yost NP, Santoso JT, McIntire DD, Iliya FA. Postpartum regression rates of antepartum cervical intraepithelial neoplasia II and III lesions. Obstet Gynecol. 1999;93(3):359–62.
24. Ackermann S, Gehrsitz C, Mehlhorn G, Beckmann MW. Management and course of histologically verified cervical carcinoma in situ during pregnancy. Acta Obstet Gynecol Scand. 2006;85(9):1134–7.
25. Mailath-Pokorny M, Schwameis R, Grimm C, Reinthaller A, Polterauer S. Natural history of cervical intraepithelial neoplasia in pregnancy: postpartum histo-pathologic outcome and review of the literature. BMC Pregnancy Childbirth. 2016;16:74. https://doi.org/10.1186/s12884-016-0861-8.
26. Sadler L, Saftlas A, Wang W, Exeter M, Whittaker J, McCowan L. Treatment for cervical intraepithelial neoplasia and risk of preterm delivery. JAMA. 2004;291(17):2100–6.
27. Kyrgiou M, Athanasiou A, Paraskevaidi M, Mitra A, Kalliala I, Martin-Hirsch P, Arbyn M, Bennett P, Paraskevaidis E. Adverse obstetric outcomes after local treatment for cervical preinvasive and early invasive disease according to cone depth: systematic review and meta-analysis. BMJ. 2016;354:i3633. https://doi.org/10.1136/bmj.i3633.
28. Chevreau J, Mercuzot A, Foulon A, Attencourt C, Sergent F, Lanta S, Gondry J. Impact of age at conization on obstetrical outcome: a case-control study. J Low Genit Tract Dis. 2017;21(2):97–101.
29. D'Agostini C, de Oliveira M, D'Souza-Li L. Comparison of cervical length in adult and adolescent nulliparae at mid-gestation. J Pediatr Adolesc Gynecol. 2013;26(4):209–11.
30. Mariya T, Nishikawa A, Sogawa K, Suzuki R, Saito M, Kawamata A, Shimizu A, Nihei T, Sonoda T, Saito T. Virological and cytological clearance in laser vaporization and conization for cervical intra-epithelial neoplasia grade 3. J Obstet Gynaecol Res. 2016;42(12):1808–13.
31. Kim M, Ishioka S, Endo T, Baba T, Saito T. Obstetrical prognosis of patients with cervical intraepithelial neoplasia (CIN) after "coin-shaped" conization. Arch Gynecol Obstet. 2016;293(3):651a–7.
32. Kawano K, Tsuda N, Nishio S, Yonemoto K, Tasaki K, Tasaki R, Ushijima K. Identification of appropriate cone length to avoid positive cone margin in high grade cervical intraepithelial neoplasia. J Gynecol Oncol. 2016;27(5):e54. https://doi.org/10.3802/jgo.2016.27.e54.
33. Bigrigg A, Haffenden DK, Sheehan AL, Codling BW, Read MD. Efficacy and safety of large-loop excision of the transformation zone. Lancet. 1994;343(8888):32–4.
34. Nobbenhuis MA, Meijer CJ, van den Brule AJ, Rozendaal L, Voorhorst FJ, Risse EK, Verheijen RH, Helmerhorst TJ. Addition of high-risk HPV testing improves the current guidelines on follow-up after treatment for cervical intraepithelial neoplasia. Br J Cancer. 2001;84(6):796–801.
35. Tanaka Y, Ueda Y, Kakuda M, Kubota S, Matsuzaki S, Iwamiya T, Okazawa A, Matsuzaki S, Hashimoto K, Kobayashi E, Mabuchi S, Sawada K, Tomimatsu T, Yoshino K, Kimura T. Predictors for recurrent/persistent high-grade intraepithelial lesions and cervical stenosis after therapeutic conization: a retrospective analysis of 522 cases. Int J Clin Oncol. 2017;22(5):921–6. https://doi.org/10.1007/s10147-017-1124-z.

36. Park JY, Lee SM, Yoo CW, Kang S, Park SY, Seo SS. Risk factors predicting residual disease in subsequent hysterectomy following conization for cervical intraepithelial neoplasia (CIN) III and microinvasive cervical cancer. Gynecol Oncol. 2007;107(1):39–44.
37. Lu CH, Liu FS, Tseng JJ, Ho ES. Predictive factors for residual disease in subsequent hysterectomy following conization for CIN III. Gynecol Oncol. 2000;79(2):284–8.
38. Zhu M, He Y, Baak JP, Zhou X, Qu Y, Sui L, Feng W, Wang Q. Factors that influence persistence or recurrence of high-grade squamous intraepithelial lesion with positive margins after the loop electrosurgical excision procedure: a retrospective study. BMC Cancer. 2015;15:744. https://doi.org/10.1186/s12885-015-1748-1.
39. Giannella L, Fodero C, Boselli F, Rubino T, Mfuta K, Prandi S. Age-related changes in pre- and post-conization HPV genotype distribution among women with high-grade cervical intraepithelial neoplasia. Int J Gynaecol Obstet. 2017;137(1):72–7.
40. Bickers W. Postoperative cervical-vaginal healing in relation to postoperative treatment. Am J Obstet Gynecol. 1950;59(5):1045–52.
41. Girardi F, Heydarfadai M, Koroschetz F, Pickel H, Winter R. Cold-knife conization versus loop excision: histopathologic and clinical results of a randomized trial. Gynecol Oncol. 1994;55(3 Pt 1):368–70.
42. Kartsiounis C, Koutlaki N, Evaggelinos D, Skafida P, Kafetzis D, Kartsiounis V, Dinas K, Dimitraki M, Liberis V. Comparison of the ultrasonic scalpel to CO(2) laser in cervical conization. Minim Invasive Ther Allied Technol. 2011;20(3):185–8.
43. dos Santos L, Odunsi K, Lele S. Clinicopathologic outcomes of laser conization for high-grade cervical dysplasia. Eur J Gynaecol Oncol. 2004;25(3):305–7.
44. Diakomanolis E, Haidopoulos D, Rodolakis A, Messaris E, Sakellaropoulos G, Calpaktsoglou C, Michalas S. Treating intraepithelial lesions of the uterine cervix by laser CO2. Evaluation of the past, appraisal for the future. Eur J Gynaecol Oncol. 2002;23(5):463–8.
45. Hagen B, Skjeldestad FE, Bratt H, Tingulstad S, Lie AK. CO2 laser conization for cervical intraepithelial neoplasia grade II-III: complications and efficacy. Acta Obstet Gynecol Scand. 1998;77(5):558–63.
46. Santesso N, Mustafa RA, Wiercioch W, Kehar R, Gandhi S, Chen Y, Cheung A, Hopkins J, Khatib R, Ma B, Mustafa AA, Lloyd N, Wu D, Broutet N, Schünemann HJ. Systematic reviews and meta-analyses of benefits and harms of cryotherapy, LEEP, and cold knife conization to treat cervical intraepithelial neoplasia. Int J Gynaecol Obstet. 2016;132(3):266–71.
47. Oyesanya OA, Amerasinghe CN, Manning EA. Outpatient excisional management of cervical intraepithelial neoplasia. A prospective, randomized comparison between loop diathermy excision and laser excisional conization. Am J Obstet Gynecol. 1993;168(2):485–8.
48. Varras M, Akrivis C, Anastasiadis A, Lekkas G, Diakakis G. Peritonitis due to iatrogenic colpotomy after large loop excision of the transformation zone (LLETZ) in a patient with cervical intraepithelial neoplasia III: our experience of a rare case with review of the literature. Eur J Gynaecol Oncol. 2012;33(2):214–6.
49. Nannapaneni P, Naik R, de Barros Lopes A, Monaghan JM. Intra-abdominal bleed following LLETZ. J Obstet Gynaecol. 2002;22(1):99–100.
50. Moon G, Jeon S, Nam KH, Choi S, Sunwoo J, Ryu A. Pseudoaneurysm of uterine artery causing intra-abdominal and vaginal bleeding after cervical conization. Obstet Gynecol Sci. 2015;58(3):256–9.
51. Ghassani A, Andre B, Simon-Toulza C, Tanguy le Gac Y, Martinez A, Vidal F. Vaginal evisceration: an unexpected complication of conization. Case Rep Obstet Gynecol. 2014;2014:983682. https://doi.org/10.1155/2014/983682.
52. Andikyan V, Khoury-Collado F, Denesopolis J, Park KJ, Hussein YR, Brown CL, Sonoda Y, Chi DS, Barakat RR, Abu-Rustum NR. Cervical conization and sentinel lymph node mapping in the treatment of stage I cervical cancer: Is less enough? Int J Gynecol Cancer. 2014;24(1):113–7.
53. Biliatis I, Kucukmetin A, Patel A, Ratnavelu N, Cross P, Chattopadhyay S, Galaal K, Naik R. Small volume stage 1B1 cervical cancer: Is radical surgery still necessary? Gynecol Oncol. 2012;126(1):73–7.

54. Fagotti A, Gagliardi ML, Moruzzi C, Carone V, Scambia G, Fanfani F. Excisional cone as fertility-sparing treatment in early-stage cervical cancer. Fertil Steril. 2011;95(3):1109–12.
55. Reade CJ, Eiriksson LR, Covens A. Surgery for early stage cervical cancer: how radical should it be? Gynecol Oncol. 2013;131(1):222–30.
56. Feng Y, Cao T, Wang Y, Huang H, Xie Y, Liu J. Neoadjuvant chemotherapy followed by conization to spare fertility in cases of locally advanced cervical cancer: a case report and review of the literature. Mol Clin Oncol. 2016;5(4):411–6.

Abdominal Hysterectomy

5

Kiyoshi Hasegawa, Mariko Watanabe, and Kaori Kiuchi

Abstract

Hysterectomy is the most common major operation performed by gynecologic surgeons. There are many indications for abdominal simple (extrafascial) hysterectomy. In high-grade squamous intraepithelial lesion (HSIL), especially cervical intraepithelial neoplasia (CIN) 3, more conservative treatments such as laser conization or the loop electrosurgical excision procedure have been introduced and are effective, making hysterectomy unnecessary in most women. However, for patients with recurrent HSIL (CIN3) who do not wish to preserve fertility, hysterectomy may be an appropriate treatment option. This decision must be made after a thorough discussion between the patient and her physician. Currently, the indications for abdominal hysterectomy are recurrence following conservative treatment for HSIL (CIN3); HSIL (CIN3) with residual disease; adenocarcinoma in situ, with or without a positive surgical margin; International Federation of Gynecology and Obstetrics (FIGO) stage IA1 disease without lymphovascular space invasion (LVSI); FIGO stage IA1 with LVSI; and central recurrent or residual cervical disease in patients with locally advanced cervical cancer treated with radiotherapy or chemoradiotherapy. The ovaries and fallopian tubes may or may not be removed along with the uterus, depending on the patient's age and a variety of other factors, such as a high risk of ovarian cancer with an identified *BRCA* 1/2 germline mutation. Gynecologic surgeons must be aware of the potential complications of hysterectomy: infection, venous thromboembolism, urinary tract injury, bowel injury, bleeding, and vaginal cuff dehiscence. Based on the results of several prospective trials, patients with low-risk, early-stage cervical cancer, a tumor size <2 cm, stromal invasion <10 mm, and no LVSI may be appropriate candidates for less radical surgery, including simple hysterectomy, simple trachelectomy, or cervical conization, with or without sentinel lymph node biopsy or pelvic lymphadenectomy.

K. Hasegawa (✉) · M. Watanabe · K. Kiuchi
Department of Obstetrics and Gynecology, Dokkyo Medical University, Mibu, Tochigi, Japan
e-mail: hasek@dokkyomed.ac.jp

M. Mikami (ed.), *Surgery for Gynecologic Cancer*, Comprehensive Gynecology and Obstetrics, https://doi.org/10.1007/978-981-13-1519-0_5

Keywords
Abdominal hysterectomy · HSIL · CIN · Microinvasive cervical cancer · Complications

5.1 History

Hysterectomy is the most common major operation performed by the gynecologist. There are many indications for hysterectomy, including uterine leiomyoma, adenomyosis, abnormal uterine bleeding, and gynecologic malignancy. The uterus can be removed using a variety of techniques; the approaches include abdominal, vaginal, laparoscopic, and, most recently, robotic.

Vaginal hysterectomy for cervical cancer has been performed in Europe since the 1810s, with the techniques undergoing systematic development until the late nineteenth century. The first attempted abdominal hysterectomy was reported in 1825; however, at that time, abdominal surgery was commonly complicated by often-lethal postoperative hemorrhage. In the mid-nineteenth century, ligation of the uterine arteries during abdominal hysterectomy was first introduced; this technique gradually became common practice. In 1878, Freund introduced an abdominal hysterectomy method that employed anesthesia and antiseptic technique. His operation consisted of ligating the ligaments and major vessels, separating the bladder from the uterus, and amputating the cardinal and uterosacral ligaments. From this point until the late nineteenth century, further improvements were made by several surgeons, and the mortality rate gradually declined to about 5%. In the early decades of the twentieth century, abdominal hysterectomy became more commonly used for the treatment of gynecologic diseases. Surgery became safer, and gynecologic surgeons contributed to developing new surgical procedures. Accurate diagnostic techniques, the use of blood transfusion and antibiotics, and the development of anesthetic techniques greatly reduced overall morbidity.

The indication for abdominal hysterectomy is a benign uterine condition in nearly 90% of patients; the remaining indications are for malignant disease. The former includes leiomyoma, adenomyosis, endometriosis, abnormal bleeding, pelvic organ prolapse, pelvic inflammatory disease, and pregnancy-related conditions, and the latter includes high-grade squamous intraepithelial lesion (HSIL), especially high-grade cervical intraepithelial neoplasm (CIN3), microinvasive cervical cancer, atypical endometrial hyperplasia, endometrial cancer, ovarian cancer, tubal carcinoma, peritoneal cancer, and gestational trophoblastic tumors. Since the introduction of laparoscopic hysterectomy in 1989, this minimally invasive approach has been increasingly employed. However, the most common route of surgery remains abdominal, despite the longer hospital stay, greater postoperative pain, higher rate of infection, and slower return to normal activity [1].

Historically, international trends of treatment for HSIL (CIN3) have changed along with the improvement in medical techniques and instruments, the medical economy, and the accumulation of evidence [2]. In the 1950s, HSIL (CIN3) was traditionally treated using hysterectomy; in the 1960s–1970s, cold knife conization was performed on an inpatient basis. In the 1980s, outpatient cryotherapy or laser conization and vaporization was used, and from 1990 to the present, either the loop electrosurgical excision procedure (LEEP) or large loop excision of the transformational zone (LLETZ) has been employed most frequently [2].

In the past, hysterectomy was performed as primary treatment for SIL (CIN). The introduction of effective, more conservative treatments such as laser conization or LEEP has made hysterectomy unnecessary in most women with this condition. However, hysterectomy remains a popular and accepted method of management for patients with HSIL (CIN3), especially in those who do not desire future fertility. The decision for the type of treatment must be made following a thorough discussion of the risks and benefits between the patient and her physician.

Removal of the upper part of the vagina was previously advocated for the treatment of CIN3, yet there is no basis for this recommendation. In a study by Creasman and Rutledge [3], the recurrence rate of CIN3 of the cervix did not depend on the amount of vagina removed with the uterus. Unless vaginal extension is identified colposcopically, there is no reason for routine removal of the upper vagina.

Although hysterectomy is considered definitive therapy for CIN3, patients must be followed in essentially the same manner as those who opt for conservative treatment. The chance of recurrence of invasive disease is small, but recurrence is not impossible, and these patients must be followed indefinitely.

5.2 Principles and Indications

Definitive pathological evaluation after cervical cone biopsy for HSIL (CIN3), adenocarcinoma in situ (AIS), and International Federation of Gynecology and Obstetrics (FIGO) stage IA cervical cancer is essential for designing an appropriate treatment strategy. Cone biopsy is recommended if a cervical biopsy is inadequate to evaluate for invasive disease or if accurate assessment of microinvasive disease (IA1 or IA2) is required. The choice of therapy should be influenced by the patient's desire to maintain fertility. The indications for simple (extrafascial) abdominal hysterectomy for HSIL (CIN3), AIS, and early cervical cancer are described in Table 5.1.

Table 5.1 Indication of simple hysterectomy in HSIL (CIN3), AIS, and cervical cancer

1. Recurrence following conservative treatment for HSIL (CIN3)
2. HSIL (CIN3) with residual disease
3. AIS with or without positive surgical margin
4. FIGO stage IA1 without LVSI
5. FIGO stage IA1 with LVSI
6. Central recurrent or residual disease existed in the cervix in patients with locally advanced cervical cancer treated with radiotherapy or chemoradiotherapy

FIGO International Federation of Gynecology and Obstetrics, *HSIL* high-grade squamous intraepithelial lesion, *CIN* cervical intraepithelial neoplasia, *AIS* adenocarcinoma in situ, *LVSI* lymph vascular space invasion

5.2.1 Recurrence Following Conservative Treatment (Laser Conization or LEEP) for HSIL (CIN3)

Reconization is appropriate for patients with recurrent HSIL (CIN3) who desire future fertility. For the patients who do not want to preserve fertility, simple hysterectomy may be an appropriate treatment option if the absence of invasive cancer is confirmed.

5.2.2 HSIL (CIN3) with Residual Disease after Conization

For patients with HSIL (CIN3) and positive surgical margins after cone biopsy who have residual disease (CIN3) pathologically confirmed, either reconization or simple hysterectomy may be offered [4].

5.2.3 AIS, with or without Positive Surgical Margins

Simple hysterectomy is recommended for patients with AIS diagnosed by conization, regardless of the status of the surgical margins. Patients with positive surgical margins have a 19% chance of experiencing recurrent disease [5]; simple hysterectomy is therefore recommended. However, patients with negative margins have only a 2.6% chance of recurrent disease [5] and may be treated conservatively if they strongly desire preservation of fertility. The incidence of residual disease in patients with negative margins after conization is low but not negligible [6]. Therefore, conservative management in these patients is possible, but careful surveillance is required.

5.2.4 FIGO Stage IA1 without Lymphovascular Space Invasion (LVSI)

Cervical cancer of FIGO stage IA1 without LVSI has a less than 1% incidence of lymph node metastasis; therefore, if patients do not desire future fertility, simple hysterectomy is an appropriate therapy option. In such cases, lymphadenectomy is not recommended. It is possible to preserve the uterus by performing only cervical conization in patients who strongly desire fertility preservation. However, these patients must have no LVSI, negative surgical margins, and negative histological results from endocervical curettage. For patients with positive margins after conization, options include repeat conization to better evaluate the depth of invasion or radical trachelectomy.

5.2.5 FIGO Stage IA1 with LVSI

For patients with stage IA1 disease with LVSI, simple hysterectomy with pelvic lymphadenectomy, including sentinel lymph node biopsy, is indicated [7]. The

National Comprehensive Cancer Network (NCCN) guideline on cervical cancer [8] recommends modified radical hysterectomy with pelvic lymphadenectomy. Radical trachelectomy with pelvic lymphadenectomy, including sentinel lymph node biopsy, is an option if patients strongly desire fertility preservation. In some patients with stage IA1 disease and LVSI, conization (with negative margins) plus laparoscopic pelvic lymphadenectomy, including sentinel lymph node biopsy, may be a reasonable strategy. These patients may also undergo elective para-aortic lymph node sampling. Observation after conization with negative margins is recommended for patients who are medically inoperable or who refuse surgery.

5.2.6 Central Recurrent or Cervical Residual Disease in Patients with Locally Advanced Cervical Cancer Treated with Radiotherapy or Chemoradiotherapy

In patients with central pelvic recurrent disease after radiation or chemoradiation, pelvic exenteration can be considered after a thorough preoperative evaluation. Surgical mortality is generally 5% or less, with survival rates approaching 50% in carefully selected patients. Radical hysterectomy may be an option in carefully selected patients with small central lesions (<2 cm) [8]. Simple hysterectomy is an option for patients with cervical residual disease after radiation therapy [9]. Reportedly, adjuvant extrafascial hysterectomy after chemoradiation in patients with locally advanced cervical adenocarcinoma improves survival outcomes compared with the current standard of care, and severe complications are rare [10].

5.3 Preoperative Evaluation

The preoperative evaluation should be thorough, taking into account the patient's general medical condition and prior surgical history. The risks, benefits, and potential complications of hysterectomy should be precisely explained to the patient and her family.

5.3.1 Medical History and Physical Examination

Surgery should be undertaken after obtaining a thorough understanding of the patient's medical history and performing a complete physical examination.

Specifically, careful attention should be paid to:

1. Medical history.
2. Current medications.
3. Allergies to medications, food, or environmental agents.
4. Previous surgical procedures.
5. Family history.
6. Others.

5.3.2 Laboratory Evaluation

There are no routinely recommended laboratory tests, although individual hospitals may have their own requirements.

5.3.3 Informed Consent

The preoperative discussion should include a description of the surgical procedure and its expected outcomes and risks; this is the basis for obtaining signed informed consent.

Alternative management options, if any exist, should be presented. The expected or likely results of no treatment should also be presented if the patient does not desire treatment.

5.3.4 Others

5.3.4.1 Venous Thromboembolism (VTE)

Patients should be evaluated for risk factors associated with VTE events such as age, medical history, inherited or acquired thrombophilias, obesity, smoking, and hormonal medications including oral contraceptives. The manifestations of this serious and potentially fatal condition include pulmonary embolism (PE) and deep vein thrombosis (DVT). All patients undergoing hysterectomy are at moderate risk for VTE and require prophylaxis [11].

5.3.4.2 Prophylactic Bilateral Salpingo-Oophorectomy or Prophylactic Bilateral Salpingectomy

The ovaries or fallopian tubes may or may not be removed along with the uterus, depending on the patient's age and a variety of other factors. There is a strong argument in favor of removing both ovaries at the time of hysterectomy in women who have a high risk of developing cancer. In women at high risk for ovarian cancer with an identified *BRCA* 1/2 germline mutation, bilateral salpingo-oophorectomy offers an 80–96% risk reduction [12, 13]. One meta-analysis also showed a reduced risk of subsequent ovarian cancer in average-risk women who have had their fallopian tubes removed [14].

However, a recent large, retrospective study indicated that patients who retain their ovaries have a significantly lower risk of all-cause mortality compared with those who have bilateral ovarian removal; the former population also has lower death rates from ischemic heart disease and cancer [15]. Although removal of both ovaries protects against subsequent development of ovarian cancer, premenopausal women should be advised that this benefit comes at the cost of an increased risk for cardiovascular disease and for other, more prevalent, cancers, along with higher overall mortality. Therefore, salpingectomy with delayed oophorectomy, particularly in premenopausal women, may be a more effective strategy that could overcome the menopause-related quality of life issues associated with oophorectomy [16].

If abdominal hysterectomy is planned, then counseling about the risks and benefits of bilateral salpingo-oophorectomy or bilateral salpingectomy should be included in the informed consent discussion.

5.4 Surgical Technique

The Querleu and Morrow surgical classification system [17] describes the degree of resection and nerve preservation for radical hysterectomy in three-dimensional planes and updates the previously used Piver-Rutledge classification [18]. The types of hysterectomy include simple (extrafascial; type A), modified radical (type B), and radical (type C) using the Querleu and Morrow system. Simple (extrafascial) hysterectomy is equivalent to a type I hysterectomy using the Piver-Rutledge classification system.

Although it is important to learn a basic technique for standard abdominal hysterectomy, every gynecologic surgeon should be interested in learning new and different techniques or modifications to apply when appropriate.

5.4.1 Skin Incision

After confirming that anesthesia is complete, the skin is opened with a scalpel, and the incision is carried down through the subcutaneous tissue and fascia using an electric scalpel. The peritoneum is opened in a similar fashion.

5.4.2 Abdominal Exploration

The upper abdomen and pelvis are explored systematically. The stomach, liver, gallbladder, kidneys, large and small intestines, and pelvic- and para-aortic lymph nodes should be examined and palpated. Particular attention should be paid to the uterus, bilateral ovaries and fallopian tubes, all ligaments, bladder, and rectosigmoid colon, and the presence of any adhesions between these organs should be carefully evaluated.

5.4.3 Wound Retraction

A variety of retractors designed for abdominal and pelvic surgery have been developed, although not all are available at every hospital. Gynecologic surgeons should choose an appropriate retractor for each patient; adjustable retractors may be necessary for obese patients.

5.4.4 Ligation of the Round Ligament

The uterus is elevated by placing clamps on the broad ligament, providing traction and securing the field of view. The round ligament is grasped with forceps at its proximal and distal portion and transected using suture ligation (Fig.5.1). The broad ligament is then incised to separate the anterior and posterior leaves. These steps are repeated on the contralateral side. The anterior leaf of the broad ligament is then incised using an electrical scalpel along the vesicouterine fold, separating the bladder from the lower uterine segment.

5.4.5 Ligation of the Infundibulopelvic Ligament, Utero-Ovarian Ligament, and Fallopian Tube

The ureter may be identified in the retroperitoneal space. If the ovaries are to be preserved, the utero-ovarian ligament and fallopian tube are grasped with forceps, cut, and suture ligated (Fig. 5.2). If the ovaries are to be removed, the peritoneal opening (window) is enlarged sufficiently to properly expose the ovarian vessels within the infundibulopelvic ligament, the uterine artery, and the ureter. The infundibulopelvic ligament is grasped with forceps, cut, and suture ligated; the ovarian vessels are doubly ligated. The bladder is dissected off of the lower uterine segment using an electrical scalpel. The connective tissue around the cardinal ligament is removed, and the posterior leaf of the broad ligament is divided inferiorly toward the uterosacral ligament to aid in uterine mobilization.

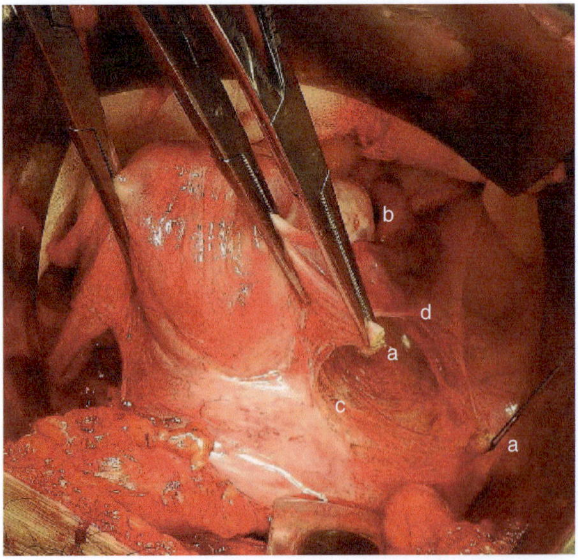

Fig. 5.1 Ligature of the round ligament. The round ligament is grasped with forceps at its proximal and distal portion and transected using suture ligation. The broad ligament is then incised to separate the anterior and posterior leaves. *a*, Stump of left round ligament; *b*, left ovary; *c*, anterior leaf of broad ligament; *d*, anterior leaf of broad ligament

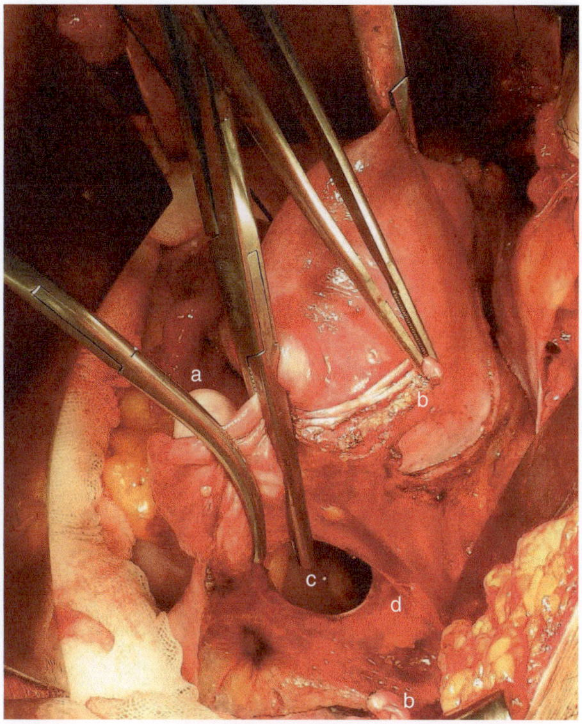

Fig. 5.2 Ligature of utero-ovarian ligament and fallopian tube. The ureter may be identified in the retroperitoneal space. If the ovaries are to be preserved, the utero-ovarian ligament and fallopian tube are grasped with forceps, cut, and suture ligated. *a*, Right ovary; *b*, stump of right round ligament; *c*, window in broad ligament; *d*, anterior leaf of broad ligament

5.4.6 Ligation of the Cardinal Ligament

The uterine artery and vein are dissected and clamped using two curved forceps at the level of the internal os of the cervix. The vessels are then cut and suture ligated (Fig. 5.3). The remaining cardinal ligament is then clamped, cut, and suture ligated. These steps are repeated two or three times, until the level of the cervicovaginal junction is reached (Fig. 5.4). The bladder and rectum are inspected to be sure they are clear of the surgical specimen. At this point, the anterior and posterior vaginal walls are exposed.

5.4.7 Removal of the Uterus

The uterus is placed on traction in a cephalad direction, and the portio vaginalis of the cervix is palpated. An incision is made in the vaginal wall, just beneath the cervicovaginal junction, using an electrical scalpel (Fig. 5.5). The uterus is then removed.

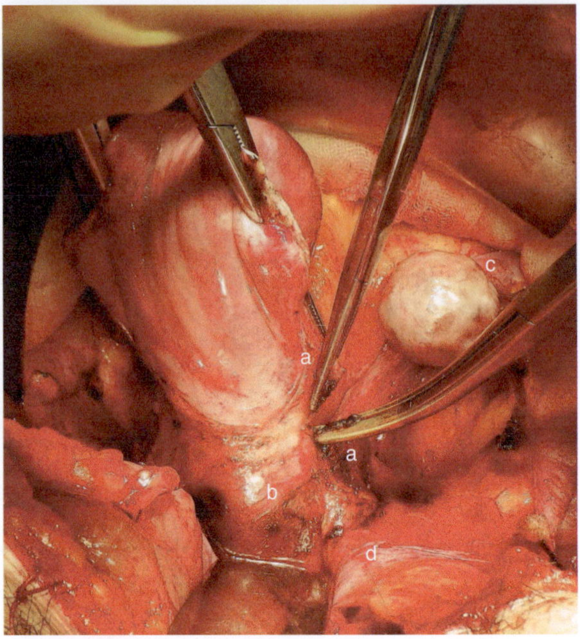

Fig. 5.3 Ligature of the uterine artery and vein. The uterine artery and vein are dissected and clamped using two curved forceps at the level of the internal os of the cervix. The vessels are then cut and suture ligated. *a*, Stump of left uterine vessels; *b*, uterine cervix; *c*, left ovary; *d*, bladder

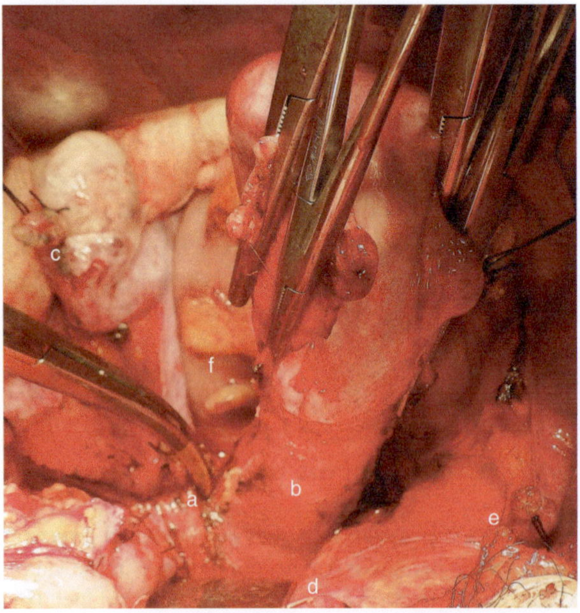

Fig. 5.4 Ligature of the cardinal ligament. After the ligature of uterine vessels, the remaining cardinal ligament is then clamped, cut, and suture ligated. These steps are repeated two or three times, until the level of the cervicovaginal junction is reached. *a*, Right cardinal ligament; *b*, uterine cervix; *c*, right ovary; *d*, bladder; *e*, stump of left round ligament; *f*, rectum

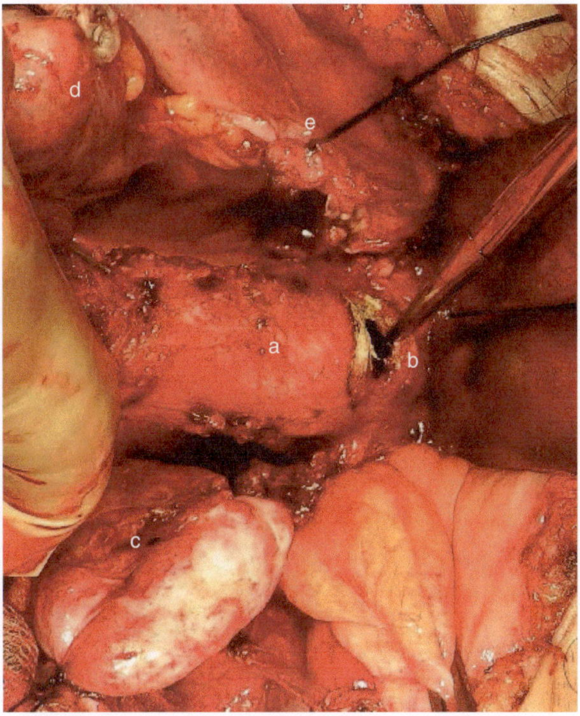

Fig. 5.5 Removal of the uterus. The uterus is placed on traction in a cephalad direction, and the portio vaginalis of the cervix is palpated. An incision is made in the vaginal wall, just beneath the cervicovaginal junction, using an electrical scalpel. The uterus is then removed. *a*, Cervix; *b*, vaginal wall; *c*, right ovary; *d*, left ovary; *e*, stump of left round ligament

5.4.8 Closure of the Vaginal Cuff

After checking to be sure the bladder and rectum are clear of the operative field, the vaginal cuff is cross-clamped using forceps to achieve hemostasis and provide traction. The vaginal cuff is typically closed by suturing (Fig. 5.6).

5.4.9 Irrigation and Hemostasis

The pelvis is thoroughly irrigated with warm saline. Complete hemostasis, particularly of the vascular pedicles, should be carefully ensured. Electrocautery or suture ligation is used to control small areas of bleeding. The bladder, ureter, and rectosigmoid colon should be checked to confirm that they are intact. Antiadhesive material is sometimes used to prevent adhesion formation, especially in patients who already have intraperitoneal adhesions from previous surgery, pelvic inflammatory disease, or endometriosis.

5.4.10 Fascia and Skin Closure

The fascia is closed using interrupted or continuous suturing. The subcutaneous tissue should be irrigated and inspected carefully for hemostasis. The risk of wound disruption seems to be decreased with closure of the subcutaneous fat layer or with

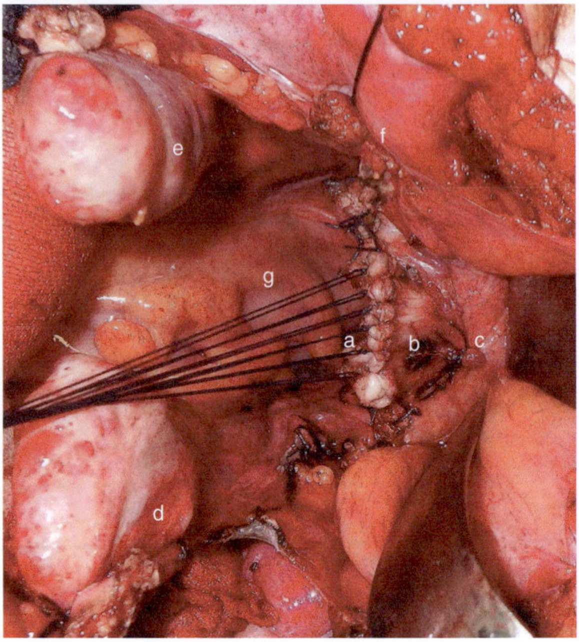

Fig. 5.6 Closure of the vaginal cuff. After checking to be sure the bladder and rectum are clear of the operative field, the vaginal cuff is cross-clamped using forceps to achieve hemostasis and provide traction. The vaginal cuff is typically closed by suturing. *a*, Vaginal stump; *b*, vaginal wall; *c*, bladder; *d*, right ovary; *e*, left ovary; *f*, stump of left round ligament; *g*, rectum

continuous low-pressure suction for draining subcutaneous hemorrhage or exudate in obese women. Skin closure is performed using either staples or subcuticular sutures with adhesive tape.

5.5 Morbidity

Several intraoperative and postoperative complications associated with abdominal hysterectomy have been reported. As trends in surgical techniques change, the complications of surgery may vary.

The rate of complications has often been compared between abdominal, vaginal, and laparoscopic approaches to hysterectomy. The major complications and their rates of reporting [19] are shown in Table 5.2.

5.5.1 Infectious Complications

The rate of infectious complications after hysterectomy is reportedly 10.5% for abdominal, 13.0% for vaginal, and 9.0% for laparoscopic hysterectomy [20]. The most common infections are vaginal cuff cellulitis, an infected hematoma or abscess, wound infection, urinary tract infection, and respiratory infection. The incidence of vaginal cuff cellulitis ranges from 0% to 8.3% [21], with no difference in rate by surgical approach. Prevention involves the use of skillful aseptic surgical technique,

Table 5.2 Complications of hysterectomy

Complications	Abdominal	Vaginal	Laparoscopic	Unclassified
Infections	10.5%	13.0%	9.0%	
Venous thromboembolism				1–12%
Urinary tract injury				
Bladder injury	1%	1.2%	2.1%	
Ureteral injury				0.05–0.5%
Bowel injury	0.3%	0.1–1.0%	0.2%	
Bleeding (mL)	238–660.5	215–287	156–568	
Vaginal cuff dehiscence	0.15%	0.08%	1.35%	0.39%

proper tissue handling, hemostasis, limiting surgical dead space, using appropriate irrigation, and proper antimicrobial prophylaxis. Perioperative antimicrobial prophylaxis is indicated for all types of hysterectomy. Antibiotics should be administered a maximum of 1 h before the time of skin incision. Readministration is recommended for procedures lasting more than 3 h and in patients with an estimated intraoperative blood loss of more than 1500 mL.

There is no difference in the rate of hematoma or abscess formation based on the approach to hysterectomy. If there is obvious purulent or bloody discharge from the vaginal cuff, opening the cuff sutures can be both diagnostic and therapeutic for an infected hematoma or abscess. Transvaginal ultrasound or computed tomography (CT) can diagnose a fluid collection and determine whether drainage is necessary for an infected hematoma or abscess.

The incidence of urinary tract infection after hysterectomy ranges from 0% to 13.0% [21]. A Cochrane meta-analysis found no difference in the rate based on surgical approach [21].

5.5.2 VTE Complications

Postoperative VTE is a serious and potentially fatal condition. Therefore, preoperative evaluation and prevention are extremely important. The precise incidence of VTE, including PE and DVT, after hysterectomy is unclear. The clinical diagnosis rate is 1%, but the rate of events detected by more sensitive laboratory methods may be up to 12% [22]. According to a Cochrane meta-analysis, there is no difference in the rate of VTE based on surgical approach to hysterectomy [21].

The high-risk factors for VTE in general surgery are reportedly increasing age, previous VTE, malignancy, surgery, treatment for cancer (chemotherapy or radiotherapy), duration of anesthesia, nonwhite ethnicity, leg edema, varicose veins, hormone use (e.g., oral contraceptives, hormone replacement therapy, or selective estrogen receptor modulators), inherited or acquired thrombophilias, major lower extremity trauma, obesity, smoking, prolonged immobility or paralysis, pulmonary or cardiac failure, inflammatory bowel disease, and central venous catheterization [22, 23]. All patients undergoing hysterectomy are at moderate risk for VTE and require prophylaxis [21]. However, there have been no clinical trials specifically focused on reducing postoperative VTE in hysterectomy patients. For moderate- or high-risk patients undergoing surgery for benign gynecologic disease, low-dose unfractionated heparin, low-molecular-weight heparin, intermittent pneumatic leg compression, and graded compression stockings have all demonstrated benefit [11].

5.5.3 Urinary Tract Injury

The rate of bladder injury is reportedly 1% for abdominal, 1.2% for vaginal, and 2.1% for laparoscopic hysterectomy [24]. There is an increased risk of combined bladder and ureteral injury during laparoscopic hysterectomy compared with abdominal and vaginal hysterectomy (odds ratio [OR], 2.41; 95% confidence interval [CI], 1.24–4.82, and OR, 3.69; CI, 1.11–12.24, respectively) [21]. Ureteral injury occurs less frequently than bladder injury, with an estimated incidence of 0.05–0.5% for gynecologic surgery. The laparoscopic approach has the highest rate and the vaginal approach the lowest rate [25]. The risk factors associated with ureteral injury are previous pelvic surgery, hemorrhage, endometriosis, cancer, a large pelvic mass or leiomyoma, and obesity.

5.5.4 Bowel Injury

Bowel injury is a less common complication of hysterectomy, with a reported rate of 0.1–1% [20]. A Cochrane review gives a rate of 0.3% rate for abdominal, 0.1–1% for vaginal, and 0.2% for laparoscopic hysterectomy, with no statistically significant difference in the rate of bowel injury by approach [21]. There are three major types of bowel injury that can occur during hysterectomy: thermal injury, direct mechanical damage, and indirect injury through interruption of the vascular supply.

5.5.5 Bleeding Complications

From the results of randomized trials comparing two or more approaches to hysterectomy, the range of blood loss is 238–660.5 mL for abdominal, 215–287 mL for vaginal, and 156–568 mL for laparoscopic hysterectomy [21]. A Cochrane review showed that laparoscopic hysterectomy has a significantly lower estimated blood loss than abdominal hysterectomy (OR, 45.26), and vaginal hysterectomy has a significantly lower estimated blood loss than laparoscopic hysterectomy (OR, 9.72). However, there is no difference in the rate of blood transfusion between the three approaches. There are many variables associated with increased bleeding, including obesity; a poor field of view due to endometriosis, adhesions, or the presence of a large mass; distorted anatomy; uterine fibroids; and the skill of the surgeons.

5.5.6 Vaginal Cuff Dehiscence

Although vaginal cuff dehiscence is a rare complication, with a rate of 0.39%, it can lead to serious morbidity. It is more common after laparoscopic hysterectomy (rate, 1.35%) than abdominal hysterectomy (rate, 0.15%; OR, 9.1; CI, 4.1–20.3) or vaginal hysterectomy (rate, 0.08%; OR, 17.2; CI, 3.5–75.9) [26]. Several risk factors have been postulated: direct trauma from sexual intercourse, chronic cough, constipation, obesity, straining, smoking, malnutrition, anemia, diabetes, immunosuppression, menopausal status, previous pelvic surgery, previous vaginoplasty, and corticosteroid use [27].

5.6 Future Prospects

The standard treatment for patients with early-stage cervical cancer (IA2-IB1) remains radical hysterectomy with pelvic lymphadenectomy. For patients desiring to preserve fertility, radical trachelectomy with pelvic lymphadenectomy is considered a viable option. However, both radical hysterectomy and radical trachelectomy require removal of the parametria and may be associated with significant morbidity. If patients have low-risk, early-stage cervical cancer, determined by a tumor size <2 cm, stromal invasion <10 mm, and no LVSI, the rate of parametrial involvement is reportedly 0–0.6% [28–30]. The retrospective studies that determined this rate suggest the possibility that less radical surgery may be appropriate for patients with low-risk, early-stage cervical cancer. These patients may be offered simple hysterectomy, simple trachelectomy, or cervical conization, with or without sentinel lymph node biopsy or pelvic lymphadenectomy.

Several small, retrospective series have provided initial data suggesting the feasibility and safety of conservative surgery in patients with low-risk, early-stage cervical cancer. The ongoing, prospective ConCerv trial, the SHAPE trial, and the Gynecologic Oncology Group (GOG) 278 study are expected to provide important information on the role of conservative surgery in such patients.

References

1. Aarts JW, Nieboer TE, Johnson N, Tavender E, Garry R, Mol BW, et al. Surgical approach to hysterectomy for benign gynaecological disease. Cochrane Database Syst Rev. 2015;(8):CD003677.
2. Strander B, Hällgren J, Sparén P. Effect of ageing on cervical or vaginal cancer in Swedish women previously treated for cervical intraepithelial neoplasia grade 3: population based cohort study of long term incidence and mortality. BMJ. 2014;348:f7361.
3. Creasman WT, Rutledge F. Carcinoma in situ of the cervix: an analysis of 861 patients. Obstet Gynecol. 1972;39:373.
4. Ghaem-Maghami S, Sagi S, Majeed G, Soutter WP. Incomplete excision of cervical intraepithelial neoplasia and risk of treatment failure: a meta-analysis. Lancet Oncol. 2007;8: 985–93.

5. Salani R, Puri I, Bristow RE. Adenocarcinoma in situ of the uterine cervix: a metaanalysis of 1278 patients evaluating the predictive value of conization margin status. Am J Obstet Gynecol. 2009;200:182.e1-5.
6. Kim JH, Park JY, Kim DY, Kim YM, Kim YT, Nam JH. The role of loop electrosurgical excisional procedure in the management of adenocarcinoma in situ of the uterine cervix. Eur J Obstet Gynecol Reprod Biol. 2009;145:100–3.
7. Lee JY, Kim HS, Kim K, Chung HH, Kim JW, Park NH, et al. Safety of less aggressive surgery for stage IA1 squamous cell carcinoma of the cervix. J Obstet Gynaecol Res. 2014;40:1382–8.
8. Cervical Cancer Guideline (Version1, 2017). NCCN Clinical Practice Guideline in Oncology.
9. Ota T, Takeshima N, Tabata T, Hasumi K, Takizawa K. Adjuvant hysterectomy for treatment of residual disease in patients with cervical cancer treated with radiation therapy. Br J Cancer. 2008;99:1216–20.
10. Yang J, Shen K, Wang J, Yang J, Cao D. Extrafascial hysterectomy after concurrent chemoradiotherapy in locally advanced cervical adenocarcinoma. J Gynecol Oncol. 2016;27:e40.
11. Clarke-Pearson DL, Abaid LN. Prevention of venous thromboembolic events after gynecologic surgery. Obstet Gynecol. 2012;119:155–67.
12. Rebbeck TR, Kauff ND, Domchek SM. Meta-analysis of risk reduction estimates associated with risk-reducing salpingo-oophorectomy in BRCA1 or BRCA2 mutation carriers. J Natl Cancer Inst. 2009;101:80–7.
13. Domchek SM, Friebel TM, Singer CF, Evans DG, Lynch HT, Isaacs C, et al. Association of risk-reducing surgery in BRCA1 or BRCA2 mutation carriers with cancer risk and mortality. JAMA. 2010;304:967–75.
14. Yoon SH, Kim SN, Shim SH, Kang SB, Lee SJ. Bilateral salpingectomy can reduce the risk of ovarian cancer in the general population: a meta-analysis. Eur J Cancer. 2016;55:38–46.
15. Mytton J, Evison F, Chilton PJ, Lilford RJ. Removal of all ovarian tissue versus conserving ovarian tissue at time of hysterectomy in premenopausal patients with benign disease: study using routine data and data linkage. BMJ. 2017;356:j372.
16. Kwon JS, Tinker A, Pansegrau G, McAlpine J, Housty M, McCullum M, et al. Prophylactic salpingectomy and delayed oophorectomy as an alternative for BRCA mutation carriers. Obstet Gynecol. 2013;121:14–24.
17. Querleu D, Morrow CP. Classification of radical hysterectomy. Lancet Oncol. 2008;9:297.
18. Piver MS, Rutledge F, Smith JP. Five classes of extended hysterectomy for women with cervical cancer. Obstet Gynecol. 1974;44:265–72.
19. Clarke-Pearson DL, Geller EJ. Complications of hysterectomy. Obstet Gynecol. 2013;121:654–73.
20. Mäkinen J, Johansson J, Tomás C, Tomás E, Heinonen PK, Laatikainen T, et al. Morbidity of 10 110 hysterectomies by type of approach. Hum Reprod. 2001;16:1473–8.
21. Nieboer TE, Johnson N, Lethaby A, Tavender E, Curr E, Garry R, et al. Surgical approach to hysterectomy for benign gynaecological disease. Cochrane Database Syst Rev. 2009;(3):CD003677.
22. Clarke-Pearson DL, DeLong ER, Synan IS, Coleman RE, Creasman WT. Variables associated with postoperative deep venous thrombosis: a prospective study of 411 gynecology patients and creation of a prognostic model. Obstet Gynecol. 1987;69:146–50.
23. Geerts WH, Pineo GF, Heit JA, Bergqvist D, Lassen MR, Colwell CW, et al. Prevention of venous thromboembolism: the Seventh ACCP Conference on Antithrombotic and Thrombolytic Therapy. Chest. 2004;126:338S–400S.
24. Johnson N, Barlow D, Lethaby A, Tavender E, Curr E, Garry R. Surgical approach to hysterectomy for benign gynaecological disease. Cochrane Database Syst Rev. 2006;(2):CD003677.
25. Gilmour DT, Das S, Flowerdew G. Rates of urinary tract injury from gynecologic surgery and the role of intraoperative cystoscopy. Obstet Gynecol. 2006;107:1366–72.
26. Kho RM, Akl MN, Cornella JL, Magtibay PM, Wechter ME, Magrina JF. Incidence and characteristics of patients with vaginal cuff dehiscence after robotic procedures. Obstet Gynecol. 2009;114:231–5.

27. Robinson BL, Liao JB, Adams SF, Randall TC. Vaginal cuff dehiscence after robotic total laparoscopic hysterectomy. Obstet Gynecol. 2009;114:369–71.
28. Covens A, Rosen B, Murphy J, Laframboise S, DePetrillo AD, Lickrish G, et al. How important is removal of the parametrium at surgery for carcinoma of the cervix? Gynecol Oncol. 2002;84:145–9.
29. Wright JD, Grigsby PW, Brooks R, Powell MA, Gibb RK, Gao F, et al. Utility of parametrectomy for early stage cervical cancer treated with radical hysterectomy. Cancer. 2007;110:1281–6.
30. Frumovitz M, Sun CC, Schmeler KM, Deavers MT, Dos Reis R, Levenback CF, et al. Parametrial involvement in radical hysterectomy specimens for women with early-stage cervical cancer. Obstet Gynecol. 2009;114:93–9.

Modified Radical Hysterectomy

6

Yasuyuki Hirashima, Munetaka Takekuma, Nobutaka Takahashi, Masakazu Abe, Nobuhiro Kado, Yuka Kasamatsu, Ayako Mochizuki, and Emi Yoshioka

Abstract

Modified radical hysterectomy (MRH) is thought to be equivalent to class II (Piver classification) or type B (Querleu classification) radical hysterectomy (RH) and identical to the original method of the Wertheim operation. MRH is a method of hysterectomy defined as being intermediate between simple hysterectomy and RH and enabling almost full preservation of the pelvic splanchnic nerves and hypogastric plexus. This surgical procedure entails the cutting of the anterior leaf, not the posterior one, of the vesicouterine ligament of the uterus. The ureter is mobilized laterally, part of the parametrial tissue is transected at the level of the ureteral tunnel, and at least 10 mm of the vaginal wall from the uterine cervix is removed. The indication of MRH (with pelvic lymphadenectomy) in cervical cancer is International Federation of Gynecology and Obstetrics stage IA1 with lymphovascular space invasion or stage IA2. MRH is associated with a very low (≤1%) rate of significant postoperative complications, and compared with RH, it reduces the rate of adverse effects on the urinary tract, such as fistula formation and severe voiding dysfunction. The mortality rate for those undergoing this procedure is 0.4–0.5%. The possibility of MRH for low-risk FIGO stage IB1 patients has been considered, and clinical trials are ongoing.

Keywords

Modified radical hysterectomy · Cervical cancer · FIGO stage IA1 · FIGO stage IA2

Y. Hirashima (✉) · M. Takekuma · N. Takahashi · M. Abe
N. Kado · Y. Kasamatsu · A. Mochizuki · E. Yoshioka
Division of Gynecology, Shizuoka Cancer Center, Shizuoka, Japan
e-mail: y.hirashima@scchr.jp

M. Mikami (ed.), *Surgery for Gynecologic Cancer*, Comprehensive Gynecology and Obstetrics, https://doi.org/10.1007/978-981-13-1519-0_6

6.1 History

After Clark of Johns Hopkins University reported the first radical hysterectomy (RH) in 1895, Wertheim performed 500 cervical cancer operations; reported the associated histological examinations, mortality rate, operability rate, and 5-year cure rate; and established RH as a new operative method [1, 2]. Several modifications were subsequently made to RH. For example, Latzko [3] and Okabayashi [4] made great contributions to this surgery by designing operative procedures. They defined the pararectal and paravesical spaces in the parametria, which were divided by three ligaments, and the concepts of their two procedures were very similar. However, in the Okabayashi method [4], the posterior leaf of the vesicouterine ligament is separated and divided intentionally, and then the paracolpium is isolated and divided. The Okabayashi procedure enables the surgeon to separate the bladder with the ureter completely away from the lateral side of the cervix and vagina and allows easy resection of any vaginal length with paracolpium deemed appropriate for the optimization of RH. Therefore, the Okabayashi method is the standard approach to RH in Japan.

Owing to the numerous modifications that have been established, the term "RH" actually connoted many different operations among surgeons. There was also confusion regarding evaluation of the results and morbidity of RH for patients with cervical cancer because of the lack of definitions of the procedures involved. In this context, Piver-Rutledge-Smith reported five classes of extended hysterectomy and defined the extent of radicality of each procedure, as outlined in Table 6.1 [5].

However, it came to be thought that this classification was insufficient. Reasons for this include a lack of clear anatomical landmarks or international anatomical definitions, the degree of vaginal resection being systematically associated with the pericervical extent and overly aggressive and rarely necessary, and the failure

Table 6.1 Piver-Rutledge-Smith classification of hysterectomy for cervical cancer

Class	Description
I	Extrafascial hysterectomy Complete removal of the cervix
II	Modified radical hysterectomy Removal of medial cardinal, uterosacral ligaments, and upper one-third vagina The uterine vessels are divided medial to the ureter
III	Equivalent to the classical Meigs, Latzko, or Okabayashi operation Wide radical resection of the parametrium and paravaginal tissues with ligation of uterine artery as it originates from the internal iliac artery Ureter dissected completely to bladder entry Uterosacral ligaments divided at origin Cardinal ligaments divided at pelvic sidewall One-half of the vagina removed
IV	Extended radical hysterectomy Ureter divided from vesicouterine ligament. Superior vesical artery ligated and upper three-fourths of the vagina excised
V	Partial exenteration Resection of portion of bladder or ureter with reimplantation

Table 6.2 Querleu-Morrow classification of RH, 2008

Type	Description
A	Extrafascial hysterectomy Paracervix medial to ureter <10 mm vagina
B	Partial uterosacral and vesicouterine ligaments Paracervix at the ureter 10 mm vagina B1: without lateral paracervical lymph nodes B2: with lateral paracervical lymph nodes
C	Uterosacral ligaments at the rectum Vesicouterine ligaments at the bladder Paracervix at the internal iliac vessels 15–20 mm vagina C1: with hypogastric nerve preservation C2: without hypogastric nerve preservation
D	Complete paracervical resection D1: with hypogastric vessels D2: with hypogastric vessels and adjacent fascia and muscular structures

to take into account the idea of nerve-sparing RH, which was introduced in the 1950s [6]. This latter procedure was subsequently refined by Japanese surgeons [7–9] and adopted by European surgeons [10, 11]. To overcome these limitations, Querleu and Morrow published a new classification in 2008, which describes four types of RH with various subcategories; this is called the Kyoto classification and is outlined in Table 6.2 [12]. In this classification, not only the therapeutic effect of the techniques but also the postoperative adverse effects are taken into account. This system can be applied to conservative operations aiming for the preservation of fertilization or to cases of vaginal, abdominal open, laparoscopic, and robotic approaches.

At an early stage of the history of RH for invasive cervical cancer, as mentioned above, the surgery was intended to be radical, and focus was placed on aggressiveness and the appropriate technique for maximizing survival, with less consideration of the patient's quality of life. However, during the latter half of the twentieth century, class III (Piver) or type C (Querleu) RH generally became relegated to the treatment of patients with earlier invasive cervical cancer, many of whom had a low risk of parametrial involvement, owing to efforts to find a better balance of cure rate and morbidity [13–18]. In addition, as cancer screening by the Papanicolaou test spread, the proportion of patients with earlier invasive cervical cancer increased [19–22]. Therefore, the policy of applying less radical procedures for these patients received wide support. In this context, Nelson [23] and Piver [5] reevaluated the original operation of Wertheim as being suitable for microinvasive cervical cancer, and Piver classified this method as type II RH. These efforts are regarded as being the source of the modern procedure of modified radical hysterectomy (MRH). MRH is now thought to be equivalent to class II (Piver) or type B (Querleu) RH and identical to the original method of the Wertheim operation.

6.2 Principle and Indication

6.2.1 Principle

MRH is a method of hysterectomy defined as being intermediate between simple hysterectomy and RH, and enabling almost full preservation of the pelvic splanchnic nerves and hypogastric plexus, which reduces the frequency of bladder dysfunction compared with RH [24–26]. The MRH surgical procedure entails cutting of the anterior leaf, not the posterior one, of the vesicouterine ligament of the uterus. The ureter is mobilized laterally, part of the parametrial tissue is transected at the level of the ureteral tunnel, and at least 10 mm of the vaginal wall from the uterine cervix is removed.

6.2.2 Indication

The indication of MRH (with pelvic lymphadenectomy) in cervical cancer with non-fertility-sparing approaches is International Federation of Gynecology and Obstetrics (FIGO) stage IA1 with lymphovascular space invasion (LVSI) or stage IA2 in the guidelines of both the National Comprehensive Cancer Network [27] and the Japan Society of Gynecological Oncology [28].

The incidence of pelvic lymph node metastasis in stage IA1 is very low at 0–1%, but some reports have described that lymph node metastasis is common in cases with LVSI, so both MRH and pelvic lymphadenectomy are performed for stage IA1 patients with LVSI [29–31]. However, it has been asserted that extraction of the uterus is sufficient in simple hysterectomy (SH) for stage IA1 patients with LVSI, including adenocarcinoma [32, 33].

On the other hand, in stage IA2, the incidence of pelvic lymph node metastasis is 0–10% and that of LVSI, which is a risk factor of lymph node metastasis, is 2–30%. The risk of parametrial invasion is very low because no such invasion was revealed in a review of 20 articles on 103 stage IA2 cases [34] or in recent reports of 142 cases [35–37]. This background suggests that MRH with pelvic lymphadenectomy should be considered for stage IA2 disease.

6.3 Preoperative Evaluation

The current official staging system for cervical cancer is based on the FIGO classification [38, 39]. The procedures for this evaluation are limited to the results of the doctor's physical examination under anesthesia, colposcopy, endocervical curettage, hysteroscopy, cystoscopy, proctoscopy, intravenous urography, barium enema, and radiography of the lungs and skeleton [40]. Especially in cases suspected of being stage IA by cervical cytology and biopsies with colposcopy, pathological diagnosis by conization sampling is basically recommended [27, 28]. When conization is omitted in cases of elderly patients with severe uterine atrophy, it is necessary to perform either hysterectomy among SH, MRH, or RH appropriate to the estimated stage after sufficient preoperative cytological examination and using the result of biopsy with colposcopy [28]. In these cases, magnetic resonance imaging (MRI) is also applied for the purpose to decide operative method.

In the revised FIGO staging, incorporation of cross-sectional imaging is encouraged where available, but it is not accepted for formal staging purposes. In addition, no cross-sectional imaging is necessary for stage IA1 patients without LVSI because the risk of metastatic disease is negligible. For patients who have LVSI or more invasive lesions, the use of computed tomography (CT), MRI, and combined positron emission tomography (PET) may aid in treatment planning, and in fact these tomographic imaging techniques play an essential role in preoperative evaluation to guide the selection of treatment in developed countries [27, 41–43].

6.4 Technique

Abdominal MRH is performed in a logical stepwise fashion as below.

6.4.1 Division of the Round Ligaments

The round ligaments are clamped and divided, and from this point, the peritoneum of the iliac fossa is dissected laterally to expose the psoas major muscle.

6.4.2 Development of Pelvic Retroperitoneal Space

Pelvic retroperitoneal space is developed with dissection of the loose avascular tissue; then, not only the external iliac artery and vein but also the internal iliac artery to the lateral umbilical ligament are identified (Fig. 6.1).

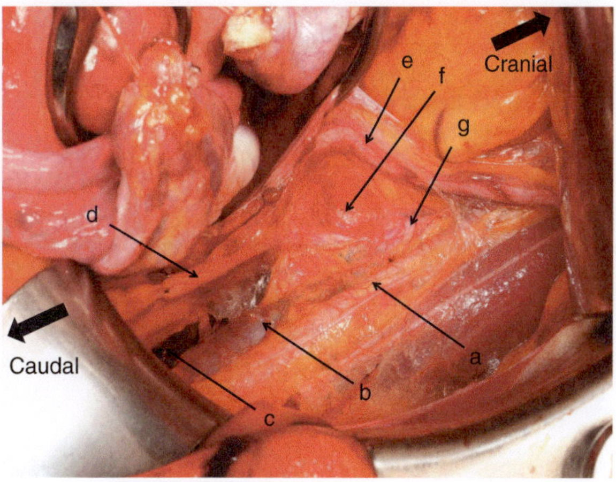

Fig. 6.1 Development of pelvic retroperitoneal space (left side). *a*, External iliac artery; *b*, external iliac vein; *c*, entrance of paravesical space; *d*, lateral umbilical ligament; *e*, ureter; *f*, entrance of pararectal space; *g*, internal iliac artery

6.4.3 Development of Paravesical Space

The lateral umbilical ligament is clamped by Kelly forceps and pulled ventrally; paravesical space is developed from a point of more medial than external iliac vessel and more lateral than the lateral umbilical ligament. If the procedure is carried out precisely, the internal obturator muscle is identified.

6.4.4 Development of (Latzko's) Pararectal Space

The pararectal space is developed from a point of more medial than the internal iliac vessel and along the lateral side of the mesoureter and the line of the pelvic axis by separating the connective tissues (Fig. 6.2).

6.4.5 Pelvic Lymphadenectomy

When pelvic lymphadenectomy or sentinel lymph node mapping is planned, they are performed at this time.

6.4.6 Separation of the Bladder from the Cervix

The bladder flap is cut by grasping the peritoneum of the vesicouterine fold just below its reflection onto the uterus. The cut end of the peritoneum is clamped by two Mikulicz forceps and pulled ventrally, and then the avascular connective tissue between the bladder and cervix is separated by electrocautery. Blunt separation with gauze or another suitable implement is not recommended in this procedure.

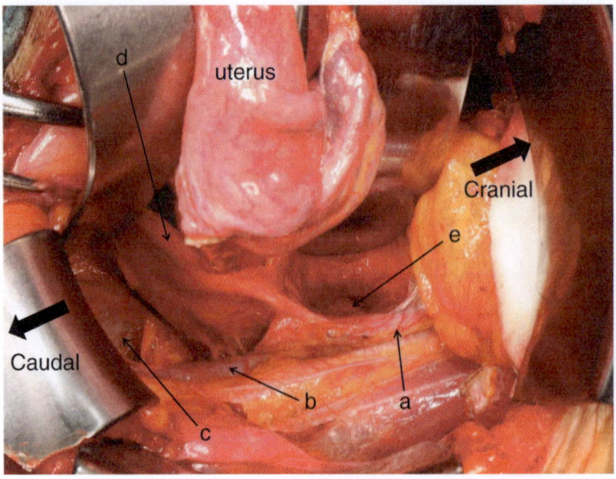

Fig. 6.2 Development of paravesical and pararectal space (left side). *a*, Internal iliac artery; *b*, external iliac vein; *c*, paravesical space; *d*, lateral umbilical ligament; *e*, pararectal space

6.4.7 Isolation and Division of the Uterine Artery

The lateral umbilical ligament is clamped by Kelly forceps, pulled ventrally, and dissected free proximally; then, the superior vesical artery and the uterine artery, which are branches of the internal iliac artery, are identified. The uterine artery is isolated (Fig. 6.3), ligated, and divided at the origin from the internal iliac artery. The medial cut end of the uterine artery is pulled ventrally, and the uterine artery is dissected free to the crossing with the ureter.

As another method, the uterine artery is divided just medial from where it crosses the ureter (Fig. 6.4). This method might preserve the distal ureteric blood supply and reduce the incidence of avascular necrosis and subsequent fistula formation of the ureter.

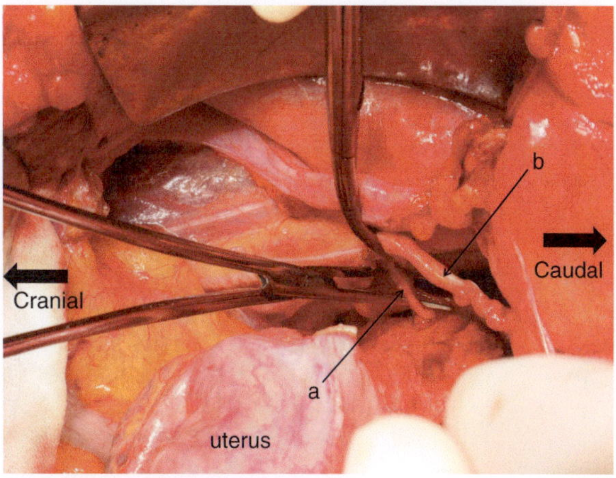

Fig. 6.3 Isolation of uterine artery (left side). *a*, Uterine artery; *b*, lateral umbilical ligament

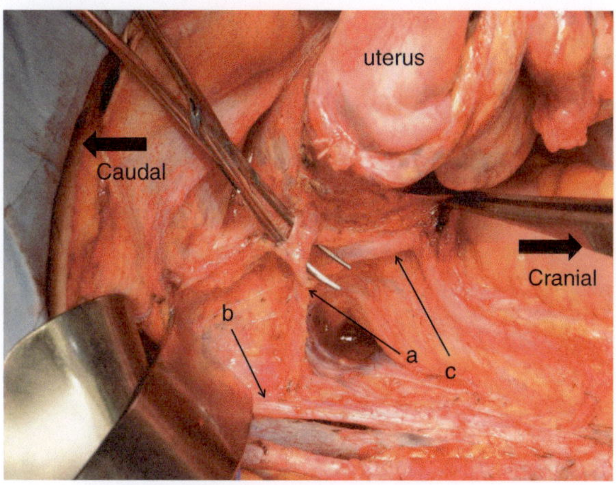

Fig. 6.4 Division of the uterine artery in another method (left side). *a*, Uterine artery; *b*, lateral umbilical ligament; *c*, ureter

6.4.8 Isolation of the Ureter

The ureter is dissected free from the peritoneum of the posterior broad ligament into the pelvis to the level where the uterine artery crosses over it.

6.4.9 Division of the Peritoneum of the Douglas Pouch and Development of the Rectovaginal Space

The uterus is pulled caudally, and the rectum is pulled cranially, and then the peritoneum of the Douglas pouch is stretched and divided. Next, avascular physaliform loose connective tissue of the rectovaginal space is separated by electrocautery (Fig. 6.5). Blunt separation is not recommended in this procedure.

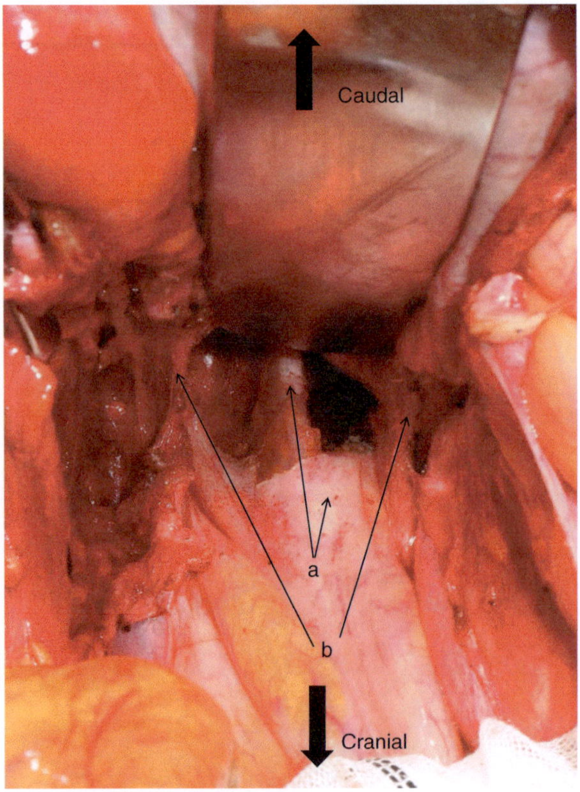

Fig. 6.5 Development of the rectovaginal space. *a*, Rectum; *b*, uterosacral ligaments

6.4.10 Division of Uterosacral Ligaments

While ensuring the same tension of the uterus and the rectum as in the above procedures, uterosacral ligaments are divided by electrocautery by releasing the sheet of the ligaments one by one. Because bleeding rarely occurs in association with this procedure, the clamping, division, and ligation of uterosacral ligaments seem to be unnecessary.

6.4.11 Division of Anterior Leaf of the Vesicouterine Ligament

The cut end of the uterine artery of the uterine side is pulled ventrally, and the ureter is pulled laterally, and after the connective tissue between them is separated carefully, the ureteral branch of the uterine artery is identified, ligated, and divided. Then, the entrance of the so-called ureteral tunnel is clearly identified. Metzenbaum scissors are inserted into the ureteral tunnel pushing the ureter latero-caudally by its back face; in this way, the tunnel is extended (Fig. 6.6). The anterior leaf of the vesicouterine ligament is clamped, divided, and ligated two to three times with the insertion of two Kelly forceps. It is very useful to use a small vessel sealing device in this division. However, the distance between the ureter and the cutting line must be sufficient to avoid heat damage to the ureter. Next, the connective tissue of the dorsal side of the ureter is separated easily, so the ureter is free and mobile to enter the bladder (Fig. 6.7).

Recently, Fuji et al. [44] reported a new anatomical knowledge and a new operative procedure for the anterior leaf of the vesicouterine ligament. They identified a new pair of small blood vessels that cross over the ureter from the lateral cervix to the urinary bladder and named them the cervicovesical blood vessels (Fig. 6.8). In this article, instead of developing the ureteral tunnel, the connective tissue of the anterior leaf of the vesicouterine ligament is carefully divided. The cervicovesical

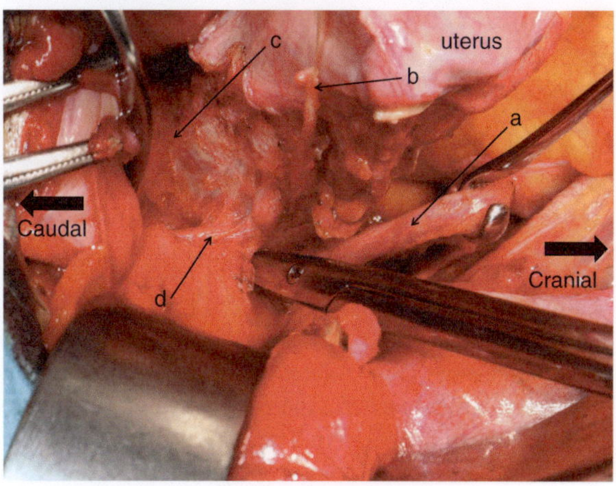

Fig. 6.6 Division of anterior leaf of the vesicouterine ligament (left side). Metzenbaum scissors is inserted into the ureteral tunnel. *a*, Ureter; *b*, cut end of uterine artery; *c*, cervix; *d*, a part of anterior layer of vesicouterine ligament

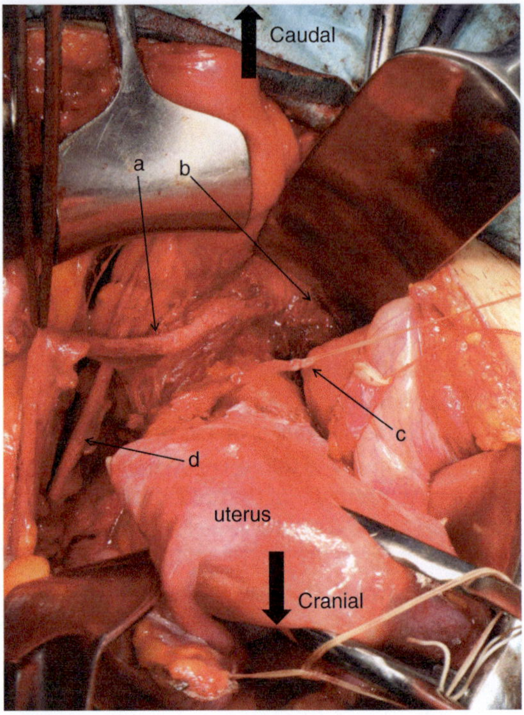

Fig. 6.7 After division of anterior leaf of the vesicouterine ligament (left side). *a*, Ureter; *b*, bladder; *c*, cut end of uterine artery; *d*, lateral umbilical ligament

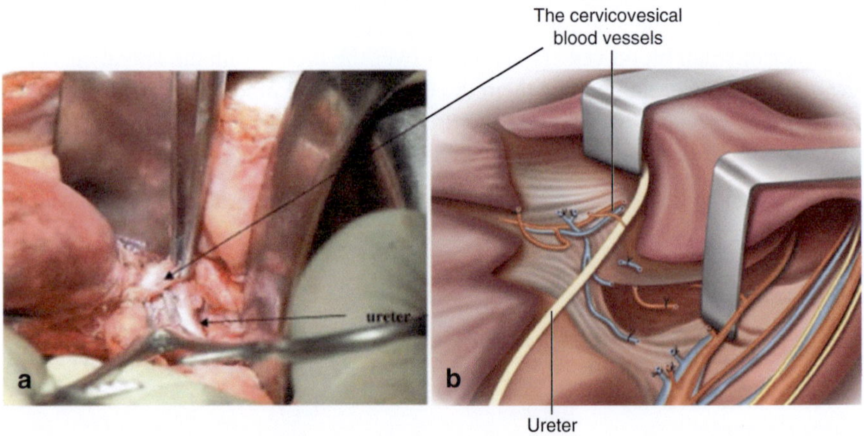

Fig. 6.8 (**a**) Division of the cervicovesical vessels. (**b**) Illustration of the division of the cervicovesical vessels. Reuse with permission [44]

blood vessels are then isolated, doubly clamped, divided, and ligated. After cutting the cervicovesical vessels, the connective tissues between the ureter and the cervix are meticulously separated. They reported that this method enabled division of the anterior leaf of the vesicouterine ligament without any blood loss.

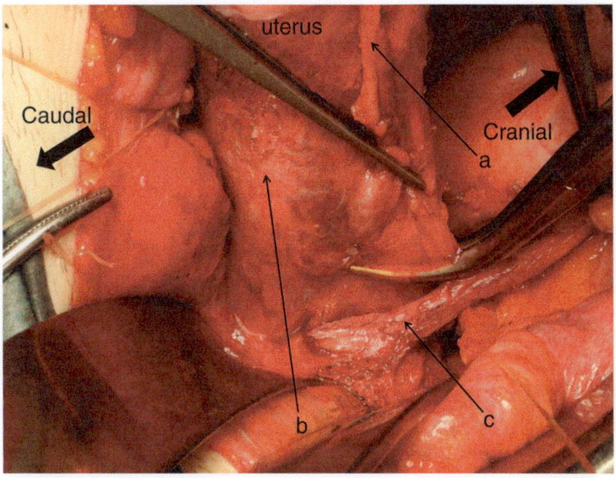

Fig. 6.9 Clamping of parametrial tissue. *a*, Uterine artery; *b*, cervix; c, ureter

6.4.12 Division of Parametrial Tissue

The parametrial tissue is clamped (Fig. 6.9), divided, and doubly ligated at the level of the ureteral tunnel to remove at least 10 mm of the vaginal wall. The divided parametrial tissue contains uterine side origins of cardinal ligament and posterior leaf of the vesicouterine ligament.

6.4.13 Amputation of Vaginal Wall

The vaginal wall is cut from the anterior wall by electrocautery, and the uterus is finally removed. The top of the vagina is closed with absorbable suture.

6.5 Morbidity and Mortality

MRH is reported to be associated with low morbidity and mortality. Magrina et al. [24] reported the morbidity and mortality of 375 MRH cases in detail during the entire length of the follow-up period averaging 8.4 years. In this previous study, pelvic and para-aortic lymphadenectomy was performed concomitantly with MRH in 55% and 10% of cases, respectively. Forty-five patients (12%) had a history of pelvic irradiation, and postoperative irradiation was administered to 120 (32%) patients. The operative mortality was 0.5%. The most common postoperative complications were urinary tract infection, inability to void, wound infection, atelectasis, and ileus. The researchers reported that MRH was associated with a very low ($\leq$1%) rate of significant postoperative complications and functional changes of the urinary tract. A comparison of complications associated with MRH from other literatures [25, 26] is shown in Table 6.3. Furthermore, urinary tract fistula occurred in 6 (0.5%) of 1190 collected patients from a review of the literature, and operative mortality was 0.4% (5 of 1190) [24].

Table 6.3 Comparison of morbidity with MRH: series from literature

Type	Magria *n*: 375 (%)	Landoni *n*: 119 (%)	Yang *n*: 39 (%)
Wound			
Infection	4	–	2.6
Dehiscence	0.5	–	2.6
Hematoma	2	–	–
Intestinal			
Ileus	4	–	2.6
Obstruction	1.3	1.7	0
Fistula	0.3	–	0
Constipation	–	–	43.6
Urinary			
Infection	10	–	–
Fistula	0.3	0	0
Voiding difficulty (atonic bladder)	5	6.7	15.4
Pulmonary			
Pneumonia	0.8	–	–
Embolism	0.8	1.7	–
Cardiovascular			
Deep vein thrombosis	0.3	0	–
Lymphatic			
Lymphocysts	1.6	3.4	0
Lymphoedema	16	13	–

Findings have shown that, compared with RH, MRH reduces the rate of adverse effects on the urinary tract, such as fistula formation and severe voiding dysfunction [24–26, 45]. Plotti et al. also reported that MRH was related to better sexual function than RH [46].

6.6 Future Prospects

The worldwide standard operative treatment for FIGO stage IB1 cervical cancer is RH [27, 28]. However, RH is associated with high morbidity and complications depending on the extent of necessary resection of the parametrium or paracolpium [47]. Therefore, the possibility of less radical procedures for FIGO stage IB1 patients has been considered. In a prospective randomized study by Landoni et al. [26], the 5-year overall survival (OS) rates of MRH and RH for FIGO stage IB and IIA patients were 81% and 77%, respectively, and late morbidity was significantly lower in patients in the MRH arm. In addition, Michalas et al. retrospectively reported that the 5-year OS of MRH for FIGO stage IA to IIA patients (IB, 86.7%) was 88.7% [48].

On the other hand, a patient population at low risk of parametrial involvement and good prognosis has been identified in order to determine the indication of less radical surgery [49–53]. In these reports, tumor diameter (TD) < 2 cm was commonly identified as a criterion of low risk, along with other factors such as no LVSI, superficial invasion, and negative lymph node metastasis. The rate of parametrial invasion in each low-risk group was reported to be very low (0–0.6%). Recently,

Kato et al. [54] also retrospectively reported about parametrial involvement and 5-year OS in patients with FIGO stage IB1 who underwent RH. Parametrial involvement was present in 1.9% of those with TD ≤ 2 cm and 12.9% with TD > 2 cm, and the 5-year OS was 95.8% in those with TD ≤ 2 cm and 91.9% with TD > 2 cm.

The satisfactory effectiveness of MRH for FIGO IB1 patients in the low-risk group mentioned above has also been reported retrospectively [25, 45, 55, 56]. A prospective non-randomized confirmatory trial is also currently ongoing in Japan to evaluate the efficacy of MRH in patients with TD ≤ 2 cm and FIGO stage IB1 [57].

References

1. Wertheim E. Die erweiterte abdominale Operation bei Carcinoma colli Uteri (auf Grund von 500 Fallen). Berlin: Urban & Schwarzenberg; 1911.
2. Wertheim E. The extended abdominal operation for carcinoma uteri (based on 500 operative cases). Am J Obstet Dis Women Child. 1912;66:169–232.
3. Latzko W, Schiffmann J. Klinisches und Anatomisches zur Radikaloperation des Geba¨rmutterkrebses (nach einem am 24. Juni 1919 gehaltenen Vortrag). Diskussinsbemerkungen, Weibel W und Wertheim E Zbl Gyna¨k. 1919;43:715–9.
4. Okabayashi H. Radical abdominal hysterectomy for cancer of the cervix uteri, modification of the Takayama operation. Surg Gynecol Obstet. 1921;33:335–41.
5. Piver MS, Rutledge F, Smith JP. Five classes of extended hysterectomy for women with cervical cancer. Obstet Gynecol. 1974;44(2):265–72.
6. Kobayashi T. Abdominal radical hysterectomy with pelvic lymphadenectomy for cancer of the cervix. Tokyo: Nanzando; 1961.
7. Yabuki Y, Asamoto A, Hoshiba T, Nishimoto H, Satou N. A new proposal for radical hysterectomy. Gynecol Oncol. 1996;62(3):370–8. https://doi.org/10.1006/gyno.1996.0251.
8. Sakuragi N, Todo Y, Kudo M, Yamamoto R, Sato T. A systematic nerve-sparing radical hysterectomy technique in invasive cervical cancer for preserving postsurgical bladder function. Int J Gynecol Cancer. 2005;15(2):389–97. https://doi.org/10.1111/j.1525-1438.2005.15236.x.
9. Fujii S. Anatomic identification of nerve-sparing radical hysterectomy: a step-by-step procedure. Gynecol Oncol. 2008;111(2 Suppl):S33–41. https://doi.org/10.1016/j.ygyno.2008.07.026.
10. Trimbos JB, Maas CP, Deruiter MC, Peters AA, Kenter GG. A nerve-sparing radical hysterectomy: guidelines and feasibility in Western patients. Int J Gynecol Cancer. 2001;11(3):180–6.
11. Raspagliesi F, Ditto A, Fontanelli R, Solima E, Hanozet F, Zanaboni F, et al. Nerve-sparing radical hysterectomy: a surgical technique for preserving the autonomic hypogastric nerve. Gynecol Oncol. 2004;93(2):307–14. https://doi.org/10.1016/j.ygyno.2004.01.048.
12. Querleu D, Morrow CP. Classification of radical hysterectomy. Lancet Oncol. 2008;9(3):297–303. https://doi.org/10.1016/s1470-2045(08)70074-3.
13. Hoskins WJ, Ford JH Jr, Lutz MH, Averette HE. Radical hysterectomy and pelvic lymphadenectomy for the management of early invasive cancer of the cervix. Gynecol Oncol. 1976;4(3):278–90.
14. Webb MJ, Symmonds RE. Wertheim hysterectomy: a reappraisal. Obstet Gynecol. 1979;54(2):140–5.
15. Underwood PB Jr, Wilson WC, Kreutner A, Miller MC 3rd, Murphy E. Radical hysterectomy: a critical review of twenty-two years' experience. Am J Obstet Gynecol. 1979;134(8):889–98.
16. Powell JL, Burrell MO, Franklin EW 3rd. Radical hysterectomy and pelvic lymphadenectomy. Gynecol Oncol. 1981;12(1):23–32.
17. Artman LE, Hoskins WJ, Bibro MC, Heller PB, Weiser EB, Barnhill DR, et al. Radical hysterectomy and pelvic lymphadenectomy for stage IB carcinoma of the cervix: 21 years experience. Gynecol Oncol. 1987;28(1):8–13.

18. Kenter GG, Ansink AC, Heintz AP, Aartsen EJ, Delemarre JF, Hart AA. Carcinoma of the uterine cervix stage I and IIA: results of surgical treatment: complications, recurrence and survival. Eur J Surg Oncol. 1989;15(1):55–60.
19. Christopherson WM, Scott MA. Trends in mortality from uterine cancer in relation to mass screening. Acta Cytol. 1977;21(1):5–9.
20. Kim K, Rigal RD, Patrick JR, Walters JK, Bennett A, Nordin W, et al. The changing trends of uterine cancer and cytology: a study of morbidity and mortality trends over a twenty year period. Cancer. 1978;42(5):2439–49.
21. Eddy DM. Screening for cervical cancer. Ann Intern Med. 1990;113(3):214–26.
22. Lees BF, Erickson BK, Huh WK. Cervical cancer screening: evidence behind the guidelines. Am J Obstet Gynecol. 2016;214(4):438–43. https://doi.org/10.1016/j.ajog.2015.10.147.
23. Jr NJ. Atlas of radical pelvic surgery. New York: Appelton-Century-Crofts; 1969.
24. Magrina JF, Goodrich MA, Weaver AL, Podratz KC. Modified radical hysterectomy: morbidity and mortality. Gynecol Oncol. 1995;59(2):277–82. https://doi.org/10.1006/gyno.1995.0022.
25. Yang YC, Chang CL. Modified radical hysterectomy for early Ib cervical cancer. Gynecol Oncol. 1999;74(2):241–4. https://doi.org/10.1006/gyno.1999.5434.
26. Landoni F, Maneo A, Cormio G, Perego P, Milani R, Caruso O, et al. Class II versus class III radical hysterectomy in stage IB-IIA cervical cancer: a prospective randomized study. Gynecol Oncol. 2001;80(1):3–12. https://doi.org/10.1006/gyno.2000.6010.
27. Cervical Cancer Guideline (version 1. 2017) [database on the Internet]. NCCN Clinical Practice Guidelines in Oncology. 2017.
28. Ebina Y, Yaegashi N, Katabuchi H, Nagase S, Udagawa Y, Hachisuga T, et al. Japan Society of Gynecologic Oncology guidelines 2011 for the treatment of uterine cervical cancer. Int J Clin Oncol. 2015;20(2):240–8. https://doi.org/10.1007/s10147-015-0806-7.
29. Sevin BU, Nadji M, Averette HE, Hilsenbeck S, Smith D, Lampe B. Microinvasive carcinoma of the cervix. Cancer. 1992;70(8):2121–8.
30. Takeshima N, Yanoh K, Tabata T, Nagai K, Hirai Y, Hasumi K. Assessment of the revised International Federation of Gynecology and obstetrics staging for early invasive squamous cervical cancer. Gynecol Oncol. 1999;74(2):165–9. https://doi.org/10.1006/gyno.1999.5473.
31. Elliott P, Coppleson M, Russell P, Liouros P, Carter J, MacLeod C, et al. Early invasive (FIGO stage IA) carcinoma of the cervix: a clinico-pathologic study of 476 cases. Int J Gynecol Cancer. 2000;10(1):42–52.
32. Bouchard-Fortier G, Reade CJ, Covens A. Non-radical surgery for small early-stage cervical cancer. Is it time? Gynecol Oncol. 2014;132(3):624–7. https://doi.org/10.1016/j.ygyno.2014.01.037.
33. Lee JY, Kim HS, Kim K, Chung HH, Kim JW, Park NH, et al. Safety of less aggressive surgery for stage IA1 squamous cell carcinoma of the cervix. J Obstet Gynaecol Res. 2014;40(5):1382–8. https://doi.org/10.1111/jog.12330.
34. van Meurs H, Visser O, Buist MR, Ten Kate FJ, van der Velden J. Frequency of pelvic lymph node metastases and parametrial involvement in stage IA2 cervical cancer: a population-based study and literature review. Int J Gynecol Cancer. 2009;19(1):21–6. https://doi.org/10.1111/IGC.0b013e318197f3ef.
35. Mahawerawat S, Charoenkwan K, Srisomboon J, Khunamornpong S, Suprasert P, Sae-Teng CT. Surgical outcomes of patients with stage IA2 cervical cancer treated with radical hysterectomy. Asian Pac J Cancer Prev. 2013;14(9):5375–8.
36. Qian Q, Yang J, Cao D, You Y, Chen J, Shen K. Analysis of treatment modalities and prognosis on microinvasive cervical cancer: a 10-year cohort study in China. J Gynecol Oncol. 2014;25(4):293–300. https://doi.org/10.3802/jgo.2014.25.4.293.
37. Yoneda JY, Braganca JF, Sarian LO, Borba PP, Conceicao JC, Zeferino LC. Surgical treatment of microinvasive cervical cancer: analysis of pathologic features with implications on radicality. Int J Gynecol Cancer. 2015;25(4):694–8. https://doi.org/10.1097/igc.0000000000000416.
38. Creasman WT. New gynecologic cancer staging. Gynecol Oncol. 1995;58(2):157–8. https://doi.org/10.1006/gyno.1995.1203.
39. Pecorelli S. Revised FIGO staging for carcinoma of the vulva, cervix, and endometrium. Int J Gynaecol Obstet. 2009;105(2):103–4.

40. Pecorelli S, Odicino F. Cervical cancer staging. Cancer J. 2003;9(5):390–4.
41. Siegel CL, Andreotti RF, Cardenes HR, Brown DL, Gaffney DK, Horowitz NS, et al. ACR Appropriateness Criteria(R) pretreatment planning of invasive cancer of the cervix. J Am Coll Radiol. 2012;9(6):395–402. https://doi.org/10.1016/j.jacr.2012.02.021.
42. Patel S, Liyanage SH, Sahdev A, Rockall AG, Reznek RH. Imaging of endometrial and cervical cancer. Insights Imaging. 2010;1(5–6):309–28. https://doi.org/10.1007/s13244-010-0042-7.
43. Bourgioti C, Chatoupis K, Moulopoulos LA. Current imaging strategies for the evaluation of uterine cervical cancer. World J Radiol. 2016;8(4):342–54. https://doi.org/10.4329/wjr.v8.i4.342.
44. Fujii S, Takakura K, Matsumura N, Higuchi T, Yura S, Mandai M, et al. Precise anatomy of the vesico-uterine ligament for radical hysterectomy. Gynecol Oncol. 2007;104(1):186–91. https://doi.org/10.1016/j.ygyno.2006.07.041.
45. Photopulos GJ, Zwaag RV. Class II radical hysterectomy shows less morbidity and good treatment efficacy compared to class III. Gynecol Oncol. 1991;40(1):21–4.
46. Plotti F, Nelaj E, Sansone M, Antonelli E, Altavilla T, Angioli R, et al. Sexual function after modified radical hysterectomy (Piver II/Type B) vs. classic radical hysterectomy (Piver III/Type C2) for early stage cervical cancer. A prospective study. J Sex Med. 2012;9(3):909–17. https://doi.org/10.1111/j.1743-6109.2011.02581.x.
47. Zullo MA, Manci N, Angioli R, Muzii L, Panici PB. Vesical dysfunctions after radical hysterectomy for cervical cancer: a critical review. Crit Rev Oncol Hematol. 2003;48(3):287–93.
48. Michalas S, Rodolakis A, Voulgaris Z, Vlachos G, Giannakoulis N, Diakomanolis E. Management of early-stage cervical carcinoma by modified (type II) radical hysterectomy. Gynecol Oncol. 2002;85(3):415–22. https://doi.org/10.1006/gyno.2002.6633.
49. Kinney WK, Hodge DO, Egorshin EV, Ballard DJ, Podratz KC. Identification of a low-risk subset of patients with stage IB invasive squamous cancer of the cervix possibly suited to less radical surgical treatment. Gynecol Oncol. 1995;57(1):3–6. https://doi.org/10.1006/gyno.1995.1091.
50. Covens A, Rosen B, Murphy J, Laframboise S, DePetrillo AD, Lickrish G, et al. How important is removal of the parametrium at surgery for carcinoma of the cervix? Gynecol Oncol. 2002;84(1):145–9. https://doi.org/10.1006/gyno.2001.6493.
51. Stegeman M, Louwen M, van der Velden J, ten Kate FJ, den Bakker MA, Burger CW, et al. The incidence of parametrial tumor involvement in select patients with early cervix cancer is too low to justify parametrectomy. Gynecol Oncol. 2007;105(2):475–80. https://doi.org/10.1016/j.ygyno.2007.01.016.
52. Wright JD, Grigsby PW, Brooks R, Powell MA, Gibb RK, Gao F, et al. Utility of parametrectomy for early stage cervical cancer treated with radical hysterectomy. Cancer. 2007;110(6):1281–6. https://doi.org/10.1002/cncr.22899.
53. Frumovitz M, Sun CC, Schmeler KM, Deavers MT, Dos Reis R, Levenback CF, et al. Parametrial involvement in radical hysterectomy specimens for women with early-stage cervical cancer. Obstet Gynecol. 2009;114(1):93–9. https://doi.org/10.1097/AOG.0b013e3181ab474d.
54. Kato T, Takashima A, Kasamatsu T, Nakamura K, Mizusawa J, Nakanishi T, et al. Clinical tumor diameter and prognosis of patients with FIGO stage IB1 cervical cancer (JCOG0806-A). Gynecol Oncol. 2015;137(1):34–9. https://doi.org/10.1016/j.ygyno.2015.01.548.
55. Magrina JF, Goodrich MA, Lidner TK, Weaver AL, Cornella JL, Podratz KC. Modified radical hysterectomy in the treatment of early squamous cervical cancer. Gynecol Oncol. 1999;72(2):183–6. https://doi.org/10.1006/gyno.1998.5245.
56. Cai HB, Chen HZ, Zhou YF, Lie DM, Hou HY. Class II radical hysterectomy in low-risk IB squamous cell carcinoma of cervix: a safe and effective option. Int J Gynecol Cancer. 2009;19(1):46–9. https://doi.org/10.1111/IGC.0b013e318197f847.
57. Kunieda F, Kasamatsu T, Arimoto T, Onda T, Toita T, Shibata T, et al. Non-randomized confirmatory trial of modified radical hysterectomy for patients with tumor diameter 2 cm or less FIGO Stage IB1 uterine cervical cancer: Japan Clinical Oncology Group Study (JCOG1101). Jpn J Clin Oncol. 2015;45(1):123–6. https://doi.org/10.1093/jjco/hyu168.

Abdominal Nerve-Sparing Radical Hysterectomy

7

Tomoyasu Kato

Abstract

Damage to the autonomic nerves during radical hysterectomy is a major cause of postoperative bladder dysfunction. Japanese gynecologists established nerve-sparing radical hysterectomy in 1961. Although a reduction of voiding dysfunction was observed, it was a problem of compromising radicality. Based on our anatomical study, we showed that there was the possibility of improving its radicality by correcting the concept of nerve topography that leads to over-preservation of the cardinal ligament. We devised a new method of nerve-sparing radical hysterectomy with more extensive and deeper dissection of the cardinal ligament. Moreover, we focused on the ureterohypogastric fascia including the ureter and autonomic nerves. This fascia serves as an index during surgery of nerve-sparing technique. Our operative method of nerve-sparing radical hysterectomy consists of four points as follows:

1. The ureterohypogastric fascia including the ureter is separated from the posterior leaf of the broad ligament, and then the hypogastric nerves running along the rectum within the ureterohypogastric fascia are identified.
2. The cardinal ligaments above the middle rectal artery are dissected to raise radicality at pelvic sidewall.
3. For complete preservation of the pelvic plexus, the medial stump of the cardinal ligament is mobilized ventrally above the hypogastric nerve before the dissection of the uterosacral and rectovaginal ligaments.
4. To maximize preservation of bladder branches, rectovaginal ligaments are clamped with right angle forceps.

T. Kato (✉)
Department Gynecology, National Cancer Center Hospital, Chuo-ku, Tokyo, Japan
e-mail: tokato@ncc.go.jp

M. Mikami (ed.), *Surgery for Gynecologic Cancer*, Comprehensive Gynecology and Obstetrics, https://doi.org/10.1007/978-981-13-1519-0_7

Keywords
Nerve-sparing radical hysterectomy · Autonomic nerves · Hypogastric nerves Pelvic splanchnic nerves · Pelvic plexus · Bladder branches · Ureterohypogastric fascia

7.1 History

Abdominal radical hysterectomy was developed by Wertheim in 1912 [1]. But for its high mortality, radiation therapy became the favored approach in the early twentieth century. Meigs made the surgical approach focus again with modification of Wertheim operation with removal of all pelvic nodes [2]. In Japan, Radium was hard to obtain. So Okabayashi made a different improvement from Meigs with wider resection of surrounding tissues of primary lesion and completed Okabayashi radical hysterectomy [3].

Although the treatment outcome was improved, the pelvic nerve plexus was cut, so that postoperative urinary voiding dysfunction occurred frequently. Autonomic nerve damage during surgery was thought to play a crucial role in the etiology of bladder dysfunction, sexual dysfunction, and colorectal motility disorders that are seen in patients after radical hysterectomy [4]. Bladder dysfunction is present in 70–85% of patients for up to 12 months postoperatively, including urinary or anal incontinence or retention [4]. In order to prevent these complications, Japanese gynecologists introduced a surgical technique with preservation of the pelvic autonomic nerves in 1961 [5]. The most important concept of nerve-sparing radical hysterectomy is that the cardinal ligament is divided into two parts as shown in Fig. A. The superficial vascular part is dissected, while the deep neural part that contains the pelvic splanchnic nerves is preserved in non-touch status [6]. Thereafter Japanese doctors had learned and modified this procedure. In the twentieth century,

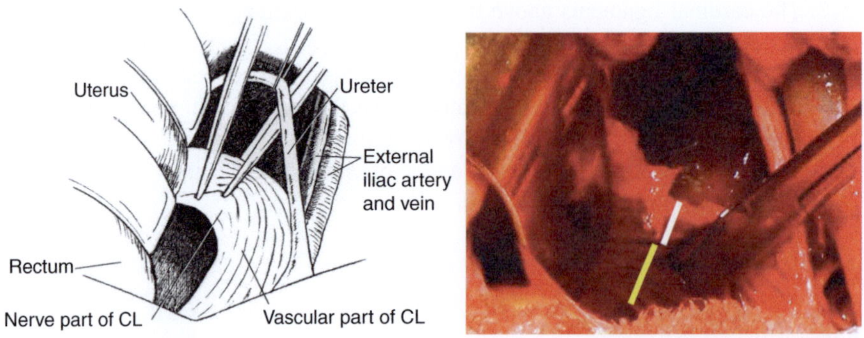

Fig. A Nerve-sparing radical hysterectomy. During nerve-sparing radical hysterectomy, the cardinal ligament is divided into two parts. The superficial vascular part is dissected, while the deep neural part that contains the pelvic splanchnic nerves is preserved **in non-touch status**

there were few articles reported in English [6, 7]. It is only recently that nerve-sparing radical hysterectomy has been introduced to Western [8] as well as to Asian countries [9]. As the postoperative QOL was noted, studies on precise neuroanatomical studies [4, 10] as well as the technique of nerve-sparing radical hysterectomy were reported [11]. Nowadays the concept of preservation of autonomic nerves during radical hysterectomy has become standard in many gynecological cancer centers in the world [12].

7.2 Principle and Indication

7.2.1 Neural Control of the Lower Urinary Tract

Pelvic organ function is organized by both central and peripheral nerve system. For instance, the lower urinary tract is innervated by three sets of peripheral nerves involving the parasympathetic, sympathetic, and somatic nervous systems: pelvic parasympathetic nerves arise at the sacral level of the spinal cord, excite the bladder, and relax the urethra. Lumbar sympathetic nerves inhibit the bladder body and excite the bladder base and urethra. Pudendal nerves excite the external urethral sphincter. These nerves contain afferent sensory as well as efferent motor axons.

7.2.2 Running of the Autonomic Nerves

These autonomic nerves are running and distributed by cadaver study as shown in Fig. 7.1. These autonomic nerves related to bladder function can be dissected during the different phases of radical hysterectomy (Fig. 7.2). The hypogastric nerves were cut when the sacral uterine ligaments were cut, the pelvic splanchnic nerves were cut when the cardinal ligaments were cut, the pelvic plexus and the bladder branches were damaged during dissection of the recto-vaginal ligaments, the bladder branches were injured by disseciton of vesicouterine ligaments.

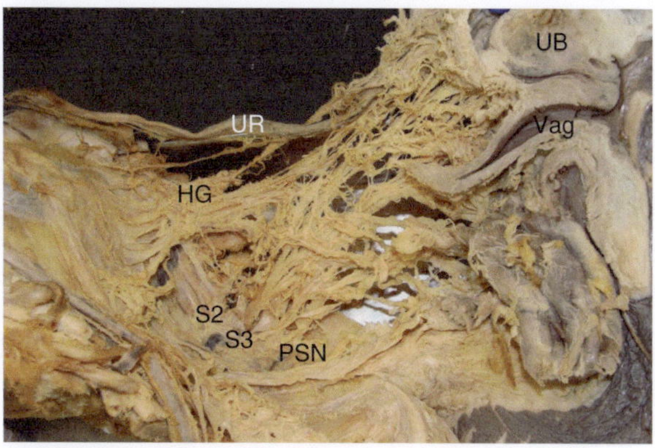

Fig. 7.1 Distribution of the left side of autonomic nerves from medial view by cadaver dissection. *UR* ureter, *Vag* vagina, *UB* urinary bladder, *HGN* hypogastric nerve, *PSN* pelvic splanchnic nerve

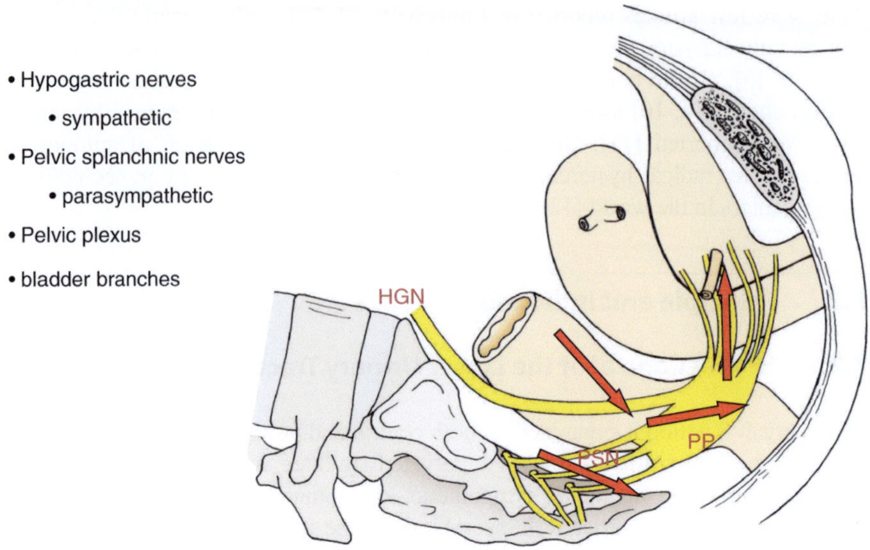

Fig. 7.2 Autonomic nerves related to voiding function. These autonomic nerves can be dissected during the different phases of radical hysterectomy

7.2.3 Principal of Autonomic Nerves During Radical Hysterectomy

A level of nerve preservation is classified into four levels: non-touch, exposure, partial preservation, and dissection. From a point of view on nerve preservation, non-touch preservation provides high quality of life. Simple and modified radical hysterectomy can archive non-touch preservation of autonomic nerves; however, they compromise radicality for invasive cervical cancer. To achieve a good balance between radicality and retaining pelvic function, we conducted to perform exposure or partial preservation of these autonomic nerves.

7.2.4 Indication

7.2.4.1 Indication

The most common indication for radical hysterectomy is early-stage invasive cancer of the cervix, FIGO stage IB1–IIA2. The cancer of the endometrium FIGO stage II or that of upper vagina is also an indication for radical hysterectomy. In Japan, radical hysterectomy is performed according to Okabayashi's method which removes paracolpium widely than Meigs' method. Therefore, the cancer of cervix stage IIB has been included in an indication for Okabayashi's radical hysterectomy.

7.2.4.2 Differences Between the Two Techniques (Meigs vs. Okabayashi)

After dissecting of the anterior layer of the vesicouterine ligament, the paracolpium and the posterior layer of the vesicouterine ligament were clamped by long forceps together and cut and ligated by the procedure of Meigs' radical hysterectomy. In contrast, by the procedure of Okabayashi's radical hysterectomy, the paracolpium was separated from the posterior layer of the vesicouterine ligament [3, 13]. This separation can lead to dissect the bladder thoroughly and resect the paracolpium and vagina wider and longer. Due to the higher local control, Okabayashi radical hysterectomy have been performed even in stage IIB cervical cancer in Japan.

7.3 Preoperative Evaluation

7.3.1 Physical Examination

The physical examination should evaluate the primary lesion and potential sites of metastatic nodes, such as the left supraclavicular fossa and groin. Inspection by naked eye or colposcope of the distal vagina and ectocervix is warranted to determine stage II diseases. The presence of parametrial extension is particularly important for determining the clinical stage and treatment modality by rectal examination. The shortening of fornix of the vagina indicates the invasion into the muscle of the vagina nevertheless the intact mucosa of the vagina. With this finding, the pTNM classification is likely to be pT2BN0, 1 M0.

7.3.2 CT Scan

Computed tomography (CT) scanning has been widely used in the preoperative evaluation of significant lymphadenopathy.

CT findings may provide delineating anatomic variances that alter surgical management, such as ureteral duplication or the presence of a duplicate of infra vena cava. Three-dimensional CT angiography may be helpful in identifying these variances. CT scanning and MRI are equally accurate (~84%) in detecting para-aortic metastasis [14].

7.3.3 MR Imaging

MRI is essential for evaluating the tumor, because MRI can discriminate tumor-containing tissue from non-tumor-containing tissue. Preoperative evaluation includes the size and shape of the primary tumor, depth of stromal invasion, and vaginal or parametrial extension as well as nodal involvement [15, 16].

7.4 Technique

7.4.1 Extended Nerve-Sparing Radical Hysterectomy

Based on the previous anatomical study, we showed that there was the possibility of improving its radicality by correcting the concept of nerve anatomy that leads to over-preservation of the cardinal ligament [10, 17]. Therefore, we devised a new method of nerve-sparing radical hysterectomy more extensive and deeper dissection of the cardinal ligament to increase radicality [18].

7.4.2 Procedures

Each step of our procedures is noted as follows.

7.4.2.1 Opening of Retroperitoneal Spaces

The round ligament is divided, and the broad ligament is opened to expose the retroperitoneal structure including the ureter and ovarian vessels attached to the medial aspect.

7.4.2.2 Identification of the Hypogastric Nerves During the Development of the Pararectal Space

Developing the pararectal space between the ureter and the internal iliac vessels, the hypogastric nerves (HGN) running along the rectum are to be identified. The ureter is separated from the retroperitoneum, and this tissue plane is kept facing downward. The ureter should not be free from the posterior layer of the broad ligament. HGN are found to be running in parallel under 3–4 cm of the ureter. The ureter and the hypogastric nerve are covered with the same fascia. It is important to keep the peeling layer until the hypogastric nerve can be seen without scooping only the ureter. This tissue plane is corresponded to the ureterohypogastric fascia (UHF), which includes the HGN and the pelvic plexus (Fig. 7.3).

7.4.2.3 Developing the Vesicouterine Spaces

Sharp dissection of bladder peritoneum is employed to create vesicouterine spaces. The bladder is separated from the anterior cervix with dissecting correct tissue plane.

7.4.2.4 Pelvic Lymphadenectomy

The systemic pelvic lymphadenectomy is started from the center height of the common iliac vessels. The dissection of the external and internal iliac vessel continues caudally until the deep circumflex vein. Great care need to preserve the obturator nerve and vessels.

7.4.2.5 Preserving the Pelvic Splanchnic Nerves During Dividing of the Cardinal Ligament

The uterine artery is ligated close to its origin at the internal iliac artery. The cardinal ligament (CL) is identified with developing both of the paravesical and

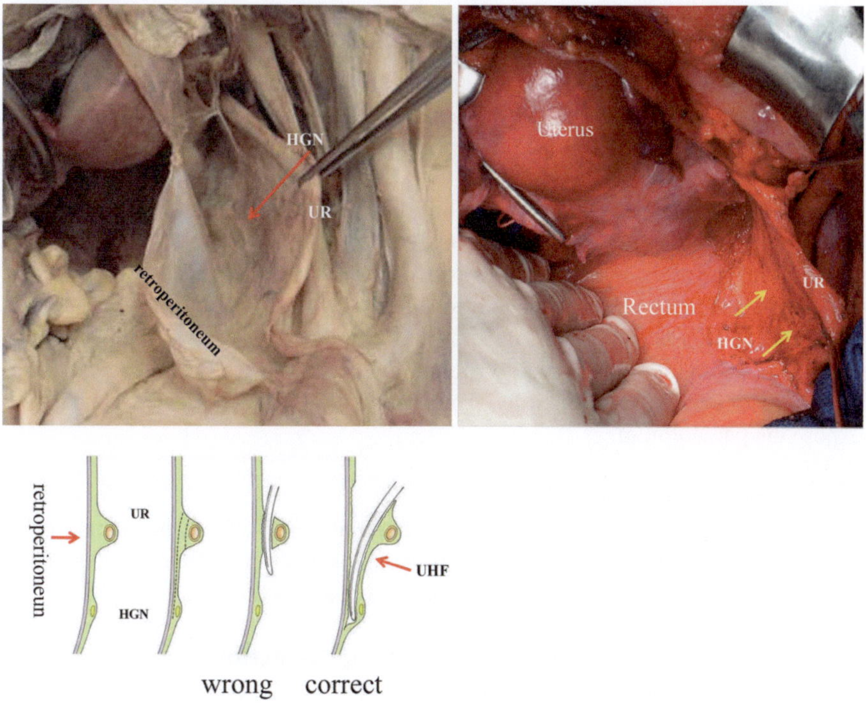

Fig. 7.3 Separation of the ureter hypogastric fascia. This fascia on the dorsal side of the ureter is thin and easy to break. It is gentle with formalin fixation, but it is difficult with actual surgery. This tissue plane is corresponded to the ureter hypogastric fascia, which includes the *hypogastric nerve* (HGN) and the pelvic plexus (PP)

pararectal spaces. According to the original procedure of nerve-sparing radical hysterectomy [5, 6], the CL is divided into two parts. The superficial vascular part is dissected, while the deep neural part that contains the PSN is preserved. Because the surgical margin of the CL might compromise radicality, the indication of this method is limited to cervical cancer with early stage. In order to raise radicality of nerve-sparing radical hysterectomy, we demonstrated that the pelvic splanchnic nerves (PSN) arise from the dorsomedial portion of the neural part of the CL, based on operative findings as well as fresh cadaver studies [10].

In order to increase the margin, the CL is dissected immediately above the middle rectal artery as close as possible to the pelvic sidewall. The PSN originating from S3 run to the pelvic plexus dorsal to the middle rectal artery. Deeply putting retractors in the paravesical space and pararectal space, the cardinial ligament is strained. As the connective tissue on the dorsal side of the deep uterine vein is incised, middle rectal artery is identified. The landmark of middle rectal artery are vessels that run under 1–2 cm of the deep uterine vein and pierce the pelvic plexus.

7.4.2.6 Developing the Rectovaginal Space

The ureter is further separated from the posterior layer of the broad ligament to clarify the entrance of ureteric tunnel, and the broad ligament is incised. Connecting both ends, the peritoneum of cul-de-sac is incised. As the rectum is being pulled cranially with gauze, the rectovaginal space is developed.

7.4.2.7 Dissection of the Anterior Layer of Vesicouterine Ligaments (VUL) with Keeping the Ureterohypogastric Fascia (UHF)

The ureteral tunnel is deroofed, allowing exposure of the uterus. The uterine artery is ligated close to its origin at the internal iliac artery. Keeping the ureterohypogastric fascia (UHF) is important to avoid bleeding during dissection of the anterior layer of vesicouterine ligament. Division of the cervicovesical vessels leads to roll the ureter downward and laterally. The bladder is further dissected caudally to expose the paracolpium.

7.4.2.8 Incision of the UHF

The UHF is incised at midline between the ureter and HGN. Then the medial stump of the cardinal ligaments is re-clamped from the inside of the UHF. So far, the UHF is maintained as an index where autonomic nerves are located.

7.4.2.9 Preserving the Pelvic Plexus During Dissection of the Uterosacral Ligaments

The UHF is incised at midline between the HGN and the ureter. The HGN entered the pelvic plexus at the anterosuperior corner. Deep uterine vein is located below the HGN. The HGN and the pelvic plexus were frequently damaged during dissection of the uterosacral ligaments (USL). To diminish these nerve injuries, the medial stump of the CL should be fully mobilized above the HGN before dissecting the USL (Fig. 7.4). In the case of the tumor with deep myometrial or parametrial

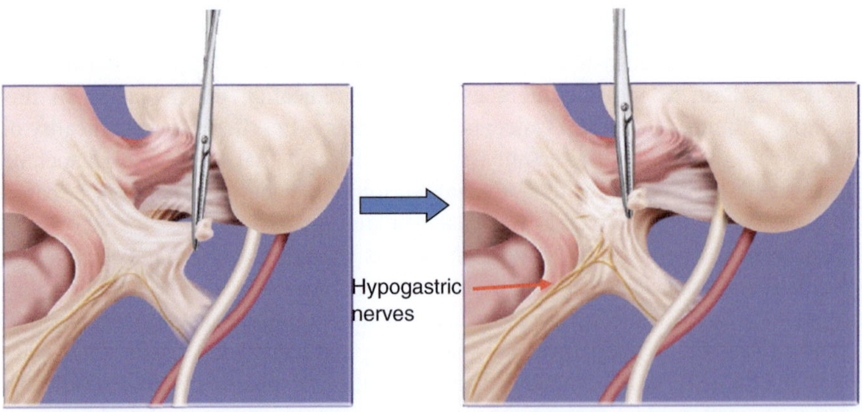

Fig. 7.4 Mobilization of the visceral stump of the cardinal ligament. For total preservation of the pelvic plexus, this stump should be mobilized ventrally above the hypogastric nerves before dissection of the uterosacral and rectovaginal ligaments

invasion, we dissect the USL just below the medial stump of the CL. Then dorsal area of the pelvic plexus is preserved.

7.4.2.10 Preserving the Bladder Branches During the Dissection of the Rectovaginal Ligaments

The ventral half of bladder branches to the ureter are more likely to be injured in dissection of the posterior leaf of the vesicouterine ligaments for wide resection of the paracolpium and the vagina. In order to maximize preservation of the dorsal half of bladder branches, the rectovaginal ligaments should be clamped using right angle forceps so as not to involve them.

7.4.2.11 Dissection of the Posterior Layer of Vesicouterine Ligaments

Further rolling the ureter allows the clearance of the boundary between the posterior layer of the vesicouterine ligaments and the paracolpium. Forceps are inserted into this boundary.

7.4.2.12 Dividing the Paracolpium and the Vagina

Separating the paracolpium from the posterior layer of the vesicouterine ligament to extend the resection field of the paracolpium is an original point of Okabayashi's hysterectomy [3, 13]. This procedure allows us wider and longer resection of the paracolpium and vagina. Then the paracolpium is divided by two steps. The specimen is removed by dividing the vagina. The vagina vault is closed with a Z-figure suture Fig. 7.5 and 7.6.

7.4.2.13 The Level of Preservation of Autonomic Nerves After Nerve-Sparing Radical Hysterectomy

Dissection line of autonomic nerves by our procedures is indicated by a red line in Fig. 7.7. According to our method, the HGN are found to be preserved in exposure,

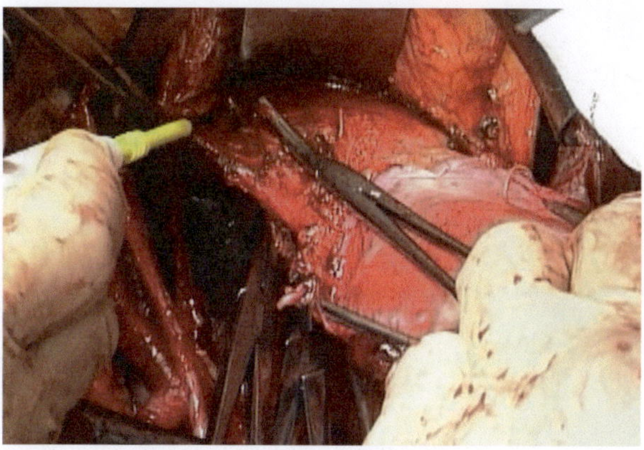

Fig. 7.5 Rolling the ureter. The top of electric cautery indicates the boundary between the paracolpium and the posterior layer of the vesicouterine ligaments

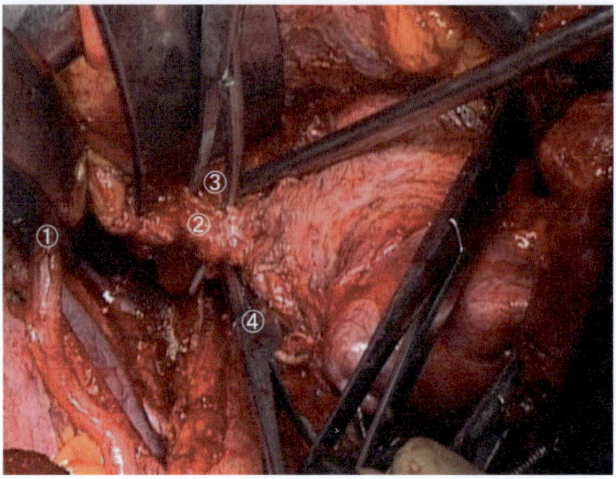

Fig. 7.6 Division of the posterior layer of the vesicouterine ligaments. The forceps are inserted into this boundary and the posterior layer of the vesicouterine ligaments is divided. *1* Ureter, *2* posterior layer of the vesicouterine ligaments, *3* paracolpium, *4* medial stump of the cardinal ligaments

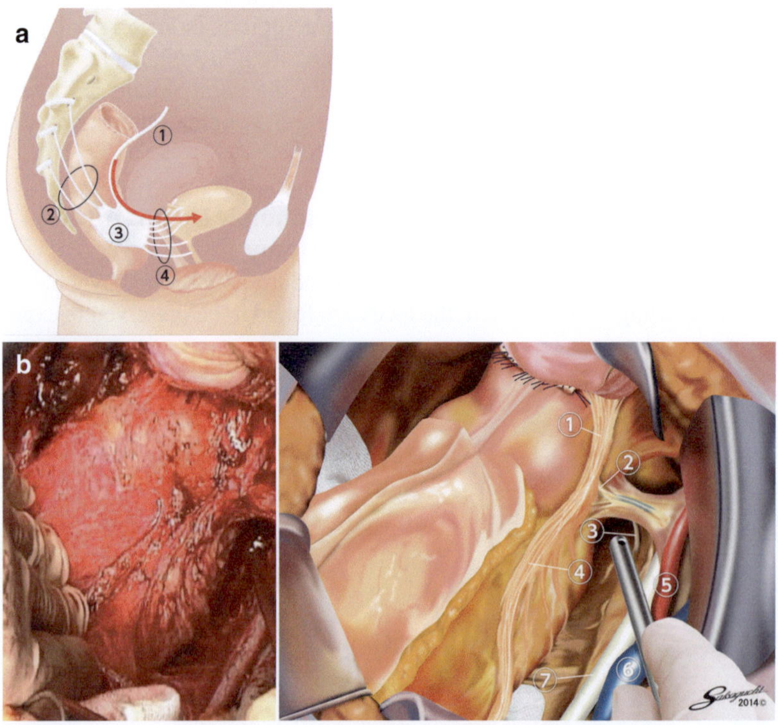

Fig. 7.7 (**a**) Red line indicates the cutting line of total preservation of pelvic plexus and hypogastric nerves and dorsal half preservation of vesical branches. *1* Hypogastric nerves, *2* pelvic splanchnic nerves (S2–4), *3* pelvic plexus, *4* vesical branches. (**b**) Completion of nerve-sparing RH. Hypogastric nerve and bladder branches are found to be preserved. *1* Bladder branches, *2* pelvic plexus, *3* pelvic splanchnic nerves, *4* hypogastric nerves, *5* internal iliac artery, *6* external iliac artery, *7* ureter

the PSN in non-touch or exposure, pelvic plexus in exposure or partial, and bladder branches in partial preservation. The difference of dissection line between radical hysterectomy and nerve-sparing radical hysterectomy is also shown in Fig. 7.7.

7.5 Morbidity

7.5.1 Five-Year Overall Survival

FIGO annual reported showed that 5-year overall survival of 3010 patients with cervical cancer stage IB1 was 89.1% [19]. In contrast, Japanese study demonstrated that a 5-year OS was 93.3% [20]. The difference could be explained by the wider resection of the paracolpium according to Okabayashi's procedure.

7.5.2 Postoperative Complication

The major postoperative complication of radical hysterectomy is the bladder dysfunction due to damage of autonomic nerves in the pelvis. Bladder function recovery by procedure of hysterectomy is shown in Table 7.1 [18]. The degree of nerve

Table 7.1 Bladder function recovery

Method	HGN	PSN	P Plexus	bladder braches	PVR<50mL
Simple Hx	◎	◎	◎	◎	<5POD
class II RH	◎	◎	◎	○	7-16POD
class III RH	×	◎(S2,3,4)	△	△	CIC: 10%
Nerve-sparing ARH (Tokyo)	○	◎(S2,3,4)	○	△	18POD
Extended NS ARH (total)	○	× (S2)○(S3,4)	○	△	18POD
NS ARH (partial)	×	× (S2)○(S3,4)	△	△	24POD

◎ non-touch preservation
○ exposure preservation
△ partial preservation
× dissection

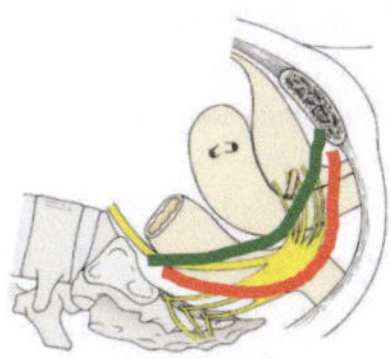

This table summarizes a degree of preservation of each autonomic nerves according to procedure of hysterectomy
Needles to say, preservation of bladder branches is important
This concept is also shown in this figure

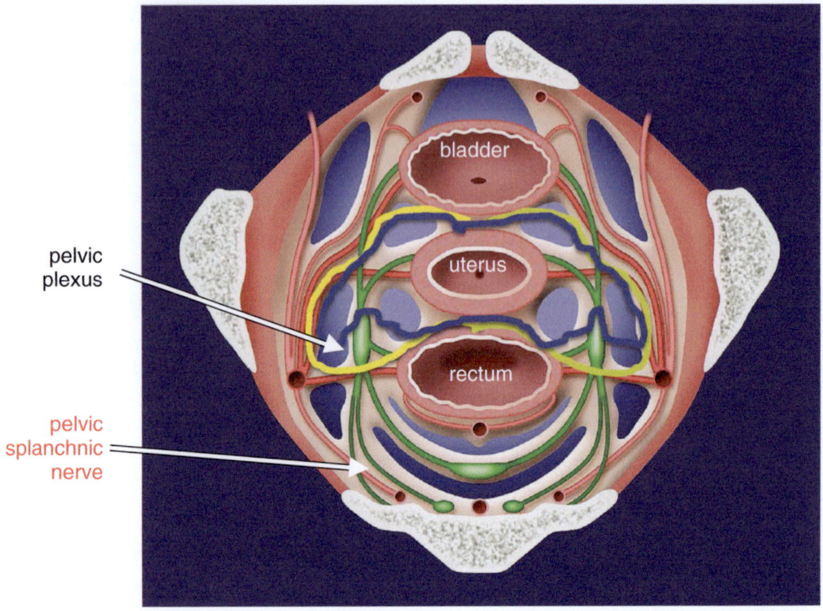

Fig. 7.8 Dissection line by class III and nerve-sparing radical hysterectomy. Scheme of the axial section of the female pelvis is shown. Green line, a nerve system; yellow line, the cut line of the radical hysterectomy (RH); blue line, the cut line of nerve-sparing RH

preservation is divided into four levels such as non-touch, exposure, partial, and non-preserved.

7.6 Future Prospect

A growing literature supports (robot-assisted) laparoscopic radical hysterectomy in early-stage cervical cancer. One review shows that robot-assisted radical hysterectomy is associated with minimal blood loss, a shortened hospital stay, and few operative complications [21].

Even when these minimally invasive surgeries are widespread, locally advanced tumors such as stages IB2, IIA2, and IIB, especially adenocarcinoma, will continue to be indicated for abdominal radical hysterectomy. The abdominal approach is the basis of radical hysterectomy, and we need to master it (Fig. 7.8).

References

1. Wertheim E. The extended abdominal operation for carcinoma of the cervix. Am J Obstet Gynecol. 1912;66:169–232.
2. Meigs JV. Radical hysterectomy with bilateral pelvic lymph node dissections; a report of 100 patients operated on five or more years ago. Am J Obstet Gynecol. 1951;62:854–70.

3. Okabayashi H. Radical hysterectomy for cancer of the cervix uteri. Surg Gynecol Obstet. 1921;33:335–43.
4. Zullo MA, Manci N, Angioli R, et al. Vesical dysfunctions after radical hysterectomy for cervical cancer: a critical review. Crit Rev Oncol Hematol. 2003;48:287–93.
5. Kobayashi T. Radical hysterectomy. Tokyo: Nanzando; 1961. (in Japanese)
6. Sakamoto S, Takizawa K. An improved radical hysterectomy with fewer urological complications and with no loss of therapeutic results for invasive cervical cancer. Ballieres Clin Obstet Gynecol. 1988;2:953–62.
7. Yabuki Y, Asamoto A, Hoshiba T, et al. Radical hysterectomy: an anatomic evaluation of parametrial dissection. Gynecol Oncol. 2000;77:155–63.
8. Trimbos JB, Maas CP, Deruiter MC, Peters AA, Kenter GG. A nerve-sparing radical hysterectomy: guidelines and feasibility in Western patients. Int J Gynecol Cancer. 2001;11:180–6.
9. Lee YN, Wang KL, Lin MH, Liu CH, Wang KG, Lan CC, et al. Radical hysterectomy with pelvic lymph node dissection for treatment of cervical cancer: a clinical review of 954 cases. Gynecol Oncol. 1989;32:135–42.
10. Kato T, Murakami G, Yabuki Y. A new perspective on nerve-sparing radical hysterectomy: nerve topography and over-preservation of the cardinal ligament. Jpn J Clin Oncol. 2003;33:589–91.
11. Sakuragi N, Todo Y, Kudo M, Yamamoto R, Sato T. A systematic nerve-sparing radical hysterectomy technique in invasive cervical cancer for preserving postsurgical bladder function. Int J Gynecol Cancer. 2005;15:389–97.
12. Querleu D, Morrow CP. Classification of radical hysterectomy. Lancet Oncol. 2008;9:297–303.
13. Fujii S. Anatomic identification and functional outcomes of the nerve sparing Okabayashi radical hysterectomy. Gynecol Oncol. 2007;107:4–13.
14. Scheidler J, Hricak H, Yu KK, et al. Radiological evaluation of lymph node metastases in patients with cervical cancer. A meta-analysis. JAMA. 1997;278:1096–101.
15. Mitchell DG, Snyder B, Coakley F, Reinhold C, Thomas G, Amendola M. Early invasive cervical cancer: tumor delineation by magnetic resonance imaging, computed tomography, and clinical examination, verified by pathologic results, in the ACRIN 6651/GOG 183 Intergroup Study. J Clin Oncol. 2006;24:5687–94.
16. Sahdev A, Sohaib SA, Wenaden AE, Shepherd JH, Reznek RH. The performance of magnetic resonance imaging in early cervical carcinoma: a long-term experience. Int J Gynecol Cancer. 2007;17:629–36.
17. Kato T, Murakami G, Yabuki Y. Does the cardinal ligament of the uterus contain a nerve that should be preserved in radical hysterectomy? Anat Sci Int. 2002;77:16–8.
18. Kato T. Extended nerve-sparing radical hysterectomy. Acta Obstet Gynaecol Jpn. 2004;56:1369–76. in Japanese
19. Quinn MA, Benedet JL, Odicino F, Maisonneuve P, Beller U, Creasman WT, et al. Carcinoma of the cervix uteri. FIGO 6th Annual Report on the Results of Treatment in Gynecological Cancer. Int J Gynaecol Obstet. 2006;95:Sd43–103.
20. Kato T, Takashima A, Kasamatsu T, et al. Clinical tumor diameter and prognosis of patients with FIGO stage IB1 cervical cancer (JCOG0806-A). Gynecol Oncol. 2015;137:34–9.
21. Lowe MP, Chamberlain DH, Kamelle SA, Johnson PR, Tillmanns TD. A multi-institutional experience with robotic-assisted radical hysterectomy for early stage cervical cancer. Gynecol Oncol. 2009;113(2):191–4.

Radical Vaginal Hysterectomy

8

Tsuyoshi Saito

Abstract

Radical vaginal hysterectomy (RVH) was first described by Shauta in 1908. At that time, RVH was performed more often than abdominal radical hysterectomy for cervical carcinoma due to its lower surgical invasiveness. However, RVH was selected only for early cases because lymphadenectomy was impossible to perform. Recently, RVH has developed into laparoscopically assisted radical vaginal hysterectomy (LARVH), which is associated with the laparoscopic procedure, and it is applied as radical vaginal trachelectomy and semi-radical vaginal hysterectomy. In this chapter, we commented on LARVH. LARVH is indicated for patients with stage IB1 and IIA1 cervical carcinoma, especially those with a tumor size of less than 2 cm, because the cardinal ligaments cannot be resected widely. Pergialiotis et al. reported that LARVH provided equal recurrence-free rates to abdominal radical hysterectomy when it is performed in patients with tumors that do not exceed 2 cm in the greatest diameter. Although RVH that is associated with laparoscopic pelvic lymphadenectomy is the most used surgical procedure, radical trachelectomy may be performed either abdominally or vaginally (laparoscopic or robotic). One report found that the pregnancy rate was higher in patients who underwent minimally invasive or radical vaginal trachelectomy than in those who underwent radical abdominal trachelectomy.

Keywords

Cervical cancer · Trachelectomy · Laparoscopically assisted radical vaginal hysterectomy · Fertility · Laparoscopy · Minimal invasiveness

T. Saito (✉)
Department of Obstetrics and Gynecology, Sapporo Medical University, Sapporo, Japan
e-mail: tsaito@sapmed.ac.jp

M. Mikami (ed.), *Surgery for Gynecologic Cancer*, Comprehensive Gynecology and Obstetrics, https://doi.org/10.1007/978-981-13-1519-0_8

8.1 History

Radical vaginal hysterectomy (RVH) was first described by Shauta in 1908 [1]. After making several improvements, Amreich reported a surgical procedure in which the parametrial ligament was resected radically according to new anatomical knowledge [2]. In these RVH procedures, there was a wide surgical field, and the vagina, perineum, and levator ani muscle were incised. At that time, RVH was performed more often than abdominal radical hysterectomy for cervical carcinoma due to its lower surgical invasiveness. However, RVH was selected only for early cases because lymphadenectomy was impossible to perform. Later, Navratil [3] presented RVH with extraperitoneal lymphadenectomy, in which incisions were made on both sides of the abdomen. In Japan, Akashi [4] demonstrated an RVH procedure that was a modification of the Mitra method [5], in which extraperitoneal lymphadenectomy and interruption of the parametrium vessels were performed after a vaginal procedure. RVH is adopted in some European countries such as Germany and Austria; however, its use has been limited. To increase the application of RVH, Dargent [6] proposed replacing the bilateral abdominal incision method with laparoscopy for systematically dissecting the pelvis, which has been part of the radical hysterectomy procedure since Meigs's study. Recently, RVH has developed into laparoscopically assisted radical vaginal hysterectomy (LARVH), which is associated with the laparoscopic procedure [7], and it is applied as radical vaginal trachelectomy [8] and semi-radical vaginal hysterectomy [9]. In this chapter, we commented on LARVH.

8.2 Principle and Indication

LARVH is indicated for patients with stage IB1 and IIA1 cervical carcinoma, especially those with a tumor size of less than 2 cm, because the cardinal ligaments cannot be resected widely.

8.3 Preoperative Evaluation

Cervical carcinoma is diagnosed based on a histologic examination of tissues that are obtained after conization or from a biopsy under colposcopy. As usual for cervical carcinomas, the tumor progression is evaluated routinely with a digital rectal examination, computed tomography scan, and magnetic resonance imaging. In patients in whom the tumor invades the parametrium, those with a large tumor more than 2 cm, and those with a narrow vagina, abdominal hysterectomy is selected. To determine the incision areas, the surgeon must perform colposcopy precisely. The vaginal orifice is stretched; a Schuchardt episiotomy is usually not performed, unless the vagina is especially narrow.

8.4 Technique

8.4.1 Pelvic Lymphadenectomy

Previously, this procedure was performed extraperitoneally, but recently, it has been performed laparoscopically using the classical peritoneal route. The round ligaments and ovary-specific ligaments are sealed and cut using energy modalities. After the retroperitoneum is expanded, the pelvic lymph nodes are dissected. The medial aspect of the iliac vessels is easily cleaned. The lateral aspect is a little more difficult to clean; however, it can be achieved laparoscopically as effectively as during laparotomy.

8.4.2 Interruption of the Cardinal Ligament

The next step is to divide the uterine arteries and prepare the cardinal ligament. Following laparoscopic lymphadenectomy, the pararectal and paravesical spaces are expanded. The fatty tissue-bearing lymph nodes around the cardinal ligament are dissected radically, and the different vessels of the vascular part of the cardinal ligament are transected laterally down to the level of the pelvic splanchnic nerves, which are kept intact.

8.4.3 Vaginal Retractors and Decision of the Incision Site

The procedure is initiated by suturing the labia to the medial aspect of the thigh. Vaginal retractors are positioned at four points in the vagina. Relatively short vaginal retractors (2.0 × 6.0 cm) are set anteriorly and posteriorly, whereas midsized vaginal retractors (2.5 × 8.5 cm) are set laterally. After the retractors are placed, the site of the incision into the vaginal wall to remove the lesion is determined. The incision line varies little between individual cases. The incision areas are determined with preoperative colposcopy and the Schiller iodine test in the vaginal wall, and the incision line is made about 2 cm distant from the borderline of the abnormal epithelium. In almost all cases in which the epithelium is located at the cervix without lateral invasion to the vaginal cuff, the length of the vaginal resection from the portio is about 1.0 cm. Vaginal resection has been performed intraoperatively for traction to prevent vaginal vault recurrence.

8.4.4 Incision of the Vaginal Wall

After determining the resection site, the surgeon clamps and lifts the vaginal wall using short Kocher hemostatic forceps at 6–8 points, according to a line circumscribing the cervix. Epinephrine (0.1% diluted in 100 mL of saline solution) is injected at the side of the incision and into the planes between the bladder and vagina (Fig. 8.1). The forceps are brought forward simultaneously, and a circular incision is made to a depth of about 5 mm (Fig. 8.2).

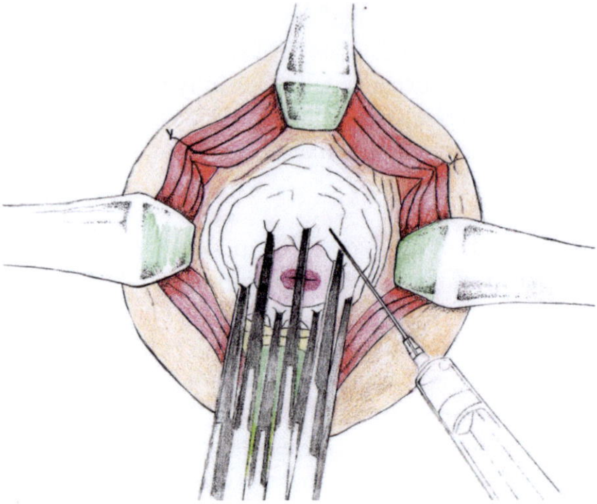

Fig. 8.1 The vaginal wall is clamped and lifted by short Kocher hemostatic forceps at 6–8 points according to a line circumscribing the area of the cervix. Epinephrine (0.1% diluted in 100 mL saline solution) is injected at the side of the incision and into the planes of the separation between the bladder and the vagina

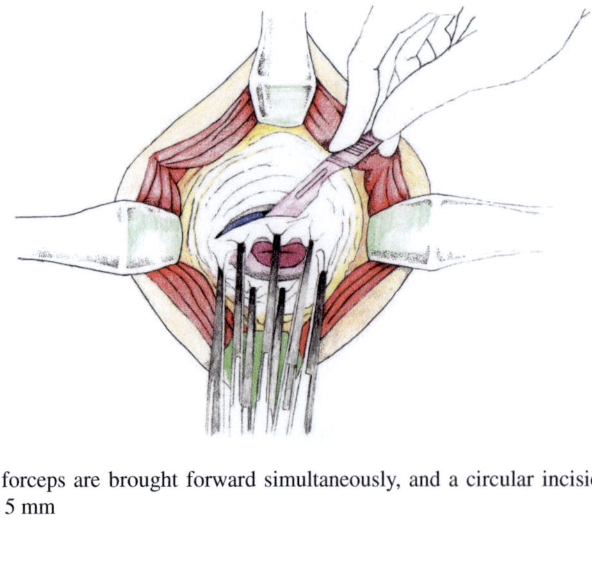

Fig. 8.2 The forceps are brought forward simultaneously, and a circular incision is made to a depth of about 5 mm

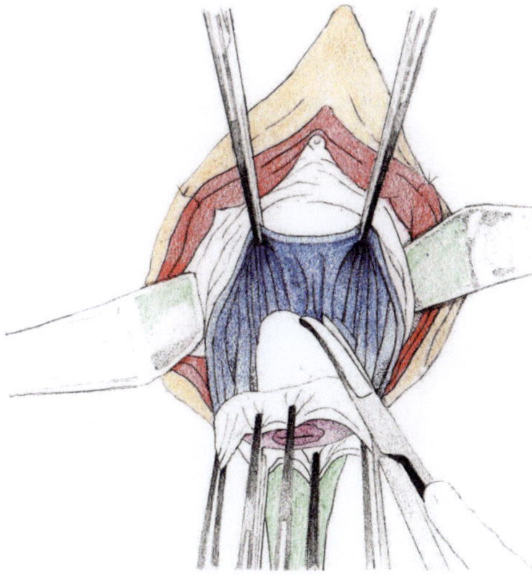

Fig. 8.3 The upper edge of the vaginal wall is clamped at two positions by Kocher hemostatic forceps and retracted upward. Using curved operating scissors, the fascia vaginalis is divided, and the vesicovaginal space is opened

8.4.5 Opening the Vesicovaginal Space

The upper edge of the vaginal wall is clamped at two positions using Kocher hemostatic forceps and retracted upward. Using curved operating scissors, the surgeon divides the fascia vaginalis and opens the vesicovaginal space (Fig. 8.3). The surgeon separates the bladder by inserting the forefinger into the space between the bladder and peritoneum, covering the uterus. The posterior fascia is divided in a similar fashion using scissors. Traction sutures are placed close to the fascial incision, covering the fascia in front and behind and including the lateral portions of the cuff as the integument (Fig. 8.4). The sutures are left long, knotted together, and used to retract the uterus.

8.4.6 Opening the Paravesical Space

To expose the left side, the surgeon retracts the traction sutures laterally to the lower right. The vaginal wall is clamped with Kocher forceps at the two o'clock position and retracted to the upper left. Using a pair of curved scissors, the surgeon divides the lateral side of the vesicouterine ligament from the vaginal wall (Fig. 8.5a–c). The surgeon then opens the paravesical space by inserting a forefinger or scissors, penetrating the space horizontally and to a point at the upper left of the cutting area (Fig. 8.6).

The paracolpos is hooked with the forefinger or curved forceps to penetrate the paravesical and retrovaginal spaces, and a midsized vaginal retractor (2.5 × 8.5 cm)

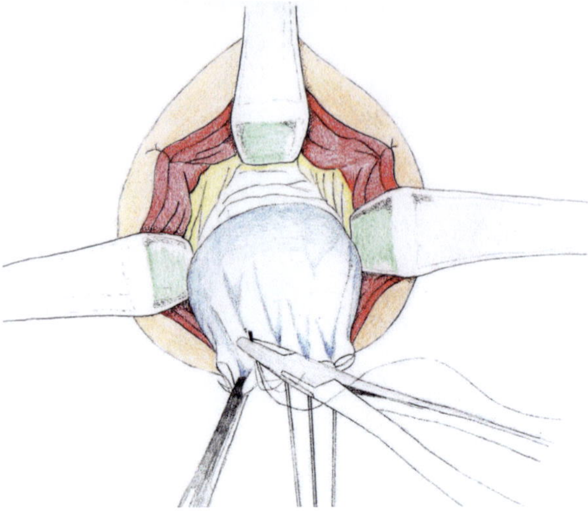

Fig. 8.4 Traction sutures are placed close to the fascial incision, covering the fascia in front and behind and including the lateral portions of the cuff as the integument

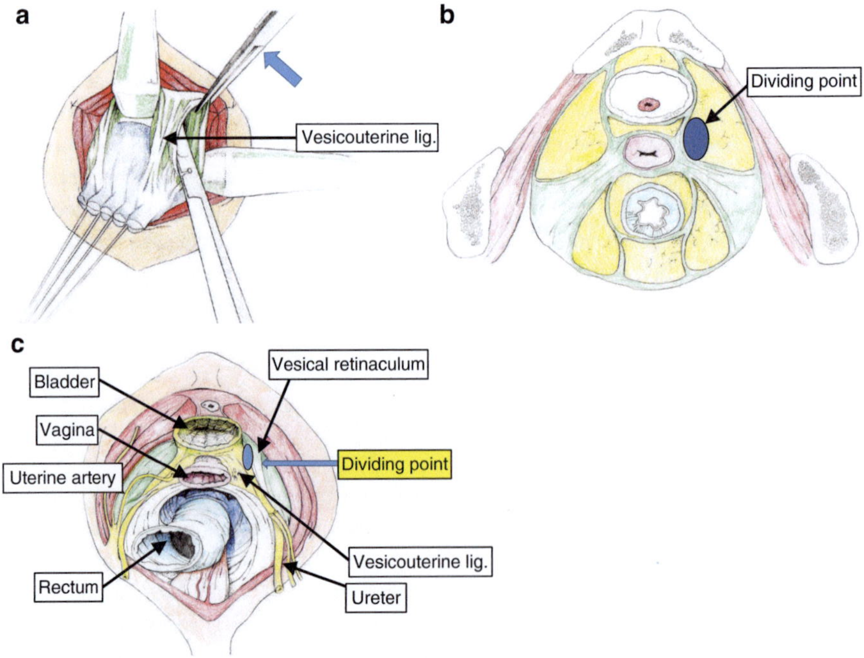

Fig. 8.5 (**a**) The vaginal wall is clamped with Kocher forceps at the two o'clock position and retracted to the upper left (arrow). Using a pair of curved scissors, the surgeon divides the lateral side of the vesicouterine ligament from the vaginal wall. (**b**) Shema of dividing point. (**c**) The dividing point viewing form of the abdomen

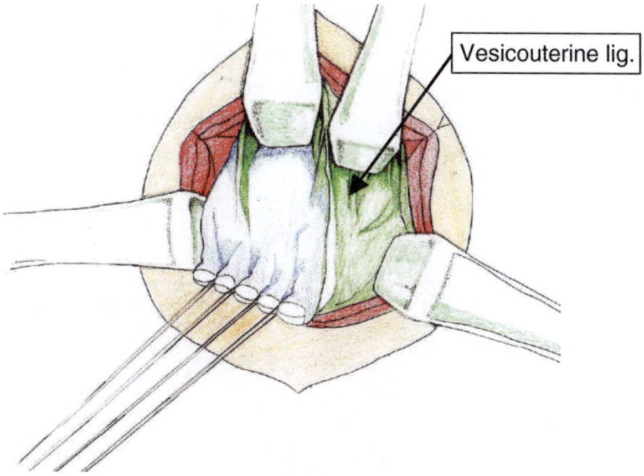

Fig. 8.6 The surgeon then opens the paravesical space by inserting a forefinger or scissors, penetrating the space horizontally and to a point at the upper left of the cutting area

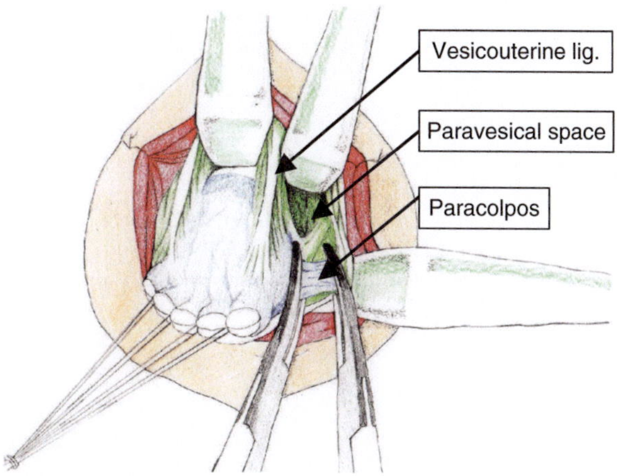

Fig. 8.7 The paracolpos is hooked with the forefinger or curved forceps to penetrate the paravesical and retrovaginal spaces, and a midsized vaginal retractor (2.5 × 8.5 cm) is inserted into the paravesical space

is inserted into the paravesical space (Fig. 8.7). The paracolpos is clamped, divided, and transfixion sutured with a 2–0 polyglycolic acid suture.

8.4.7 Division of the Inner Vesicouterine Ligament

The surgeon extends the uterus firmly to the lower right by retracting the bladder and stretching the vesicouterine ligament longitudinally. The ureter can be felt and touched between the forefinger and middle finger to establish its position (Fig. 8.8). The outer top of the external vesicouterine ligament is clamped in two places and divided using curved scissors, and the clamps are replaced with a 2–0 polyglycolic acid transfixion suture. Curved scissors are passed into the ureteric tunnel from the divided area using gentle dissection (Fig. 8.9), and the inner vesicouterine ligament

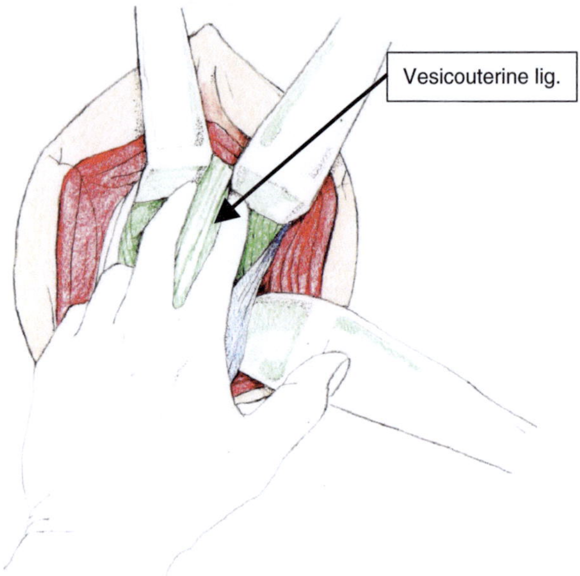

Fig. 8.8 The ureter can be felt and touched between the forefinger and middle finger to establish its position

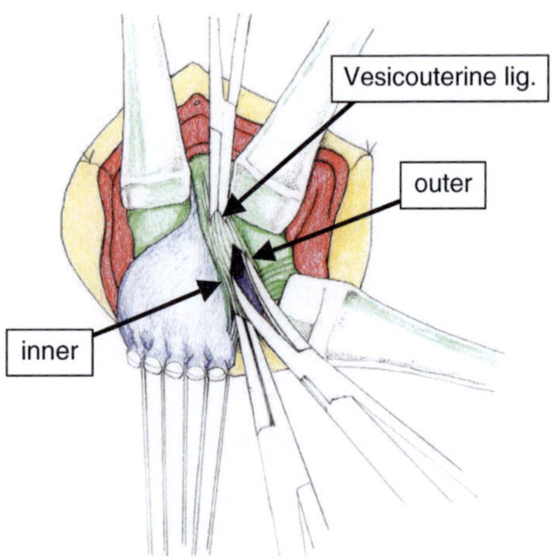

Fig. 8.9 The outer top of the external vesicouterine ligament is clamped at two places and divided by curved scissors. From divided area, curved scissors are passed into the ureteric tunnel by gentle dissection; the inner vesicouterine ligament is divided

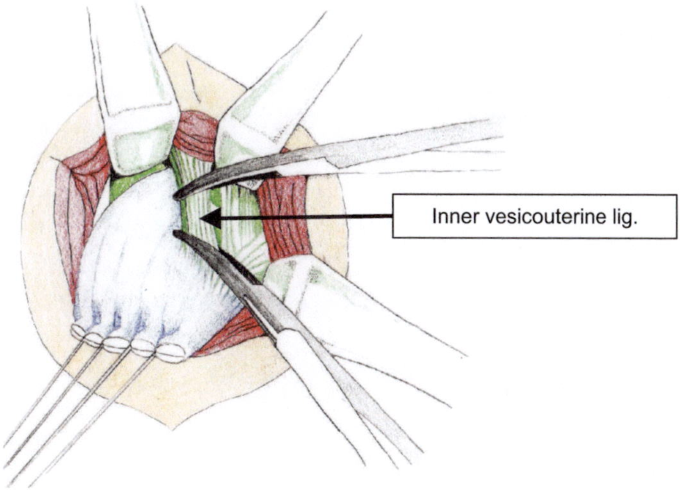

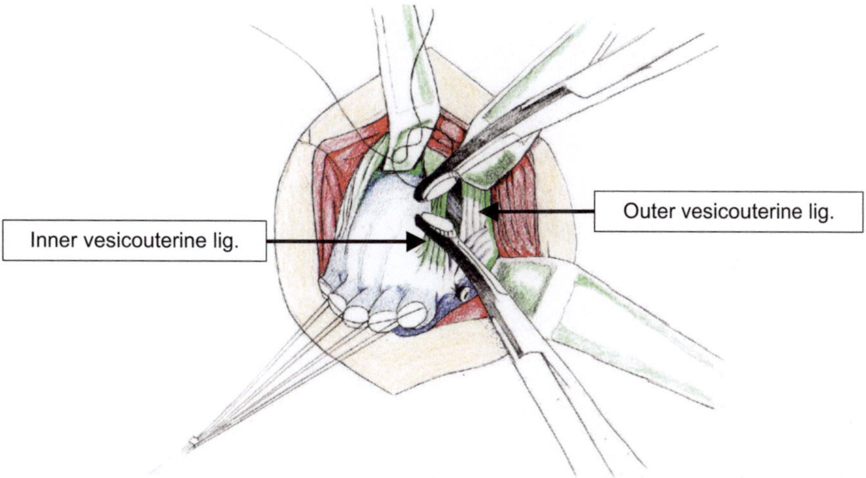

Figs. 8.10 and 8.11 The inner vesicouterine ligament is divided in two or three separate stages using the same maneuver

is divided in two or three separate stages using the same maneuver (Figs. 8.10 and 8.11). Upon separation and ligation of the inner vesicouterine ligament, the site at which the uterine artery crosses the ureter is seen clearly (Fig. 8.12). The uterine artery, which has already been divided laparoscopically, is pulled out. Then, the outer vesicouterine ligaments, which contain the bladder branch of the pelvic splanchnic nerve, are preserved to exclude them at the dorsal side and are partially divided using curved operating scissors (Fig. 8.13). In that sense, the procedure corresponds to levels II and III of the Piver classification [10].

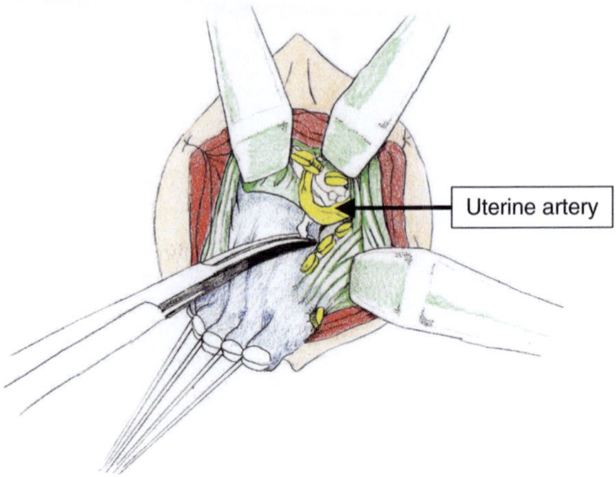

Fig. 8.12 Upon separation and ligation of the inner vesicouterine ligament, the site at which the uterine artery crosses the ureter is seen clearly

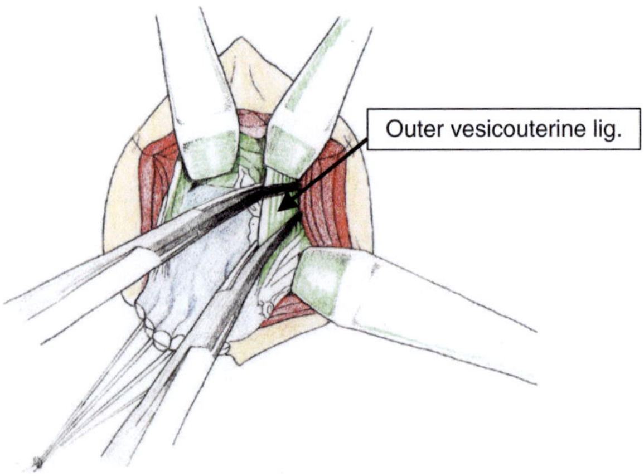

Fig. 8.13 The outer vesicouterine ligaments, which contain the bladder branch of the pelvic splanchnic nerve, are preserved to exclude them at the dorsal side and are partially divided using curved operating scissors

8.4.8 Division of the Cardinal Ligament

After opening the peritoneum of the vesicouterine pouch, the surgeon pulls the uterine corpus using Muzeaux uterine tenaculum forceps, and 3–4 traction sutures are placed on top of the uterine corpus. The uterine corpus is pulled forward to expose the Douglas pouch, which is opened by dividing the peritoneum (Fig. 8.14). The uterosacral ligament is resected using a suture midway between the uterus and the sacral attachment of the ligament. A curved clamp (or finely serrated multipurpose forceps) is placed approximately 2 cm from the edge of the cervix. The cardinal ligament is divided and resected (Fig. 8.15). The resection is located near where the uterine artery and ureter cross.

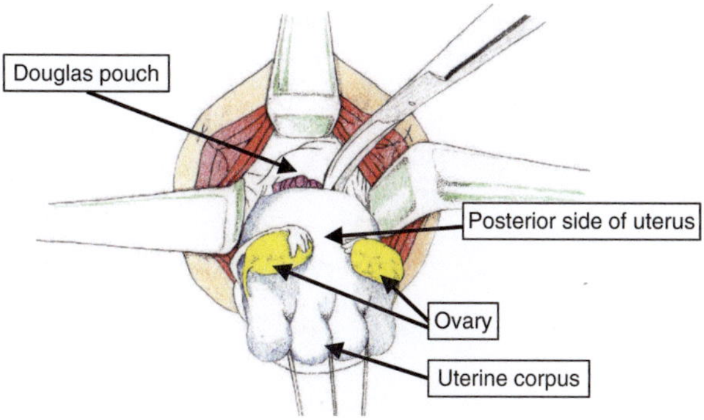

Fig. 8.14 The uterine corpus is pulled forward to expose the Douglas pouch, which is opened by dividing the peritoneum

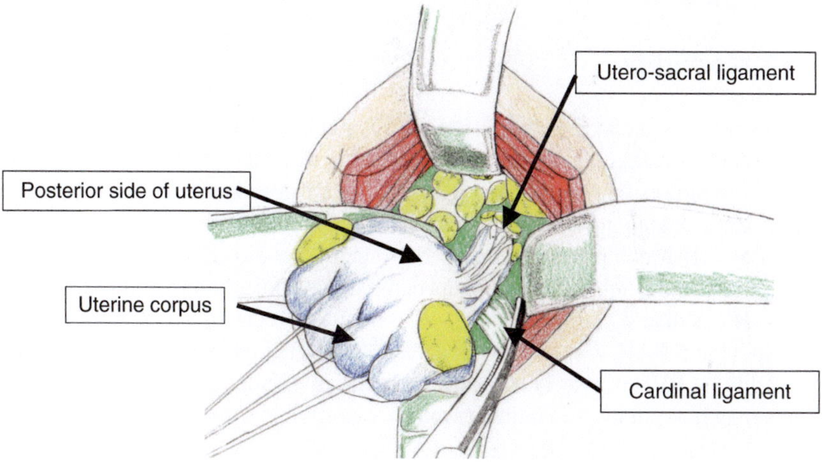

Fig. 8.15 The cardinal ligament is divided and resected

The same procedure is used for the right side. However, the cardinal ligament can be resected after the anterior part of the peritoneum is opened.

8.4.9 Resection of the Uterus and Closing the Vagina

The anterior peritoneal pouch is opened, and the uterine fundus is drawn forward using uterine vulsellum forceps, after which sutures are placed in three to four positions. These sutures are used for retracting the uterine body. The pelvic peritoneal cavity is closed using continuous sutures of 2–0 polyglycolic acid on both sides, each suture starting in the midline. Silicon drains are placed intraperitoneally on each side, and the vaginal wall is united using interrupted sutures (Fig. 8.16).

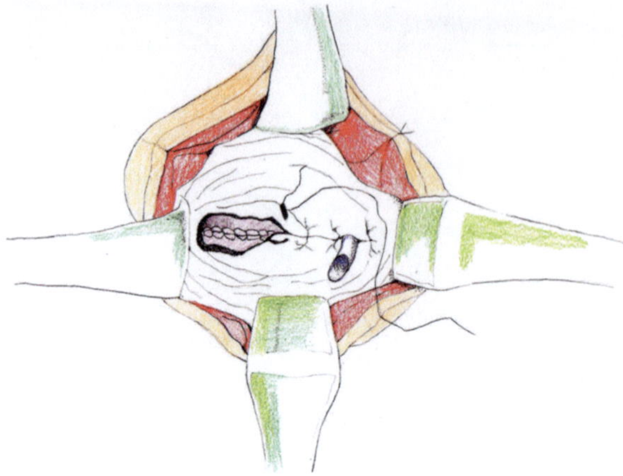

Fig. 8.16 Silicon drains are placed intraperitoneally on each side, and the vaginal wall is united using interrupted sutures

8.4.10 Morbidity

Pergialiotis et al. searched Medline (1966–2013) and Scopus (2004–2013) and reported that LARVH provided equal recurrence-free rates to RAH when it is performed in patients with tumors that do not exceed 2 cm in the greatest diameter [11]. Kucukmetin et al. reviewed that there was no statistically significant difference in the risk of intra- and postoperative complications between women who received LARVH and those who received RAH, although women appeared to have lost more blood if they underwent RAH (median 400 mL (IQR 325–1050 mL) and 1000 mL (IQR 800–1025 mL) for LARVH and RAH, respectively (*P* value = 0.05) [12]. However, Steed et al. commented that LARVH is associated with an increase in intraoperative complications and patients may have an increased time to return to normal bladder function [13].

8.4.11 Future Prospects

RVH is a fertility-sparing technique that was first described by Daniel Dargent in 1994, in which the cervix, parametrium, and vaginal cuff are removed while maintaining the patient's uterine fundus and adnexae [14]. This procedure, combined with laparoscopic pelvic lymphadenectomy, is the most common and accepted fertility-sparing procedure for patients with early cervical cancer [15]. Although RVH that is associated with laparoscopic pelvic lymphadenectomy is the most used surgical procedure, radical trachelectomy may be performed either abdominally or vaginally (laparoscopic or robotic) [16–18]. One report found that the pregnancy rate was higher in patients who underwent minimally invasive or radical vaginal trachelectomy than in those who underwent radical abdominal trachelectomy [19].

References

1. Schauta F. Die erweiterte vaginal total Exsirpation des Uterus bei Collumcarcinoma Safer Wien-Lepzig. 1908.
2. Amreich I. Zur Anatomie und Technik der erweiterten vaginalen Carcinomoreration. Arch Gynakol. 1924;122:497–553.
3. Navratil E. Radical vaginal panhysterectomy and pelvic lymphadenectomy. In congress on obstetrics and gynecology. St Louis: CV Mosby; 1951.
4. Akashi K. The extraperitoneal vaginal ultra radical surgery of cancer of the collum. Arch Gynakol. 1967;204:25–6.
5. Mitta S. Extraperitoneal lymphadenectomy and radical vaginal hysterectomy for cancer of cervix. (Mitta technique). Am J Obstet Gynecol. 1959;78:191–6.
6. Dargent D, Mathevet P. Radical laparoscopic vaginal hysterectomy. J Gynecol Obstet Biol Reprod. 1992;21:709–10.
7. Pergialiotis V, Rodolakis A, Christakis D, Thomakos N, Vlachos G, Antsaklis A. Laparoscopically assisted vaginal radical hysterectomy: systematic review of the literature. J Minim Invasive Gynecol. 2013;20:745–53.
8. Ishioka S, Endo T, Hayashi T, Baba T, Umemura K, Saito T. Pregnancy-related complications after vaginal radical trachelectomy for early-stage invasive uterine cervical cancer. Int J Clin Oncol. 2007;12:350–5.
9. Kudo R, Ito E, Kusanagi T, Hashimoto M. Vaginal semiradical hysterectomy: a new operative procedure for microinvasive carcinoma of the cervix. Obstet Gynecol. 1984;64:810–5.
10. Piver MS, Rutledge F, Smith JP. Five classes of extended hysterectomy for women with cervical cancer. Obstet Gynecol. 1974;44:265–72.
11. Marchiole P, Benchaib M, Buenerd A, Lazlo E, Dargent D, Mathevet P. Oncological safety of laparoscopic-assisted vaginal radical trachelectomy (LARVT or Dargent's operation): a comparative study with laparoscopic-assisted vaginal radical hysterectomy (LARVH). Gynecol Oncol. 2007;106:132–41.
12. Kucukmetin A, Biliatis I, Naik R, Bryant A. Laparoscopically assisted radical vaginal hysterectomy versus radical abdominal hysterectomy for the treatment of early cervical cancer. Cochrane Database Syst Rev. 2013;(10):CD006651.
13. Steed H, Rosen B, Murphy J, Laframboise S, De Petrillo D, Covens A. A comparison of laparoscopic-assisted radical vaginal hysterectomy and radical abdominal hysterectomy in the treatment of cervical cancer. Gynecol Oncol. 2004;93:588–93.
14. Fagherazzi S, Longone M, Vendemiati L, D'Antona D, Nardelli GB. Radical trachelectomy: the first step of fertility preservation in young women with cervical cancer (review). Oncol Rep. 2013;30:2545–54.
15. Dargent D, Mathevet P. Schauta's vaginal hysterectomy combined with laparoscopic lymphadenectomy. Baillieres Clin Obstet Gynaecol. 1995;9:691–705.
16. Burnett AF, Stone PJ, Duckworth LA, Roman JJ. Robotic radical trachelectomy for preservation of fertility in early cervical cancer: case series and description of technique. J Minim Invasive Gynecol. 2009;16:569–72.
17. Mejia-Gomez J, Feigenberg T, Arbel-Alon S, Kogan L, Benshushan A. Radical trachelectomy: a fertility-sparing option for early invasive cervical cancer. Isr Med Assoc J. 2012;14:324–8.
18. Ramirez PT, Schmeler KM, Soliman PT, Frumovitz M. Fertility preservation in patients with early cervical cancer: radical trachelectomy. Gynecol Oncol. 2008;110:S25–8.
19. Gizzo S, Ancona E, Saccardi C, Patrelli TS, Berretta R, Anis O, Noventa M, Bertocco A, Bentivegna E, Maulard A, Pautier P, Chargari C, Gouy S, Morice P. Fertility results and pregnancy outcomes after conservative treatment of cervical cancer: a systematic review of the literature. Fertil Steril. 2016;106:1195–211.

9 Indication, Technique, and Outcome of Super-Radical Hysterectomy for Cervical Cancer

Mikio Mikami, László Ungár, and Koji Matsuo

Abstract

Mibayashi invented super-radical hysterectomy, and his operative method was intended for radical surgery in patients with stage IIIB cervical cancer. However, the combination of intracavitary and external radiation currently provides a good outcome with good quality of life in patients with advanced cervical cancer. However, the survival rate of patients with stage IIIB cancer is approximately 50–65%, and further efforts to improve the outcome should be continued. As described by Mibayashi himself, a parametrial lymph node metastasis fixed to the origin of the cardinal ligament can be identified at laparotomy in some patients with clinical stage IB–IIB disease, and super-radical hysterectomy is a useful surgical approach in such patients. Regarding the safety of this operative method, because the internal iliac vessels can be clearly visualized after lymph node dissection during current curative surgery for cervical cancer, it is possible to perform super-radical hysterectomy safely. Although super-radical hysterectomy is not a surgical procedure of routine use for cervical cancer, it is an important operative method that should be used in a flexible manner as indicated, depending on the tumor findings at laparotomy.

M. Mikami (✉)
Department of Obstetrics and Gynecology, Tokai University School of Medicine, Isehara, Kanagawa, Japan
e-mail: mmikami@is.icc.u-tokai.ac.jp

L. Ungár
Department of Obstetrics, Gynecology and Gynecologic Oncology, St. Stephen Hospital, Budapest, Hungary

K. Matsuo
Division of Gynecologic Oncology, Department of Obstetrics and Gynecology, University of Southern California, Los Angeles, CA, USA

Norris Comprehensive Cancer Center, University of Southern California, Los Angeles, CA, USA

M. Mikami (ed.), *Surgery for Gynecologic Cancer*, Comprehensive Gynecology and Obstetrics, https://doi.org/10.1007/978-981-13-1519-0_9

Keywords
Super-radical hysterectomy · Mibayashi · Okabayashi · Laterally extended parametrectomy (LEP)

9.1 History

Before describing the history of super-radical hysterectomy for cervical cancer, we should describe the history of standard radical hysterectomy itself. The usefulness of the radical hysterectomy was demonstrated by Wertheim, who performed it in many patients with cervical cancer and reported the detailed outcomes of 500 cervical cancer patients in the early 1900s. However, Wertheim reported that the operative mortality rate was as high as 30%, being approximately 15% for the first 100 patients and also for the last 100 patients [1]. Moreover, the outcomes were not particularly good. Therefore, the suitability of performing radical hysterectomy for cervical cancer was questioned. In 1895, X-rays were discovered by Roentgen, and radium was discovered by Curie in 1898. In 1903, Cleaves in New York performed treatment of cervical cancer by using small radium sources. At that time, definitive radiation therapy was shown to be as effective as surgery for cervical cancer. Since studies of radium therapy for cervical cancer found no treatment-related deaths and few complications along with good outcomes, advocacy of radical hysterectomy for cervical cancer subsided, and the standard treatment shifted toward radiation therapy, especially in the United States [2]. Depending on the timing of introduction of radiation therapy and the treatment trends, the role of radical hysterectomy has varied widely among the United States, Japan, and Europe. It is important to understand that radical hysterectomy has evolved uniquely in each region.

Latzko (Austria) and Okabayashi (Kyoto University) subsequently modified Wertheim's operation to increase the curability and radicality of operative treatment [3]. In 1921, Okabayashi published an article about the so-called Okabayashi method [4]. While Okabayashi's method is similar to Latzko's operation, there is a fundamental difference between the two approaches with regard to handling the anterior part of the vesicouterine ligament. In Okabayashi's method, the anterior and posterior layers of the vesicouterine ligament are handled separately. This procedure allows the vaginal wall and paracolpium connective tissues to be removed adequately. In Japan, Okabayashi's method is the most commonly used approach for radical hysterectomy [4]. In 1941, Mibayashi (Kyoto University) advocated super-radical hysterectomy for the treatment of stage IIIB disease [5]. Super-radical hysterectomy is an operative method in which the cardinal ligament infiltrated by cancer is completely removed together with the tumor in the pelvic sidewall and adjacent blood vessels, including the internal iliac artery and vein. Mibayashi's method is intended to cure stage IIIB cervical cancer without radiation therapy. The readers of this chapter can understand that our predecessors have worked enormously on developing this surgical method by reviewing and learning textbooks which described the vascular anatomy in detail.

In this chapter, we made a strenuous effort to describe Mibayashi's method as accurately as possible so that our description approximates the information provided by Mibayashi at that time, since he did not publish any articles about his surgical method in English literature. We also describe Ungar's method of laterally extended parametrectomy (LEP) [6], which is classified as Type D: laterally extended resection according to the classification of radical hysterectomy advocated by Querleu and Morrow [7], as well as the procedure we employ for lateral parametrial resection after radical hysterectomy for patients with cervical cancer involving pelvic lymph nodes.

9.2 Mibayashi's Method

9.2.1 Super-Radical Hysterectomy

Radical hysterectomy is offered as a curative surgical treatment approach for stage IB–IIB cervical cancer. It includes comprehensive pelvic lymphadenectomy, and the cardinal ligament is to be resected just medial to the internal iliac vessels. Theoretically, the pelvic attachment of the cardinal ligament is not removed by this operative method, remaining in the patient. Therefore, a novel method was developed to improve the curability of surgical treatment. This operative method is called super-radical hysterectomy, and the surgery requires an en bloc complete resection of the cardinal ligament infiltrated by tumor together with the internal iliac vessels (i.e., the pelvic attachment site). Super-radical hysterectomy was originally developed for the surgical treatment of women with stage IIIB advanced cervical cancer with a curative intent [5].

9.2.2 Regional Anatomy Relevant to Super-Radical Hysterectomy (Figs. 9.1 and 9.2)

The common iliac artery gives off the two main branches: external iliac artery and internal iliac artery. Immediately past this bifurcation point, the superior gluteal artery arises from the posterior division of internal iliac artery on the dorsal side and runs through the supra-piriform foramen to exit the pelvis. Then the obturator artery branches from the internal iliac artery and runs laterally, after which the common trunk of the internal pudendal artery and inferior gluteal artery arises from the internal iliac artery and runs inferiorly. The vaginal artery and the uterine artery also branch from the anterior division of internal iliac artery, after which the internal iliac artery reaches the obliterated umbilical ligament. The obturator artery runs through the obturator foramen to exit the pelvis, while the common trunk of the internal pudendal artery and the inferior gluteal artery passes through the infra-piriform foramen and also leaves the pelvis. As landmarks for the arterial system, the origin of the internal iliac artery, the obliterated umbilical ligament distal to the origin of the uterine artery, and the obturator artery can be usually be identified easily, while the other arteries can be identified by thoroughly removing the surrounding connective tissue from the vessels. When performing super-radical hysterectomy, the internal iliac artery is manipulated from its origin of the main trunk (Fig. 9.1).

Similar to the arterial system, immediately past the bifurcation of the internal iliac vein and external iliac vein, the superior gluteal vein runs dorsally into the internal iliac vein. Then the internal iliac vein branches into the superficial uterine vein, deep uterine vein, vaginal veins, etc. toward the cardinal ligament medially, while it also branches to form the common trunk of the internal pudendal vein and the inferior gluteal vein inferiorly. The internal iliac vein eventually leads to the obturator vein (Fig. 9.2).

Because the venous vasculature runs closer to the pelvic sidewall than the arterial system, the internal iliac venous system can be visualized by adequately ablating and removing the surrounding connective tissues of the pelvic sidewall. When performing radical hysterectomy, the vessels in the cardinal ligament are ligated and cut just before the anatomical point where several veins, including the deep uterine vein, run into the internal iliac vein from the uterus. However,

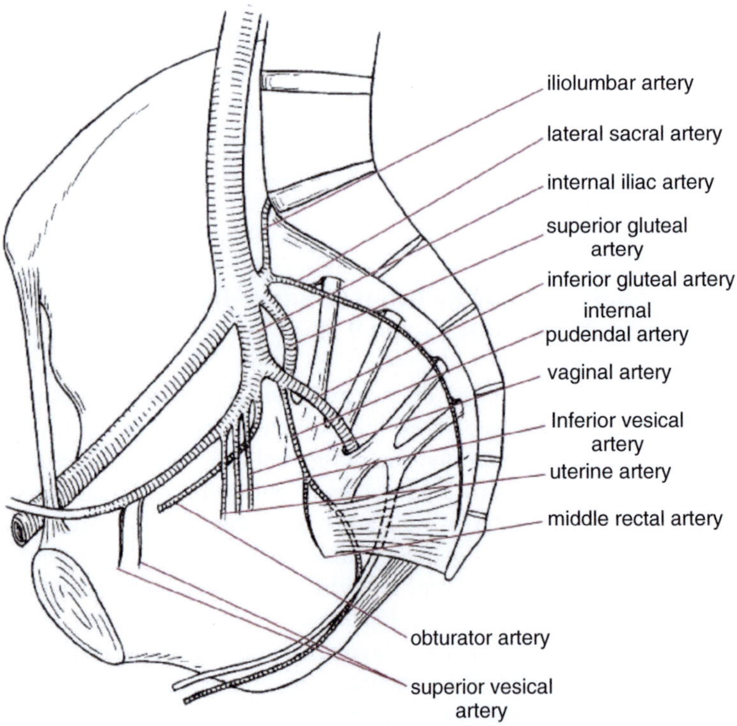

Fig. 9.1 Internal iliac artery and its branches (Mibayashi T; Modern Handbook of Obstetrics and Gynecology8E, Cervical cancer, 1970, Nakayama Shoten, Tokyo). Reprinted by courtesy of Nakayama Shoten and translated by Mikio Mikami

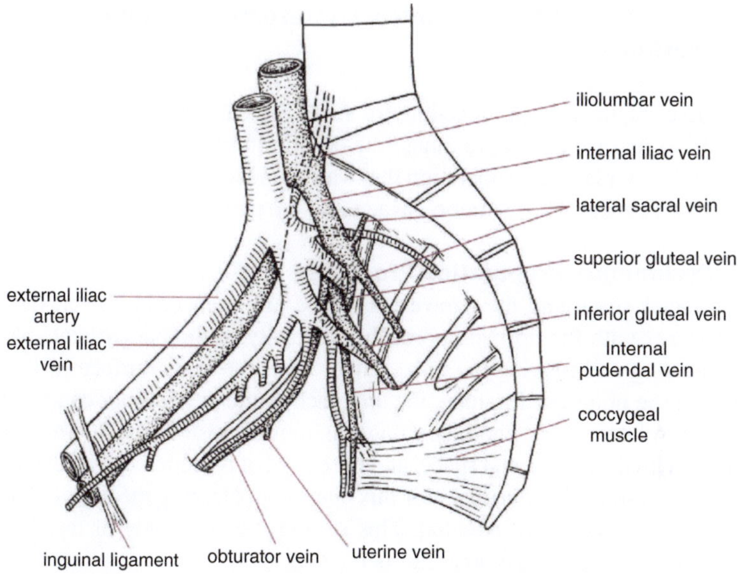

Fig. 9.2 Relation between internal iliac artery and vein (Mibayashi T; Modern Handbook of Obstetrics and Gynecology8E, Cervical cancer, 1970, Nakayama Shoten, Tokyo). Reprinted by courtesy of Nakayama Shoten and translated by Mikio Mikami

the internal iliac vein is also removed in super-radical hysterectomy. Thus, the vessels in the cardinal ligament can be theoretically removed widely, including their basal parts, by performing the following three manipulations after transection of the superior gluteal blood vessels cranially: (1) manipulation of the internal iliac artery and vein, (2) manipulation of the obturator artery and vein running to the obturator foramen, and (3) manipulation of the common trunk of the internal pudendal and the inferior gluteal arteries and veins running to the infra-piriform foramen. This is the essential step in super-radical hysterectomy (Fig. 9.3).

However, it should be noted that the anatomical course of the internal iliac blood vessels shows a variety of variations, especially for the venous system. Regarding the arterial system, the arteries follow the abovementioned pattern in majority of the female pelvis, but the internal pudendal artery and inferior gluteal artery sometimes do not form a common trunk and branch independently from the internal iliac artery. Although it is rare, the obturator artery can arise from the superior gluteal artery. Regarding the venous system, the middle iliac vein sometimes runs into the external iliac vein past the confluencc of the internal and external iliac veins, or the internal iliac vein and middle iliac vein form an anastomosis into which the deep uterine vein runs into. The obturator vein does not always follow the same anatomical course either. Not only the internal pudendal vein and inferior gluteal vein run up to the internal iliac vein, but many other veins also run toward it from the pelvic floor. In the final step of super-radical hysterectomy, careful attention is required for the bleeding from these veins as above.

9.2.3 Procedure of Super-Radical Hysterectomy (Mibayashi's Method)

Here we describe the typical procedure for super-radical hysterectomy as faithfully as possible so that we can approximate the description written by Mibayashi himself. Mibayashi explained an operation that was intended to be performed in patients with advanced cancer whose tumors invade into the cardinal ligament.

9.2.3.1 Preliminary Preparation Procedure

The para-rectal space and the paravesical space are opened. However, the tumor mass interferes with the normal approach, especially to the paravesical space. By bluntly inserting and moving the index finger from the inner surface of the pubic bone toward the obturator foramen, the approach to the pelvic floor can be accomplished with relative ease. The index finger is moved posteriorly to create a communication with the para-rectal space, and the extent of resection can be determined. Among the preliminary procedures for this operation, clearing the adjacent adipose tissues and lymph nodes is essential. This step reveals the body of the ilium, the anterior pubic ramus, and the obturator nerve (Fig. 9.3).

9.2.3.2 First Ligation

Using the obturator nerve as a landmark, the obturator artery and vein can be dissected easily. Then the obturator artery and vein are ligated and transected at the site where they enter into the obturator foramen (Figs. 9.3 and 9.4). Ligation and transection of the

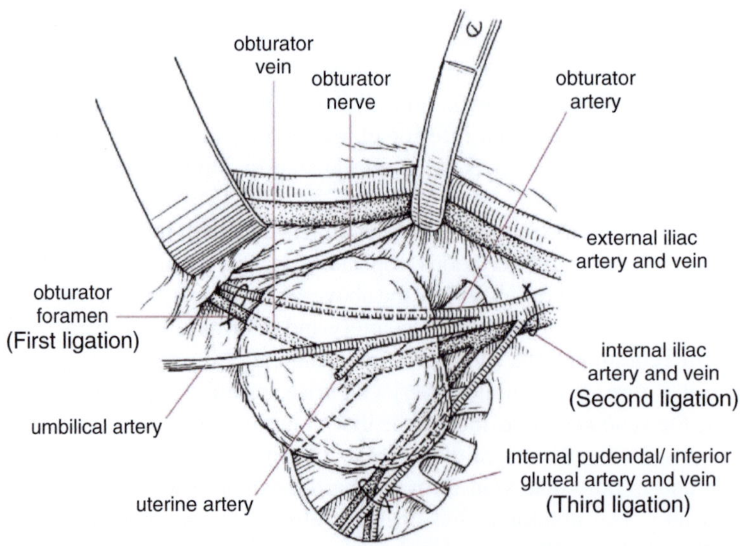

Fig. 9.3 Three ligations of vessels in super-radical hysterectomy (Mibayashi T; Modern Handbook of Obstetrics and Gynecology8E, Cervical cancer, 1970, Nakayama Shoten, Tokyo). Reprinted by courtesy of Nakayama Shoten and translated by Mikio Mikami

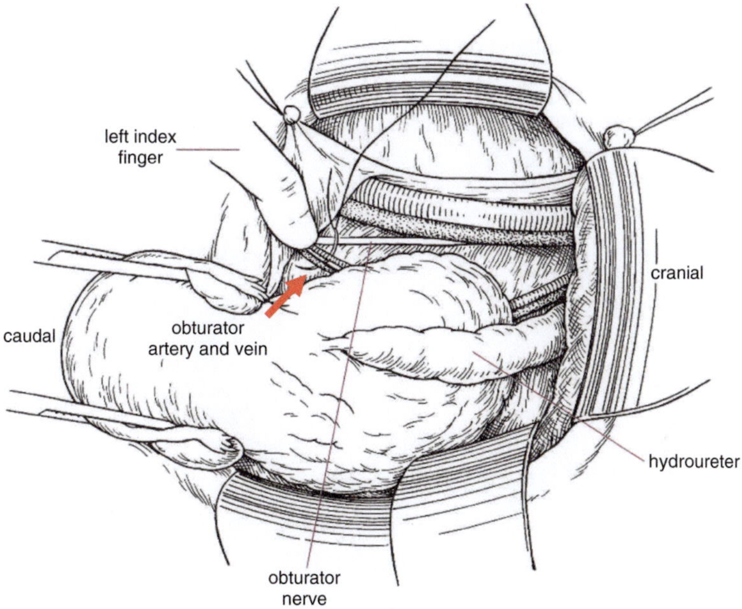

Fig. 9.4 First ligation of vessels in super-radical hysterectomy (Mibayashi T; Modern Handbook of Obstetrics and Gynecology8E, Cervical cancer, 1970, Nakayama Shoten, Tokyo). Reprinted by courtesy of Nakayama Shoten and translated by Mikio Mikami

obturator artery and vein is called the "first ligation" in this operation. Next, the cardinal ligament is dissected from the lateral sidewall using Cooper scissors and the index finger.

9.2.3.3 Second Ligation

The internal iliac artery and vein in the cranial part of the cardinal ligament, which has been heavily infiltrated by the tumor, are identified using the index finger. In particular, the internal iliac vein is located outside the membranous tissue. Then the internal iliac artery and vein are bluntly lifted away from the lateral pelvic sidewall by the index finger, and both vessels are ligated and cut (Fig. 9.5). This is the "second ligation" of the operation. In patients with advanced cancer, the ureter is usually involved by the tumor, leading to hydroureter. Therefore, the ureter is also transected at this time, and urinary diversion is performed later.

9.2.3.4 Third Ligation

Performance of the abovementioned manipulations completes the procedures for handling thc blood vessels in the cranial and caudal parts of the cardinal ligament, which has become involved by the tumor. In addition, it is necessary to deal with the internal pudendal and inferior gluteal arteries and veins running into the infra-piriform foramen inferoposterior to the cardinal ligament. The tumor is pulled forward and upward to allow blunt dissection from the sacral plexus using Cooper scissors. Then, the connective tissue containing the internal pudendal and inferior gluteal arteries and veins is dissected, clamped with forceps, and transected (Fig. 9.6). The cardinal ligament can be excised and removed completely by performing these steps.

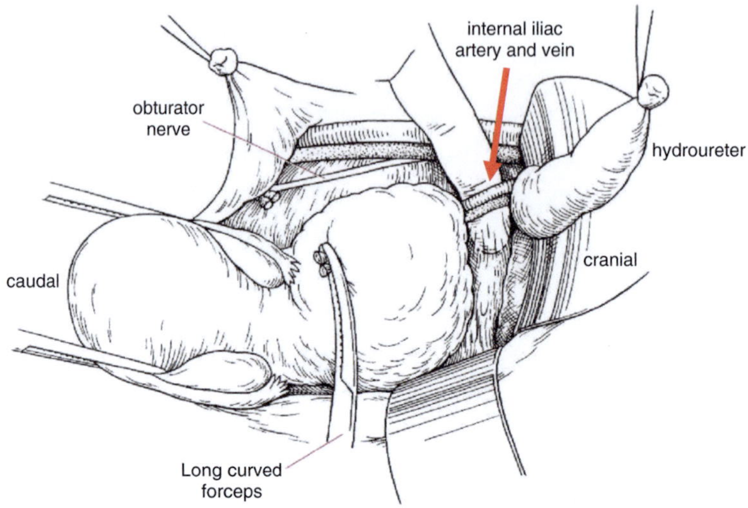

Fig. 9.5 Second ligation of vessels in super-radical hysterectomy (Mibayashi T; Modern Handbook of Obstetrics and Gynecology8E, Cervical cancer, 1970, Nakayama Shoten, Tokyo). Reprinted by courtesy of Nakayama Shoten and translated by Mikio Mikami

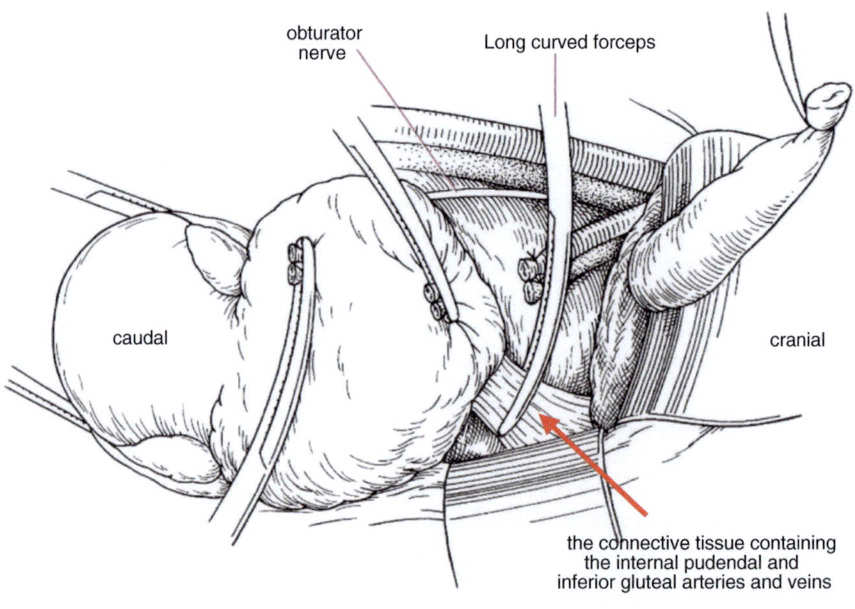

Fig. 9.6 Third ligation of vessels in super-radical hysterectomy (Mibayashi T; Modern Handbook of Obstetrics and Gynecology8E, Cervical cancer, 1970, Nakayama Shoten, Tokyo). Reprinted by courtesy of Nakayama Shoten and translated by Mikio Mikami

The abovementioned procedures comprise the basic method of Mibayashi's super-radical hysterectomy, with the three ligations reflecting the anatomical courses of the main vessels in the basal part of the cardinal ligament. For practical reasons, the arteries and veins should be handled separately and individually in an actual procedure. Because there is usually an enough distance between the arterial and venous systems, the arterial system is generally handled first to improve the visualization of the venous system, after which the venous system is treated. While paying attention to variations of vascular anatomy across patients, the vessels to be resected are determined according to the sites of tumor infiltration and individual circumstances.

9.2.4 Outcome of Treating Cervical Cancer at the Kyoto University Department of Obstetrics and Gynecology (1953–1955) [8]

The 5-year survival rates after surgical treatment are shown in Table 9.1. The rate was similar between stages I, II, and III although the outcome of early-stage disease is somehow higher than expected compared to the current era. This unusual outcome was obtained by a treatment strategy in which Okabayashi's method was modified according to the tumor size in individual patients and super-radical hysterectomy was performed if necessary. When a specific operation is uniformly performed in all patients, the 5-year survival rate would usually decrease as the stage advances (i.e., the 5-year survival rate is lower for stage II disease than stage I disease), and the 5-year survival rate would not be similar for patients across different disease stages.

Outcomes of definitive radiation therapy at that time are shown in Table 9.2. Although radiation therapy was only performed in patients ineligible for surgery, the 5-year survival rate improved over 3 years: the rate was 25.7% in 1953,

Table 9.1 5-year survival rate by surgery (5 years observation)

	Stage				
Year	Stage I	Stage II	Stage III A	Stage III B	Total
1953	75.0%	78.1%	56.4%	60.0%	67.5%
1954	89.2%	67.6%	50.0%	75.0%	66.9%
1955	76.0%	85.0%	74.0%	60.0%	76.6%

Table 9.2 5-year survival rate by radiation

	Stage I	Stage II	Stage III A	Stage III B	Stage IV	Total
1953 (35)	0 (0)	50.0% (2)	33.3% (6)	25.0% (23)	0 (4)	25.7%
1954 (41)	100% (1)	100% (1)	20.0% (5)	29.0% (31)	0 (3)	29.2%
1955 (43)	0 (0)	50.0% (4)	28.5% (14)	41.6% (24)	0 (1)	37.2%

Number of patients

increased to 29.2% in 1954, and rose dramatically to 37.2% in 1955. The same treatment approach was used to deliver radiotherapy throughout the 3-year period, which was rotatory irradiation using a large radiation port invented by the physicians at their institution. However, the dose rate was increased each year, suggesting that the 5-year survival rate increased along with the increasing dose rate. In 1953, rotatory irradiation was first performed using a large radiation port invented by them, allowing the entire cavity of the lesser pelvis to be irradiated almost equally and evenly at a dose of approximately 700 gamma and achieving a 5-year survival rate of 25.7% for 35 patients with stage II–IV disease. Later, the dose was gradually increased. With dose escalation, the 5-year survival rate increased markedly to 37.2% for 43 patients with stage II–IV disease. It is expected that the outcome could have been improved further by continuing to increase the dose. Based on these results, it is obvious to state that outcomes in the super-radical hysterectomy group were superior to the definitive radiotherapy group.

9.2.5 History of Controversy About Super-Radical Hysterectomy in Japan

Not all surgeons thought that Mibayashi's super-radical hysterectomy was a safe and curative surgical approach, with some surgeons doubting both the curability and safety. However, Ogino conducted an additional study on Mibayashi's method and concluded that the approach should be preferably used to the case where lymph node metastasis is fixed to the origin of the cardinal ligament, stating that Okabayashi's method allowed resection of the cardinal ligament, whereas Mibayashi's method achieved extirpation of the cardinal ligament [9]. Kobayashi evaluated the significance of super-radical hysterectomy according to disease stage. He stated that instead of performing the third ligation in Mibayashi's original method, the blood vessels should be separated into an anterior set (internal pudendal artery and vein and the surrounding connective tissue), a middle set (inferior gluteal artery and vein and the surrounding connective tissue), and a posterior set (trunks of the internal iliac artery and vein or common trunks of the arteries and veins peripheral to the internal iliac vessels and surrounding connective tissue), which should be ligated and transected individually. Because the middle set, including the inferior gluteal artery and vein, runs vertically and deeply toward the sacrum, manipulation is most difficult; so Kobayashi also suggested that it was reasonable to handle the anterior set, posterior set, and middle set in this sequence order [10]. Tojo later agreed upon that the anterior and middle sets should be separated and ligated individually in some patients, as advocated by Kobayashi. However, because there were variations in the vascular anatomy, the internal pudendal vein and inferior gluteal vein (which generally form a confluence near the infra-piriform foramen) may be injured by forcible separate manipulation, so the original third ligation of Mibayashi's method should be performed in many patients [11].

9.3 Type D: Laterally Extended Resection (Classification of Radical Hysterectomy by Denis Querleu, C Paul Morrow) [7]

This group of rare operations features additional ultra-radical procedures, mostly indicated at the time of pelvic exenteration. Type D1 is defined as the resection of the entire para-cervix at the pelvic sidewall along with the hypogastric vessels, exposing the roots of the sciatic nerve. There is total resection of the vessels of the lateral part of the para-cervix; these vessels (i.e., inferior gluteal, internal pudendal, and obturator vessels) arise from the internal iliac vascular system. Type D2 is defined as Type D1 plus resection of the entire para-cervix with the hypogastric vessels and adjacent fascial or muscular structures. This resection corresponds to the LEER (laterally extended endopelvic resection) procedure. Because Type D2 is an operation for pelvic sidewall recurrence, Type D1 is mainly described in this chapter.

9.3.1 History and Introduction of Laterally Extended Parametrectomy (LEP) [12, 13]

Various technical variations were described in the initial procedure. A grading system for the radicality of the operation was proposed by Piver and colleagues in 1974. Survival outcomes did not improve substantially for several decades after this, until the introduction of concomitant chemotherapy with irradiation. Local control remained a problem, however, as most of the tumor recurrences occurred in the pelvis with the majority of patients dying from local recurrence. Thus, it is evident that improving local control in the treatment of cervical cancer could also improve survival. In 1993 Ungar introduced a more extensive surgical technique for the treatment of lymph node-involving stage IB cervical cancers and all cancers of stage IIB disease. The intervention, which we call "laterally extended parametrectomy" (LEP), is aimed to remove all the lymphatic tissue from the pelvic sidewall. This procedure removes the parametrial tissue not usually removed by the conventional class III–IV Wertheim hysterectomy by means of extending the lateral limits of the dissection to the true boundaries of the pelvic sidewall rather than the medial surface of the internal iliac vessels.

The LEP procedure is based on three theoretical considerations, namely, that (1) most of the treatment failures in cervical cancer are due to pelvic sidewall recurrences, that (2) lymph node metastases can occur anywhere in the parametrium or pelvic sidewall lymph nodes, and that (3) the connective tissue containing lymph nodes situated lateral to the internal iliac vessels was considered technically inaccessible in most gynecologic oncology centers. This region is the mid part of the pelvic sidewall, corresponding to the lateral insertion of the parametrium, exactly where the superior gluteal, inferior, and pudendal lymph nodes are located. Incomplete resection of this region is a limitation of the classical radical hysterectomy. Several studies have described the anatomical location of tumor metastasis in the parametrial lymph nodes. These studies have found that there is no uniform distribution of lymph node metastasis in the area with an almost equal incidence of metastasis across the parametrial lymph nodes in the medial and lateral parametria.

9.3.2 Surgical Technique [12, 13]

The dissection of the pelvic sidewall begins with a meticulous pelvic lymphadenectomy. In order to remove all lymphatic adipose tissue surrounding the vessels, we mobilize the external iliac vessels from the psoas muscle, displacing them medially, preserving the genitor-femoral nerve. Connective tissue between the vessels is dissected, so that the entire circumference of the external and common iliac arteries and veins are mobilized. As the vessels are retracted from the psoas muscle (a small vascular branch from the iliac vessels to the muscle can be usually divided here) (Fig. 9.7), the lateral or "deep" common iliac nodes can be dissected. In fact the nodal tissues include the superior gluteal and iliolumbar lymph nodes. There is no well-defined limit between the "lateral common iliac" nodes and the cranial part of the obturator nodes. In this way the adipose tissue between the common iliac vein and the sacrum can also be removed. This part of the pelvic adipose tissue is a bridge between the "deep" or lateral common iliac lymph nodes and the presacral lymph nodes. Without discussing the anatomical terminology of the different lymph node stations, the pelvic lymphadenectomy is complete when the vessels are totally free all around their circumferences, the obturator nerve is visualized posteriorly until its retro-psoas portion, and the adipose tissue around the obturator nerve has been removed such that the superior branch of the sacral plexus is visible.

The key essence of the LEP is to use different dissection planes compared to that of the conventional radical hysterectomy. Not only the visceral branches of the internal iliac vessels are sectioned, but the parietal branches are also clipped and divided at the point where they leave or enter into the pelvis (Fig. 9.7). Thus the entire hypogastric system is removed, and no connective tissue is left behind on the pelvic sidewall. The technique is the following: after completing the lymphadenectomy, we clip and divide the iliolumbar vessels, and the superior gluteal vessels, and dissect free the superior branch of the sacral plexus. Anteriorly, the obturator vessels are also ligated and divided on the surface of the obturator internus muscle. We

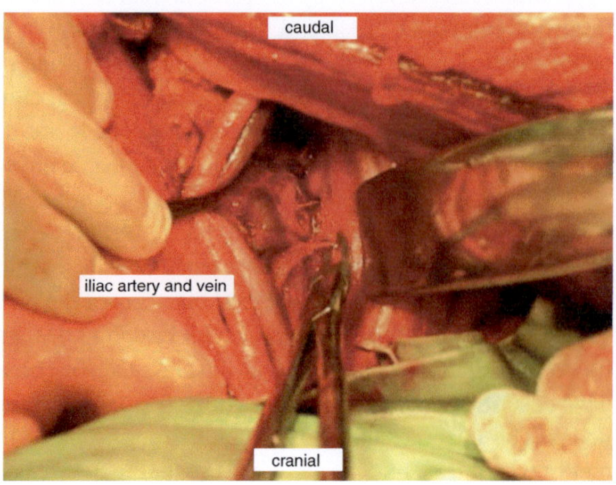

Fig. 9.7 The first step of the LEP operation. The branches of the hypogastric vessels are clipped and divided above the lumbar branch of the lumbosacral nerve

ligate and divide the internal iliac artery and vein at their origin. With slight medial traction on the dissected internal iliac vessels, the sacral plexus with the piriformis muscle between and under its branches can be dissected free, using hemoclips for the various number of parietal vessels in this region. Finally, we clip and divide the pudendal and inferior gluteal vessels at their entrance/exit from the pelvis. At the end of this procedure, the following structures of the pelvic sidewall can be seen clearly from the anteroinferior to posterosuperior direction, with no connective tissue intervening: the levator ani and the internal obturator muscles, the linea arcuata, above it the psoas muscle, under it the piriformis muscle with the convergent branches of the sacral plexus, posterior the sacrum (Fig. 9.8). The main technical difficulty of the procedure results from the various number and calibers of the pelvic sidewall veins. Heavy bleeding may occur and electrocautery cannot be used because of the nerve plexus. Suture ligation or the application of hemoclips to control bleeding vessels may be required. The resected specimen was shown in Fig. 9.9. Packing the small pelvis might be necessary in order to stop bleeding.

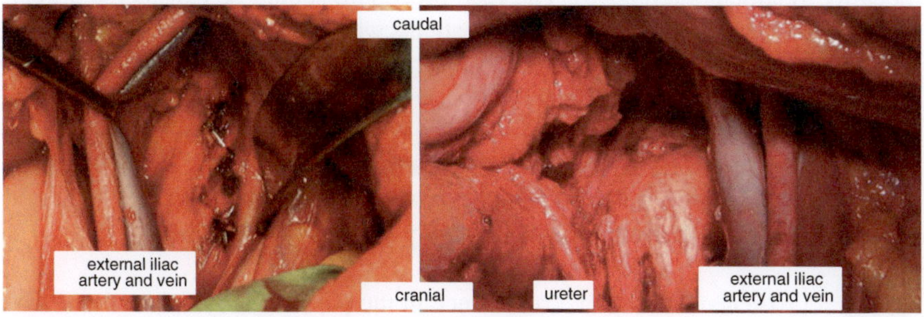

Fig. 9.8 The clearance of the lumbar branch of the lumbosacral nerve. At the end of LEP procedure, the following structures of the pelvic sidewall can be seen clearly from the anteroinferior to posterosuperior direction, with no connective tissue intervening: the levator ani and the internal obturator muscles, the linea arcuata, above it the psoas muscle, under it the piriformis muscle with the convergent branches of the sacral plexus, posterior the sacrum

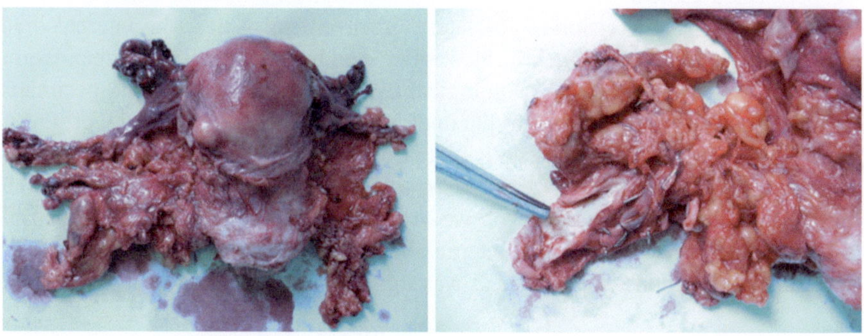

Fig. 9.9 The extent of the parametrium on the surgical specimen

9.3.3 Outcome of the LEP Procedure [14]

Here, the outcome of the LEP procedure will be shown with a completed 5-year follow-up. In 70 (66%) out of 106 patients who underwent the LEP-Wertheim surgery, no adjuvant treatment was used. In the remaining 36 (34%) patients, where histology results suggested tumor spread beyond the threshold of our surgery, adjuvant chemoradiotherapy was advised. The 5-year follow-up was completed without any patient who lost to follow-up for the whole cohort. In 70 patients treated by the LEP procedure alone, the overall 5-year survival was 91.4%. For those 36 patients who received adjuvant therapy and who were excluded due to disease spread above study criteria, 5-year survival was 44%. Complications encountered in 10% of the cases necessitated the second operation. Apart from transient hyper continence and one case of permanent incontinence, no severe quality of life consequence of the operation was observed. These results suggest that in two-thirds of pelvic lymph node-positive, stage IB cervical cancer cases, surgery alone could provide equal or superior survival without the toxicity of chemoradiotherapy than any kind of multimodality treatment alternatives. The LEP procedure should be considered a treatment option for stage IB cervical cancer patients with pelvic lymph node metastases if no adjuvant therapy is intended after surgery.

9.4 Complete Resection of the Cardinal Ligament and Para-aortic Lymph Node Dissection Immediately After Ordinal Radical Hysterectomy (Mikami Methods) [15]

Among 35 patients with the first recurrence in the para-aortic lymph nodes (PAN) after radical hysterectomy whose data we collected, approximately 40% had simultaneous recurrence in the PAN and at other sites. In these patients with multiple recurrent tumors, metastases outside the PAN involved cervical and mediastinal lymph nodes (50%) or sites within the pelvis (20%). Based on these findings, we hypothesized that patients with PAN metastasis probably often had pelvic recurrence because of residual cancer in the stump of the cardinal ligament. Therefore, we performed radical hysterectomy using Okabayashi's method combined with PAN dissection and excision of the lateral involvement of near the internal iliac origin if pelvic lymph node metastasis was detected by intraoperative frozen section diagnosis, and we performed pathological evaluation of the resected specimens (Fig. 9.10). This study shows that parametrial tumor involvement at the origin of internal iliac vessels was significantly associated with increased risk of PAN metastasis: of 14 patients with PAN metastasis, 8 (57%) had tumor involvement of the origin of internal iliac vessels. Then we examined the risk factors for parametrial tumor involvement at the origin of internal iliac vessels. On univariate analysis, only bilateral pelvic lymph node metastasis was significantly associated with parametrial

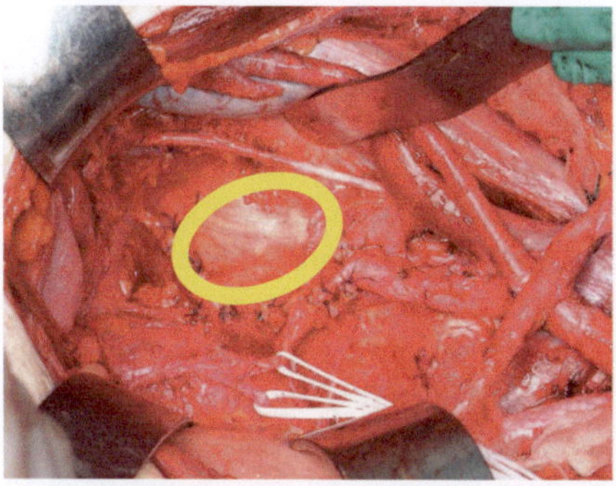
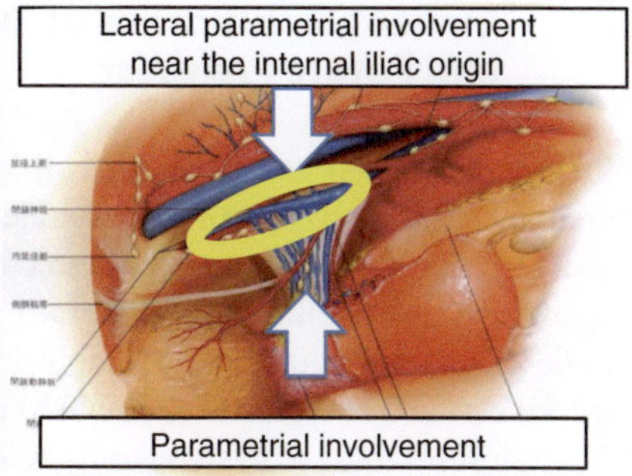

Fig. 9.10 Resection of the lateral parametrial involvement near the internal iliac origin. We performed radical hysterectomy using Okabayashi's method combined with PAN dissection and excision of the lateral parametrial involvement near the internal iliac origin if pelvic lymph node metastasis was detected by intraoperative frozen section diagnosis, and we performed pathological evaluation of the resected specimens

tumor involvement at the origin of internal iliac vessels (50 vs. 9.1%, odds ratio 10.0, 95% confidence interval 1.10–90.8, $P = 0.027$). When there was a tumor involvement in the parametrial tissue near the uterine cervix, there was an increased risk of parametrial tumor involvement at the origin of internal iliac vessels although it did not reach statistical significance (57.1 vs.23.8%, odds ratio 4.27, 95% confidence interval 0.99–18.4, $P = 0.075$). A clinically meaning interpretation of this study was that more than half of cases with parametrial tumor involvement near the uterine cervix had tumor involvement in the parametrial tissue near the internal iliac origin (57.1%). Tumor involvement in this anatomical location was also associated with pelvic and para-aortic lymph node metastasis. This association not only supports a hypothesis of lymphatic tumor spread via the anatomical sequence of parametria, pelvic, and para-aotic lymph nodal chains but also translates into the treatment intervention in women with stage IIB cervical cancer. That is, if systemic chemotherapy is considered as postoperative therapy rather than radiotherapy for high-risk group given comparable effectiveness on survival [16], (1) assessment of tumor involvement in the lateral parametrial at the origin of internal iliac vessels and (2) complete resection in necessary case would be paramount because chemotherapy alone may not have adequate local control in the pelvis in high-risk group [16]. Morbidity related to this extended surgical procedure was not available in our study, and further study is warranted to assess the risks and benefits related to this procedure. We are now planning to launch a clinical trial for stage IIB patients with positive pelvic nodes with the size being larger than 1 cm. Our treatment proposal is to perform radical surgery followed by PAN dissection, after which complete resection of the cardinal ligament (at the origin of internal iliac vessels) is added. Postoperative adjuvant chemotherapy, as opposed to radiotherapy, is to be given in an attempt to avoid the complications related to radiotherapy.

9.5 Current Significance of Super-Radical Hysterectomy and Future Prospect

When pelvic lymph node metastasis fixed to the origin of the cardinal ligament is found at the time of laparotomy conducted for women with clinical stage IB–IIB cervical cancer, super-radical hysterectomy may be a useful surgical approach. Regarding the feasibility of this operative method, because the internal iliac vessels can be clearly visualized after lymph node dissection during current curative surgery for cervical cancer, it is possible to perform super-radical hysterectomy safely. Although super-radical hysterectomy would not be a routine choice of surgical procedure for cervical cancer, it is an important operative method that should be used in a flexible manner on demand, depending on the findings at laparotomy. As our data on super-radical hysterectomy were obtained from retrospective observations in limited institutions, the interpretation remains limited. Being said, it will be paramount to state the above utility of super-radical hysterectomy based upon the results from prospective studies. However, such trials for super-radical hysterectomy might be difficult to conduct in reality. Our philosophy is that once the surgeons start surgery for the complete eradication of tumor from the patient, the surgeon should do the very best for the patient. Do no harm: if this won't be achievable otherwise, the surgeon should stop surgery as soon as they possibly can. However, we feel that the most important concept of the super-extensive parametrectomy is that this surgical procedure is aimed for the curative intent by itself for pelvic sidewall recurrences following chemoradiotherapy [17]. This group of patients with pelvic sidewall recurrence after concurrent chemoradiotherapy has no other choice for cure unless the extensive pelvic sidewall resection with clear surgical margins is to be achieved by this surgery.

References

1. Mikuta JJ. Historical development of radical surgery for cancer of the cervix. In: Rubin SC, Hoskins WJ, editors. Cervical cancer and preinvasive neoplasia. Philadelphia, PA: Lippincott-Raven; 1996. p. 183–8.
2. Wertheim E. The extended abdominal operation for carcinoma uteri(based on 500 operative cases). Am J Obstet Gynecol. 1912;66:169.
3. Ogura T, Nakano R. Okabayashi radical hysterectomy for cervical cancer. Osaka: Nagai Shoten Co., Ltd.; 1983. p. 1–9.
4. Okabayashi H. Radical abdominal hysterectomy for cancer of the cervix uteri. Modification of the Takayama operation. Surg Gynecol Obstet. 1921;33:335–43.
5. Mibayashi R. Mibayashi super-radical hysterectomy. Modern handbook of obstetrics and gynecology 8E, Cervical cancer. Tokyo: Nakayama Shoten Co., Ltd.; 1970. p. 269–79.
6. Ungár L, Pálfalvi L, Tarnai L, Nechushkina V, Lintner B, Novák Z, FACOG Committee on Practice Bulletins. Surgical treatment of stage IB cervical cancer. Int J Gynecol Cancer. 2012;22:1597–603. https://doi.org/10.1097/IGC.0b013e3182725ecd.
7. Querleu D, Morrow CP. Classification of radical hysterectomy. Lancet Oncol. 2008;9:297–303. https://doi.org/10.1016/S1470-2045(08)70074-3.
8. Mibayashi R. Outcome of patients with cervical cancer treated in Kyoto University (1953). Acta Obstetrica et Gynecol Jpn. 1959;11:1003–6.

9. Ogino K. Radical hysterectomy performed by me (modified Okabayashi method). Surgery. 1950;4:160–73.
10. Kobayashi T. Surgery for cervical cancer. Tokyo: Nanzanndo; 1961.
11. Tojo S. Basic surgery for cervical cancer. Osaka: Nagaishoten; 1981.
12. Ungar L, Pálfalvi L. Surgical treatment of lymph node metastases in stage IB cervical cancer: the laterally extended parametrectomy (LEP) procedure. Int J Gynecol Cancer. 2003;13:647–51.
13. Pálfalvi L, Ungár L. Laterally extended parametrectomy (LEP), the technique for radical pelvic side wall dissection: feasibility, technique and results. Int J Gynecol Cancer. 2003;13:914–7.
14. Ungár L, Pálfalvi L, Tarnai L, Horányi D, Novák Z. Surgical treatment of lymph node metastases in stage IB cervical cancer. The laterally extended parametrectomy (LEP) procedure: experience with a 5 year follow-up. Gynecol Oncol. 2011;123:337–41.
15. Matsuo K, Grubbs BH, Mikami M. Quality and quantity metrics of pelvic lymph node metastasis and risk of para-aortic lymph node metastasis in stage IB-IIB cervical cancer. J Gynecol Oncol. 2018;29(1):e10. https://doi.org/10.3802/jgo.2018.29.e10.
16. Matsuo K, Shimada M, Aoki Y, Sakamoto M, Takeshima N, Fujiwara H, Matsumoto T, Mikami M, Sugiyama T. Comparison of adjuvant therapy for node-positive clinical stage IB-IIB cervical cancer: systemic chemotherapy versus pelvic irradiation. Int J Cancer. 2017;141:1042–51.
17. Kim HS, Kim R, Lee M. Super-radical hysterectomy for recurrent cervical cancer. Surg Oncol. 2017;26(4):331–2.

Laparoscopic Radical Hysterectomy

10

Eiji Kobayashi, Tsuyoshi Takiuchi, Shinya Matsuzaki, Yuri Matsumoto, Michiko Kodama, Kae Hashimoto, Seiji Mabuchi, Yutaka Ueda, Kenjiro Sawada, Takuji Tomimatu, Kiyoshi Yoshino, and Tadashi Kimura

Abstract

Radical hysterectomy is the currently accepted treatment for early-stage cervical cancer. Various radical hysterectomy techniques have been demonstrated in the literature, based predominantly around abdominal radical hysterectomy but more recently on laparoscopic radical hysterectomy. Over the last two decades, many studies have indicated laparoscopic radical hysterectomy's safety and feasibility for early-stage cervical cancer. The proven benefits, in the appropriately selected cancer patient, of laparoscopy over laparotomy for radical hysterectomy have been significant reductions in blood loss, pain, duration of hospital stay, wound complications, etc. However, until just recently, there had been few studies comparing laparoscopic radical hysterectomy and abdominal radical hysterectomy regarding recurrence and survival rates over a long follow-up period. In this chapter, we review previous reports of laparoscopic radical hysterectomy, having relatively large number of patients, that described perioperative morbidity, tumor recurrence, and survival rate. We present our view of laparoscopic radical hysterectomy's bright prospects for the future.

Keywords

Laparoscopy · Radical hysterectomy · Cervical cancer

E. Kobayashi (✉) · T. Takiuchi · S. Matsuzaki · Y. Matsumoto · M. Kodama · K. Hashimoto · S. Mabuchi · Y. Ueda · K. Sawada · T. Tomimatu · K. Yoshino · T. Kimura
Faculty of Medicine, Graduate School of Medicine, Osaka University, Osaka, Japan
e-mail: ekobayashi@gyne.med.osaka-u.ac.jp

M. Mikami (ed.), *Surgery for Gynecologic Cancer*, Comprehensive Gynecology and Obstetrics, https://doi.org/10.1007/978-981-13-1519-0_10

10.1 History

A protocol for laparoscopic radical hysterectomy (LRH) combined with pelvic and aortic lymph node dissection was first described by Nazhat in 1992 [1]. This technically challenging procedure was initially received with reticence by gynecologic oncologists more familiar with the traditional abdominal radical hysterectomy (ARH). Regardless, there are now hundreds of published reports of successful LRH, supporting its safety and efficacy. Remarkably, with the recent introduction of computer-assisted robotic platforms, complex laparoscopic radical hysterectomy is no longer a procedure limited only to surgeons with advanced laparoscopic skills. Just recently, the results of Laparoscopic Approach to Carcinoma of the Cervix (LACC) trial were reported, and there is big debate concerning the oncological safety of LRH [2].

10.2 Principles and Indications

The ideal candidates for LRH are young thin women with no concurrent medical problems who are highly motivated toward a rapid return to normal life activity, in contrast to those who would select undertaking an extended course of radiation therapy.

In traditional ARH, the most common indication for radical hysterectomy and pelvic lymphadenectomy is early-stage invasive cancer of the cervix, i.e., International Federation of Gynecology and Obstetrics (FIGO) stages IB and IIA. The 5-year overall and disease-free survival rates for a solely primary surgical approach to treatment of these stages are similar to those of radiation therapy (83% and 74%, respectively) [3]. Although the therapeutic efficacies of a radical hysterectomy and radiation therapy are equivalent, most patients with early-stage cervical cancer undergo radical hysterectomy because the procedure has been associated with fewer long-term complications and a superior quality of life and sexual function, compared with radiation therapy. Like for ARH, the indication stage for LRH is FIGO stages IB–IIA.

Among early-stage cervical cancers, treatment for bulky IB cervical cancer is controversial. Common treatments include radical surgery followed by either radiation or concurrent chemoradiation, primary concurrent chemoradiation, and neoadjuvant chemotherapy/concurrent chemoradiation before surgery. The majority of previous LRH studies limited their patient enrollments to those with cancers of stage IB1 or less, predisposing a favorable prognosis. To date, only rare LRH studies have included patients with a tumor size greater than 4 cm. Kong et al. reported a comparison study of LRH vs. ARH regarding the feasibility, morbidity, and recurrence rate when used for stage IB and IIA cervical cancers with tumor diameters of 3 cm or greater [4]. Among 88 patients, 40 received LRH, whereas 48 underwent ARH. The mean tumor diameter was 44.4 mm in the LRH group and 45.3 mm for ARH ($p = 0.194$). For the ARH group compared with the LRH group, the mean blood loss was 588 vs. 449 mL ($p < 0.001$), mean operating time was similar (246.0

vs. 254.5 min, $p = 0.042$), and disease-free survival rates were 97.9 vs. 97.5% ($p = 0.818$). Although further studies that could add support to this approach are still necessary, LRH appears to be a feasible therapeutic procedure for the management of bulky FIGO stage IB and IIA cervical cancers.

10.3 Preoperative Evaluation

In most cases, the suspicion of cervical cancer arises through a Pap test, followed by a secondary examination and a colposcopy and/or biopsy. Despite the critical impact that the stage of the disease should have on the primary treatment plan, cervical cancer is still based primarily on a clinical assessment. Thus, the extent of the disease is evaluated by a bimanual gynecological examination under anesthesia and, only in selected cases, other tests, such as cystoscopy and proctoscopy. Lymph node status and tumor spread within the abdominal cavity and peritoneal surface are certainly the most difficult variables to evaluate by clinical examination, with respect to a possible infiltration of the paracervix, vagina, and rectovaginal and vesicovaginal septa.

Although not recognized by FIGO for staging, CT and MRI are widely used for therapeutic decisions for patients with cervical cancer. The National Comprehensive Cancer Network (NCCN) recently added the MRI evaluation for clinical evaluation of FIGO stages higher than IB1 disease. Some authors have proposed a lymph node laparoscopic staging to determine the extent of the disease outside the cervix, vagina, and paracervix. Presently among authors, there is a general consensus that dichotomizes cervical cancer into two categories: early stage and locally advanced stage. Early-stage cervical cancer is an invasive carcinoma that is strictly confined to the cervix, or it involves the vagina—but not the lower third. It is no greater than 4 cm in diameter, and it has no obvious paracervical involvement or spread of the growth to adjacent or distant organs. Locally advanced cervical cancer is defined as all FIGO stages higher than IIA1.

10.4 Technique

Radical hysterectomy refers to the excision of the uterus en bloc with the parametrium (i.e., with the round, broad, cardinal, and uterosacral ligaments) and the upper one-third to one-half of the vagina. The surgeon usually also performs a bilateral pelvic lymph node dissection. The procedure requires a thorough knowledge of pelvic anatomy, meticulous attention to sharp dissection, and careful technique to allow dissection of the ureters and mobilization of both the bladder and rectum from the vagina. Particular care must be taken with the vasculature of the pelvic sidewalls and the venous plexuses at the lateral corners of the bladder to avoid excessive blood loss. Removal of the ovaries and fallopian tubes is not a required part of a radical hysterectomy; they may be preserved, if judged clinically appropriate.

The most reported LRH technique is a reproduction of the ARH procedure, but via laparoscopic surgery. LRH-specific equipment and instrumentation are used, which the surgeon should sufficiently know how to set up. The operating room setup and a supply of dedicated instruments are essential for every kind of surgery but are even more important for laparoscopic radical hysterectomy.

Generally, the patient's arms are blocked at her side. She is placed in a steep Trendelenburg position after pneumoperitoneum is completed (Fig. 10.1). A 10 mm 0° high-definition video laparoscope is placed at the level of umbilicus, either by open technique or under direct visualization. An alternative 5 mm 0° video laparoscope can be adopted. In general, three additional 5 mm trocars are placed—one in each lower quadrant and one 4 cm below the umbilicus. The surgeon should not hesitate to place additional trocars to perform the surgery safely.

Intra-abdominal pressure is maintained at 10–12 mm Hg. The small bowel is mobilized to the upper abdomen, and, if necessary, the sigmoid is fixed to the abdominal wall to free the Douglas pouch. The round ligaments are transected bilaterally along their lateral section. After opening the wide ligament cranially, the infundibulopelvic ligament is stretched medially to identify the ureter. The pelvic retroperitoneum opening is performed in the following sequence: lateral pararectal space (Latzko), paravesical space, and medial pararectal space (Okabayashi) (Figs. 10.2 and 10.3). A pelvic lymphadenectomy is then performed from the level of the iliac or aortic bifurcation to the circumflex iliac vein (according to the tumor staging). The obturator lymph nodes are removed, with care taken to identify the obturator nerve and avoid injuring it. Para-aortic lymphadenectomy is not routinely performed. If bilateral salpingo-oophorectomy is being performed, the infundibulopelvic ligament is transected. Fallopian tubes are always removed. The bladder is then mobilized inferiorly by a lateral approach to ensure adequate vaginal margins. The posterior peritoneum is incised using monopolar or bipolar forceps, and the

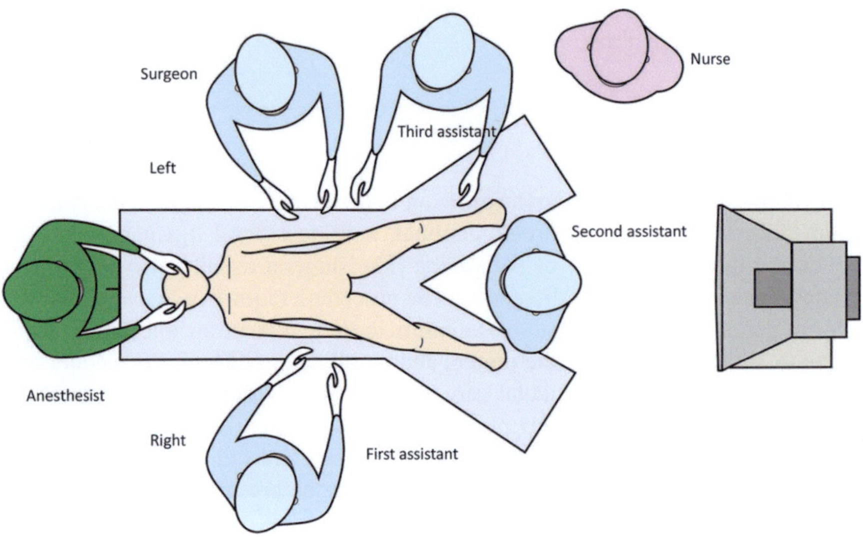

Fig. 10.1 Ideal position of surgical team for laparoscopic surgery

rectovaginal space is entered. After clipping and dissection of the uterine artery at its origin, the connective tissue between the ureter and the uterine artery is dissected. At this point, the course of the ureter is usually clearly exposed up to the entrance of the ureteral tunnel. After sufficient dissection of the bladder, the anterior vesicouterine ligament (VUL) is transected, followed by transection of the cardinal ligament and posterior VUL (Figs. 10.4, 10.5, 10.6, and 10.7).

The tumor specimen is completely separated from the upper vagina and removed. Intracorporeal colpotomy under CO_2 pneumoperitoneum is said to be an independent risk factor for recurrence after LRH in previous study [5]. We routinely select

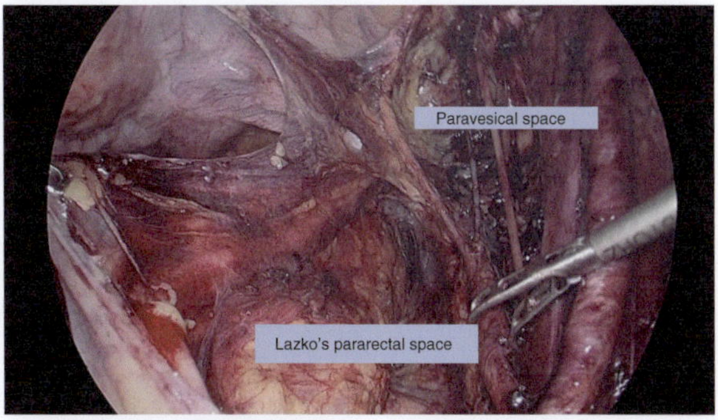

Fig. 10.2 The surgical view of paravesical and pararectal space (right side)

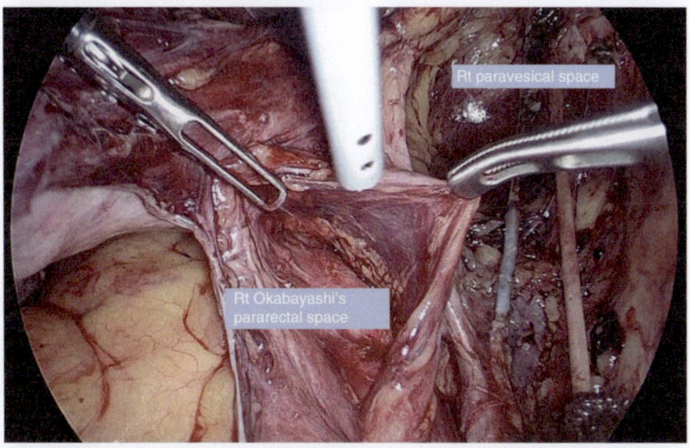

Fig. 10.3 The view of Okabayashi's pararectal space (right side)

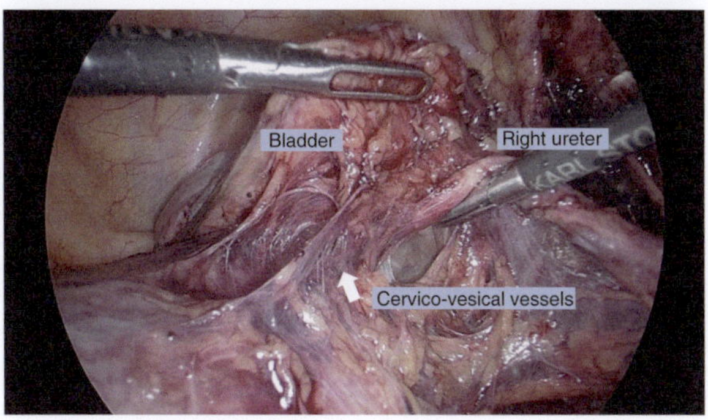

Fig. 10.4 Visualization of cervico-vesical vessels (right side)

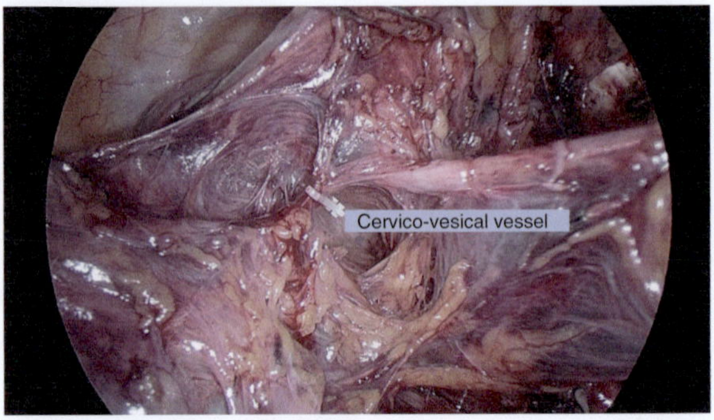

Fig. 10.5 The view of clipping the cervico-vesical vessels (right side)

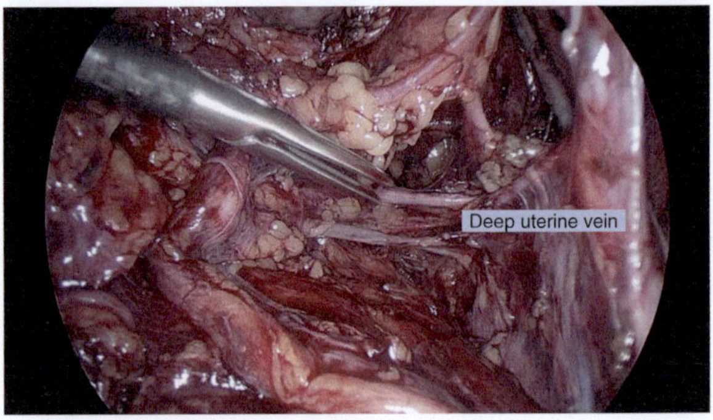

Fig. 10.6 Visualization of the deep uterine vein (right side)

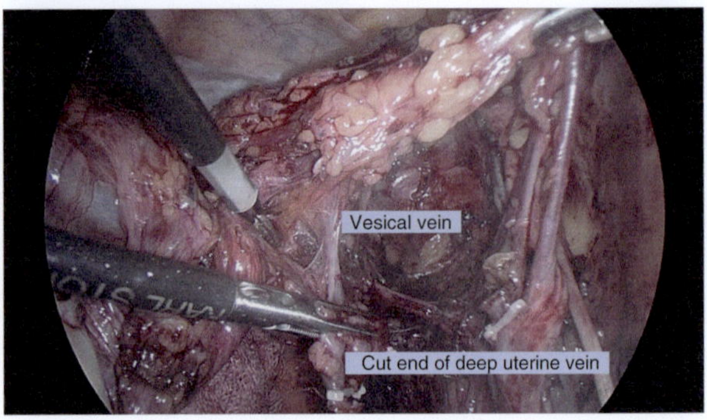

Fig. 10.7 Visualization of the vesical vein (posterior leaf of the vesicouterine ligament) (right side)

vaginal colpotomy with supine position to prevent tumor seeding to peritoneal cavity (Fig. 10.8). The vaginal cuff is laparoscopically or vaginally sutured (according to the surgeon's preference). Finally, before completing surgery, the vagina and all port sites are washed with 5% povidone-iodine solution.

In November 2018, the results of Laparoscopic Approach to Carcinoma of the Cervix (LACC) trial were reported [2]. The main objective of this trial was to compare disease-free survival at 4.5 years among patients who underwent a total laparoscopic or robotic radical hysterectomy (TLRH/TRRH) vs. ARH for early stage cervical cancer. The main result was that TLRH/TRRH was associated with higher

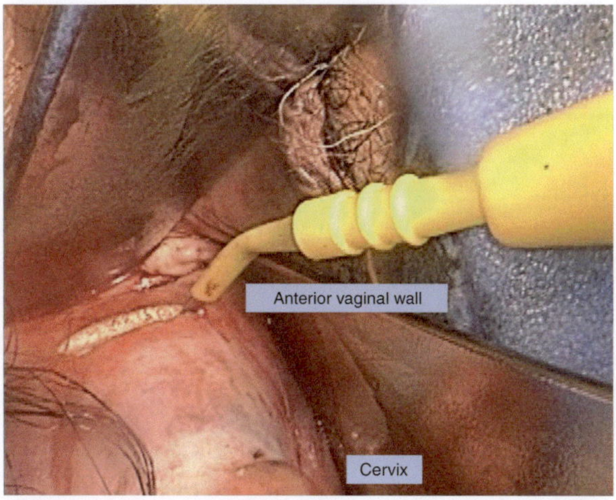

Fig. 10.8 The view of vaginal colpotomy procedure

recurrence rates and worse overall survival compared to ARH. Park et al. refuted the result [6]. They claimed the high recurrence rate of the MIS (minimally invasive surgery) group may be due to surgical technique or inattentiveness of the operator. During the LRH, the use of the uterine manipulator during MIS RH can cause tumor breakdown and fragmentation. They speculate the use of the uterine manipulator and intracorporeal colpotomy may predispose the patient's intrapelvic recurrence shortly after surgery. And they also alleged, in the LACC trial, this factor was not considered and the recurrences after MIS RH were mainly pelvic recurrences which occurred shortly after surgery. They emphasized that in order to reduce the incidence of peritoneal seeding from broken tumor fragments during MIS RH, the stiff Trendelenburg position should be changed to a supine position, and vaginal cuff resection and repair should be performed by vaginal approach. Irrigation of the vagina and pelvic cavity should be performed rigorously before closure of the vaginal stump. Although it seems that the discussion on this result will continue for a while, we consider that the surgeons should be cautious with the procedure of colpotomy during the LRH.

10.5 Morbidity

Significant amounts of non-comparative morbidity data from large series of LRH are available. In 2002, Spirtos et al. reported on 78 patients with stage IA2–IB cervical cancer [7]. In their series, 93.5% of the procedures were completed laparoscopically (i.e., LRH). The mean operative time was 205 min, and the mean blood loss was 225 mL. 1.3% of the procedure required a blood transfusion. Three patients had unintended cystotomies, two patients required laparotomy to control bleeding, and one patient suffered an ureterovaginal fistula. There were four documented recurrences (5.1%) after a minimum of 3 years of follow-up (Table 10.1).

Table 10.1 Studies of LRH for cervical cancer

Author	Country	Year	No of patients	FIGO stage	Operative time (min)[a]	Blood loss (mL)[a]	Duration of hospital stay (day)[a]	Follow up (month)[a]	Recurrence (%)	Survival (%)
Spirtos NM [7]	USA	2002	78	IA2-IB	205	225	2.9	66.8	10.3	93.6
Pomel C [8]	France	2003	50	IA1-IB1	258	200	7.5	44	6	96.8
Zakashansky K [19]	USA	2007	30	IA1-IIA	318	200	3.8	20	0	100
Xu H [9]	China	2007	317	IA2-IIB	NA	NA	12	NA	NA	NA
Puntambekar SP [10]	India	2007	248	IA2-IB1	92	165	3	36	2.8	100
Li G [16]	China	2007	90	IB-IIA	262	369	13.8	26	13.8	90
Frumovitz M [15]	USA	2007	35	IA1-IB1	344	319	2	7.2	2.8	100.0
Pellegrino A [11]	Italy	2009	107	IB1<3 cm	305	200	4	30	10	95
Malzoni M [17]	Italy	2009	65	IA1-IB1	196	55	4	52.5	7.6	NA
Lee CL [12]	Taiwan	2010	139	IA2-IIA	231	666	16	92.1	9	92.7
Lee EJ [31]	Korea	2011	24	IA2-IIA	334	414	10.7	78	8.3	90.5
Yan X [13]	China	2011	237	IA2-IIB	264	255	13	35	17.2	82.0
Hwang JH [14]	Korea	2012	70	IA-IIA	287	389	15.7	NA	4.2	99.0
Pareja R [21]	Colombia	2012	50	IA2-IB2	235	79	1	12	0	100.0
Nam J-H [18]	Korea	2012	263	IA2-IIA	246	379	12.5	63	7.2	95.2
Kong TW [4]	Korea	2014	40	IB-IIA	254	449	14.8	28	2.5	100

NA not applicable
[a]Average or mean

In 2003, Pomel et al. reported on 50 patients with stage IA1–IB1 cervical cancer [8]. The median LRH operating time was 258 min. No conversion to laparotomy was required. Ten patients had an early complication (arising within 2 months after surgery); two required reoperation. Three patients had late complications (more than 2 months after surgery); two of them required reoperation. Three patients experienced recurrence after a median follow-up time of 44 months. Overall survival was 100% for stage IA1 and 96.8% for stages IA2 and IB1.

In 2007, Xu et al. reported on a large series of patient population [9]. Among 317 candidates for LRH with lymph adenectomy, 313 procedures were fully completed laparoscopically. The patients were all with stages IA2–IIB. A major intraoperative complication was experienced by 14 patients (4.4%), with only 4 patients (1.3%) requiring conversion to an open procedure. Five cystotomies and five vascular injuries were repaired laparoscopically. Postoperative complications occurred in 5% of patients, including five ureterovaginal fistulas, one with stenosis of the ureter, and four with vesicovaginal fistula. In the same year, Puntambekar et al. reported on 248 patients with stage IA2–IB1 cervical cancer [10]. No patients were converted to laparotomy. Fifteen intraoperative complications were managed laparoscopically: four with urinary tract injury, nine with vascular injury, and two with bowel injury. Seventeen had early postoperative complications within 2 months of surgery: five had bladder dysfunction, two had urinary tract injury, three had wound infection, four had ureterovaginal fistula, two had bowel obstruction, and 1 had secondary hemorrhage. Seven patients (2.8%) experienced recurrent disease after a median follow-up of 36 months.

In 2009, Pellegrino et al. reported on LRH surgical outcomes in a series of 107 patients with stage IB1 cervical cancer [11]. Conversion to laparotomy was necessary in six patients. Median duration of surgery was 305 min, and median blood loss was 200 mL. Intraoperative complications were registered in two patients: one patient had a cystotomy repaired laparoscopically and the second had an obturator nerve injury. Five patients needed a second surgery for intraoperative complications: two patients had a vaginal cuff resuture for bowel evisceration, and three patients required ureteral implantation because of ureteral stenosis or fistula. After a median follow-up of 30 months, 11 patients had a recurrence; the survival rate was 95%.

In 2010, Lee et al. published on a series of 139 patients with stage IA–IIA cervical cancer [12]. Mean operation time was 231.1 min, and mean blood loss was 666 mL. Major LRH intraoperative complications included one great vessel injury, one ureteral injury, one colon injury, and six cystotomies. After a median follow-up of 92.1 months, disease-free survival and overall survival rates were 91% and 93%, respectively. In 2011, Yan et al. evaluated the morbidity and oncological outcome in a large series of 240 cervical cancer patients treated with LRH and pelvic lymphadenectomy [13]. The conversion rate was 1.25%. Mean operative time was 264 min. Median operative blood loss was 255 mL. Intraoperative and postoperative complications occurred in 7% and 9% patients, respectively. During a median follow-up of 92.1 months, the mean disease-free and overall survival rates were 91.1% and 92.8%, respectively.

Hwang et al. performed meta-analysis of 20 LRH studies [14]. They found that the odds ratio (OR) for the risk of intraoperative urologic complications of LRH compared to ARH was 1.97 [95% confidence interval (CI) 1.23–3.13]. Urologic structures are at significant risk for injuries during the LRH and pelvic lymphadenectomy procedures. In particular, this injury is mainly related to an injury of the bladder or ureter because part of the vesicouterine ligament was dissected laparoscopically by an energy sources.

A relatively larger number of retrospective comparative studies are available; we will discuss only those series with over 20 LRH patients. For example, in 2007 Frumovitz et al. compared 54 patients with stage IA–IB cervical cancer undergoing ARH with 35 patients undergoing LRH [15]. Mean estimated blood loss was 548 mL with ARH compared with 319 mL with LRH ($p = 0.009$). The mean operative time was 307 min for ARH compared with 344 min for LRH ($p = 0.03$), but the median hospital stay was significantly shorter for LRH (2 vs. 5 days). Although there was no difference in overall noninfectious postoperative morbidity between the two groups, infectious morbidity was substantially less frequent (18 vs. 53%) after the laparoscopic approach. The median duration of follow-up for all patients was 13 months (15.2 months for ARH, 7.2 months for LRH), during which 2.8% of LRH and 3.7% of ARH patients experienced recurrence.

In 2007, Li et al. reported on a series of 90 LRH that were compared to 35 ARH performed for stage IB–IIA cervical cancer during the same period of time [16]. Two cases were converted to laparotomy. Consistent with other reports, the operating time was significantly longer in the LRH group (262 vs. 217 min, $p = 0.001$). However, the blood loss during operation in LRH was similar to that in ARH group (369 vs. 455 mL, $p = 0.125$). The incidence of intraoperative complication was not significantly different between the two groups (8.89 vs. 8.57%, $p = 0.955$). Interestingly, the time to recover bowel movement was significantly reduced after LRH (1.96 vs. 2.40 days). However, the recurrence rate (13.75 vs. 12%, $p > 0.05$) and the mortality rate (10 vs. 8%, $p > 0.05$) were similar between the two groups.

In 2009, Malzoni et al. compared two series of laparoscopic ($n = 65$) and open ($n = 62$) radical hysterectomy for stage IA1–IB1 cervical cancer patients [17]. Consistent with other reports above, there was less blood loss (55 vs. 145 mL), median operating time was longer (196 vs. 152 min), and hospital stay was shorter (4 vs. 7 days) in the laparoscopy group. The median follow-up was 71.5 months in the ARH group and 52.5 months in the LRH group. There was no difference in disease-free survival between the two groups: 93.6% remained free of disease in the ARH group vs. 92.4% in the LRH group.

In 2012, Nam et al. compared 263 patients undergoing ARH with 263 patients undergoing LRH for stage IA2–IIA cervical cancer patients [18]. They reported that the intraoperative complication rates were similar in the two groups (6.8 vs. 5.7%, $p = 0.711$), but the postoperative complication rate was lower in the LRH than in the ORH group (9.2 vs. 21%, $p = 0.001$). LRH did not have a higher risk of recurrence (HR = 1.28; 95% confidence interval (CI) 0.62–2.64) or death (HR = 1.46; 95% CI 0.62–3.43). Even in patients with tumors >2 cm in diameter, the risk of recurrence

(HR = 0.82; 95% CI 0.31–2.16) or death (HR = 1.01; 95% CI0.35–2.95) were not higher for LRH than for ARH.

The LRH technique is thus feasible, with a high success rate for a trained gynecologic oncologist with laparoscopic skills, and can be taught by experienced proctors. However, a steep learning curve is observed that prevents widespread use of the LRH technique, despite its obvious merits. The training cutoff is generally set at 25–50 cases. In 2007, Zakashansky et al. specifically examined the use of total LRH in a fellowship program [19]. They demonstrated that greater node counts, decreased hospital stay, and less blood loss are possible, without increased morbidity, in their LRH training program.

In 2007, Stefano et al. compared the incidence of complications in 50 patients, where the LRH was conducted in either the early or late stages of surgeon training, and also compared results with a previous laparotomy series with urinary complications [20]. There was no significant difference ($p = 0.09$) between urinary tract complications during training, it occurred in 6/25 of the first 25 cases and 1/25 in the latter 25 cases, but it tended to occur more in the first half of training. The results, when compared with a control group of 48 laparotomy cases, showed that complications were significantly higher (6/25 vs. 2/48; $p = 0.02$) in the 25 patients in the first half compared with laparotomies, compared with laparotomy in 25 late-stage training cases (1/25 vs. 2/48; $p = 1.00$); they concluded that surgical outcome was significantly improved with experience, as the complication rate was higher earlier in training. There was no significant difference in survival between the two groups.

Provided that the necessary efforts to improve the skills of the surgeon have been made, excellent results can be achieved. This statement applies even to the so-called developing countries. In 2012, Pareja et al. compared the surgical and oncologic outcomes of patients undergoing LRH at a large comprehensive cancer center in the United States versus a cancer center in Colombia [21]. The first 50 cases performed in Colombia were as successful as the first 50 cases performed at the MD Anderson Cancer Center. This adds to the evidence that, with adequate teaching and proctorship and willingness to learn, the technique of manual laparoscopic radical hysterectomy can be implemented in any place in the world, critical knowledge where the additional cost of robotic surgery is not affordable.

Despite the inherent limitations of LRH's learning curve, the procedure conveys many documented advantages over the open technique, mainly in terms of blood loss and hospital stay. The outcome balance, combining improved quality of life (QOL) without compromising survival, is in favor of adopting minimally invasive LRH surgery as the gold standard for radical hysterectomy.

10.6 Nerve-Sparing Radical Hysterectomy

Nerve-sparing radical hysterectomy (NSRH) has been designed to prevent the frequent urinary dysfunctions associated with classical (type C) radical hysterectomy [22]. The concept of NSRH was first proposed Kobayashi in the 1960s and Sakamoto and Takizawa in the 1980s and named the "Tokyo method" [23, 24]. However, the

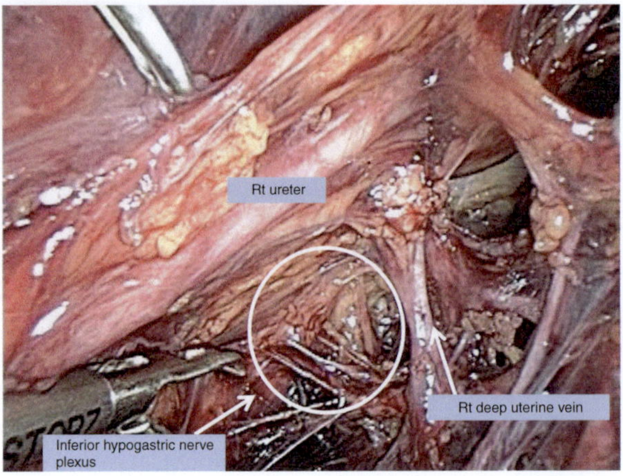

Fig. 10.9 The view of deep uterine vein and inferior hypogastric nerve plexus (Right side)

complexity of pelvic anatomy, including vessels and autonomic nerves around the uterus and bladder, and the insufficient visual representation of pelvic space during ARH have been barriers to better understanding of this technique. Logically, the magnification and lighting provided by the laparoscope has been used to achieve a precise dissection of the pelvic autonomic nerves (Fig. 10.9). This technique has been shown to achieve similar results to open surgery, and its feasibility and safety have been widely recognized. Also, a meta-analysis of 20 individual studies concluded that NSRH was associated with a reduced incidence of intraoperative complications in comparison with conventional radical surgery. The incidences of urinary incontinence or frequency and constipation were also less frequent with NSRH, and there were no adverse effects on survival or sexual function [25].

The technique was pioneered by Possover et al., who identified the middle rectal artery as a landmark separating the neural part from the vascular part of the paracervix [26]. Following the nerve-sparing technique, patients regained bladder function significantly quicker compared with a control group ($n = 28$) in which the neural part of the cardinal ligament was not preserved: suprapubic drainage occurred in 11.2 days versus 21.4 days ($p = 0.0007$).

Since 2010, several investigators reported on full laparoscopic nerve-sparing radical hysterectomy (LNSRH). Liang et al. reported on 163 patients with cervical cancer who underwent laparoscopic radical hysterectomy and pelvic lymphadenectomy, of whom 82 women underwent LNSRH [27]. The average time taken to obtain a post-void residual urine volume of less than 50 mL after removal of the ureteral catheter was 7.4 days in the NSRH group compared to 16.75 days. The bladder function recovered, with no or minor symptoms, in 94% of the LNSRH group compared to 73% for the LRH group. Kavallaris et al. published a series of 32 patients who underwent LNSRH with pelvic lymphadenectomy [28]. The average operating time was 221 min. The authors reported that in all patients spontaneous voiding was possible on the third postoperative day, with a median residual urine volume of <50 mL. Park et al. [29] carried out a retrospective study of 125 patients with cervical cancer stages IB1 ($n = 105$) and IB2 ($n = 20$). In this series, a high rate of urological complications (13/125, 10.4%) was observed. However, these surgical morbidities were corrected with increased experience. Patients were able to self-void at a mean of 10.3 days postoperatively. The return rates to normal voiding function at postoperative 14 and 21 days were 92.0% and 95.2%, respectively. Shi et al. evaluate histopathology of autonomic verve removal within the cardinal ligaments, patient's postoperative urinary function, and feasibility and safety of LNSRH for the treatment of early-stage cervical cancer [30]. Patients who underwent LNSRH had significantly earlier return of bladder and bowel function, with an average time to achieve residual urine of 50 mL or less of 10.22 days and mean first defecation time of 3.58 days. Nerves were observed mainly in the cardinal ligaments of the LRH group. Disease-free survival rate did not differ between the LNSRH (90.6%) and LRH (88.1%) groups ($p = 0.643$). The authors concluded that an LNSRH for stage IB cervical cancer is comparable to the corresponding open procedure in terms of early recovery of bladder function. To summarize, nerve-sparing techniques are feasible laparoscopically.

10.7 Future Prospects

MIS approaches in gynecologic oncology have greatly evolved since the introduction of laparoscopy to the field. The advantages of laparoscopy over laparotomy in the appropriately selected cancer patient have proven beneficial to the patient, both intra- and postoperatively, and with similar outcomes. With our current knowledge and experience, it appears that laparoscopy should be the gold standard in the management of ECC. However, LRH and lymph adenectomy are complex surgeries, and should be performed by skilled physicians and dedicated surgical centers.

After the report of the LACC trial, we, and many other Japanese oncologists who have been promoting LRH, saw the potentially discouraging LACC results, of higher recurrence with LRH, and were deeply concerned. Since the current situation in Japan is exactly the same as when the LACC trial was started about ten years ago in the USA, could the same detrimental outcome happen here? Many institutions are now conflicted as to whether or not they should promote the introduction of MIS for cervical cancer. But many large retrospective studies contradict the initial LACC results, and find no recurrence differences. Therefore, with this swirling controversy in mind, we have to establish the safe LRH procedure and collect data concerning the safety and efficacy of LRH performed in our country in the future.

Acknowledgment We would like to thank Ms. Hazuki Abe for creating the figures.

References

1. Nazhat CR, et al. Laparoscopic radical hysterectomy with paraaortic and pelvic node dissection. Am J Obstet Gynecol. 1992;166:864–5.

2. Ramirez PT, et al. Minimally invasive versus abdominal radical hysterectomy for cervical cancer. N Engl J Med. 2018;379:1895–904.
3. Landoni F, et al. Randomised study of radical surgery versus radiotherapy for stage Ib-IIa cervical cancer. Lancet. 1997;350:535–40.
4. Kong TW, et al. Comparison of laparoscopic versus abdominal radical hysterectomy for FIGO stage IB and IIA cervical cancer with tumor diameter of 3 cm or greater. Int J Gynecol Cancer. 2014;24:280–8.
5. Kong TW, et al. Pattern of recurrence and survival after abdominal versus laparoscopic/robotic radical hysterectomy in patients with early cervical cancer. J Obstet Gynaecol Res. 2016;42:77–86.
6. Park JY, et al. How should gynecologic oncologists react to the unexpected results of LACC trial? J Gynecol Oncol. 2018;29:e74.
7. Spirtos NM, Eisenkop SM, Schlaerth JB, Ballon SC. Laparoscopic radical hysterectomy (type III) with aortic and pelvic lymphadenectomy in patients with stage I cervical cancer: Surgical morbidity and intermediate follow-up. Am J Obstet Gynecol. 2002;187(2):340–8.
8. Pomel C, Atallah D, Le Bouedec G, Rouzier R, Morice P, Castaigne D, Dauplat J. Laparoscopic radical hysterectomy for invasive cervical cancer: 8-year experience of a pilot study. Gynecol Oncol. 2003;91(3):534–9.
9. Xu H, Chen Y, Li Y, Zhang Q, Wang D, Liang Z. Complications of laparoscopic radical hysterectomy and lymphadenectomy for invasive cervical cancer: experience based on 317 procedures. Surg Endosc. 2007;21(6):960–4.
10. Puntambekar SP, Palep RJ, Puntambekar SS, Wagh GN, Patil AM, Rayate NV, Agarwal GA. Laparoscopic total radical hysterectomy by the Pune technique: Our experience of 248 cases. J Minim Invasive Gynecol. 2007;14(6):682–9.
11. Pellegrino A, Vizza E, Fruscio R, Villa A, Corrado G, Villa M, Dell'Anna T, Vitobello D. Total laparoscopic radical hysterectomy and pelvic lymphadenectomy in patients with Ib1 stage cervical cancer: analysis of surgical and oncological outcome. Eur J Surg Oncol. 2009;35(1):98–103.
12. Lee CL, et al. Long-term survival outcome of laparoscopically assisted radical hysterectomy in treating early stage cervical cancer. Am J Obstet Gynecol. 2010;203:165.1–7.
13. Yan X, Li G, Shang H, Wang G, Han Y, Lin T, Zheng F. Twelve-year experience with laparoscopic radical hysterectomy and pelvic lymphadenectomy in cervical cancer. Gynecol Oncol. 2011;120(3):362–7.
14. Hwang JH. Urologic complication in laparoscopic radical hysterectomy: Meta-analysis of 20 studies. Eur J Cancer. 2012;48(17):3177–85.
15. Frumovitz M, dos Reis R, Sun CC, Milam MR, Bevers MW, Brown J, Slomovitz BM, Ramirez PT. Comparison of total laparoscopic and abdominal radical hysterectomy for patients with early-stage cervical cancer. Obstet Gynecol. 2007;110(1):96–102.
16. Li G, Yan X, Shang H, Wang G, Chen L, Han Y. A comparison of laparoscopic radical hysterectomy and pelvic lymphadenectomy and laparotomy in the treatment of Ib-IIa cervical cancer. Gynecol Oncol. 2007;105(1):176–80.
17. Malzoni M, Tinelli R, Cosentino F, Fusco A, Malzoni C. Total laparoscopic radical hysterectomy versus abdominal radical hysterectomy with lymphadenectomy in patients with early cervical cancer: our experience. Ann Surg Oncol. 2009;16(5):1316–23.
18. Nam J-H, Park J-Y, Kim D-Y, Kim J-H, Kim Y-M, Kim Y-T. Laparoscopic versus open radical hysterectomy in early-stage cervical cancer: long-term survival outcomes in a matched cohort study. Ann Oncol. 2012;23(4):903–11.
19. Zakashansky K, Chuang L, Gretz H, Nagar NP, Sheth J, Rahaman FRN. A case-controlled study of total laparoscopic radical hysterectomy with pelvic lymphadenectomy versus radical abdominal hysterectomy in a fellowship training program. Int J Gynecol Cancer. 2007;17(5):1075–82.
20. Uccella S, Laterza R, Ciravolo G, Volpi E, Franchi M, Zefiro F, Donadello N, Ghezzi F. A comparison of urinary complications following total laparoscopic radical hysterectomy and laparoscopic pelvic lymphadenectomy to open abdominal surgery. Gynecol Oncol. 2007;107(1):S147–9.

21. Pareja R, Nick AM, Schmeler KM, Frumovitz M, Soliman PT, Buitrago CA, Borrero M, Angel G, dos Reis R, Ramirez PT. Quality of laparoscopic radical hysterectomy in developing countries: A comparison of surgical and oncologic outcomes between a comprehensive cancer center in the United States and a cancer center in Colombia. Gynecol Oncol. 2012;125(2):326–9.
22. Cibula D, Abu-Rustum NR, Benedetti-Panici P, Köhler C, Raspagliesi F, Querleu D, Morrow CP. New classification system of radical hysterectomy: Emphasis on a three-dimensional anatomic template for parametrial resection. Gynecol Oncol. 2011;122(2):264–8.
23. Kobayashi T. Abdominal radical hysterectomy with pelvic lymphadenectomy for cancer of cervix. 2nd ed. Tokyo: Nanzando; 1961.
24. Sakamoto S, Takizawa K. An improved radical hysterectomy with fewer urological complications and with no loss of therapeutic results for invasive cervical cancer. Baillieres Clin Obstet Gynaecol. 1988;2(4):953–62.
25. Kim HS, Kim K, Ryoo S-B, Seo JH, Kim SY, Park JW, Kim MA, Hong KS, Jeong CW, Song YS. Conventional versus nerve-sparing radical surgery for cervical cancer: a meta-analysis. J Gynecol Oncol. 2015;26(2):100.
26. Possover M, et al. Identification and preservation of the motoric innervation of the bladder in radical hysterectomy type III. Gynecol Oncol. 2000;79:154–7.
27. Liang Z, et al. Laparoscopic nerve-sparing radical hysterectomy with fascia space dissection technique for cervical cancer: description of technique and outcomes. Gynecol Oncol. 2010;119:202–7.
28. Kavallaris A, et al. Laparoscopic nerve-sparing radical hysterectomy: description of the technique and patient's outcome. Gynecol Oncol. 2010;119:198–201.
29. Park NY, Chong GO, Hong DG, Cho YL, Il SP, Lee YS. Oncologic results and surgical morbidity of laparoscopic nerve-sparing radical hysterectomy in the treatment of FIGO Stage IB cervical cancer. Int J Gynecol Cancer. 2011;21(2):355–62.
30. Shi R, Wei W, Jiang P. Laparoscopic nerve-sparing radical hysterectomy for cervical carcinoma. Int J Gynecol Cancer. 2016;26(1):192–8.
31. Lee E-J, Kang H, Kim D-H. A comparative study of laparoscopic radical hysterectomy with radical abdominal hysterectomy for early-stage cervical cancer: a long-term follow-up study. Eur J Obstet Gynecol Reprod Biol. 2011;156(1):83–6.

Robotic Surgery for Gynecologic Cancer 11

Masaki Mandai, Tsukasa Baba, Kaoru Abiko,
and Akifumi Horie

Abstract

Since FDA approval of the da Vinci system for general laparoscopic surgery in 2000, application of robotic surgery has been spread rapidly to include gynecological laparoscopic surgical procedures worldwide. In Japan, da Vinci S system was first approved in 2009 for urology, gynecology, general surgery, and thoracic surgery. However, mostly due to lack of cost coverage by public health insurance in Japan, robotic surgery is not popular in gynecologic field. Meantime, in the USA and some other European countries, robotic surgery has been shown to be superior to laparotomy and even to laparoscopy and has already become a standard in uterine cervix and endometrial cancer surgery. Robotic surgery is basically defined as "computer-mediated surgery," which enables it to integrate various computer-based technologies, such as remote surgery, image-guided surgery, and surgical education in future, leading to a drastic change in the field of surgery. Healthy development of robotic surgery in Japan is an urgent issue.

Keywords

Robotic surgery · Gynecologic cancer · Minimally invasive · Remote surgery · Image-guided surgery

M. Mandai (✉) · T. Baba · K. Abiko · A. Horie
Department of Gynecology and Obstetrics, Kyoto University Graduate School of Medicine, Kyoto, Japan
e-mail: mandai@kuhp.kyoto-u.ac.jp

M. Mikami (ed.), *Surgery for Gynecologic Cancer*, Comprehensive Gynecology and Obstetrics, https://doi.org/10.1007/978-981-13-1519-0_11

11.1 History

Robotic surgical systems were initially developed to improve the accuracy and precision of surgical techniques in the fields of neurosurgery and orthopedic surgery. In the early 1990s, the US Army launched projects to develop remote surgical systems by which wounded soldiers could be operated on by surgeons in remote places. These technologies were transferred for civilian use to facilitate minimally invasive approaches. One of the first surgical robots to be approved by the FDA (in 1994) was the AESOP (automated endoscopic system for optimal positioning) by Computer Motion Inc. In this surgical system, surgeons could control the endoscope either by voice commands or a foot pedal [1].

The ZEUS robotic system (Computer Motion Inc.), the successor of the AESOP, employed a "master-slave" system. A surgeon could manipulate robot arms by moving the controller in the remote console. The reliability of the remote control of the Zeus system was proven in 2001 when remote surgery was performed across the Atlantic Ocean. In 2003, Computer Motion Inc. and Intuitive Surgical Inc. merged and developed the da Vinci surgical system, the prototype of today's da Vinci system. It had four arms for one endoscopy and three surgical instruments. The camera had dual lenses and could generate 3D vision. The FDA approved the da Vinci system for general laparoscopic surgery in 2000, followed by approval for radical prostatectomy, gynecological laparoscopic surgical procedures, general thoracoscopic surgical procedures, and thoracoscopically assisted cardiotomy procedures [1]. In Japan, da Vinci S system was first approved in 2009 for urology, gynecology, general surgery, and thoracic surgery. Subsequently, the da Vinci Si system was approved, followed by the da Vinci Xi system (Fig. 11.1). In 2012, radical

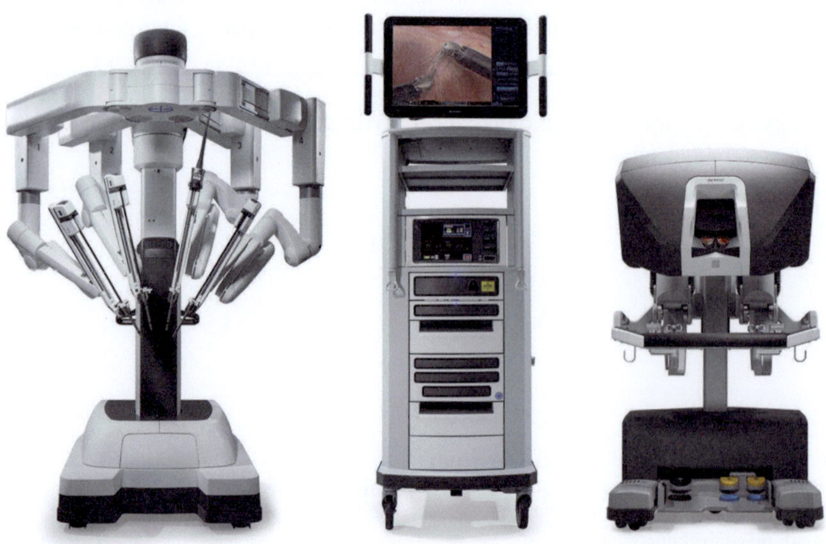

Fig. 11.1 da Vinci Si system. Images are duplicated with an authorization for publications to make duplicate copies for editorial use only. © [year] Intuitive Surgical, Inc.

prostatectomy was covered by national health insurance. As of 2013, more than 200 da Vinci systems were introduced in Japan, making it the second largest da Vinci-possessing country after the USA. However, no gynecologic surgery is covered by the national health insurance, and few robotic gynecologic surgeries have been performed in Japan.

11.2 Principles and Indication

Surgeons should realize both the merits and demerits of robotic surgery before they determine the indication of robotic surgery. Worldwide, more than half of all robotic surgeries are being performed in the field of gynecology, both for benign and malignant disease. This fact indicates that, in general, robotic surgery is suitable for gynecologic surgery. The pelvic cavity is narrow and complicated, and the clear 3D view and freely accessible arm movement of robotic instruments enable surgeons to perform precise and safe surgery as intended. These are the apparent advantages of robotic surgery over laparotomy and even over laparoscopic surgery. In the USA, robotic surgery has overtaken laparotomy and laparoscopy in a short period of time, as stated above, which clearly indicates the superiority of robotic surgery in the gynecologic field, especially in gynecologic oncology surgery. As mentioned later, the obvious advantage of robotic surgery over laparoscopy is that the training period for robotic surgery (so-called learning curve) is much shorter than that of laparoscopy. On the other hand, it has been recognized that the main disadvantages of robotic surgery include high cost and long operation time. However, recent reports from robot-advanced countries suggest that robotic surgery is not significantly expensive, if not less expensive, compared with laparotomy and laparoscopy, as the cost of the disposal of instruments decreases. Likewise, as surgeons treat many cases and develop their surgical skills, the operation time has become shorter, making it not significantly different from laparotomy and laparoscopy.

11.2.1 Endometrial Cancer

Primary surgery for endometrial cancer is a major indication for robotic surgery. A recent meta-analysis of 24 studies comparing robotic hysterectomy to open hysterectomy and 24 comparing robotic to laparoscopic surgery for endometrial cancer shows that no significant difference was found in survival outcomes. Compared to open surgery, robotic surgery showed less estimated blood loss, a lower rate of complications and readmission, a lower rate of transfusion, and a shorter length of hospital stay. However, robotic hysterectomy showed a longer operation time and a higher incidence of vaginal cuff dehiscence. Compared to laparoscopic hysterectomy, robotic surgery showed less blood loss, less conversion to laparotomy, and fewer intraoperative complications, including urinary tract injury. Additionally, several patient-reported outcomes were favorable to robotic surgery. The authors concluded that robotic hysterectomy for endometrial cancer may be safer and better than open or laparoscopic hysterectomy [2]. Another systematic review including 589 robotic, 396 laparoscopic, and 606 open surgeries for endometrial cancer indicated that robotic and laparoscopic surgeries are superior to open surgery in terms of estimated blood loss and length of stay but inferior in operation time. Other parameters, such as the resected number of lymph nodes and complications, were similar [3]. In a randomized controlled trial comparing robotic and laparoscopic surgery for endometrial cancer, the operation time was significantly shorter in robotic surgery. The conversion rate was significantly lower in robotic surgery. There was no difference in the number of removed lymph nodes, blood loss, and length of hospital stay. The authors concluded that robotic surgery offers an effective and safe alternative in the treatment of endometrial cancer [4].

11.2.2 Uterine Cervical Cancer

There are several systematic reviews on robotic radical hysterectomy for uterine and cervical cancer. Park et al. included 15 studies comparing robotic and open radical hysterectomy and 11 comparing robotic and laparoscopic radical hysterectomy in their systematic review [5]. Compared to the open approach, overall complications, urinary infection, wound infection, and fever were significantly less common in robotic surgery. Estimated blood loss was also reduced in robotic surgery. The length of stay and transfusion rate were lower with robotic surgery compared to open or laparoscopic surgery. Patient-reported outcomes were better in robotic surgery. Another systematic review analyzed 26 nonrandomized studies: 10 comparing robotic and open radical hysterectomy and 10 comparing robotic and laparoscopic radical hysterectomy. Robotic surgery was associated with less blood loss and shorter hospital stay than open surgery. Robotic surgery was also associated with a lower rate of febrile morbidity, blood transfusion, and wound-related complications over open surgery. Robotic surgery was comparable to laparoscopic surgery in all outcomes [6]. Zhou et al. compared robotic and laparoscopic radical hysterectomy in their meta-analysis [7]. Compared to laparoscopic radical hysterectomy, robotic surgery was associated with less blood loss and shorter hospital stay. There were no significant differences in operative time, complications, mortality, transfusion, conversion, number of retrieved lymph nodes, recurrence, or disease-free survival between the two groups.

A retrospective Canadian study including 383 patients compared MIS (laparoscopy or robotic) and laparotomy. Overall survival was not different between the two groups. The rate of complications was not different. The mean number of resected lymph nodes was significantly higher in the MIS group. Median estimated blood loss was significantly higher in the laparotomy group, and the transfusion rate was also higher [8].

11.2.3 Post-NAC Surgery

Neoadjuvant chemotherapy (NAC) is often used as a treatment for locally advanced cervical cancer. The feasibility of robotic surgery after NAC has been reported in several studies. Zanagnolo et al. retrospectively compared robotic and open radical hysterectomy in patients with stage IB2–IIB cervical cancer who underwent NAC

[9]. The mean operative time was significantly longer in the robotic group. In contrast, estimated blood loss was significantly less, and the length of stay was shorter in the robotic group. The incidence of perioperative complications and the prognosis were similar. Likewise, Minig et al. compared various clinical parameters between 30 patients with stage IB2–IIB cervical cancer who underwent robotic radical hysterectomy after NAC with 176 patients who underwent robotic radical hysterectomy with stage IA2–IB1 disease [10]. Although the operative time, type of radical hysterectomy (type C1), and mean tumor size were different between the groups, estimated blood loss and length of hospital stay were similar. There was no difference in perioperative complications. Another report by Corrado et al. enrolled 41 patients with locally advanced cervical cancer who underwent robotic radical hysterectomy after successful NAC and compared surgical and oncologic outcomes with the laparoscopy and laparotomy group [11]. The estimated blood loss, operative time, and length of stay were significantly in favor of the robotic group. There were no significant differences in 3-year overall and disease-free survival. The authors in these reports concluded that robotic radical hysterectomy is feasible and safe.

11.2.4 Quality of Life

Several studies investigated whether robotic surgery is feasible in terms of patients' quality of life. Herling et al. conducted a prospective cohort study using patient-reported outcome measures to detect short-term health-related QOL after robotic hysterectomy for endometrial cancer [12]. A total of 139 women answered the EORTC C-30, EN-24, and EQ-5D-3 L preoperatively, as well as 1 week, 5 weeks, and 4 months after the operation. Overall, HR-QOL returned to the preoperative level 5 weeks after the operation. Negatively affected symptoms included fatigue, pain, constipation, gastrointestinal symptoms, appetite, ability to perform work and hobbies, change of taste, and sexually related problems. In a comparison of robotic and laparoscopic radical hysterectomy, there were no significant differences in the SF-36 and EORTC C-30 between the two groups [13]. However, regarding postoperative pain in patients who underwent surgery for endometrial cancer, robotic surgery was associated with significantly lower levels of postoperative pain and required pain medication compared to laparoscopic surgery [14]. Thus, robotic surgery seems equal or superior in terms of postoperative QOL compared to laparoscopy.

11.2.5 Obese Patients

Indications for robotic surgery in obese women have been discussed in several reports. Hinshaw et al. evaluated the surgical and pathological outcomes of robotic versus open hysterectomy for obese women with endometrial cancer [15]. Among 136 women (56 robotic and 80 abdominal) with BMI >35, the robotic group had fewer postoperative complications, shorter hospital stays, and lower blood loss compared to the abdominal group. A subset group with BMI >40 had similar findings. The oncologic outcome was similar in both groups. Another study analyzed a total of 128 obese women who underwent robotic surgery mainly with endometrial cancer or fibroids by dividing them into three groups (group 1, BMI 30–34.9; group 2, 35–39.9; group 3, >40) [16]. Conversions were more common in groups 2 and 3, with a positive correlation with BMI. These reports indicate that robotic surgery is useful for obese women, who have greater perioperative risks.

11.2.6 Elderly Patients

A retrospective, multi-institutional study including endometrial cancer patients 70 years or older was conducted with 89 robotic cases and 93 open surgery cases [17]. The robotic surgery group had a higher incidence of pelvic lymphadenectomy and decreased levels of blood loss, a lower incidence of blood transfusion, and less overall complications compared to laparotomy. Additionally, the robotic surgery group had a shorter median hospital stay with no increase in readmission. Other clinical parameters were similar in both groups. Robotic surgery may be beneficial for elderly patients.

11.3 Preoperative Evaluation

Basically, the preoperative evaluation for robotic surgery is the same as that for open surgery. Needless to say, an accurate diagnosis of cancer histology and stage is important to determine the type of surgery. The patient's status should be properly evaluated to avoid operative complications. There are several points to be evaluated, especially in robotic surgery. First, operability by robotic surgery should be carefully assessed. Repeated laparotomies, including C-sections, may be a risk factor for intra-abdominal adhesion. Obesity itself may not be a contraindication for robotic surgery. There are reports indicating the superiority of robotic surgery in obese women as stated above. Nevertheless, obesity is apparently a risk of surgery, even in robotics, considering that the patient should be maintained in a steep Trendelenburg position during robotic surgery. Robotic surgery may also be advantageous in elderly women as mentioned earlier. However, again, advanced age itself may be a risk factor for robotic surgery.

Second, the risk of robotic-specific complications should be assessed. Although very rare, it has been reported that intraocular high pressure caused by a steep Trendelenburg position may be associated with postoperative visual loss, and glaucoma may increase the risk. Therefore, careful history taking and consultation with the ophthalmologist in suspicious cases are necessary.

11.4 Technique

No principal modifications of laparotomy are needed for general robotic surgery procedures for cervical and endometrial cancer. Compared to laparoscopy, robotic surgery provides clearer vision with the 3D camera and more free movement with multiple joints, which enables the surgical procedure to be more similar to laparotomy. However, there are several limitations to robotic surgery. First, there is no tactile sensation in the robotic arm, and it is almost impossible to obtain operative information by touching the tissues, as can be done in laparotomy. Second, the number of arms is limited compared to laparotomy, in which any number of assistants is possible. Usually, in robotic surgery, the operator can use three hands, and one to two laparoscopic assistants are available, allowing a maximum of five hands to be used for surgery. Therefore, a device such as a uterine manipulator is a useful substitute for intra-abdominal uterine traction.

In robotic surgery, it is easier to operate in a deep and narrow area. Therefore, the surgeon can start the procedure from a deeper area than is possible for laparotomy. For example, in laparotomy, it is relatively difficult to isolate the deep uterine vein until the uterine artery and superficial uterine vein are dissected. However, in robotic surgery, the surgeon can easily access the deep uterine vein while leaving the uterine artery intact. In contrast, massive ligation of thick tissue is not easy in robotic surgery. Therefore, the skeletonization of vessels by isolating each vessel and their individual dissection is typically employed in robotic surgery.

Another difference between laparotomy and robotic surgery is that robotic surgery uses more electric devices. A vessel-sealing system is often used instead of ligation. With these devices, surgeons can save time and can perform safer surgery.

The biggest difference between robotic surgery and laparoscopic surgery is that training for robotic surgery is easier than that for laparoscopy. In training for laparoscopy, the greatest barrier for surgeons is to develop their hand-eye coordination. In contrast, robotic surgery offers 3D visualization, as well as almost free angulation of the robotic arms, which enables surgeons to develop surgical skills more quickly than laparoscopy.

Lim et al. conducted a case-control study to compare the learning curve of robotic and laparoscopic hysterectomy with lymph node dissection and compared it with that of laparotomy and laparoscopy. Although some bias cannot be excluded, they concluded that robotic hysterectomy with lymphadenectomy has a faster learning curve in comparison to laparoscopic hysterectomy with lymphadenectomy for the management of endometrial cancer [18].

11.5 Morbidity Rate

As stated above, the general incidence of perioperative complications was reported to be lower in robotic surgery compared with laparotomy and possibly with laparoscopy. Barrie et al. classified postoperative complications in robotic surgery compared to laparoscopic hysterectomy for endometrial cancer [19]. All complications were categorized using the Clavien-Dindo classification system. In a comparison of 745 robotic and 688 laparoscopic hysterectomies, the overall intraoperative complications or major postoperative complications were not significantly different. However, there were significantly fewer minor postoperative complications with robotic surgery. The median operative time, length of stay, estimated blood loss, conversions to laparotomy, and median number of lymph nodes retrieved were superior in robotic surgery.

11.6 Future Prospects

11.6.1 Cost

Recent reports suggest that robotic surgery is not as expensive as it used to be. Herling et al. reported a cost analysis of robotic hysterectomy vs. abdominal hysterectomy for endometrial cancer and atypical endometrial hyperplasia [20]. The average cost of consumables was more expensive in robotic surgery. In contrast, when including all cost drivers such as complications, duration of surgery, and duration of hospital stay, robotic hysterectomy was 17% less expensive than laparotomy. When the robotic instruments were included, the cost was still less expensive (7%) for robotic surgery.

Desille-Gbaguidi et al. reported that conventional laparoscopy was less expensive in their institution than robotic-assisted surgery for surgery for endometrial (1:2.7) and cervical (1:2.6) cancers [21]. However, when considering overall medical care, the difference was lower: the use of robotic-assisted surgery was found to be 1.6 times more expensive than conventional surgery.

Reynisson et al. reported that the cost for robotic radical hysterectomy is apparently higher for the first 30 cases compared to open radical hysterectomy but slightly lower for the last 30 cases, indicating that after a substantial implementation period, it is feasible to perform robotic-assisted radical hysterectomy at an equal hospital cost compared with open surgery [22].

11.6.2 Status of Robotic Surgery in Gynecologic Oncology in Japan

Although Japan has introduced the second most da Vinci systems after the USA in the world, at present, robotic surgery is not actively employed in gynecologic cancer surgery. To date, less than 200 gynecologic oncology surgeries have been performed per year in Japan. This is mainly because robotic surgery in the gynecologic field is not covered by public health insurance in Japan. As a result, the patient must pay more than $10,000 to undergo robotic surgery. Laparoscopy for gynecologic cancer surgery is also not popular in Japan because of technical difficulties. To facilitate minimally invasive surgery in this field, the short learning curve of robotic surgery may be advantageous. The approval for robotic gynecologic cancer surgeries to be covered by health insurance is awaited.

The establishment of a nationwide system for registration, certification, and education to monitor and warrant the safety of robotic surgery is also mandatory because it is still in the introductory phase in Japan.

There is no domestic surgery robot system in Japan. It is expected that, in the near future, several Japanese companies, in cooperation with academic groups, will develop original robotic surgery instruments, which may lead to a significant decrease in cost and may widen the application of robotic surgery in the oncology field, including gynecologic oncology.

11.6.3 Technical Development of Robotic Surgery in the Future

A fundamental difference between robotic surgery and laparoscopy is that, in the former, surgical manipulation is mediated by a computer. In this respect, robotic surgery is defined as "computer-mediated surgery" rather than "minimally invasive surgery." This enables robotic surgery to integrate various computer-based technologies.

First, remote surgery is already technically available with robotic surgery. As early as 2001, the first remote surgery was performed across the Atlantic Ocean using a Zeus robotic system. A surgeon in New York performed a cholecystectomy on a female patient in a hospital in Strasbourg, France. It was named "the Lindbergh operation" after Charles Lindbergh's transatlantic flight. Thus, remote surgery is really a practical technique once social issues are addressed. In the future, remote surgery will be used in such cases that the expert surgeon would support a less-experienced surgeon operating on his patient, enabling patients to receive the best care in their hometown.

Second, the development of imaging techniques may lead to effective image-guided robotic surgery (Fig. 11.2). Preoperative imaging of a variety of vessels, ureters, and tumors should promote safer and effective cancer surgery. The integration of real-time images into the robotic surgery field may further require technical solutions on how to obtain intraoperative images and how to visualize them in the surgical field. The accurate localization of an anatomical reference point is essential to create reproducible organ images [23].

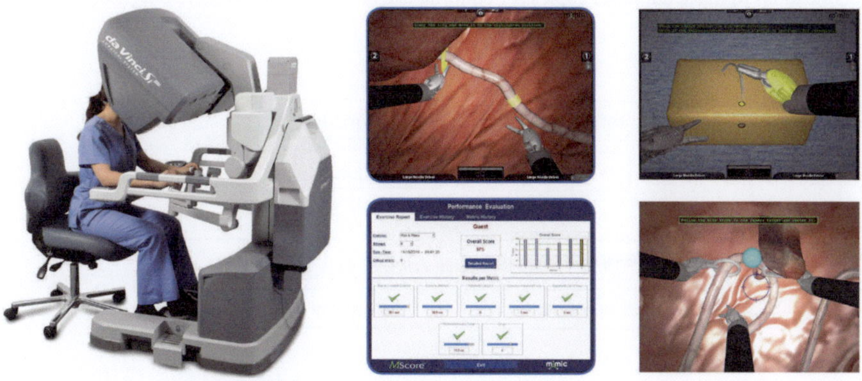

Fig. 11.2 Virtual training using the da Vinci Skills Simulator. Images are duplicated with an authorization for publications to make duplicate copies for editorial use only. © [year] Intuitive Surgical, Inc.

Third, the most drastic change that robotic surgery will bring about is surgical education. Learning a robotic surgery procedure is easier than learning open surgery because robotic surgery can provide a clearer view compared with open surgery. Beginners can repeatedly learn the procedure through videos of experts and of themselves. Furthermore, the future development of a VR (virtual reality)-based training system may promote full learning of the procedure using real instruments before getting into the human body (Fig. 11.3). Thus, the trainee can develop their surgical skills step by step using an appropriate training module according to their skills and the type of surgery that they want to perform.

11.7 Summary

Robotic surgery has the potential to change gynecologic cancer surgery drastically in the future. Leading to safer and more effective surgery, it may introduce a new concept such as remote surgery, image-guided surgery, and VR-based surgical education, which are not available by conventional open surgery or laparoscopy (Fig. 11.4). To warrant the safe introduction of this new technology,

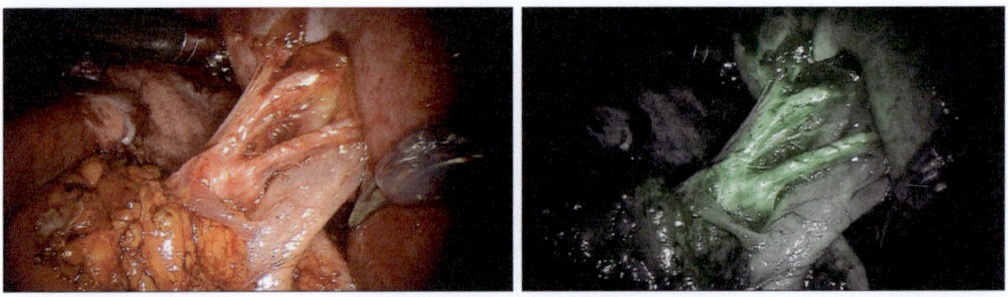

Fig. 11.3 Firefly image for vessel detection. Images are duplicated with an authorization for publications to make duplicate copies for editorial use only. © [year] Intuitive Surgical, Inc.

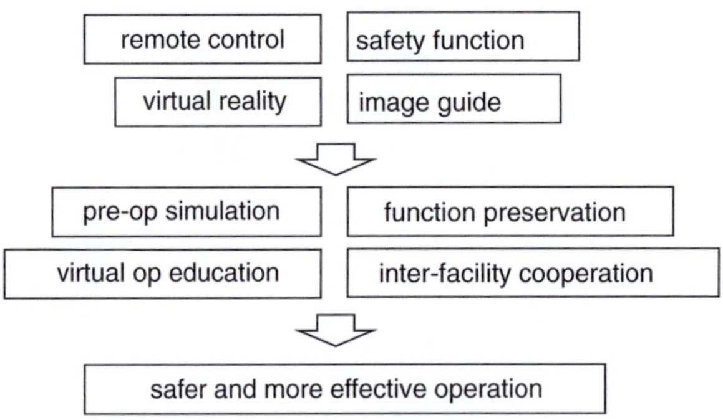

Fig. 11.4 Future direction of robotic surgery

the establishment of a nationwide system for registration, certification, and education is mandatory.

References

1. Hussain A, Malik A, Halim MU, Ali AM. The use of robotics in surgery: a review. Int J Clin Pract. 2014;68(11):1376–82.
2. Park DA, Lee DH, Kim SW, Lee SH. Comparative safety and effectiveness of robot-assisted laparoscopic hysterectomy versus conventional laparoscopy and laparotomy for endometrial cancer: A systematic review and meta-analysis. Eur J Surg Oncol. 2016;42(9):1303–14.
3. Gaia G, Holloway RW, Santoro L, Ahmad S, Di Silverio E, Spinillo A. Robotic-assisted hysterectomy for endometrial cancer compared with traditional laparoscopic and laparotomy approaches: a systematic review. Obstet Gynecol. 2010;116(6):1422–31.
4. Mäenpää MM, Nieminen K, Tomás EI, Laurila M, Luukkaala TH, Mäenpää JU. Robotic-assisted vs traditional laparoscopic surgery for endometrial cancer: a randomized controlled trial. Am J Obstet Gynecol. 2016;215(5):588.e1–7.
5. Park DA, Yun JE, Kim SW, Lee SH. Surgical and clinical safety and effectiveness of robot-assisted laparoscopic hysterectomy compared to conventional laparoscopy and laparotomy for cervical cancer: A systematic review and meta-analysis. Eur J Surg Oncol. 2017;43(6):994–1002.
6. Shazly SA, Murad MH, Dowdy SC, Gostout BS, Famuyide AO. Robotic radical hysterectomy in early stage cervical cancer: A systematic review and meta-analysis. Gynecol Oncol. 2015;138(2):457–71.
7. Zhou J, Xiong BH, Ma L, Cheng Y, Huang W, Zhao L. Robotic vs laparoscopic radical hysterectomy for cervical cancer: a meta-analysis. Int J Med Robot. 2016;12(1):145–54.
8. Diver E, Hinchcliff E, Gockley A, Melamed A, Contrino L, Feldman S, Growdon W. Minimally Invasive Radical Hysterectomy for Cervical Cancer Is Associated With Reduced Morbidity and Similar Survival Outcomes Compared With Laparotomy. J Minim Invasive Gynecol. 2017;24(3):402–6.
9. Zanagnolo V, Minig L, Cárdenas-Rebollo JM, Achilarre MT, Garbi A, Patrono MG, Colombo N, Maggioni A. Robotic Versus Open Radical Hysterectomy in Women With Locally Advanced Cervical Cancer After Neoadjuvant Chemotherapy: A Single-institution Experience of Surgical and Oncologic Outcomes. J Minim Invasive Gynecol. 2016;23(6):909–16.
10. Minig L, Zanagnolo V, Cárdenas-Rebollo JM, Colombo N, Maggioni A. Feasibility of robotic radical hysterectomy after neoadjuvant chemotherapy in women with locally advanced cervical cancer. Eur J Surg Oncol. 2016;42(9):1372–7.
11. Corrado G, Cutillo G, Saltari M, Mancini E, Sindico S, Vici P, Sergi D, Sperduti I, Patrizi L, Pomati G, Baiocco E, Vizza E. Surgical and Oncological Outcome of Robotic Surgery Compared With Laparoscopic and Abdominal Surgery in the Management of Locally Advanced Cervical Cancer After Neoadjuvant Chemotherapy. Int J Gynecol Cancer. 2016;26(3):539–46.
12. Herling SF, Møller AM, Palle C, Thomsen T. Health-related quality of life after robotic-assisted laparoscopic hysterectomy for women with endometrial cancer--A prospective cohort study. Gynecol Oncol. 2016a;140(1):107–13.
13. Kim JY, Lee YH, Chong GO, Lee YS, Cho YL, Hong DG. Comparative Study Between Total Laparoscopic and Total Robotic Radical Hysterectomy for Cervical Carcinoma: Clinical Study. Anticancer Res. 2015;35(9):5015–21.
14. Leitao MM Jr, Malhotra V, Briscoe G, Suidan R, Dholakiya P, Santos K, Jewell EL, Brown CL, Sonoda Y, Abu-Rustum NR, Barakat RR, Gardner GJ. Postoperative pain medication requirements in patients undergoing computer-assisted ("Robotic") and standard laparoscopic procedures for newly diagnosed endometrial cancer. Ann Surg Oncol. 2013;20(11):3561–7.

15. Hinshaw SJ, Gunderson S, Eastwood D, Bradley WH. Endometrial carcinoma: The perioperative and long-term outcomes of robotic surgery in the morbidly obese. J Surg Oncol. 2016;114(7):884–7.
16. Cosin JA, Brett Sutherland MA, Westgate CT, Fang H. Complications of Robotic Gynecologic Surgery in the Severely Morbidly Obese. Ann Surg Oncol. 2016;23(12):4035–41.
17. Backes FJ, ElNaggar AC, Farrell MR, Brudie LA, Ahmad S, Salani R, Cohn DE, Holloway RW, Fowler JM, O'Malley DM. Perioperative Outcomes for Laparotomy Compared to Robotic Surgical Staging of Endometrial Cancer in the Elderly: A Retrospective Cohort. Int J Gynecol Cancer. 2016;26(9):1717–21.
18. Lim PC, Kang E, Park DH. A comparative detail analysis of the learning curve and surgical outcome for robotic hysterectomy with lymphadenectomy versus laparoscopic hysterectomy with lymphadenectomy in treatment of endometrial cancer: a case-matched controlled study of the first one hundred twenty two patients. Gynecol Oncol. 2011;120(3):413–8.
19. Barrie A, Freeman AH, Lyon L, Garcia C, Conell C, Abbott LH, Littell RD, Powell CB. Classification of Postoperative Complications in Robotic-assisted Compared With Laparoscopic Hysterectomy for Endometrial Cancer. J Minim Invasive Gynecol. 2016;23(7):1181–8.
20. Herling SF, Palle C, Møller AM, Thomsen T, Sørensen J. Cost-analysis of robotic-assisted laparoscopic hysterectomy versus total abdominal hysterectomy for women with endometrial cancer and atypical complex hyperplasia. Acta Obstet Gynecol Scand. 2016b;95(3):299–308.
21. Desille-Gbaguidi H, Hebert T, Paternotte-Villemagne J, Gaborit C, Rush E, Body G. Overall care cost comparison between robotic and laparoscopic surgery for endometrial and cervical cancer. Eur J Obstet Gynecol Reprod Biol. 2013;171(2):348–52.
22. Reynisson P, Persson J. Hospital costs for robot-assisted laparoscopic radical hysterectomy and pelvic lymphadenectomy. Gynecol Oncol. 2013;130(1):95–9.
23. Herrell SD, Kwartowitz DM, Milhoua PM, Galloway RL. Toward image guided robotic surgery: system validation. J Urol. 2009;181(2):783–9. discussion 789-90

Radical Trachelectomy

12

Shintaro Yanazume and Hiroaki Kobayashi

Abstract

Due to the trends of marrying at a later age and delayed birth, cervical cancer patients who desire fertility-sparing surgery (FSS) are increasing. Radical trachelectomy (RT) which is a FSS is listed in the cervical cancer guidelines and was established as one of the cervical cancer surgery methods. When considering this procedure, oncological outcome and fertility outcome must be considered together. The data of RT and radical hysterectomy (RH) have the same results in oncological outcome. Dargent and colleagues have accumulated reports on the early beginnings of vaginal trachelectomy (VRT), and findings show abdominal trachelectomy (ART) is better recommended for a lesser recurrence rate when the tumor diameter (TD) reaches 2 cm < TD. ART has the highest curability with the RH surgical formula. On the other hand, ART research has reported problems of postoperative complications and pregnancy rates that are not necessarily low, but cannot be considered high. Less invasive surgery for tumors with a TD ≤ 2 cm has been discussed. In addition to ART and VRT, studies including the application of laparoscopic RT and robotic RT have begun. The optimum technique should be decided for each case while considering the TD and fertility result. This is a developing technique, and the accumulation of evidence and further research is warranted for the establishment and selection of adaptation and surgery.

Keywords

Radical · Trachelectomy · Cervical cancer · Fertility-sparing surgery

---

S. Yanazume · H. Kobayashi (✉)
Faculty of Medicine, Department of Obstetrics and Gynecology, Kagoshima University, Kagoshima, Japan
e-mail: hirokoba@m2.kufm.kagoshima-u.ac.jp

M. Mikami (ed.), *Surgery for Gynecologic Cancer*, Comprehensive Gynecology and Obstetrics, https://doi.org/10.1007/978-981-13-1519-0_12

12.1 History

Fertility-sparing surgery (FSS) for patients with cervical cancer is a relatively new surgical therapy with a history of only about 30 years. In 1987, Dargent et al. [1] proposed laparoscopic vaginal radical trachelectomy (VRT) which was a combination of vaginal modified radical hysterectomy and laparoscopic lymphadenectomy for young cervical cancer patients who wanted to preserve fertility, and it was reported as a tolerable surgical procedure based on 47 cases with a long-term follow-up period. Since then more than 1000 cases of radical trachelectomy (RT) have been reported. Covens [2], Roy [3], Shepherd [4], and others started similar surgical procedures, but about 80% of reported cases represented a tumor diameter (TD) ≤ 2 cm of VRT. Therefore, evidence on the surgical outcome of trachelectomy has been reported mainly on VRT data. Smith et al. [5] pointed out that resecting the cardinal ligament in the VRT via Piver class II is insufficient radicality and started to implement abdominal radical trachelectomy (ART) based on abdominal radical hysterectomy (ARH). This procedure (Piver III) was considered to be applicable on larger tumors, and a recent review proved the prognostic superiority of ART for stage IB1 for 2 cm < TD [6, 7].

The next development of FSS for cervical cancer has been examined and is led by the improvement of oncological and obstetrical outcomes followed by more non-invasive techniques. The potential of neoadjuvant chemotherapy for patients with 2 cm < TD followed by ART was reviewed, and it has been reported that the pregnancy rate (30.7%) appeared to be higher than previously reported for VRT (24%) or for ART (16.2%) [8]. Regarding the minimally invasive techniques, the first laparoscopic RT was performed in 2002 [9], and the first robotic surgery took place in 2008 [10]. Recent systematic data may indicate a higher pregnancy rate in patients with minimally invasive RT than laparotomic RT [6].

Regarding the use of RT on patients undergoing FSS, recent research indicates no significant differences in recurrence (3.6% in RT vs. 7.8% in RH) with ART [11] when comparing the nerve-sparing RT group vs. the nerve-sparing RH group. Nerve-sparing FSS is considerable for patients with stage1A–1B1 disease who desired the preservation of fertility to the same degree as RH.

12.2 Principle and Indication

Delayed childbearing is the trend in the United States as well as Japan [12]. Peaks in the age distribution of new cases of cervical cancer have been observed in patients in their 30s and 40s, and this matches the peak of the number of births in Japan [13]. In patients aged 39 years or less, stage I accounted for 79% and stage II for 14% showing that younger patients tend to be in earlier stages [14]. The term trachelectomy includes the procedures of simple trachelectomy, modified-RT, and RT. Trachelectomy is an early-stage FSS for patients in the childbearing age range that includes the procedures of removing the uterine cervix and placing a cerclage between the uterine lower segment and vaginal cuff. The importance and popularity of fertility-sparing trachelectomy are increasing annually [15]. The trend of trachelectomy in the United States has increased from 1.5% in 2004 to 3.8% in 2014 ($P < 0.001$) and 4.6% in

2004 to 17.0% in 2014 for limited patients aged 30 years or less ($P < 0.001$) [15]. The RT is defined as resecting the cervix, upper vagina, and uterine parametrium as well as pelvic lymph node removing similar to the procedure of a radical hysterectomy. The role of RT has been established as indicated in the publication of several clinical guidelines [16, 17]. The National Comprehensive Cancer Network (NCCN) guidelines for 2018 [16] and the Japanese version of the Japan Society of Gynecologic Oncology (JSGO) guidelines of cervical cancer for 2017 [17] approve RT in conjunction with lymphadenectomy procedures (with or without SLN mapping) as a treatment choice for stage 1A2 or stage 1B1 lesions of TD ≤ 2 cm.

12.3 Preoperative Evaluation

The authors have performed ART from 2005, which has been undertaken on more than 150 cases with only 1 case of recurrence. This procedure needs to be performed while guaranteeing the safety of the patient by thoroughly checking strict preoperative eligibility criteria, carefully diagnosing intraoperative frozen section samples, etc. RT is a collaborative work done by gynecological pathologist, sterility specialists, and perinatal specialists in addition to gynecological oncologists. The ultimate goal of RT treatment besides curing the patient of cervical cancer is to ensure the success of live birth after recovery. Patients who desire FSS must receive a sufficient informed explanation, including consultation with the partner and family members. In addition to the risk of the surgery itself, the explanation needs to address the issues of possible infertility, the tendency toward preterm labor, and other labor risks. FSS can be performed in almost the same manner as a usual radical hysterectomy but offers the benefits of preserving the uterine artery and anastomoses of the vaginal stump with the conserved uterus.

12.4 Indication and Contraindication

Inclusion criteria for RT is described in Table 12.1, which has been modified from the 2017 JSGO guidelines for the treatment of cervical cancer. ART has an advantage of resecting the parametrium according to the Piver class III hysterectomy. The authors permitted larger tumors (2 cm < TD) with SCC under the stipulation of

Table 12.1 Inclusion criteria for radical trachelectomy modified Japanese version of JSGO guidelines 2017 for cervical cancer

1	Desire to preserve fertility and no evidence of infertility
2	FIGO stage 1A1 with lymphovascular space involvement and stage 1B1
3	Tumor with ≤2 cm tumor diameter
4	No evidence of lymph metastases
5	Histologic type of squamous cell carcinoma, adenocarcinoma, adenosquamous carcinoma

JSGO Japan Society of Gynecologic Oncology, *FIGO* International Federation of Gynecology and Obstetrics providing a secure ≤1 cm cancer-free space between the tumor's edge and the internal os (Fig. 12.1). The inclusion criteria strategy [18] in our research application is referred to in Table 12.2. This procedure is recommended to leave at least 5 mm of

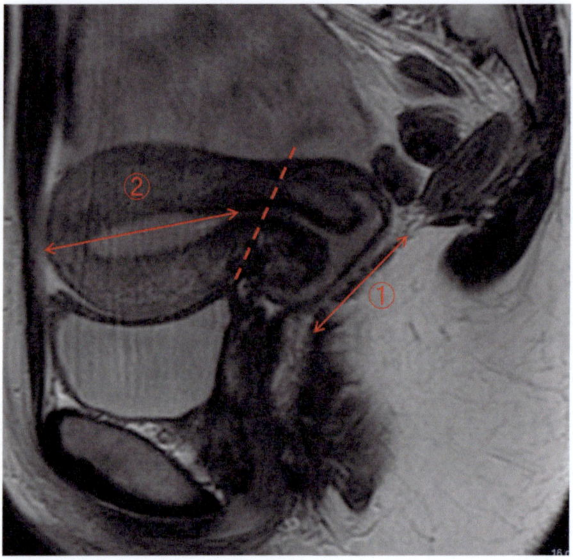

Fig. 12.1 Preoperative MRI (T2WI, a case of uterine sagittal image of squamous cell carcinoma). In a case of squamous cell carcinoma with a lateral diameter of 3 cm as shown in ①, the depth spread (progress toward the internal os) was about 1 cm. The part ② indicated by the perforated line is the bottom of the uterus to the histologic inner uterine opening 5 cm from the uterus bottom, leaving at least 5 mm of the cervical canals the line to be resected to the neck; eligibility for 10 mm or more cancer-free space has been confirmed

Table 12.2 Inclusion and exclusion criteria strategy [Ref. 16] for radical trachelectomy for cervical cancer

Preoperative inclusion criteria	
1	Desire to preserve fertility and no evidence of infertility
2	FIGO stage 1B1 or less-advanced squamous cell carcinoma with a maximum transverse diameter of ≤3 cm and ≤ 1 cm cancer-free space between the tumor's edge and the internal os
3	Stage IB1 or less-advanced adenocarcinoma/adenosquamous carcinoma with a maximum transverse diameter of ≤2 cm and with mainly superficial or exophytic growth
4	No evidence of lymph metastases
Preoperative exclusion criteria	
1	Histologic type of cancer indicative of a poor prognosis (e.g., small cell carcinoma)
2	Suspicion of extrauterine spread based on imaging findings
Intraoperative inclusion criteria	
1	The absence of lymph node metastasis by serial frozen sections of the bilateral sentinel lymph nodes
2	A ≥ 5-mm cancer-free margin in the cervical canal of the extirpated cervix

FIGO International Federation of Gynecology and Obstetrics the cervical canal; the risk of depth along the cervical canal is not considered the same as the lateral spread of the uterine cervix. Our technique is first to introduce the concept of two directions "transverse diameter and depth" [19]. Conversely in smaller, less invasive tumors, abdominal modified radical trachelectomy (AmRT) was performed which removed less parametrium than ART. The criteria of AmRT were as follows: (a) stage IB1 cancer with a maximum transverse diameter of ≤2 cm without deep stromal invasion and (b) stage IA2 cancer.

12.5 Preoperative and Postoperative Management

As a preoperative examination, contrast computed tomography (CT) and contrast magnetic resonance imaging (MRI) are performed to judge the above qualifications. As an intraoperative examination regarding the sentinel lymph node biopsy, an isotope was used as a tracer (RI method): 99 mTc-labeled phytic acid was injected just under the mucous membrane of the uterine cervical lesion on the day before surgery, followed by lymphoscintigraphy and SPECT-CT imaging. Compared to a usual hysterectomy, this procedure is prone to infections for a number of reasons: (1) the neocervix is exposed, (2) anastomosis stitches are applied between the cervix and the vaginal canal, (3) cervical sutures for preventing premature labor during pregnancy are implemented, and (4) a contraceptive ring FD-1® is placed after surgery. All of these factors are likely to cause postoperative infections, so therefore the use of antimicrobial vaginal tablets before and after surgery and frequent vaginal washing after surgery are recommended.

During outpatient follow-up periods, special attention is to be paid to the condition of the menstruation and the external os, with the prompting of cervical dilation when cervical stenosis or closure is suspected. Since cervical mucus is decreased, ascending infections such as adnexitis and PID are likely to occur. FD-1® is removed 6 months after surgery and permits the patient to become pregnant. If natural pregnancy is not established easily, promptly undertake infertility treatment intervention (considering artificial insemination and in vitro fertilization early because it is thought that the permeability of sperm is also decreased due to a decrease in cervical mucus).

12.6 Technique

12.6.1 Laparotomy: Deployment of the Pelvic Retroperitoneal Cavity

After laparotomy with a midline longitudinal incision, careful evaluation of the extent of the tumor is inspected, and palpation is performed. The uterus is retracted by holding the uterus with No. 1 Vicryl® thread sutured after cutting the bilateral round ligament and No. 1 Vicryl® thread Z-sutured at the bottom of the uterus. This procedure allows the crushing of the uterine endometrium when using uterine grasping forceps to be avoided. Expand the retroperitoneal cavity of the pelvis, and explore the paravesical space and the pararectal space.

12.6.2 Sentinel Lymph Node Biopsy

A gamma probe was used to identify a hot node, considered to be a sentinel lymph node, after consulting the image of a sequential lymphoscintigraph utilizing the injection of an isotope tracer (Fig. 12.2) around the cervical lesion on the previous day. The reason why sequential lymphoscintigraphy was selected is because it is possible to distinguish the primary node (this is the original sentinel lymph node) that is drawn first and the secondary node that is drawn thereafter (not the sentinel lymph node).

On the day of surgery, after developing the retroperitoneum of the pelvis, a scan of the pelvic lymph node region with a gamma probe was performed to identify and remove the SN. If there is no metastasis to the SN after an intraoperative pathological examination, ART will be the chosen method of treatment. The removal of the hot node is decided by the results of an intraoperative frozen section. If there is no metastasis to the sentinel lymph nodes, the operation will proceed as planned.

12.6.3 Ureter and Uterine Artery Liberation

The ureter is peeled from the posterior broad ligament with the sufficient binding weave attached around the ureter, and the ureteral plate following the

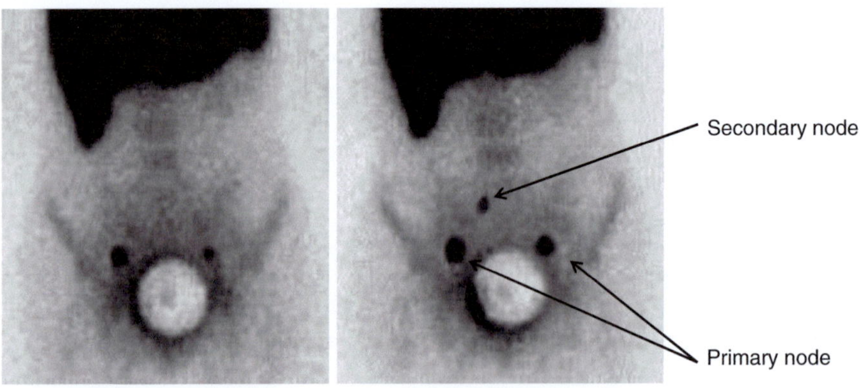

20 minutes after injection 20 minutes after injection

Fig. 12.2 Detection of sentinel lymph nodes by lymphoscintigraphy. After infusing the isotope around the lesion of the uterine vagina, sequential imaging of lymphoscintigraph is performed, and the primary node (sentinel lymph node) which is drawn first and the secondary node which is drawn after the sentinel lymph node are detected as a hot node during surgery. Tumor parts interfere with the surrounding strong radioactivity (shine-through phenomenon); the lead plate is seated ureter is placed together with the lower abdominal nerve on the pelvic floor side, from the side wall of the rectum (so-called rectal side lumen of Okabayashi). Thereafter, the ureter is fenestrated in front of the lower abdominal nerve, and the lower abdominal nerve bundle is liberated toward the vaginal side wall.

The uterine artery branching from the internal iliac artery is liberated toward the uterus until it crosses the intersection with the ureter (the middle ureteral branch is ligated). If the uterine artery can be liberated for a sufficient length, it will not interfere with the next cardinal ligament resection.

12.6.4 Cardinal Ligament Dissection

The cardinal ligament and paracolpium are divided several times and cut on the pelvic side (Piver III) and ligated. When cutting to a level exceeding the uterine vein, scrape the ligaments while preserving the pelvic nerve plexus located at the bottom of the pelvis. Scooping is executed to the level exceeding the pelvic nerve plexus while remaining conscious of the curve of the pelvis.

12.6.5 Vesicouterine Ligament Anterior Sheath/Posterior Sheath Dissection

After successively dissecting the anterior sheath of the vesicouterine ligament several times, sufficiently move the ureter to the outer side while thinning the layer of the surface to the level where blood vessels of the posterior sheath can be identified. Upon cutting of the posterior leaf, cut only the exposed blood vessel so as to preserve the bladder nerve branch near the vaginal canal.

12.6.6 Rectovaginal Ligament Dissection

Open the broad ligament along the side wall of the uterus, detach the Douglas fossa peritoneum, and sufficiently liberate the rectum from the vaginal wall. Subsequently, the uterosacral ligament and the rectovaginal ligament are cut along the upper edge of the already identified hypogastric nerve, and finally dissect the paracolpium remaining in the shallow part of the pelvic plexus (uterus side). Through the above procedure, as shown in Fig. 12.3, the T-shaped urination-related nerve restiform tissues (neural network) formed by the hypogastric nerve, the pelvic splanchnic nerve, and the bladder nerve branch centered on the pelvic nerve plexus can be preserved. Even if the vaginal canal is cut just above this pelvic plexus, it can be excised more than 2 cm, so it is sufficiently radical against stage Ib cervical cancer. Since the bladder nerve branch is located near the posterior vesicouterine ligament layer, when cutting the posterior layer, do not use a power source including bipolar scissors.

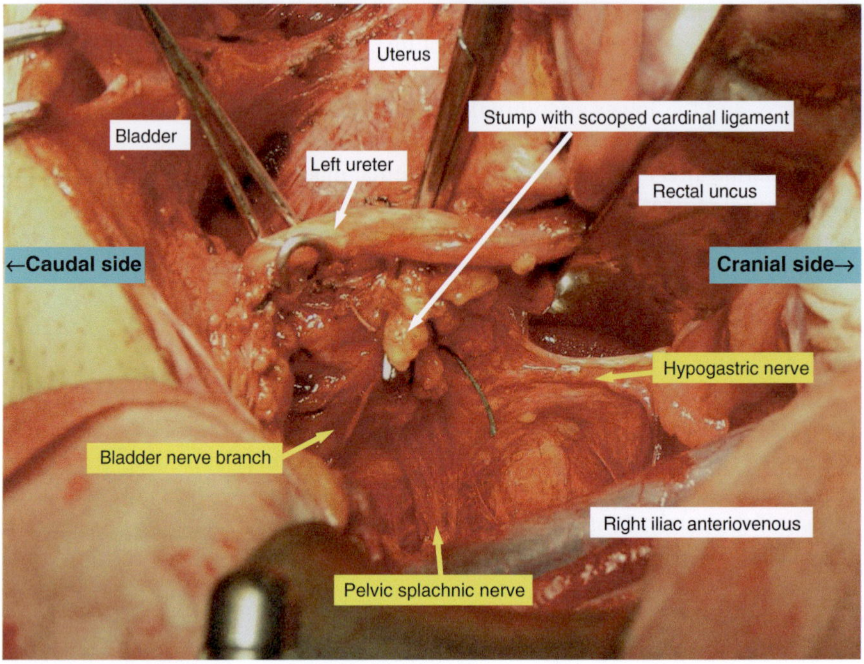

Fig. 12.3 T-shaped network of preserved urination-related nerves. The hypogastric nerve descending on the lateral side of the rectum, the pelvic splanchnic nerve located on the dorsal side of the cardinal ligament blood vessel, the pelvic plexus where both are jointed, and the bladder nerve branch that exits from junction through the dorsal side of the vesicouterine ligament layer to the bladder make the so-called T-shaped neural network consisting of nerve branches which is preserved

12.6.7 Site of Cervical Cleavage Determination and Uterine Descending Artery Cutting

Intraoperative ultrasonography is performed while referring to the preoperative MRI, and the cutting position of the cervix is determined. An ultrasound probe is placed directly on the serosal surface of the uterine anterior wall (Fig. 12.4a), and the position of the endocervical canal is confirmed (Fig. 12.4b). The incision marking is drawn so that the cervical canal remains at least 5 mm, with 10 mm producing better results, from the endocervix to the vaginal side (Fig. 12.4c). Although it is easy to confirm the position of the endometrium through a preoperative MRI sagittal image before operation, the distance (Fig. 12.1) from the uterine fundus to the cutting position is commonly to be extended about 5 mm due to the retention of the uterus during surgery. Therefore, the cutting position is finally determined by the ultrasonic probe which is applied to the uterus intraoperatively while referencing the preoperative MRI. It is impossible for VRT to be able to accurately determine the cut position by ultrasonography, hence creating what is to be considered a laparotomic advantage. Expose the uterine artery toward the uterine wall, and then cut and double ligate the descending branches.

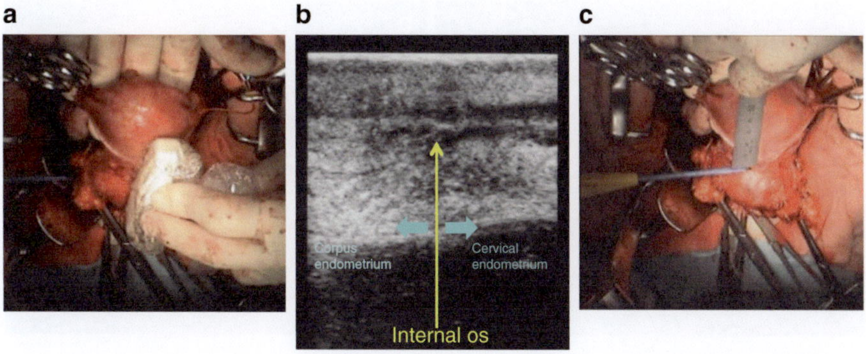

Fig. 12.4 Determination of cervical cutting level by intraoperative ultrasonography. To the serosal surface of the uterine anterior wall, apply an ultrasonic probe (**a**) and confirm the position of the endocervical canal (**b**); the incision marking is drawn so that the cervical canal remains at least 5 mm, with 10 mm producing better results, from the endocervix to the vaginal side (**c**)

12.6.8 Vaginal Canal/Cervical Canal Dissection: New Cervical (Neocervix) Formation

Cut the vaginal wall with 2–3 cm of the vagina attached to the cervix, and then ligate both ends of the vaginal stump. The cervical canal is cut with an electric scalpel at the level to be marked (Fig. 12.5a). The endocervix undergoing intraoperative pathologic diagnosis is cut with a cold knife to increase diagnostic accuracy (Fig. 12.5b). At the time of pathological examination, two sections are cut from the cervix so as to create two thin discs at intervals of 2.5 mm from the stump end of the cervix. Both slices are frozen, and sections for pathological diagnosis are prepared from a section 5 mm away from the section to be excised. Although some institutions examine only the cervical resected section intraoperatively, we are also targeting adenocarcinoma that often have skip lesions, and we want to secure a margin of at least 5 mm even in SCC, so the authors examined the surrounding 5 mm area intraoperatively. Bleeding from the cervical section is usually mild, and hemostasis and coagulation by electrocautery are sufficient. The severed cervical stump is trimmed into the shape of a normal uterine vagina in order to form a neocervix while taking note that the vascular system traveling longitudinally through the uterine sidewalls in the 3 o'clock and 9 o'clock direction is not injured.

When the uterine artery is preserved, an abnormality such as congestion occurs in the tissue around the uterine-vaginal canal anastomosis part, and formation of a varix at an inappropriate level is formed. In case of pregnancy, severe varix occurred around the cervical-vaginal canal anastomosis (it was extreme in pregnancy cases following simple cervical excision rather than RT), and it is difficult to manage. Therefore, we barely cut the bilateral uterine artery. The blood flow of uterine body parts recovers promptly via bilateral ovarian artery-uterine artery anastomosis even without preservation. Natural pregnancy after bilateral uterine artery amputation was also established, so that major disadvantages to fertility are not present.

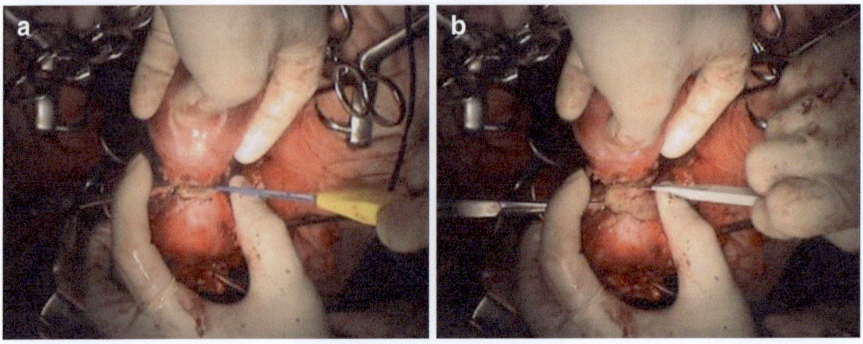

Fig. 12.5 Vaginal canal dissection. Dissect the cervical canal with an electric scalpel at the level of resection that was marked (**a**). The part of the endocervical canal which undergoes intraoperative pathologic diagnosis is cut with a cold knife (**b**)

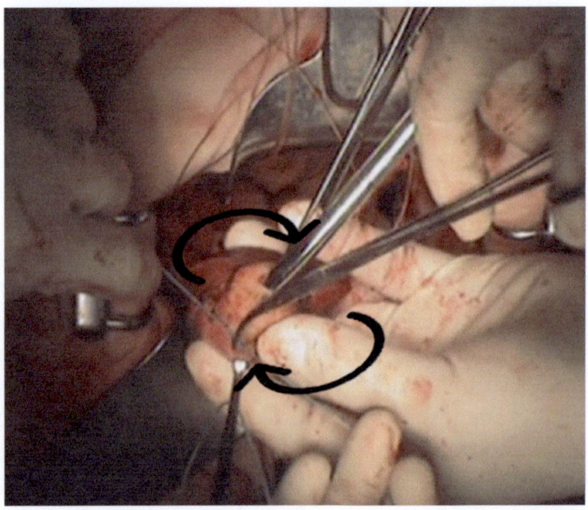

Fig. 12.6 A cerclage of the cervix. Cervical canal retraction is performed with a thick needle and nonabsorbable thread with a No. 8 Hegar Uterine dilator. It is returned 180 degrees at the level of the internal os level and is sewn very loosely so as not to tighten (in the photograph, mosquito forceps are interposed for loose suturing)

12.6.9 A Permanent Cerclage of the Cervix

We performed a cerclage of the cervix if an intraoperative frozen section did not detect a malignant lesion to prevent premature birth in the future. The cervical canal is sequentially enlarged with Hegar Uterine dilators, and cervical stitching is performed with No. 1 Prolene® (nonabsorbable monofilament stitch) with a No. 8 Hegar cervical dilator inserted. At the height of the internal os level, insert the needle from the 6 o'clock direction of the cervical canal, rotate the needle 180° in order to pull the needle in the direction of 12 o'clock one time, and then rotate the needle another 180° to move backward at 6 o'clock turning the needle toward you (Fig. 12.6). Be sure to suture loosely, and refrain from tightening in order to avoid cervical stenosis which may occur if strongly sutured. The sutured end with nonabsorbable thread is safer along the rectal side than the bladder side. A double cervical stitch is performed. In the case of VRT, cervical stitching is often performed in accordance with the McDonald surgical procedure, and a part of the suture stitch is exposed in the vagina. In contrast, cervical sutures can be implanted under the cervical serosal membrane in accordance with the Shirodkar technique in the abdominal operation, and the knot can also be retained in the retroperitoneal cavity at the time of anastomosis with the vaginal canal. Therefore, the knot is not exposed in the vagina, which is considered to be advantageous for the prevention of infection around the anastomotic region after surgery.

12.6.10 Anastomosis of Neocervix and Vaginal Stump

Regarding the anastomosis of the cervical stump and vaginal canal, a U-shaped suture in the directions of 6 o'clock and 12 o'clock is executed using 2-0 Monocryl UR6® with a strongly scored needle and then a single-knot suture in the 3 o'clock and 9 o'clock directions which is parallel to both sides of the uterus. Loosen the suture so that the stump of the vaginal canal encapsulates the neocervix while grasping the six sutures above. This technique not only allows the neocervix to protrude into the vagina like a natural uterine vagina but also assists postoperative sexual pain (Fig. 12.7).

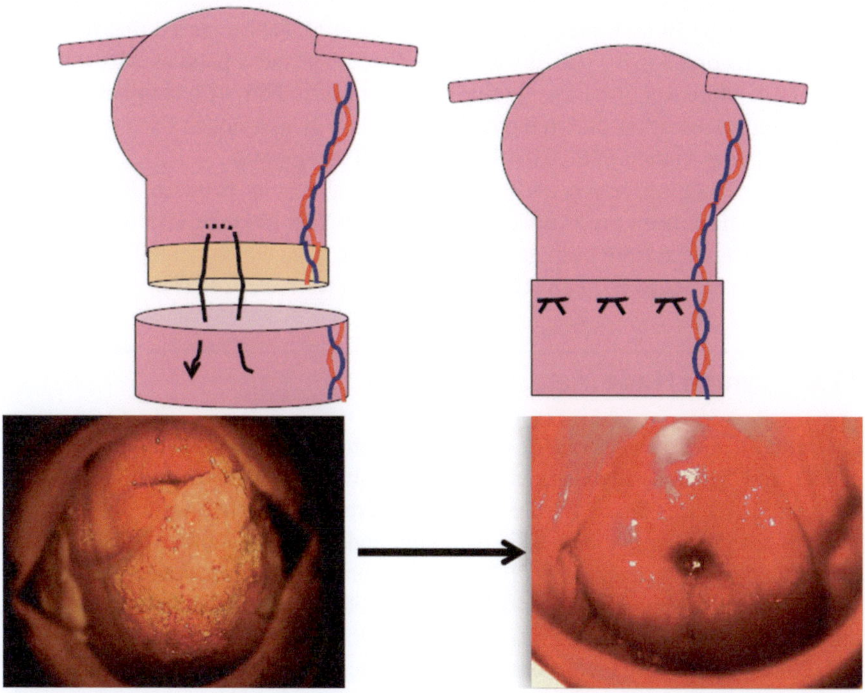

Fig. 12.7 Anastomosis of the neocervix and vaginal stump. Left figure: suturing at 12 o'clock and 6 o'clock of the vaginal canal is "reverse U-shaped suture"; 3 o'clock and 9 o'clock shall be a single ligation parallel to the blood vessel so as not to disturb the blood flow of the side wall. Performing anastomosis to wrap the neocervix in the vaginal canal like this can avoid postoperative sexual pain

12.6.11 Reconstruction of Circular Ligament: Pelvic Peritoneal Closure (Closed)

After placing the transabdominal continuous aspiration drain in the retroperitoneal cavity of the left and right pelvis, reanastomose the bilateral circular ligaments, and suture the pelvic peritoneum. After attaching the antiadhesive agent sheet to the peritoneal suture part, surroundings of the oviduct, etc., consider the possibility of future oocyte retrieval, and guide the bilateral ovary to the Douglas fossa, and close it.

12.7 Morbidity

The preferred FSS method choice for patients with stage 1A2 is RT + pelvic lymph node dissection +/− para-aortic lymph node sampling as stated in the NCCN and JSGO guidelines [16, 17]. A review [20] indicated that postoperative recurrence rates for stage 1A2 in RT including VRT, ART, or laparoscopic RT was 0–8% and not different from a series of patients treated with radical hysterectomy. Obstetrical outcomes revealed that out of a total of 210 patients who underwent RT treatment, 109 patients tried to become pregnant with 47 patients being successful. Although the frequency of preterm birth and premature rupture increases, 35 live babies were delivered out of 59 total pregnancies. Okugawa et al. [18] reported that no recurrence was recorded in 10 patients with modified ART and 7 patients with ART for stage 1A2. Moreover, the investigation of less invasive FSS with simple trachelectomy or cone resection plus removal of the pelvic lymph nodes for stage 1A2 is currently being studied (NCT01048853 and NCT01649089).

Several retrospective reports provide statistical results between RT and RH, while there have been no prospective studies [21–24]. In stage 1B1 disease, data found no difference from each group in recurrence rates which range from 0.9% to 5.0% in RT and 1.1 to 6.5% in RH, respectively [11, 18, 22, 24–27].

12.8 Lymph Node Metastasis

Lymph node metastasis is one of the most important prognostic factors in cervical cancer, and lymph node enlargement detection in preoperative imaging exams has been indicated as a factor to rule out RT. Several reports have been published in favor of the preoperative diagnosis of lymph node metastasis using MRI, CT, and positron emission tomography (PET) [7, 28]. Commonly, lymph node dissection is performed, and in cases when positive lymph node metastasis is determined by an intraoperative pathologic diagnosis, RT is abandoned and treatment is converted to RH. Some facilities are incorporating the intraoperative sentinel lymph node (SLN) biopsies [7, 29–31]. A systematic review by Selman et al. [32] described that sentinel lymph node biopsy has an observably higher metastatic diagnosis rate than imaging, including PET, in cases of early cancer. In the results of a study regarding the feasibility of employing the use of SLN to detect early cervical cancer, the intraoperative SLN detection rate was 88%, and the subgroups of patients with stage Ia–Ib1 disease and smaller tumor sizes (<or = 3 cm in maximal diameter) were 95%. Sensitivity, false-negative rate, and negative predictive value for metastasis were reported at 100%, 0%, and 100%, respectively. The application of the SLN theory for early cancer stages with smaller tumors (TD $\leq$ 3 cm) in cervical cancer is reasonable and as beneficial as its use in breast cancer and cutaneous melanoma.

This examination not only improves safety but also greatly contributes to the reduction of lower limb lymphoedema and pelvic lymphatic cysts after operation. With respect to SN biopsy theory in conjunction with ART, Du et al. [30] reported that SN was detectable in 94.1% of 68 patients with 99 mTc, and treatment for 8 out of 68 patients (12%) was converted to RH due to SN metastasis. The results of a total of 164 cases where RT was tried at Kyushu University (June 2005 to March 2014) and Kagoshima University (April 2014–November 2015) were that the SN identification rate by the RI method exceeded 95%, with only 12 cases (7%) converted into RH due to SN metastasis.

12.9 Tumor Size

As with disease stage, tumor size is an important factor after lymph node metastasis for performing RT. Most research has been aware of tumor size for performing RT [2, 7, 8, 11, 15, 19, 21, 25, 26, 33–36]. In cases with 2 cm < TD in stage 1B1, inferior outcomes have been reported [7, 8, 33, 34, 37]. In VRT, the recurrence rate increases from 12.5% to 29% when the 2 cm < TD. In a review by Rob et al. [36], the recurrence rate in VRT rises to 20.8% (only 2.9% in cases of TD $\leq$ 2 cm) in the case of 2 cm < TD, whereas it reaches 4.8% in ART. Comparing 71 patients with VRT and 55 patients with ART in a multicenter collaborative study revealed that all of the 7 relapsed cases were VRT cases [33]. In VRT cases, the recurrence rate was 4.2% in TD < 2 cm, whereas the recurrence rate was 21.7% at 2 cm < TD. This data confirms that patients with 2 cm < TD are unable to undergo radical surgery in VRT. In a review concerning 485 cases of ART (IA1 stage, 33 cases; IA2 stage, 90 cases; IB1 stage, 330 cases; IB 2 stage, 11 cases), the recurrence rate of 3.8% was recorded (observation period 31.6 months) [38]. Table 12.3 summarizes the ART of stage IB which was performed on cases with 2 cm < TD. It may show that ART has a lower recurrence rate than VRT even in cases of tumors with a 2 cm < TD. Regarding the recent reports of ART for large tumor diameters, Wethington et al. [39] analyzed and reported 29 cases of 2–4 cm TD out of 110 RT trial patients: 22 cases were ART, 6 cases were VRT, and 1 case was robotic RT. Fourteen out of 29 cases (48%) were converted into RH during surgery; the breakdown was 7 cases due to margin-positive and 7 cases of lymph node metastasis. One of the cases was positive in two lymph node metastases during the operation, so the surgery was interrupted and converted to concurrent chemoradiotherapy. Finally, only 15 patients (52%) were able to undergo RT, and only 1 patient with a TD of 3 cm (recurrence rate 3%; observation period, 44 months) showed signs of recurrence. In addition, Wellington summarized 147 cases from existing literature that 2 cm < TD verifying the

Table 12.3 The literatures of performed abdominal radical trachelectomy in stage IB cervical cancer

		Ungar 2005	Nishio H 2009	Cibula 2009	Li J 2011	Du XL 2011	Saso S 2011	Wethington SL 2012	Cao DY 2013	Lintner B 2013	Zhang D 2014	Gent 2014	Capilna 2014	Tokunaga H 2015	Vieira MA 2015	Deng 2017	Guo 2018
The number of patients		30	61	17	62	60	30	81	73	31	36	28	26	42	50	45	143
(including converted radical hysterectomy)		33	71	24	64	68		101		45			29		58	49	153
Median age (year)		30.5	33	32.4	29.5	28	32.5	31	31	32	32	31.2	32	32	29.3	28.5	31
FIGO stage 1B1 (≤2 cm)		21	48	14	22	25	20	88*	29		20	22	14*	34	42		
FIGO stage 1B1 (>2 cm)		9	13	3	14	12	5		24	17	16			3		45	
FIGO stage 1B2		0	0	0	0	0	3	2	0	14		3	1	0			0
	SCC	26	58	14	50	60	15	40	64	17	25	14	15	42	29	46	111
	Non-SCC	4	3	10	12	0	15	61	9	14	11	14	8	0	29	3	32
Median follow-up periods (months)		–	33	21.2	22.8	38	24	32	20.6	90	12	68.5	20	29.9	66	–	75.5
Recurrences		0	6/61 (9.8%)	1/17 (5.9%)	0	2/60 (3.3%)	3/30 (10%)	0	0	4 (12.9%)	0	2/28 (7.1%)	0	3/42 (7.1%)	1/50 (2%)	2/45 (4.4%)	4 (2.8%)
	≤2 cm	0	1/48 (2.1%)	1/14 (7.1%)	0	–	–	0	0		0	–	0	–	–	–	2 (2.9%)
	>2 cm	0	5/13 (38%)	0	0	–	–	0	0		0	–	0	–	–	2/45 (4.4%)	2 (2.7%)

FIGO International Federation of Gynecology and Obstetrics
*No distinction at around 2 cm

recurrence rate of VRT is 16% (12/77), while the recurrence rate of ART is only 9% (6/69). According to reports of Li et al. [34] (62 cases) and Lintner et al. [37] (45 cases), the recurrence rates of ART are 0% and 12.9%, respectively, with the 5-year survival rate at an excellent result of 100% and 93.5%. Saso et al. [40] indicated that ART is more preferable for cases of 2 cm < TD than VRT and should be performed on tumors within 4 cm TD. The safety of ART in patients with 2 cm < TD, even in cases of proven adenocarcinoma, was compared to RH in a recent large series. The result was an overall recurrence rate in 2 cm < TD of only 2.7% in ART, which is comparable to RH. Only one out of four recurrence patients relapsed with adenocarcinoma, and progression-free survival rates at 5 years were 96.8% and 97.2% in the non-SCC and SCC groups, respectively ($p = 0.999$) [25]. The efficacy of neoadjuvant chemotherapy in cases of tumors 2 cm < TD on patients who mostly underwent VRT was reviewed, and the overall recurrence rate was 7.6% with pregnancy rates being 30.7% [8].

12.10 Histology

Guidelines indicate that SCC, adenosquamous carcinoma, and adenocarcinoma are considered to be inclusive factors for RT [16, 17]. There is no evidence that adenocarcinoma has a significant recurrence rate after RT as compared with SCC. However, adaptation for adenocarcinoma should be carefully examined because there is a risk that a skip lesion is present on the inner cervical side, even if the cervical section is negative at RT [41]. Histology type of neuroendocrine tumor, gastric-type adenocarcinoma, or adenoma malignum was not suitable for fertility sparing because of insufficient data [16]. There are reports of including clear cell adenocarcinoma [39], glassy cell carcinoma [37, 40, 42], and sarcoma botryoides [34] as indications for ART, while at the present time, such special types should also be out of adaptation.

12.11 Age or History of Parity

There is no well-defined age range or determined age margin of safety for the procedure. It seems that many institutions do not have an upper age limit, but some reported literature has limited patients to 40 years old [33, 43, 44] or 45 years old or less [34]. It is a criterion that changes with the progress of infertility treatment, so it is not stipulated in our department. However, when pregnancy is established after RT, complications such as chromosomal abnormality, pregnancy-induced hypertension, or gestational diabetes are considered to increase in patients in their 40s; therefore we must fully explain the risk of pregnancy or parturition.

Although the majority of reported patients who underwent RT were unparous, the majority of reported cases have been adapted to include parous patients except for only one article [28]. However, we should avoid recommending RT lightly, and always receive written and signed consent after a thorough explanation of the risks and benefits of RT.

The most common complications regarding ART are cervical stenosis (1.6–7.8%), cervical erosion (2%), and amenorrhea (8.2%). Moreover, intra-abdominal abscess or peritonitis (1.7–24.6%) has been reported. However, uterine necrosis is rarely reported [6, 35].

Quality of life (QOL) and sexual function are other important considerations and side effects to keep in mind for post-RT patients. A few reports reveal that several patients have reported an immediate decrease in QOL and sexual function postoperatively, and there seems to be no differences in conventional surgery with RT or RH [45]. However, most patients return to normal levels around 6 months postoperatively with the exception of those suffering from poor emotional well-being who need an average of 4 years to recover [46]. The complications which occurred postoperatively such as poor healing, cervical stenosis, etc. influence these patients' scores.

Fertility results comparing FSS procedures including simple trachelectomy/cone resection, AmRT, ART, minimally invasive RT, and neoadjuvant chemotherapy have been recently reported [6]. It has been concluded that there is no difference between live birth rates. However, there was a significant difference in fertility rates between each FSS procedure: 44% in ART, 57% in VRT, and 65% in minimally invasive RT, respectively. A majority of fetal losses and premature deliveries were related to premature rupturing of membranes. The impact of fertility outcomes in FSS has still not been determined [47]. The newest detailed information regarding FSS for obstetrical outcome by Bentivegna et al. [6] has been outlined in Table 12.4.

The reason why ART has a relatively low fertility outcome is mainly attributed to poor cervical factors [48, 49]. (1) In abdominal RT, cutting levels can be more accurately determined by consulting a preoperative MR. The position of the inner uterine opening can be established by intraoperative UST. (2) In vaginal RT, which often deals with relatively small lesions, it is necessary to determine an accurate cervical cannulation site, and it is likely that a longer cervical gland will be left. Thus the remaining cervical gland after abdominal RT seems to be shorter. It is presumed that this leads to a cervical insufficiency factor and may contribute to a higher infertility rate in abdominal RT. Indeed, as mentioned above, the results of our own research show that there was no difference in the pregnancy rates between RT, mRT, and ST, and by positively introducing artificial insemination, in vitro fertilization, etc., pregnancy cases are clearly increasing [18].

12.12 Future Prospect

The information and research from various reports have stated that among stage IB1 cervical cancer patients in Japan under the age of 40 who underwent surgery, the proportion of cases with 2 cm < TD is considered to be about 1/3. If these patients are excluded based on eligibility criteria of conventional vaginal RT, a considerable number of patients will lose their uterus even if they desire fertility sparing. Reviews show that 30% of all trachelectomies were 2 cm < TD and 4% were 4 cm < TD according to the National Cancer Database [15].

Table 12.4 Details of the main fertility results of this systematic review according to FSS procedures for cervical cancer. Reuse with permission ([6])

Parameter	Simple trachelectomy/ cone resection	Dargent procedure	Radical trachelectomy, laparotomy	Radical trachelectomy, minimally invasive	Neoadjuvant chemotherapy	Total
Patients	212	1355	735	314	161	2777
Patients excluded[a]	12	150	92	22	13	289
Recurrences	4	52	28	15	7	106
Infertile patients	4	90	93	23	19	229
No. of pregnancies	103	499	175	74	93	944
Fetal loss, first trimester	9	67	18	15	12	121
Fetal loss, second trimester	5	34	8	2	5	54
Fetal loss, first or second trimester undetermined	0	0	11	0	0	11
Interruption-abortion	2	21	1	0	0	24
Ectopic pregnancy	1	6	0	0	1	8
Ongoing pregnancy	14	18	17	7	4	60
Preterm delivery (<6 WG)	8	120	59	25	11	223
Between 22 and 28 WG	1	11	8	6	2	28
Between 29 and 33 WG	3	25	15	5	5	53
Between 34 and 36 WG	0	24	26	12	2	64
Undetermined or other cutoff	4	60	10	2	2	78
Pregnancy rate[b]	22/39 (56)	241/424 (57)	135/310 (44)	57/87 (65)	60/78 (77)	515/938 (55)
Live birth rate[c]	51/69 (74)	308/460 (67)	120/175 (68)	50/64 (78)	71/93 (76)	600/861 (70)
Prematurity rate[d]	8/51 (15)	113/285 (39)	59/104 (57)	25/50 (50)	11/71 (15)	216/561 (38)

Note: Values are number (percentage)

[a]Patients excluded for oncologic reasons depriving them of FSS management

[b]Pregnancy rate determined in series with complete data on the total number of patients attempting to become pregnant and the number of them succeeding

[c]Live birth rate determined in series with complete data about the total number of pregnancies and the number of live births. Ratio between the two was then determined

[d]Prematurity rate determined in series with complete data about the number of live birth deliveries and the number of premature deliveries. Ratio between the two was then determined

ART is most likely to be recommended for larger tumors with 2–4 cm TD. However, another problem was the accurate detection of lymph node metastasis which increases in correlation with the enlargement of the tumor size. Intraoperative detection of sentinel lymph node navigations seems to decrease in 3 cm < TD [50]. Preoperative chemotherapy may be more useful for relieving complications of surgery but may not assist in the improvement of recurrence rate. If the tumor diameter is <2 cm, VRT is performed, but the possibility of more noninvasive surgery will be considered in the future for greater prospective results (UMIN000009726).

References

1. Dargent D, Martin X, Sacchetoni A, Mathevet P. Laparoscopic vaginal radical trachelectomy: a treatment to preserve the fertility of cervical carcinoma patients. Cancer. 2000;88:1877–82.
2. Covens A, Shaw P, Murphy J, et al. Is radical trachelectomy a safe alternative to radical hysterectomy for patients with stage IA-B carcinoma of the cervix? Cancer. 1999;86:2273–9.
3. Roy M, Plante M. Pregnancies after radical vaginal trachelectomy for early-stage cervical cancer. Am J Obstet Gynecol. 1998;179:1491–6.
4. Shepherd JH, Mould T, Oram DH. Radical trachelectomy in early stage carcinoma of the cervix: outcome as judged by recurrence and fertility rates. BJOG. 2001;108:882–5.
5. Smith JR, Boyle DC, Corless DJ, et al. Abdominal radical trachelectomy: a new surgical technique for the conservative management of cervical carcinoma. Br J Obstet Gynaecol. 1997;104:1196–200.
6. Bentivegna E, Maulard A, Pautier P, Chargari C, Gouy S, Morice P. Fertility results and pregnancy outcomes after conservative treatment of cervical cancer: a systematic review of the literature. Fertil Steril. 2016;106:1195–211. e1195
7. Wethington SL, Sonoda Y, Park KJ, et al. Expanding the indications for radical trachelectomy: a report on 29 patients with stage IB1 tumors measuring 2 to 4 centimeters. Int J Gynecol Cancer. 2013;23:1092–8.
8. Pareja R, Rendon GJ, Vasquez M, Echeverri L, Sanz-Lomana CM, Ramirez PT. Immediate radical trachelectomy versus neoadjuvant chemotherapy followed by conservative surgery for patients with stage IB1 cervical cancer with tumors 2cm or larger: A literature review and analysis of oncological and obstetrical outcomes. Gynecol Oncol. 2015;137:574–80.
9. Bafghi A, Castaigne D, Pomel C. Radical trachelectomy: From the laparoscopic approach to the vaginal routeJ Gynecol Obstet Biol Reprod (Paris). 2006;35:696–701.
10. Persson J, Kannisto P, Bossmar T. Robot-assisted abdominal laparoscopic radical trachelectomy. Gynecol Oncol. 2008;111:564–7.
11. van Gent MD, van den Haak LW, Gaarenstroom KN, et al. Nerve-sparing radical abdominal trachelectomy versus nerve-sparing radical hysterectomy in early-stage (FIGO IA2-IB) cervical cancer: a comparative study on feasibility and outcome. Int J Gynecol Cancer. 2014;24:735–43.
12. Hamilton BE, Martin JA, Osterman MJ, Curtin SC, Matthews TJ. Births: Final Data for 2014. Natl Vital Stat Rep. 2015;64:1–64.
13. Saito T, Takahashi F, Katabuchi H. Committee on Gynecologic Oncology of the Japan Society of O, Gynecology. Annual Report of the Committee on Gynecologic Oncology, Japan Society of Obstetrics and Gynecology: Patient Annual Report for 2014 and Treatment Annual Report for 2009. J Obstet Gynaecol Res. 2017;43:1667–77.
14. Yamagami W, Nagase S, Takahashi F, et al. Clinical statistics of gynecologic cancers in Japan. J Gynecol Oncol. 2017;28:e32.
15. Cui RR, Chen L, Tergas AI, et al. Trends in Use and Survival Associated With Fertility-Sparing Trachelectomy for Young Women With Early-Stage Cervical Cancer. Obstet Gynecol. 2018;131:1085–94.

16. NCCN Guidelines Version 2. 2018 Cervical cancer. 2018.
17. Guidelines for treatment of uterine cervical cancer: Japan Society of Gynecologic Oncology(JSGO)2017 edition. 2017.
18. Okugawa K, Kobayashi H, Sonoda K, et al. Oncologic and obstetric outcomes and complications during pregnancy after fertility-sparing abdominal trachelectomy for cervical cancer: a retrospective review. Int J Clin Oncol. 2017;22:340–6.
19. Kobayashi H. Eligibility cliterias and disease outcomes in abdominal radical trachelectomy in our institution. J Jpn Soc Gynecol Oncol. 2011;29(3):668–74.
20. Koliopoulos G, Sotiriadis A, Kyrgiou M, Martin-Hirsch P, Makrydimas G, Paraskevaidis E. Conservative surgical methods for FIGO stage IA2 squamous cervical carcinoma and their role in preserving women's fertility. Gynecol Oncol. 2004;93:469–73.
21. Beiner ME, Hauspy J, Rosen B, et al. Radical vaginal trachelectomy vs. radical hysterectomy for small early stage cervical cancer: a matched case-control study. Gynecol Oncol. 2008;110:168–71.
22. Diaz JP, Sonoda Y, Leitao MM, et al. Oncologic outcome of fertility-sparing radical trachelectomy versus radical hysterectomy for stage IB1 cervical carcinoma. Gynecol Oncol. 2008;111:255–60.
23. Marchiole P, Benchaib M, Buenerd A, Lazlo E, Dargent D, Mathevet P. Oncological safety of laparoscopic-assisted vaginal radical trachelectomy (LARVT or Dargent's operation): a comparative study with laparoscopic-assisted vaginal radical hysterectomy (LARVH). Gynecol Oncol. 2007;106:132–41.
24. Xu L, Sun FQ, Wang ZH. Radical trachelectomy versus radical hysterectomy for the treatment of early cervical cancer: a systematic review. Acta Obstet Gynecol Scand. 2011;90:1200–9.
25. Guo J, Zhang Y, Chen X, Sun L, Chen K, Sheng X. Surgical and oncologic outcomes of radical abdominal trachelectomy versus hysterectomy for stage IA2-IB1 cervical cancer. J Minim Invasive Gynecol. 2018;
26. Bentivegna E, Gouy S, Maulard A, Chargari C, Leary A, Morice P. Oncological outcomes after fertility-sparing surgery for cervical cancer: a systematic review. Lancet Oncol. 2016;17:e240–53.
27. Zhang Q, Li W, Kanis MJ, et al. Oncologic and obstetrical outcomes with fertility-sparing treatment of cervical cancer: a systematic review and meta-analysis. Oncotarget. 2017;8:46580–92.
28. Maneo A, Chiari S, Bonazzi C, Mangioni C. Neoadjuvant chemotherapy and conservative surgery for stage IB1 cervical cancer. Gynecol Oncol. 2008;111:438–43.
29. Cibula D, Slama J, Svarovsky J, et al. Abdominal radical trachelectomy in fertility-sparing treatment of early-stage cervical cancer. Int J Gynecol Cancer. 2009;19:1407–11.
30. Du XL, Sheng XG, Jiang T, et al. Sentinel lymph node biopsy as guidance for radical trachelectomy in young patients with early stage cervical cancer. BMC Cancer. 2011;11:157.
31. Rob L, Charvat M, Robova H, et al. Less radical fertility-sparing surgery than radical trachelectomy in early cervical cancer. Int J Gynecol Cancer. 2007;17:304–10.
32. Selman TJ, Mann C, Zamora J, Appleyard TL, Khan K. Diagnostic accuracy of tests for lymph node status in primary cervical cancer: a systematic review and meta-analysis. CMAJ. 2008;178:855–62.
33. Cao DY, Yang JX, Wu XH, et al. Comparisons of vaginal and abdominal radical trachelectomy for early-stage cervical cancer: preliminary results of a multi-center research in China. Br J Cancer. 2013;109:2778–82.
34. Li J, Wu X, Li X, Ju X. Abdominal radical trachelectomy: Is it safe for IB1 cervical cancer with tumors >/= 2 cm? Gynecol Oncol. 2013;131:87–92.
35. Nishio H, Fujii T, Kameyama K, et al. Abdominal radical trachelectomy as a fertility-sparing procedure in women with early-stage cervical cancer in a series of 61 women. Gynecol Oncol. 2009;115:51–5.
36. Rob L, Skapa P, Robova H. Fertility-sparing surgery in patients with cervical cancer. Lancet Oncol. 2011;12:192–200.
37. Lintner B, Saso S, Tarnai L, et al. Use of abdominal radical trachelectomy to treat cervical cancer greater than 2 cm in diameter. Int J Gynecol Cancer. 2013;23:1065–70.

38. Pareja R, Rendon GJ, Sanz-Lomana CM, Monzon O, Ramirez PT. Surgical, oncological, and obstetrical outcomes after abdominal radical trachelectomy - a systematic literature review. Gynecol Oncol. 2013;131:77–82.
39. Wethington SL, Cibula D, Duska LR, et al. An international series on abdominal radical trachelectomy: 101 patients and 28 pregnancies. Int J Gynecol Cancer. 2012;22:1251–7.
40. Saso S, Ghaem-Maghami S, Chatterjee J, et al. Abdominal radical trachelectomy in West London. BJOG. 2012;119:187–93.
41. Plante M. Vaginal radical trachelectomy: an update. Gynecol Oncol. 2008;111:S105–10.
42. Ungar L, Palfalvi L, Hogg R, et al. Abdominal radical trachelectomy: a fertility-preserving option for women with early cervical cancer. BJOG. 2005;112:366–9.
43. Robova H, Rob L, Halaska MJ, Pluta M, Skapa P. Review of neoadjuvant chemotherapy and trachelectomy: which cervical cancer patients would be suitable for neoadjuvant chemotherapy followed by fertility-sparing surgery? Curr Oncol Rep. 2015;17:446.
44. Tokunaga H, Watanabe Y, Niikura H, et al. Outcomes of abdominal radical trachelectomy: results of a multicenter prospective cohort study in a Tohoku Gynecologic Cancer Unit. Int J Clin Oncol. 2015;20:776–80.
45. Carter J, Sonoda Y, Baser RE, et al. A 2-year prospective study assessing the emotional, sexual, and quality of life concerns of women undergoing radical trachelectomy versus radical hysterectomy for treatment of early-stage cervical cancer. Gynecol Oncol. 2010;119:358–65.
46. Fleming ND, Ramirez PT, Soliman PT, et al. Quality of life after radical trachelectomy for early-stage cervical cancer: A 5-year prospective evaluation. Gynecol Oncol. 2016;143:596–603.
47. Vieira MA, Rendon GJ, Munsell M, et al. Radical trachelectomy in early-stage cervical cancer: A comparison of laparotomy and minimally invasive surgery. Gynecol Oncol. 2015;138:585–9.
48. Li J, Li Z, Wang H, et al. Radical abdominal trachelectomy for cervical malignancies: surgical, oncological and fertility outcomes in 62 patients. Gynecol Oncol. 2011;121:565–70.
49. Boss EA, van Golde RJ, Beerendonk CC, Massuger LF. Pregnancy after radical trachelectomy: a real option? Gynecol Oncol. 2005;99:S152–6.
50. Ogawa S, Kobayashi H, Amada S, et al. Sentinel node detection with (99m)Tc phytate alone is satisfactory for cervical cancer patients undergoing radical hysterectomy and pelvic lymphadenectomy. Int J Clin Oncol. 2010;15:52–8.

Role of Para-aortic Lymphadenectomy During Radical Hysterectomy for Stage IB–IIB Cervical Cancer

13

Mikio Mikami and Koji Matsuo

Abstract

The current guidelines of the Japanese Society of Gynecologic Oncology (JSGO) state that in the setting of cervical cancer, para-aortic lymph node (PAN) dissection or biopsy is only indicated when there is a high suspicion for PAN metastasis. This recommendation, however, is not based on conclusive evidence, and moreover, there is no objective strategic schema or triage system to indicate in which situations PAN dissection should be performed at the time of radical hysterectomy for stage I–II cervical cancer. In this chapter, we provide a concrete incidence table for PAN metastasis and recurrence that can be integrated into daily practice patterns. We also describe the "meticulous" and "awesome" PAN dissection procedure that is performed in Japan.

Keywords

Uterine cervical cancer · Radical hysterectomy · Para-aortic node dissection Lymph node metastasis · Lymphadenectomy · Cardinal ligament · Adjuvant chemotherapies

M. Mikami (✉)
Department of Obstetrics and Gynecology, Tokai University School of Medicine, Isehara, Kanagawa, Japan
e-mail: mmikami@is.icc.u-tokai.ac.jp

K. Matsuo
Division of Gynecologic Oncology, Department of Obstetrics and Gynecology, University of Southern California, Los Angeles, CA, USA

Norris Comprehensive Cancer Center, University of Southern California, Los Angeles, CA, USA

M. Mikami (ed.), *Surgery for Gynecologic Cancer*, Comprehensive Gynecology and Obstetrics, https://doi.org/10.1007/978-981-13-1519-0_13

13.1 Principles and Indications for Para-aortic Lymph Node Sampling

Para-aortic lymph node (PAN) metastasis is an important prognostic factor in patients with cancer of the uterine cervix [1–3]. PAN dissection is performed with the objective of diagnosing metastatic lymph nodes for the purpose of treatment planning and/or the therapeutic removal of these nodes. In Japan, PAN dissection is not routinely performed for diagnostic purposes, and instead, the decision to perform this procedure is determined on an individual basis. The National Comprehensive Cancer Network (NCCN) guidelines give the option for PAN biopsy in patients for stage IA1 disease with lymphovascular space invasion or more advanced disease. In patients with positive PAN metastasis by biopsy and imaging, the current guidelines recommend extraperitoneal or laparoscopic PAN dissection and concurrent chemoradiotherapy (CCRT) with the radiation field extending to the renal vessels provided that other distant metastases are excluded [4]. Preoperative imaging has been compared with biopsy and dissection of these lymph nodes in various studies, and these have shown that imaging has high specificity but lower sensitivity. The current NCCN guidelines recommend PET/CT for patients with stage IB2 or more advanced disease [4–6]; however, a retrospective study performed in 462 patients with stage IB1–IVA disease revealed PAN metastasis in resected nodes from patients who had been negative for PAN metastasis by preoperative PET/CT. In this study, 9% of the patients who were negative for pelvic lymph node metastasis and 22% of those positive for pelvic lymph node (PLN) metastasis by PET/CT actually had PAN metastasis, suggesting that PAN biopsy should be performed proactively in patients with positive PLN metastasis by PET/CT and, in many cases, even if imaging is negative for PAN metastasis [5].

An investigation of patients with stage IB2, IIA2, or IIB disease conducted by the Japanese Gynecologic Oncology Group (JGOG) showed that PAN dissection was performed at the time of radical hysterectomy in some of these patients at 101 out of 166 medical institutions (61%). At these 101 institutions, the main criteria for performing PAN biopsy or dissection included positive metastasis to the common iliac lymph nodes and/or enlargement of the PAN on imaging [7].

A prospective multicenter study was recently conducted to evaluate the therapeutic significance of PAN dissection. Laparoscopic dissection was performed on 237 patients who were negative for PAN metastasis by PET/CT, and notably, PAN metastasis was detected in 29 patients (12%), who subsequently underwent CCRT using an extended radiation field. Following treatment, survival in patients with PAN metastases measuring ≤5 mm in size was similar to those without PAN metastasis. However, CCRT with an extended field was insufficient in patients whose PAN metastases were >5 mm, suggesting that modification of the CCRT regimen or the addition of systemic chemotherapy after CCRT should be considered in the treatment of such patients [8].

There is little solid evidence that either PAN biopsy or dissection has a significant effect in determining subsequent treatment strategies. Currently, two ongoing randomized controlled trials (the EPLND for cervix study, NCT01365156, and the uterus 11 study, NCT01049100) are being conducted to assess the diagnostic and therapeutic utility of PAN dissection. In the former trial, 600 patients with suspected PLN metastasis who had been negative for PAN metastasis on PET/CT are being randomly assigned to one of the two treatment groups. The first group will undergo PAN dissection followed by individualized treatment, while the other group will receive CCRT targeting the pelvis based on the results of imaging studies. The 3-year survival rate will be compared between these groups, and it is expected that the results of these two trials will demonstrate the importance of PAN dissection for both diagnostic and therapeutic purposes.

13.2 Different Philosophies of Lymph Node Metastasis Between Japan and the USA

At present, it has yet to be demonstrated whether complete regional lymph node dissection improves the prognosis of patients with positive lymph node metastasis in cervical cancer. The situation is complicated by significant differences in the theory of lymph node metastasis mechanisms between Japan and Western countries. In Japan, it is widely accepted that solid tumors remain localized for a period of time and lymph node metastases are considered a manifestation of local disease (spectrum theory), implying that tumor can be cured by resection. In Western countries, it is generally believed that a solid tumor progresses to systemic disease at an early stage and lymph node metastases are evidence of systemic spread (Fischer theory), implying that tumor cannot be cured by resection alone. These different concepts are reflected in the differences in the number of resected lymph nodes reported between Japan and Western countries [9]. These differences in philosophy lead to differences in the completeness of PAN dissection between different surgeons and centers and are primarily due to the differing goals of diagnosis vs therapy. The presence of lymph node metastasis has been integrated into the International Federation of Gynecology and Obstetrics (FIGO) cancer stage classification of endometrial cancer, ovarian cancer, and vulvar cancer. In particular, the size of the metastatic lymph nodes is factored for staging in vulvar cancer (FIGO 2008 criteria) and ovarian cancer (FIGO 2014 criteria). In cervical cancer, lymph node status is not currently incorporated into the FIGO staging system. However, FIGO cervical cancer staging is now being modified according to the lymph node status diagnosed by the use of any imaging modality and pathological finding.

In addition to differing frequencies in which PAN dissection is performed between different Japanese institutions, there also appears to be institutional variation in the extent of the dissection, and routine PAN dissection to the level of infrarenal vessels is rarely performed. This is despite the fact that nearly one-third of PAN metastasis can be seen in the infrarenal nodal chain in the absence of inframesenteric artery chain metastasis [10]. As PAN metastasis is not an uncommon clinical entity in early-stage cervical cancer [11, 12], identification of PAN metastasis is crucial in its management, as it impacts not only patient prognosis but also the surgical approach and choice for adjuvant therapy [12, 13].

13.3 PAN Dissection and CCRT

The Meta-analysis Group (Medical Research Council Clinical Trials Unit, London, UK) reported that the addition of chemotherapy to standard radiotherapy for stage IIB–IVA disease clearly improves both overall and disease-free survival. This was based on the results of 18 trials performed in 11 countries (including five studies that formed the basis of the 1999 National Cancer Institute [NCI] alert), comprising the assessment of 4818 women from the 15 trials in the main analysis [14]. These analyses reinforce the recommendations of the 1999 NCI alert regarding the benefits of chemoradiotherapy, but with far greater reliability and precision. The report provides strong evidence supporting the value of CCRT for patients with stage IIB–IVA disease; however, three of these trials excluded women with PAN involvement, while PAN were either uninvolved (48%) or the status was unknown (51%) in the vast majority of women from the remaining trials. This suggests that the benefits of the treatment of PAN-positive patients by current CCRT protocols may be less clear. In the United States, treatment planning is dependent on PLN and PAN status, which is mainly determined by imaging [4]. The 3- and 5-year survival rates for patients with stage I–IV diseases and positive PAN following extended field concurrent chemoradiotherapy (EF-CCRT) were reported to be 69% and 39%, respectively [15]. These results are not satisfactory, and better treatments are needed for patients with positive PAN, a surrogate marker for systemic disease spread. Herein, we propose a treatment approach which includes radical hysterectomy and PAN dissection followed by systemic chemotherapy for cases with PAN metastasis. The goal of this treatment would be disease cure, and the benefit of this chemotherapy-based approach would be to avoid the morbidity related to adjuvant radiotherapy.

13.4 Risk Stratification Models for PAN Metastasis and Recurrence in Stage IB–IIB Cervical Cancer [16]

We conducted a study to examine the surgical-pathological factors associated with the presence of PAN metastasis at the time of radical hysterectomy and to identify predictors for PAN recurrence among women who did not undergo PAN dissection at radical hysterectomy. This is a retrospective analysis of a nationwide cohort study of surgically treated stage IB–IIB cervical cancer in Japan ($N = 5620$). Multivariable models were used to identify independent surgical-pathological predictors for PAN metastasis/recurrence. There were 120 (2.1%) cases of PAN metastasis at the time of radical hysterectomy. Parametrial involvement of the tumor (adjusted odds ratio [aOR] 1.65), deep stromal invasion (aOR 2.61), ovarian metastasis (aOR 3.10), and pelvic nodal metastasis (single-node aOR 5.39 and multiple-node aOR 33.5) were all independent risk factors for PAN metastasis (all, $P < 0.05$; Table 13.1). Without any risk factors, the incidence of PAN metastasis was 0.9%, while women exhibiting certain risk factor patterns (>20% of the study population) had PAN metastasis incidences of ≥4% (Table 13.2). PAN recurrence was seen in 22.5% of cases with

Table 13.1 Independent risk factors for para-aortic lymph node metastasis

Characteristic	Adjusted OR (95% CI)	*P*-value
Tumor size (cm)		
≤4	1	
>4	0.96 (0.33–2.78)	0.93
Parametrial involvement		
No	1	
Yes	1.65 (1.01–2.70)	0.046
Deep stromal invasion		
No	1	
Yes	2.61 (1.05–6.46)	0.038
LVSI		
Absence	1	
Presence	0.97 (0.47–2.03)	0.94
Corpus invasion		
No	1	
Yes	0.95 (0.57–1.60)	0.85
Ovarian metastasis		
No	1	
Yes	3.10 (1.33–7.23)	0.009
Cytology results		
No malignancy	1	
Malignancy	1.61 (0.71–3.68)	0.26
Not performed	0.72 (0.44–1.17)	0.18
Pelvic lymph node		
No metastasis	1	
Single metastasis	5.39 (1.74–16.6)	0.003
Multiple metastasis	33.5 (13.7–81.8)	<0.001

Adopted and modified from the original table [16]. A multivariable logistic regression model for para-aortic lymph node metastasis. All the listed covariates were entered in the final model. *OR* odds ratio, *CI* confidence interval, and *LVSI* lymphovascular space invasion

PAN metastasis present at the time of surgery, 4.2% among clinically PAN-negative cases at the time of surgery, and 2.5% among histologically PAN-negative cases at the time of surgery.

Among 4663 clinically PAN-negative cases at the time of surgery, parametrial involvement (aHR 1.67), lymphovascular space invasion (aHR 1.95), ovarian metastasis (aHR 2.60), and pelvic lymph node metastasis (single-node aHR 2.49 and multiple-node aHR 8.11) were independently associated with PAN recurrence (all, $P < 0.05$; Table 13.3). Without any of these risk factors, the 5-year PAN recurrence risk was 0.8%; however, women demonstrating certain risk factor patterns (>15% of the clinically PAN-negative population) had 5-year PAN recurrence risk of ≥8% (Table 13.4). Surgical-pathological risk factors proposed in this study will be useful in the identification of women with an increased risk of PAN metastasis/recurrence. Currently, the JSGO guidelines only state that PAN dissection is recommended when there is a high suspicion for PAN metastasis [17]. However, this is not based on thoroughly evaluated evidence, and moreover, there is no objective schema or

Table 13.2 Risk factor-based incidence of para-aortic lymph node metastasis

Parametrial involvement	Deep invasion	Ovarian mets	Single PLN	Multiple PLN	No.	PAN (+)
No	No	No	No	No	2044	18 (0.9%)
Yes	No	No	No	No	46	1 (2.2%)
No	Yes	No	No	No	1308	15 (1.1%)
No	No	Yes	No	No	6	0
No	No	No	Yes	No	112	1 (0.9%)
No	No	No	No	Yes	106	7 (6.6%)
Yes	Yes	No	No	No	380	7 (1.8%)
Yes	No	No	Yes	No	10	1 (10%)
Yes	No	No	No	Yes	20	0
No	Yes	Yes	No	No	7	1 (14.3%)
No	Yes	No	Yes	No	225	9 (4.0%)
No	Yes	No	No	Yes	287	14 (4.9%)
No	No	Yes	Yes	No	1	0
No	No	Yes	No	Yes	1	0
Yes	Yes	Yes	No	No	5	0
Yes	Yes	No	Yes	No	155	8 (5.2%)
Yes	Yes	No	No	Yes	328	21 (6.4%)
No	Yes	Yes	Yes	No	2	0
No	Yes	Yes	No	Yes	8	1 (12.5%)
Yes	Yes	Yes	Yes	No	4	0
Yes	Yes	Yes	No	Yes	25	1 (4.0%)

Adopted and modified from the original table [16]. Among 5098 cases with available results for these four risk factors, incidence of para-aortic lymph node metastasis was examined based on patterns of risk factors. *PAN* para-aortic lymph node metastasis; *mets* metastasis; and *PLN* pelvic lymph node metastasis

Table 13.3 Independent risk factors for para-aortic lymph node recurrence

Characteristic	Adjusted HR (95% CI)	*P*-value
Histology		
Squamous	1	
Non-squamous	1.08 (0.74–1.58)	0.68
Tumor size (cm)		
≤4	1	
>4	1.22 (0.85–1.76)	0.29
Parametrial involvement		
No	1	
Yes	1.67 (1.14–2.45)	0.009
Deep stromal invasion		
No	1	
Yes	0.83 (0.53–1.31)	0.43
LVSI		
Absence	1	
Presence	1.95 (1.15–3.31)	0.014
Corpus invasion		
No	1	
Yes	1.36 (0.91–2.02)	0.14
Peritoneal cytology		
No malignancy	1	
Malignancy	1.49 (0.98–2.25)	0.06

Table 13.3 (continued)

Characteristic	Adjusted HR (95% CI)	*P*-value
Not performed	0.47 (0.13–1.71)	0.26
Ovarian metastasis		
No	1	
Yes	2.60 (1.03–6.58)	0.044
Pelvic lymph node		
No metastasis	1	
Single metastasis	2.49 (1.36–4.54)	0.003
Multiple metastasis	8.11 (5.16–12.7)	<0.001
Neoadjuvant chemotherapy		
No	1	
Yes	2.25 (1.56–3.24)	<0.001
Adjuvant treatment		
None	1	
RT-based	1.26 (0.66–2.41)	0.48
Chemotherapy	0.91 (0.45–1.86)	0.80

Adopted and modified from the original table [16]. A Cox proportional hazard regression model for multivariable analysis. All the listed covariates were entered in the final model. *SCC* squamous cell carcinoma, *LVSI* lymphovascular space invasion, *RT* whole pelvic radiotherapy, *HR* hazard ratio, and *CI* confidence interval

Table 13.4 Recurrence risk at para-aortic lymph nodes based on risk factor pattern among clinically negative para-aortic nodes at radical hysterectomy

Parametrial involvement	LVSI	Ovarian mets	Single PLN	Multiple PLN	No.	5-yr (%)*
No	No	No	No	No	1769	0.8%
Yes	No	No	No	No	70	1.6%
No	Yes	No	No	No	1198	1.9%
No	No	Yes	No	No	4	0%
No	No	No	Yes	No	57	6.0%
No	No	No	No	Yes	45	18.0%
Yes	Yes	No	No	No	276	4.8%
Yes	No	No	Yes	No	12	0%
Yes	No	No	No	Yes	19	15.0%
No	Yes	Yes	No	No	5	0%
No	Yes	No	Yes	No	218	2.5%
No	Yes	No	No	Yes	257	14.9%
No	No	Yes	No	Yes	1	0%
Yes	Yes	Yes	No	No	5	0%
Yes	Yes	No	Yes	No	117	9.0%
Yes	Yes	No	No	Yes	247	22.6%
No	Yes	Yes	Yes	No	4	0%
No	Yes	Yes	No	Yes	7	35.7%
Yes	Yes	Yes	Yes	No	3	100%
Yes	Yes	Yes	No	Yes	11	47.9%

Adopted and modified from the original table [16]. Among 4325 cases with complete information for the 5 risk factors, cumulative recurrence risk to para-aortic lymph node was examined based on the patterns of risk factors. *5-year cumulative recurrence risk of para-aortic lymph node recurrence. *LVSI* lymphovascular space invasion, *mets* metastasis, *PLN* pelvic lymph node metastasis triage system guiding performance of PAN dissection at the time of radical hysterectomy. In this study, we have provided a concrete incidence list for PAN metastasis and recurrence that can be integrated into practice patterns. The threshold to perform PAN dissection has not been determined in this study, and we used arbitrary cutoffs of 4% for PAN metastasis and 8% for PAN recurrence based on clinically meaningful significance compared to the overall PAN metastasis/recurrence found in our study (PAN metastasis ~2% and PAN recurrence ~4%). Indeed, we found that a significant proportion (nearly one in five) of women with stage IB–IIB cervical cancer was at risk for PAN metastasis. Further cost-effective studies are necessary to determine the ultimate cutoff value to determine when PAN dissection should be performed.

13.5 Quality and Quantity Metrics of PLN Metastasis and Risk of PAN Metastasis in Stage IB–IIB Cervical Cancer (Tokai University) [18]

This study was conducted to identify predictors of PAN metastasis at the time of surgery for women with stage IB–IIB cervical cancer who underwent radical hysterectomy at both Tokai University School of Medicine and National Hospital Organization Saitama Hospital between January 1976 and December 2014. Inclusion criteria were as follows: (a) histology types including squamous cell carcinoma, adenocarcinoma, and adenosquamous and (b) lymphadenectomy sites including both PLN and PAN chains. Excluded cases were those that had received neoadjuvant chemotherapy prior to radical hysterectomy and rare histology types or if lymphadenectomy had been performed in the PLN chain only. Among the eligible cases, clinicopathological characteristics were abstracted from the medical record. In this study, we also assessed the pathological findings of surgical specimens from the parametrial tissue located at the origin of internal iliac vessels (Fig. 13.1). Lymph node status included the number of sampled lymph nodes as well as the number of lymph node containing tumor cells. Lymph node ratio (LNR) was then determined as the percent proportion of tumor-positive lymph node per the total number of sampled lymph nodes per each case. Detailed qualities of PLN status were further assessed for common iliac node status, bilateral PLN status, size of PLN determined during surgery (cutoff, 1 cm), the presence of multiple PLN metastases, and high LNR (cutoff 6.6%) [19]. The primary focus of this analysis was to identify surgical-pathological factors for PAN metastasis. The secondary goal of this analysis was to examine the surgical-pathological factors predictive of the presence of parametrial tumor metastasis at the origin of internal iliac vessels.

There were 555 cases identified from the surgical tumor registry. Of these, there were 112 cases of surgically treated stage IB–IIB cervical cancer in which both PLN and PAN dissections were performed that did not receive neoadjuvant chemotherapy. The median numbers of sampled PLN and PAN were 39.5 and 30, respectively. PAN metastasis was seen in 27 (24.1%) cases in this study. On univariate analysis, the absence of PLN metastasis (proportion of PAN metastasis, yes *versus*

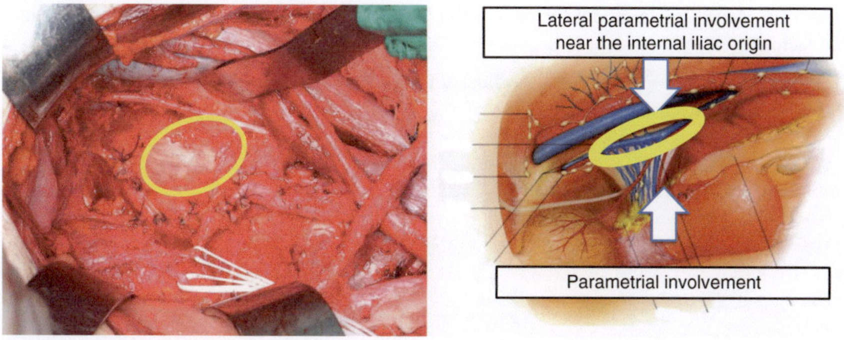

Fig. 13.1 Resection of the parametrial tissue located at the origin of internal iliac vessels. We performed radical hysterectomy using Okabayashi's method combined with PAN dissection and excision of the lateral parametrial involvement near the internal iliac origin if pelvic lymph node metastasis was detected by intraoperative frozen section diagnosis, and we performed pathological evaluation of the resected specimens

no, 31.8% *versus* 0%) demonstrated a negative predictive value of 100%, while LVSI (yes *versus* no, 29.0% *versus* 0%) and parametrial tumor involvement at the origin of internal iliac vessels (yes *versus* no, 53.8% *versus* 36.4%) were statistically significantly associated with PAN metastasis (all, $P < 0.05$). We were not able to perform multivariate analysis due to the absence of cases which were positive for PAN metastasis but negative for PLN and LVSI involvement.

In an attempt to articulate the utility of intraoperative findings to predict PAN metastasis, quality and quantity metrics of PLN status were assessed for PAN metastasis. On univariate analysis, common iliac node metastasis (proportion of PAN metastasis, yes *versus* no, 66.7% *versus* 10.6%), bilateral PLN metastasis (52.2% *versus* 4.5%), PLN size of ≥1 cm (54.8% *versus* 10.3%), the presence of multiple PLN metastases (52.1% *versus* 3.1%), and a high LNR of ≥6.6% (63.2% *versus* 4.1%) were statistically significantly associated with PAN metastasis (all, $P < 0.001$). In a multivariate model (Table 13.5), common iliac lymph node metastasis (adjusted OR 4.03), multiple PLN metastasis (adjusted OR 7.35), and PLN size of ≥1 cm (adjusted OR 8.92) remained independent predictors for PAN metastasis (all, $P < 0.05$). By utilizing these intraoperatively assessable PLN characteristics, the incidences of PAN metastasis were determined (Table 13.6). When none of these factors were present, there were no cases of PAN metastasis. If a PLN ≥1 cm or multiple PLN metastases were identified, the incidences of PAN were 16.7% and 18.2%, respectively. When two of these lymph node factors were present, the incidences of PAN metastases ranged from 28.6 to 45.5%. With all three nodal factors present, the incidence of PAN metastases exceeded 80% (84.2%) ($P < 0.001$).

Because parametrial tumor involvement at the origin of internal iliac vessels was significantly associated with an increased risk of PAN metastasis, we examined the risk factors for parametrial tumor involvement at the origin of internal iliac vessels. On univariate analysis, only bilateral PLN metastasis was significantly

Table 13.5 Multivariate model for para-aortic lymph node metastasis examining pelvic lymph node factors

Characteristic	Adjusted OR (95% CI)	*P*-value
Multiple PLN metastases		
No	1	
Yes	7.35 (1.27–42.6)	0.026
Common PLN metastasis		
No	1	
Yes	4.03 (1.04–15.7)	0.044
PLN size ≥1 cm		
No	1	
Yes	8.92 (2.30–34.6)	0.002
Not assessed	n/a	0.99

Adopted and modified from the original table [18]. A binary logistic regression model for multivariate analysis. All the listed covariates were entered in the final model. *OR* odds ratio, *CI* confidence interval, *PAN* para-aortic lymph node metastasis, and *PLN* pelvic lymph node

Table 13.6 Incidence of para-aortic lymph node metastasis based on quality and quantity of pelvic lymph node metastasis

Multiple PLN metastasis	Common iliac metastasis	Node size ≥1 cm	No.	PAN metastasis
No	No	No	20	0
Yes	No	No	11	2 (18.6%)
No	No	Yes	12	2 (16.7%)
Yes	Yes	No	7	2 (28.6%)
Yes	No	Yes	11	5 (45.5%)
Yes	Yes	Yes	19	16 (84.2%)

Adopted and modified from the original table [18]. Chi-square test, $P < 0.001$. Among cases with available results for all these factors, number and incidence of PAN metastasis are shown. *PLN* pelvic lymph node and *PAN* para-aortic lymph node

associated with parametrial tumor involvement at the origin of internal iliac vessels (50% *versus* 9.1%, odds ratio 10.0, $P = 0.027$). When there was tumor involvement in the parametrial tissue near the uterine cervix, there was an increased risk of parametrial tumor involvement at the origin of the internal iliac vessels although it did not reach statistical significance (57.1% *versus* 23.8%, OR 4.27, $P = 0.075$).

The identification of PAN metastasis impacts not only patient counseling for prognosis but also the options for postoperative treatment. Because PAN dissection during radical hysterectomy can increase surgical or postsurgical morbidity related to the procedure, selective PAN dissection targeting women at increased risk of PAN metastasis is an ideal approach for the reduction of procedure-related complications. In this study, we not only validated the location, size, and quantity of PLN metastasis as predictors of PAN metastasis, we but also provided combined quantitative and qualitative metrics to assess the incidence of PAN metastasis. All of these parameters are assessable during the surgery (Table 13.6), making the utility of this study useful in daily practice.

13.6 Technique and Strategy for Para-aortic Lymph Node Dissection: Operative Procedure

13.6.1 Entering the Retroperitoneal Space (Retroperitoneal Incision, Mobilization and Rotation of the Intestines, Identification of the Right Ureter, and Ligation and Cutting of the Right Ovarian Vein)

When performing PAN dissection, particularly when removal of metastatic lymph nodes is required, adequate exposure is of the utmost importance for the management of potential emergencies such as hemorrhage. To achieve this, an initial midline abdominal incision is extended up toward the sternum. The falciform ligament of the liver is transected to release the liver from the peritoneum. The abdominal wall should then be elevated with a Kent retractor, while a Nakayama retractor is placed in the lower abdominal region (Fig. 13.2). Next, the peritoneum is incised along the right paracolic gutter from the lateral side of the ileocecal junction to allow mobilization of the ascending colon. Following this, the incision is extended along the medial side of the right kidney to the point where the right renal vein drains into the inferior vena cava (IVC), and then, the retroperitoneum is incised

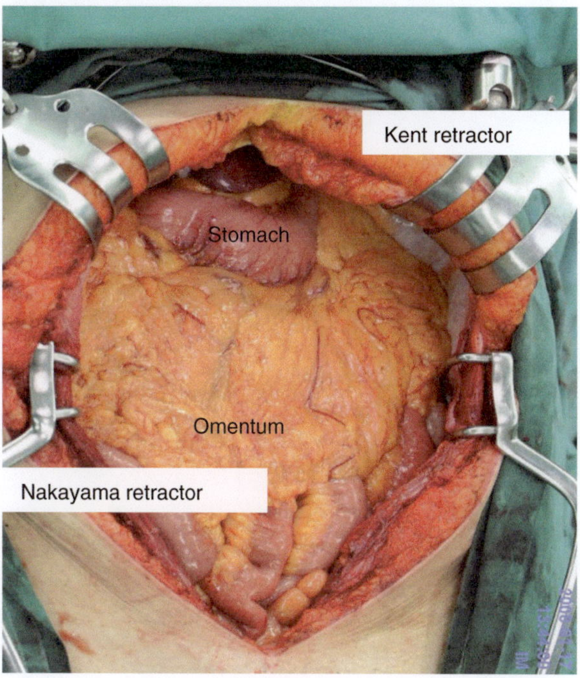

Fig. 13.2 Laparotomy. Then the abdominal wall is lifted upward with a Kent retractor, while a Nakayama retractor is placed in the lower abdominal region

from the origin of the right common iliac artery and vein toward the ligament of Treitz. This will mobilize the duodenum, the small intestine, and the ascending colon anterior to the IVC (Figs. 13.3–13.5). These organs are then placed into an intestinal bag held by an octopus retractor (Figs. 13.5 and 13.6). Lymphatic channels should now be observed in the vicinity of the left renal vein, and these must be ligated to prevent postoperative chylous ascites (Fig. 13.6). At this time, the courses of the right ureter, the right ovarian vein, and the inferior mesenteric vein should be mapped. The right ovarian vein is then isolated and ligated at the point where it enters the IVC (Fig. 13.5). Prior to starting the dissection, it is important to take note of the courses of the lumbar veins arising from the IVC/common iliac vein (Fig. 13.7).

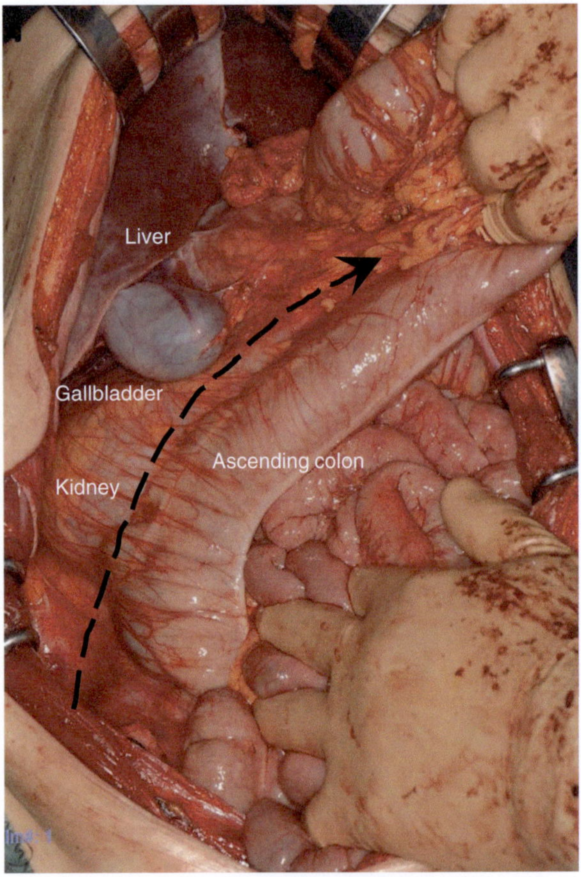

Fig. 13.3 Incision of the retroperitoneum. Incision of the peritoneum along the right paracolic gutter from the lateral side of the ileocecal junction

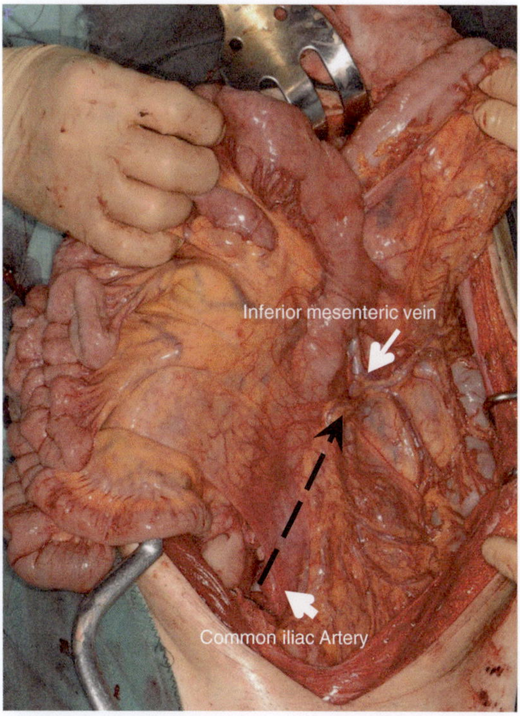

Fig. 13.4 Incision of the retroperitoneum. Retroperitoneum is incised from the origin of the right common iliac artery and vein toward the ligament of Treitz

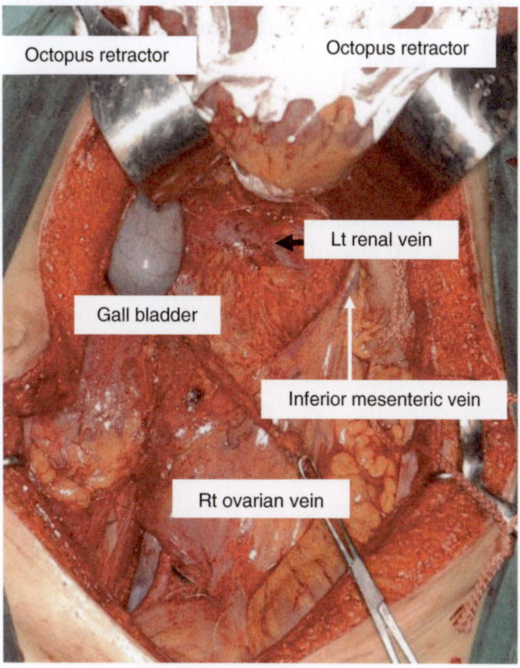

Fig. 13.5 Surgical view after mobilizing the duodenum, small intestine, and ascending colon anterior to the aorta and inferior vena cava

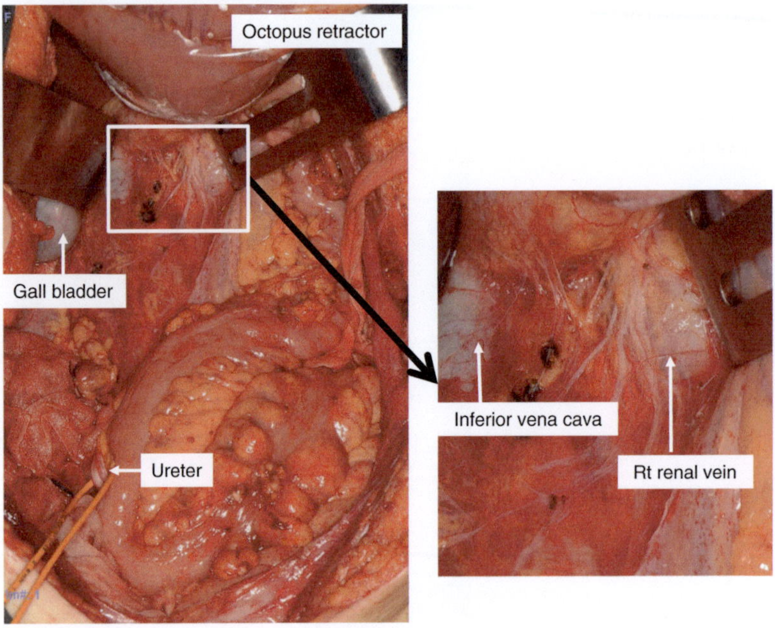

Fig. 13.6 Network of lymph vessels. A lymph vessel can be observed in the vicinity of the left renal vein, and it must be ligated to prevent postoperative chylous ascites

13.6.2 Right PAN Dissection (Residual Right Common Iliac Nodes and Right Side and Anterior Surface of the Inferior Vena Cava)

The IVC is retracted laterally by an assistant, and dissecting forceps are inserted from the right side of the IVC to separate the vascular sheath between the outer layer (tunica externa) and adipose tissue, which is ligated and transected using an ultrasonic scalpel (Fig. 13.8①). Next, the vascular sheath at the point two-thirds from the left side of the anterior surface of the IVC should be similarly separated using dissecting forceps, followed by ligation and transection using an ultrasonic scalpel (Fig. 13.8②). The right PAN can then be dissected by removal of the vascular sheath from the right half of the IVC, which allows the right side of the IVC to be clearly visualized. During the right PAN dissection, the sites where the lumbar veins enter the IVC should be checked. These veins are often symmetrical (Fig. 13.7), and their position of entry into the IVC is used as markers for the left PAN dissection. During the insertion of dissecting forceps, care should be taken to avoid injury to the lumbar veins. With adequate displacement of the IVC to the left side, the lymph nodes posterior to the IVC and between the abdominal aorta and IVC can be more easily removed.

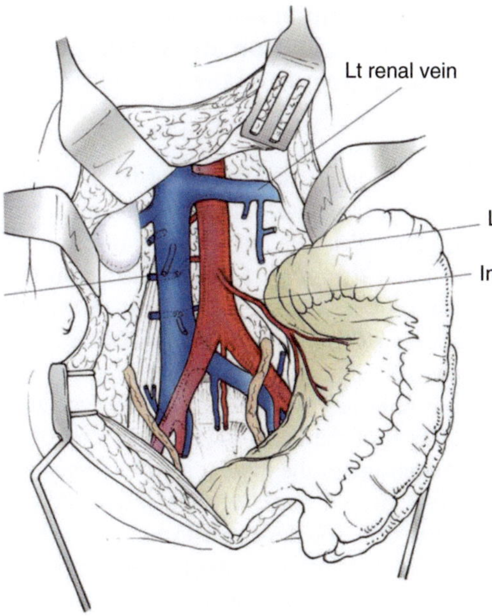

Fig. 13.7 Vessel anatomy for para-aortic node dissection (OGS NOW No.6 Surgery for Endometrial Cancer and Ovarian Cancer—Essential Procedures and Advanced Techniques for Tumor Progression). *Reprinted* by courtesy of Medical View and translated by Mikio Mikami. At the start of PAN dissection, it is important to take note of the courses of the lumbar veins arising from the inferior vena cava/common iliac vein. Especially, during right PAN dissection, the sites where the lumbar veins enter the inferior vena cava should be checked. These veins are often symmetrical. The positions of the sites of lumbar vein entry are used as markers for left PAN dissection

Fig. 13.8 Right PAN dissection (OGS NOW No.6 Surgery for Endometrial Cancer and Ovarian Cancer—Essential Procedures and Advanced Techniques for Tumor Progression). *Reprinted* by courtesy of Medical View and translated by Mikio Mikami

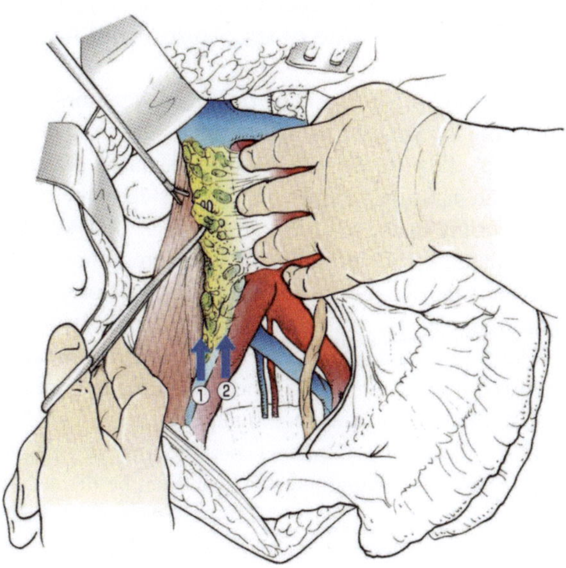

13.6.3 Exposure of the Abdominal Aorta and IVC, Exposure of the Left Renal Vein, Ligation and Cutting of the Left Ovarian Vein, and Exposure of the Inferior Mesenteric Artery (IMA)

Next, the vascular sheaths enveloping the left half of the IVC and the abdominal aorta are removed (Fig. 13.9) to the level where the left renal vein runs into the IVC. The point where the left ovarian vein meets the left renal vein is identified, and the ovarian vein is ligated and transected following isolation of 2–3 cm of the peripheral left ovarian vein (Fig. 13.10). Gerota's fascia of the left kidney should next be separated from the adipose tissues in the left PAN dissection field (above the IMA, area 326B1) which will allow for lateral displacement of the left kidney (Fig. 13.11). Next, tissue is removed from the anterior surface and left side of the abdominal aorta from the level of the IMA down to the level of the left common iliac which will allow for exposure of the lumbar arteries (Fig. 13.12). Small veins are often observed running to the IVC anteriorly at approximately 2–3 cm from the entry site of the common iliac vein, and these small veins should be transected using an ultrasonic scalpel (Fig. 13.7). Adipose tissues containing lymph nodes and the vascular sheaths covering the IVC and the abdominal aorta are removed by peeling them off while aiming to leave some of the tissue between the IVC and abdominal aorta. If the region between the abdominal aorta and IVC is dissected deeply, bleeding from the many small blood vessels in this area may occur, particularly in the region of the IMA (this region should be treated afterward [refer 14.6.5.]). Therefore, the tissues surrounding the IMA should be resected using an ultrasonic scalpel and submitted as lymph nodes from the area 326B2 (the area below the IMA; Fig. 13.12).

13.6.4 Left PAN Dissection (Residual Left Common Iliac Nodes and Left Side of the Abdominal Aorta)

The sigmoid colon should be displaced superiorly to provide an open view of the area from the left external iliac artery and vein to the common iliac artery and vein. This will allow for dissection of the residual left common iliac nodes (Fig. 13.13). Next, the paraspinal tissues on the left side of the aorta are removed up to the level of the origin of the left renal artery (Figs. 13.14 and 13.15). As mentioned above, when the left para-aortic lymph nodes are removed, suture ligation should be performed at the site immediately inferior to the origin of the left renal artery and vein to prevent chylous ascites. Prior to removal of the residual left common iliac nodes, the left ureter and left ovarian vein should be isolated and their courses mapped, followed by placement of a tape around the left ureter. Special attention should be paid to the lumbar veins running upward from the left common iliac vein and anastomosing with the lumbar veins running downward from the left renal vein (Fig. 13.6). The abdominal aorta can then be displaced to the right using a forceps

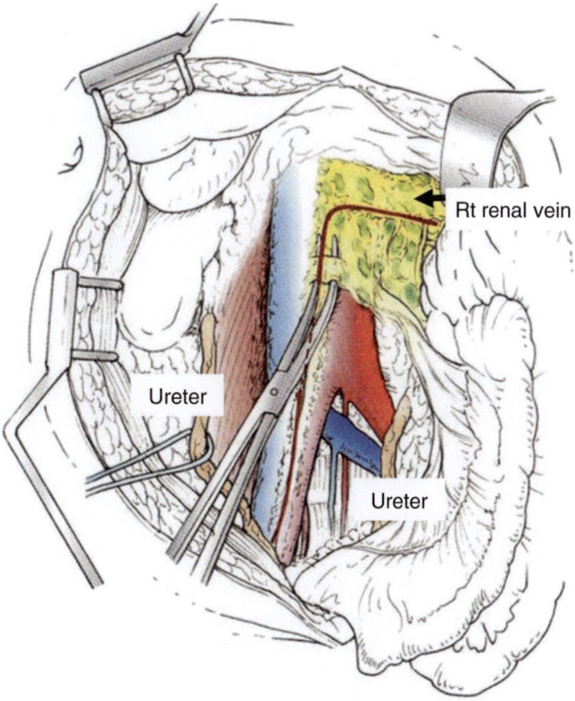

Fig. 13.9 Exposure of the abdominal aorta and vena cava (OGS NOW No.6 Surgery for Endometrial Cancer and Ovarian Cancer—Essential Procedures and Advanced Techniques for Tumor Progression). *Reprinted* by courtesy of Medical View and translated by Mikio Mikami. The vascular sheaths enveloping the left half of the inferior vena cava and the abdominal aorta are removed similarly. When the level where the left renal vein runs into the inferior vena cava is reached, the vascular sheaths are removed along the renal vein

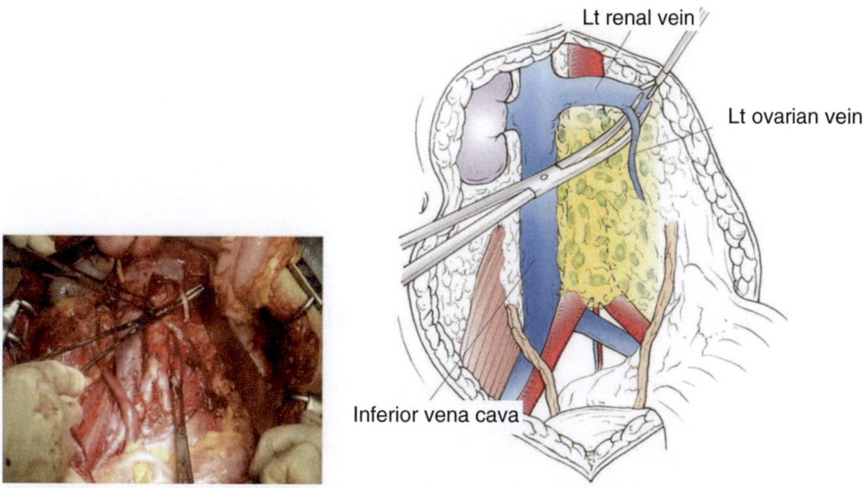

Fig. 13.10 Ligation and cut of the left ovarian vein (OGS NOW No.6 Surgery for Endometrial Cancer and Ovarian Cancer—Essential Procedures and Advanced Techniques for Tumor Progression). *Reprinted* by courtesy of Medical View and translated by Mikio Mikami

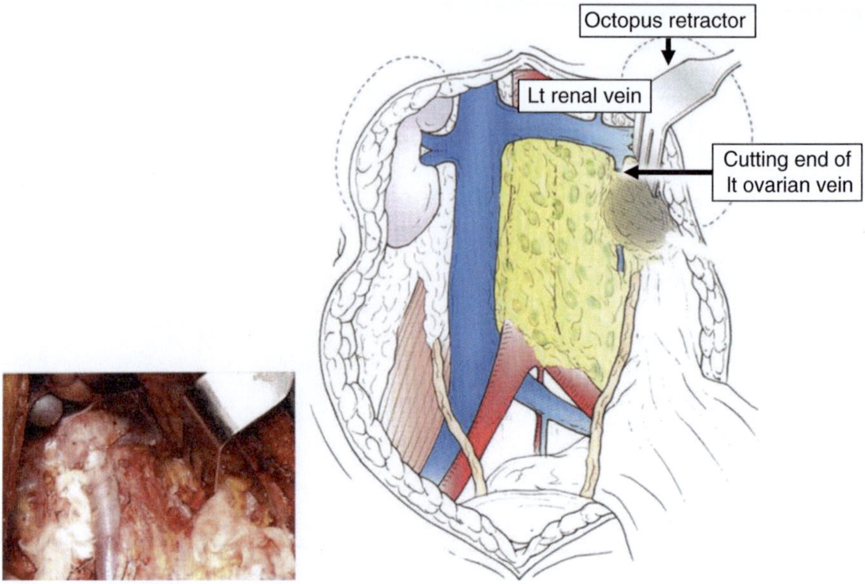

Fig. 13.11 Separation between Gerota's fascia on the left kidney and the fatty tissues in the left PAN dissection field (OGS NOW No.6 Surgery for Endometrial Cancer and Ovarian Cancer—Essential Procedures and Advanced Techniques for Tumor Progression). *Reprinted* by courtesy of Medical View and translated by Mikio Mikami. Then Gerota's fascia on the left kidney and the fatty tissues in the left PAN dissection field (above the inferior mesenteric artery, area 326B1) are separated (there is an easy dissection plane), and the left kidney is displaced laterally

with small gauze ball which allows for removal of the tissue posterior to the aorta (Fig. 13.14). Prior to removal of this lymphoid tissue, the adjacent lumbar veins should be ligated using an ultrasonic scalpel to provide a wide visual field. If ligation is not performed, lumbar veins may be torn when traction is applied to the vessels, and massive hemorrhage may occur. The sympathetic nerves which run toward the right and left sides of the spine near the iliopsoas muscle should be identified and preserved wherever possible.

13.6.5 Dissection Between the Abdominal Aorta and IVC

The abdominal aorta and IVC are displaced laterally in opposite directions through the use of forceps with small gauze ball or a finger. The lymphoid tissues between the aorta and IVC can then be removed while avoiding transection of the lumbar veins running transversely in this area. The proximal margin of tissue removal is immediately inferior to the origin of the right renal artery and extends down to the bifurcation into the left and right common iliac arteries (Fig. 13.16).

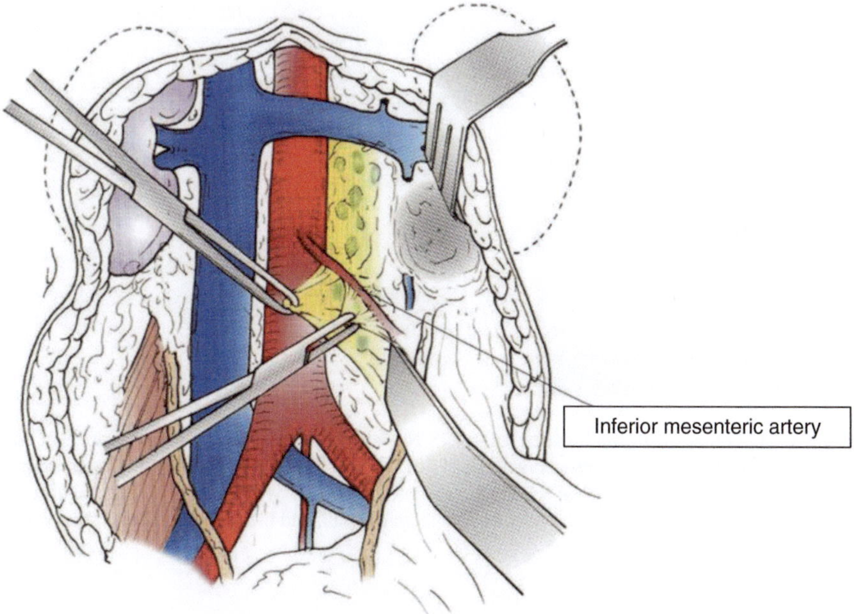

Fig. 13.12 Exposing the inferior mesenteric artery (OGS NOW No.6 Surgery for Endometrial Cancer and Ovarian Cancer—Essential Procedures and Advanced Techniques for Tumor Progression). *Reprinted* by courtesy of Medical View and translated by Mikio Mikami. There are many blood vessels in the region around the inferior mesenteric artery, and bleeding may occur easily. Therefore, the tissues surrounding the inferior mesenteric artery are resected using an ultrasonic scalpel.

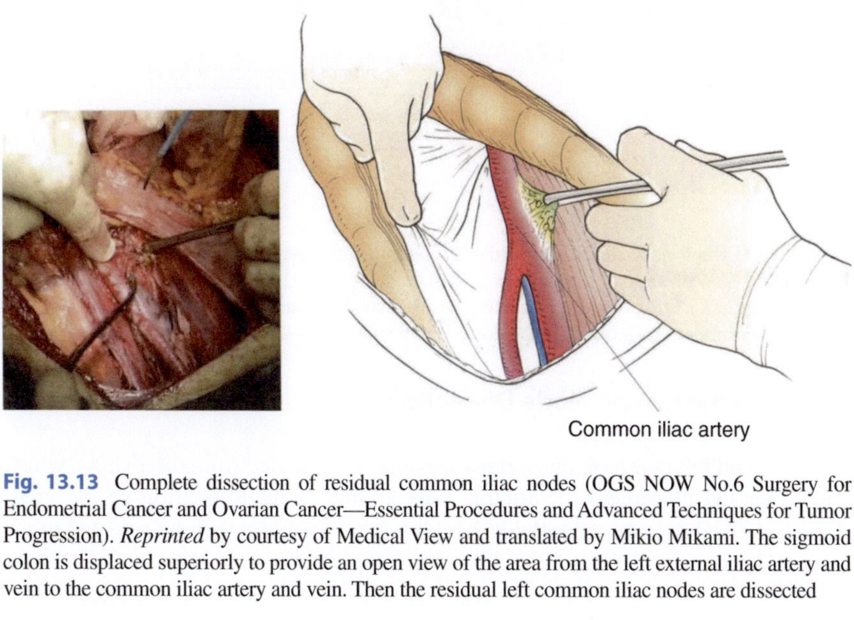

Fig. 13.13 Complete dissection of residual common iliac nodes (OGS NOW No.6 Surgery for Endometrial Cancer and Ovarian Cancer—Essential Procedures and Advanced Techniques for Tumor Progression). *Reprinted* by courtesy of Medical View and translated by Mikio Mikami. The sigmoid colon is displaced superiorly to provide an open view of the area from the left external iliac artery and vein to the common iliac artery and vein. Then the residual left common iliac nodes are dissected

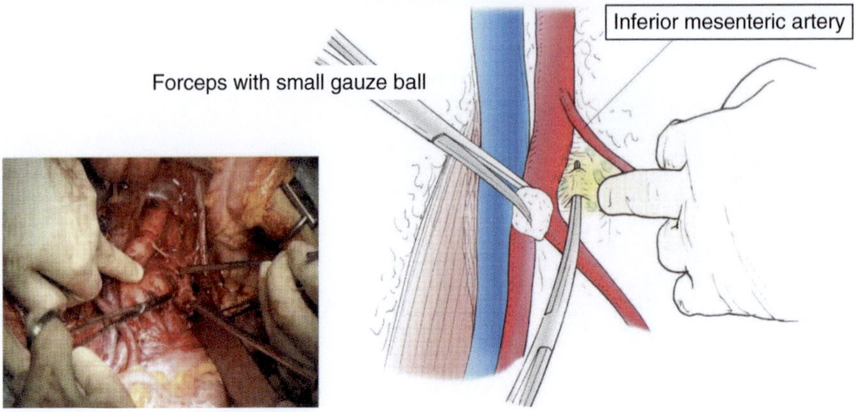

Fig. 13.14 Forceps with small gauze ball (OGS NOW No.6 Surgery for Endometrial Cancer and Ovarian Cancer—Essential Procedures and Advanced Techniques for Tumor Progression). *Reprinted* by courtesy of Medical View and translated by Mikio Mikami. The abdominal aorta is displaced to the right by using a forceps with small gauze ball, and tissues behind the aorta are also removed

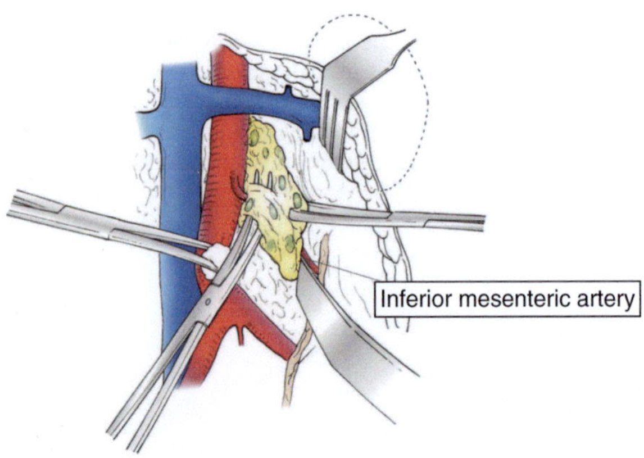

Fig. 13.15 Lymph node dissection of the left side of the aorta (OGS NOW No.6 Surgery for Endometrial Cancer and Ovarian Cancer—Essential Procedures and Advanced Techniques for Tumor Progression). *Reprinted* by courtesy of Medical View and translated by Mikio Mikami. Paraspinal tissues on the left side of the aorta are removed up to the origin of the left renal artery

13.6.6 Sacral Lymph Node Dissection

The right and left common iliac arteries should be separated from their veins, which allows for the placement of vascular tape around them. Retraction of the tapes (Fig. 13.17) exposes the underlying lymph nodes which can then be resected to the level of the sacrum.

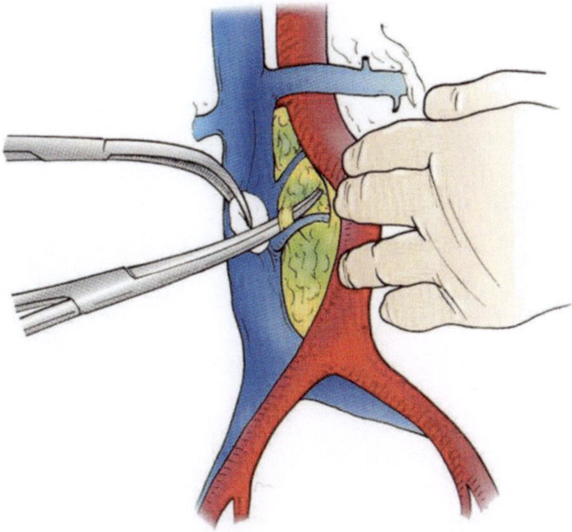

Fig. 13.16 Dissection between the abdominal aorta and inferior vena cava (OGS NOW No.6 Surgery for Endometrial Cancer and Ovarian Cancer—Essential Procedures and Advanced Techniques for Tumor Progression). *Reprinted* by courtesy of Medical View and translated by Mikio Mikami. The abdominal aorta and inferior vena cava are displaced laterally in opposite directions by using a forceps with small gaze ball or a finger, and the tissues between the aorta and vena cava are removed while paying attention to the lumbar veins running transversely

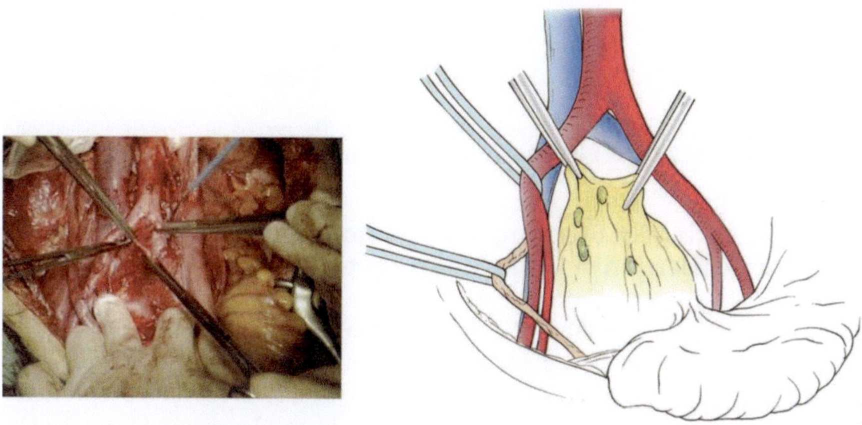

Fig. 13.17 Sacral lymph node dissection (OGS NOW No.6 Surgery for Endometrial Cancer and Ovarian Cancer—Essential Procedures and Advanced Techniques for Tumor Progression). *Reprinted* by courtesy of Medical View and translated by Mikio Mikami. The right and left common iliac arteries are separated from their veins by placing vascular tapes around the arteries and pulling on the tapes

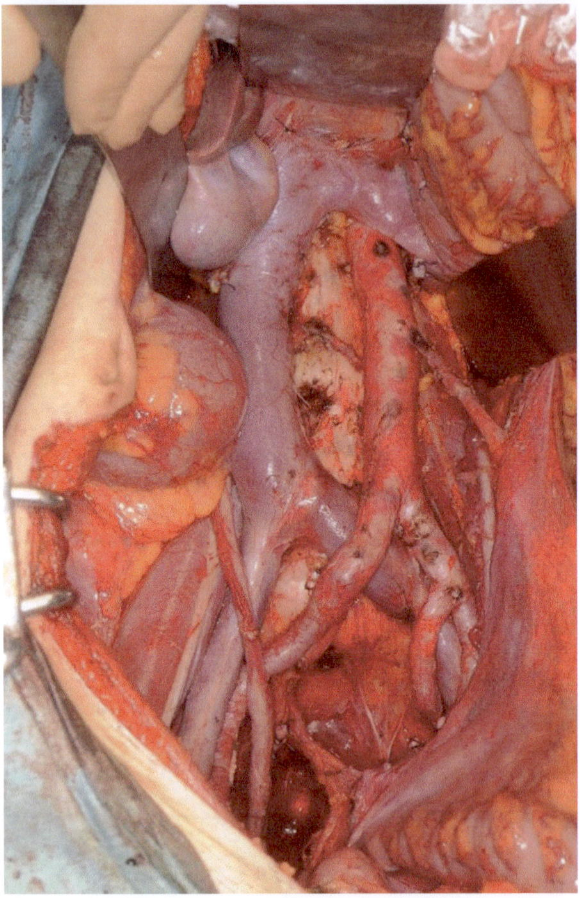

Fig. 13.18 Final view after the complete PAN dissection. The peritoneal cavity is washed with physiological saline, and checking is performed to confirm that bleeding has stopped

13.6.7 Checking for Bleeding, Intraperitoneal Irrigation, and Insertion of Drain/Measures to Prevent Adhesions

Following completion of the LND, the peritoneal cavity should be irrigated with physiological saline solution, checking to confirm hemostasis (Fig. 13.18). A drain is then inserted into the paravesical region, and the ileum and cecum are replaced to their normal anatomic position. The intestine should next be checked from the terminal ileum to the ligament of Treitz to ensure the absence of torsion. An adhesion prevention agent can then be applied to the common and external iliac arteries and veins prior to covering these vessels with the peritoneum. As the small intestine and the ascending colon have been fully mobilized, it is important to replace them to their correct anatomic position prior to abdominal closure.

13.6.8 Closure of the Abdomen

An adhesion prevention agent should be applied to the sutured sites of the peritoneum prior to closure of the abdomen. Obese patients have a higher risk of postoperative surgical wound dehiscence; therefore, it is recommended that a subcutaneous drain with continuous suction should be inserted after the subcutaneous tissues have been irrigated with physiological saline solution.

13.7 Surgical Morbidity

Recent reports suggest relatively low mortality and morbidity rates when type III radical hysterectomy is performed for early-stage cervical cancer. This includes intraoperative complications in 1–3%, grade 3–4 postoperative complications in 5.0–17%, and postoperative bladder dysfunction in 7.5–30% [20, 21]. However, the addition of PAN dissection to radical hysterectomy is associated with an increased risk of postoperative complications compared to radical hysterectomy alone. The combination of radical hysterectomy and PAN dissection with adjuvant radiotherapy further increases the risk of grade 3–4 postoperative complications to approximately 15% (JGOG1070S, Machida H, Matsuo K, Mikami M, et al., manuscript in preparation). Our study showed that adjuvant radiotherapy causes an increase in the incidence of adverse events such as lymphedema, ileus, and ureteral obstruction compared to adjuvant chemotherapy. The JGOG is currently launching a phase III clinical trial to compare postoperative CCRT with chemotherapy alone following radical hysterectomy for clinical stage IB–IIB cervical cancer (JGOG1082), and this trial will provide data regarding the effectiveness of adjuvant chemotherapy in high-risk patients with early-stage cervical cancer. The clinical implications of our results are that adjuvant chemotherapy may be used to avoid grade 3–4 complications of radical hysterectomy plus PAN dissection. We recently reported that both adjuvant radiotherapy-based therapy and chemotherapy alone have a comparable effect on survival of women with early-stage cervical cancer for both the high-risk and intermediate-risk groups [22–24].

13.8 Future Prospect

The current article provides a summary of our treatment strategy for cervical cancer patients with surgically removable primary tumor and suspected PAN metastasis. Preoperatively, we always perform a manual examination to determine the clinical tumor stage and surgical feasibility. Imaging studies are then performed to assess the tumor size, lymph nodes status, and the presence of distant metastasis. In the absence of PLN/PAN metastasis, local therapy either by definitive whole pelvic radiotherapy or surgery alone is generally sufficient curative treatment. If PLN size >1 cm is suspected, radical hysterectomy followed by PAN dissection is recommended. In such cases, complete resection of the cardinal ligament is also suggested. Postoperative adjuvant chemotherapy is then given in an attempt to avoid the complications from radiotherapy. Our proposed strategy is originally based on our experience with the treatment of a patient who underwent radical hysterectomy for cervical cancer approximately 20 years ago. This patient had widespread lymph node metastasis extending sequentially from the PLN to the PAN, and during the surgery, 48 metastatic lymph nodes were resected. Her disease was subsequently cured by adjuvant chemotherapy alone without the need for radiation. We also treated a patient with cancer of the uterine corpus who was cured by surgery without further treatment despite the presence of 102 lymph node metastases. Our strategy is founded on the concept that "some patients with lymph node metastasis can be cured by local treatment alone if the proximal limit of the involved lymph nodes is removable." We hope that surgeons will adopt our proposed strategy for patients with disease metastatic to the PLN >1 cm in the resected specimen. In the future, we hope that a prospective trial will be conducted to demonstrate the true value of the additional PAN dissection during radical hysterectomy for stage IB–IIB cervical cancer.

Acknowledgment We thank Dr. Brendan H. Grubbs for his scientific input for this chapter.

References

1. Ramirez PT, Jhingran A, Macapinlac HA, Euscher ED, Munsell MF, Coleman RL, et al. Laparoscopic extraperitoneal para-aortic lymphadenectomy in locally advanced cervical cancer: a prospective correlation of surgical findings with positron emission tomography/computed tomography findings. Cancer. 2011;117:1928–34.
2. Cosin JA, Fowler JM, Chen MD, Paley PJ, Carson LF, Twiggs LB. Pretreatment surgical staging of patients with cervical carcinoma : the case for lymph node debulking. Cancer. 1998;82:2241–8.
3. Brockbank E, Kokka F, Bryant A, Pomel C, Reynolds K. Pre-treatment surgical para-aortic lymph node assessment in locally advanced cervical cancer. Cochrane Database Syst Rev. 2013;3:CD008217.
4. Cervical Cancer Guideline (Version 1.2017). NCCN Clinical Practice Guidelines in Oncology http://www.nccn.org/professionals/physician_gls/PDF/cervical.pdf
5. Gouy S, Morice P, Narducci F, Uzan C, Gilmore J, Kolesnikov-Gauthier H, et al. Nodal-staging surgery for locally advanced cervical cancer in the era of PET. Lancet Oncol. 2012;13:e212–20.
6. Gold MA, Tian C, Whitney CW, Rose PG, Lanciano R. Surgical versus radiographic determination of para-aortic lymph node metastases before chemoradiation for locally advanced cervical carcinoma : a Gynecologic Oncology Group Study. Cancer. 2008;112:1954–63.
7. Mikami M, Aoki Y, Sakamoto M, Shimada M, Takeshima N, Fujiwara H, et al. Surgical principles for managing stage IB2,IIA2, and IIB uterine cervical cancer (Bulky Tumors) in Japan: a survey of the Japanese Gynecologic Oncology Group. Int J Gynecol Cancer. 2014;24:1333–40.
8. Gouy S, Morice P, Narducci F, Uzan C, Martinez A, Rey A, et al. Prospective multicenter study evaluating the survival of patients with locally advanced cervical cancer undergoing laparoscopic paraaortic lymphadenectomy before chemoradiotherapy in the era of positron emission tomography imaging. J Clin Oncol. 2013;31:3026–33.
9. Sakuragi N. Up-to-date management of lymph node metastasis and the role of tailored lymphadenectomy in cervical cancer. Int J Clin Oncol. 2007;12(3):165–75.

10. Gil-Moreno A, Magrina JF, Perez-Benavente A, Diaz-Feijoo B, Sanchez-Iglesias JL, Garcia A, Cabrera-Diaz S, Puig O, Martinez-Gomez X, Xercavins J. Location of aortic node metastases in locally advanced cervical cancer. Gynecol Oncol. 2012;125:312–4.
11. Benedetti-Panici P, Maneschi F, Scambia G, Greggi S, Cutillo G, D'Andrea G, Rabitti C, Coronetta F, Capelli A, Mancuso S. Lymphatic spread of cervical cancer: an anatomical and pathological study based on 225 radical hysterectomies with systematic pelvic and aortic lymphadenectomy. Gynecol Oncol. 1996;62:19–24.
12. Morice P, Castaigne D, Pautier P, Rey A, Haie-Meder C, Leblanc M, Duvillard P. Interest of pelvic and paraaortic lymphadenectomy in patients with stage IB and II cervical carcinoma. Gynecol Oncol. 1999;73:106–10.
13. Kim PY, Monk BJ, Chabra S, Burger RA, Vasilev SA, Manetta A, DiSaia PJ, Berman ML. Cervical cancer with paraaortic metastases: significance of residual paraaortic disease after surgical staging. Gynecol Oncol. 1998;69:243–7.
14. Vale C, Tierney JF, Stewart LA, Brady M, Dinshaw K, Jakobsen A, Parmar MK, Thomas G, Trimble T, Alberts DS, Chen H, Cikaric S, Eifel PJ, Garipagaoglu M, Keys H, Kantardzic N, Lal P, Lanciano R, Leborgne F, Lorvidhaya V, Onishi H, Pearcey RG, Pras E, Roberts K, Rose PG, Thomas G, Whitney CW, Chemoradiotherapy for Cervical Cancer Meta-Analysis Collaboration. Reducing uncertainties about the effects of chemoradiotherapy for cervical cancer: a systematic review and meta-analysis of individual patient data from 18 randomized trials. J Clin Oncol. 2008;26(35):5802–12. https://doi.org/10.1200/JCO.2008.16.4368.
15. Kuji S, Hirashima Y, Komeda S, Tanaka A, Abe M, Takahashi N, Takekuma M, Asakura H, Harada H, Nishimura T. Feasibility of extended-field irradiation and intracavitary brachytherapy combined with weekly cisplatin chemosensitization for IB2-IIIB cervical cancer with positive paraaortic or high common iliac lymph nodes: a retrospective review. Int J Clin Oncol. 2014;19(2):341–7. https://doi.org/10.1007/s10147-013-0551-8.
16. Matsuo K, Shimada M, Saito T, Takehara K, Tokunaga H, Watanabe Y, Todo Y, Morishige K, Mikami M, Sugiyama T. Risk stratification models for para-aortic lymph node metastasis and recurrence in stage IB-IIB cervical cancer. J Gynecol Oncol. 2018;29(1):e11. https://doi.org/10.3802/jgo.2018.29.e11.
17. Ebina Y, Yaegashi N, Katabuchi H, Nagase S, Udagawa Y, Hachisuga T, Saito T, Mikami M, Aoki Y, Yoshikawa H. Japan Society of Gynecologic Oncology guidelines 2011 for the treatment of uterine cervical cancer. Int J Clin Oncol. 2015;20:240–8.
18. Matsuo K, Grubbs BH, Mikami M. Quality and quantity metrics of pelvic lymph node metastasis and risk of para-aortic lymph node metastasis in stage IB-IIB cervical cancer. J Gynecol Oncol. 2018;29(1):e10. https://doi.org/10.3802/jgo.2018.29.e10.
19. Fleming ND, Frumovitz M, Schmeler KM, dos Reis R, Munsell MF, Eifel PJ, et al. Significance of lymph node ratio in defining risk category in node-positive early stage cervical cancer. Gynecol Oncol. 2015;136:48–53.
20. Pikaart DP, Holloway RW, Ahmad S, et al. Clinical-pathologic and morbidity analyses of Types 2 and 3 abdominal radical hysterectomy for cervical cancer. Gynecol Oncol. 2007;107:205–10.
21. Landoni F, Maneo A, Zapardiel I, Zanagnolo V, Mangioni C. Class I versus class III radical hysterectomy in stage IB1-IIA cervical cancer. A prospective randomized study. Eur J Surg Oncol. 2012;38:203–9.
22. Matsuo K, Shimada M, Aoki Y, Sakamoto M, Takeshima N, Fujiwara H, Matsumoto T, Mikami M, Sugiyama T. Comparison of adjuvant therapy for node-positive clinical stage IB-IIB cervical cancer: Systemic chemotherapy versus pelvic irradiation. Int J Cancer. 2017;141:1042–51.
23. Matsuo K, Shimada M, Yokota H, Satoh T, Katabuchi H, Kodama S, Sasaki H, Matsumura N, Mikami M, Sugiyama T. Effectiveness of adjuvant systemic chemotherapy for intermediate-risk stage IB cervical cancer. Oncotarget. 2017;15(8):106866–75.
24. Matoda M, Takeshima N, Michimae H, Iwata T, Yokota H, Torii Y, Yamamoto Y, Takehara K, Nishio S, Takano H, Mizuno M, Takahashi Y, Takei Y, Hasegawa T, Mikami M, Enomoto T, Aoki D, Sugiyama T. Postoperative chemotherapy for node-positive cervical cancer: results of a multicenter phase II trial (JGOG1067). Gynecol Oncol. 2018;149(3):513–9. https://doi.org/10.1016/j.ygyno.2018.04.009. Epub ahead of print, PMID: 29661497.

14 Laparoscopic Pelvic Exenteration for Recurrent Cervical Cancer

Hiroyuki Kanao and Nobuhiro Takeshima

Abstract

For locally advanced cervical carcinoma, the concurrent chemoradiotherapy (CCRT) ± surgery is the standard treatment. However, in some cases, even this multimodal therapy cannot prevent the recurrence, and almost 3000 women die from the cervical carcinoma every year in our country. Therefore, the treatment for the recurrent cervical cancer after CCRT is a big issue.

When the recurrent mass is localized in a pelvic cavity, a complete surgery, such as pelvic exenteration, is the most promising. However, the previous surgery and CCRT create severe adhesion and fibrosis in the pelvis, which complicates the complete tumor excision and causes the morbidity and mortality of this operation to be very high. Recently, laparoscopic pelvic exenteration is established as technically feasible, and the rate of this morbidity and mortality assumes to be low compared with an open procedure, because of the advantage of laparoscopy, better visualization, and meticulous dissection.

Keywords

Recurrent cervical cancer · CCRT · Laparoscopic pelvic exenteration · LEER

14.1 Background

Concurrent chemoradiotherapy (CCRT) is now regarded as the standard treatment for locally advanced cervical carcinoma, but this multimodal approach does not prevent recurrence. The risk of recurrence increases with increases in FIGO (International Federation of Gynecology and Obstetrics) stage and is approximately

H. Kanao (✉) · N. Takeshima
Cancer Institute Hospital, Koutou-ku, Tokyo, Japan
e-mail: hiroyuki.kanao@jfcr.or.jp

M. Mikami (ed.), *Surgery for Gynecologic Cancer*, Comprehensive Gynecology and Obstetrics, https://doi.org/10.1007/978-981-13-1519-0_14

10% for patients with stage IB disease, 17% for those with stage IIA disease, 23% for those with stage IIB disease, 42% for those with stage III disease, and 74% for those with stage IV disease [1].

When recurrence is within the original field of radiation, treatment options are limited. Re-irradiation, i.e., delivery of radiation to the field that https://rdcu.be/1I6bt was previously radiated, is contraindicated because of the possibility of severe adverse effects, and chemotherapy seems to be ineffective because previously irradiated tissue is not well vascularized [2]. Surgery is often the only option for previously irradiated recurrent cervical cancer, and the most significant prognostic factor is whether the resection margins are clear [3]. Marnitz et al. reported that postoperative survival at 2 years drops from 55.2% when margins are negative to 10.2% when margins are positive [2]. Some authors have reported that survival of patients with one or more positive margins falls to 0% after 3 years [4].

Pelvic exenteration is indicated for selected cases of cervical cancer that recurs centrally after CCRT. Pelvic exenteration is used to achieve complete resection with negative margins. Pelvic exenteration for centrally recurrent cervical cancer was described in 1948 by Dr. Alexander Brunschwig [5]. However, he received numerous criticisms due to high mortality and morbidity rates associated with the procedure in general and to doubts about the therapeutic efficacy of the procedure in such cases. After the procedure was first described, many authors reported on its technical feasibility and oncologic outcome, and it gained widespread acceptance. Reports published within the past 20 years have documented a 5-year survival rate of 35.4% [1]. However, morbidity associated with this procedure is close to 70%. Early surgical complications include a large blood loss volume, sepsis, thromboembolic accidents, and pulmonary complications [1]. Pelvic exenteration of recurrent cervical carcinoma involves previously irradiated tissue; therefore, the risk of anastomotic leakage, poor wound healing, and/or ureter and bowel obstruction increases. Long-term morbidity associated with pelvic exenteration includes but is not limited to disorders such as chronic and recurrent urinary infection, urinary tract and bowel obstruction, pyelonephritis, renal insufficiency, loss of sexual function, and pouch stones. Over the past 20 years, close to 1000 pelvic exenterations for advanced/recurrent gynecologic malignancies have been reported, and the reported intraoperative mortality rate is 4.5% [1].

Because of the technical feasibility and good oncologic outcomes, pelvic exenteration has become the treatment of choice for centrally recurrent previously irradiated cervical carcinoma.

14.2 Classification of Pelvic Exenteration

Pelvic exenteration as described by Alexander Brunschwig was originally classified into three types: anterior pelvic exenteration, posterior pelvic exenteration, and total pelvic exenteration [5]. Anterior pelvic exenteration removes the entire bladder, uterus, and vagina and is performed when the tumor invades the bladder.

Posterior pelvic exenteration removes the rectum, uterus, and vagina and is performed when the tumor invades the rectum. Total pelvic exenteration removes the entire bladder, rectum, uterus, and vagina and is performed when the tumor invades the bladder and rectum. Although this classification system is commonly used, the extent of surgical resection is unclear—whether anterior pelvic exenteration includes resection of the urethra, whether posterior pelvic exenteration includes resection of the anal canal, and whether resection of the vagina is total or partial, for example.

For further clarification, Magrina and colleagues classified pelvic exenteration in relation to the levator ani muscle as supralevator pelvic exenteration, infralevator pelvic exenteration, and infralevator pelvic exenteration plus vulvectomy [6, 7]. We use the Magrina et al. classification system to guide the discussion below of laparoscopic pelvic exenteration for recurrent cervical cancer.

14.3 Laparoscopy vs. Laparotomy

Laparoscopy optimizes visualization and thus provides for meticulous dissection. Laparoscopic pelvic exenteration has become an option for treatment of recurrent cervical carcinoma. Iavazzo et al. [8] reviewed laparoscopic pelvic exenteration and compared the advantages and disadvantages of the procedure against those of open surgery. They reported that laparoscopic exenteration seems to result in minimal intraoperative blood loss, minimal intraoperative complications, fewer postoperative complications, a shorter hospital stay, and better cosmesis. Although laparoscopic exenterations have been limited in number and longer follow-up periods are needed to compare late postoperative complications and overall survival between the laparoscopic and open procedures, the authors concluded that laparoscopic pelvic exenteration is a valid option for recurrent cervical cancer. These advantages have led us to apply laparoscopic pelvic exenteration to cases of previously irradiated centrally recurrent cervical cancer.

14.4 Preoperative Evaluation

Microscopically margin-negative resection (R0 resection) of recurrent cervical cancer is essential. Therefore, evaluating the extent of the recurrence, whether the adjacent organs are involved or the pelvic sidewall is involved, is essential to determining whether and which type of pelvic exenteration is indicated.

14.4.1 Evaluation of Local Disease

Preoperative determination of the extent of tumor spread has traditionally involved clinical examination of the patient under general anesthesia and endoscopic evaluation of the bladder and rectum. This type of evaluation is somewhat costly, and there is a risk of complications. Magnetic resonance imaging (MRI) or computed tomography (CT) is often performed to evaluate the extent of tumor spread. According to Rockall et al., MRI is more sensitive than CT for detecting spread to the bladder, rectum, parametrium, and/or lymph nodes, and they concluded that an MRI scoring system can be used to predict absence of bladder or rectal invasion with sufficient confidence to safely obviate the need for invasive cystoscopic or endoscopic staging in the majority of patients with cervical cancer [9]. This may also reduce staging costs and morbidity. Forner et al. analyzed the usefulness of preoperative MRI for identifying uninvolved surgical margins and reported a sensitivity of 85%, specificity of 52%, positive predictive value of 60%, and negative predictive value of 80%, but they concluded that surgical outcomes cannot be predicted with sufficient accuracy [10]. Jurado et al. reported resectability of approximately a third of centrally recurrent cervical cancers judged unresectable on the basis of clinical examination and imaging [11]. This is not surprising in patients who have been previously treated primarily with chemoradiation or surgery followed by adjuvant radiation because the fibrotic changes produced in the pelvic tissues are often misjudged as recurrent tumor, and these kinds of changes can be difficult to distinguish even when sophisticated imaging techniques are used. MRI is an appropriate imaging modality for assessment of the extent of tumor spread, but MRI is not always adequate, and traditional preoperative evaluation (clinical examination under general anesthesia and endoscopic evaluation of the tumor spread) is necessary in some cases.

14.4.2 Evaluation of Distant Disease

When the recurrent cervical cancer has spread beyond the local area, pelvic exenteration is not appropriate because this situation points to systemic disease. Therefore, identification of distant disease is very important in determining whether pelvic exenteration is indicated.

Positron emission tomography (PET)-CT has been shown to be superior to both MRI and CT for evaluation of distant metastasis [12]. Husain et al. reported 100% sensitivity, 73% specificity, a positive predictive value of 55%, and a negative predictive value of 100% of PET-CT for detection of distant metastases [13]. In a meta-analysis of reports that covered 1757 patients, PET-CT was found to have a sensitivity of 90% and specificity of 99% in detecting distant metastases in patients with recurrent cervical cancer and was thus shown to be valuable for assessment of recurrent cervical cancer [14].

R0 resection is the strongest prognostic factor for postoperative survival of patients with recurrent cervical cancer; thus, evaluating resectability of the recurrent tumor is important for determining the surgical indication and avoiding pelvic exenteration in cases of unresectable disease. MRI and PET-CT can provide precise information about the extent of recurrent cervical cancer, including distant metastasis, and these two imaging modalities used in combination are the standard upon which the surgical indication is determined.

14.5 Techniques

When pelvic exenteration is applied to cervical carcinoma, the patient has already undergone CCRT, and thus almost all pelvic exenterations involve the previously irradiated field. Because the pelvic anatomy in the previously irradiated field is usually distorted as a result of severe adhesion and fibrosis, the pelvic exenteration procedure performed for recurrent cervical carcinoma is very complicated. The procedure is described below in the context of three different tumor types. Only the third example is of a recurrent cervical carcinoma after CCRT; the first two examples, which are not of cervical carcinoma, are given to clarify details of the operative procedure.

14.5.1 Supralevator Anterior Pelvic Exenteration for a Recurrent Low-Grade Endometrial Stromal Sarcoma (LGESS)

14.5.1.1 Case

The patient had undergone abdominal hysterectomy for what was assumed to be a leiomyoma but was determined by pathologic examination of the surgical specimen to be an LGESS. Almost 20 years later, a recurrent LGESS was detected at the vaginal stump, and the patient underwent several rounds of chemotherapy and hormonal therapy. These treatments were inefficacious, and the tumor progressed. Abdominal CT revealed that the recurrent tumor occupied the left vaginal stump and extended to the bladder, vagina, and left pelvic sidewall; the left ureter was also involved (Fig. 14.1). To achieve complete resection with negative margins, supralevator anterior pelvic exenteration including creation of an ileal conduit was planned.

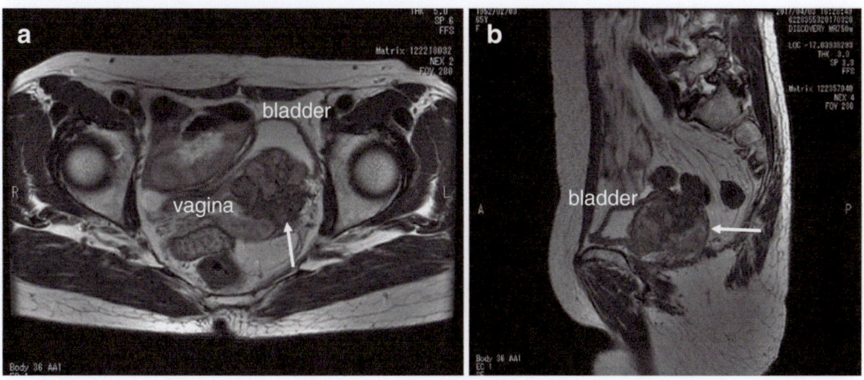

Fig. 14.1 Preoperative MRI of recurrent low-grade endometrial stromal sarcoma (LGESS). (**a**) Transverse; (**b**) Sagittal. The recurrent tumor (←) occupied the left vaginal stump and extended to the bladder, vagina, and left pelvic sidewall. The left ureter was also involved

14.5.1.2 Operative Procedure

Mobilization of the Rectum

The retroperitoneal space around the rectum was widely dissected, and the rectum was mobilized. An avascular space between the mesorectal fascia and the presacral fascia was dissected and developed. Because the patient had not undergone radiation therapy, there was no fibrosis, so the procedure was very easy. The inferior hypogastric nerves and the pelvic nerve plexus around the rectum were easily identified during the dissection and easily transected. (In cases of anterior pelvic exenteration, it is not necessary to consider postoperative bladder function.) The dissection was continued around the rectum down to the levator ani muscle, and the rectum was lifted toward the opposite side for creation of the surgical field (Fig. 14.2).

Dissection of the Ureter (Fig. 14.3)

The recurrent mass involved the left ureter, and left hydronephrosis was found. The left ureter was identified at its entrance into the pelvic cavity, dissection was performed around the ureter down to the bladder, and the ureter was transected. A temporary urinary stent was placed to preserve left renal function during the operation.

Detachment of the Tumor from the Pelvic Sidewall

The recurrent tumor involved the internal iliac artery and vein and was fixed to the pelvic sidewall. To detach the tumor from the pelvic sidewall, the internal iliac

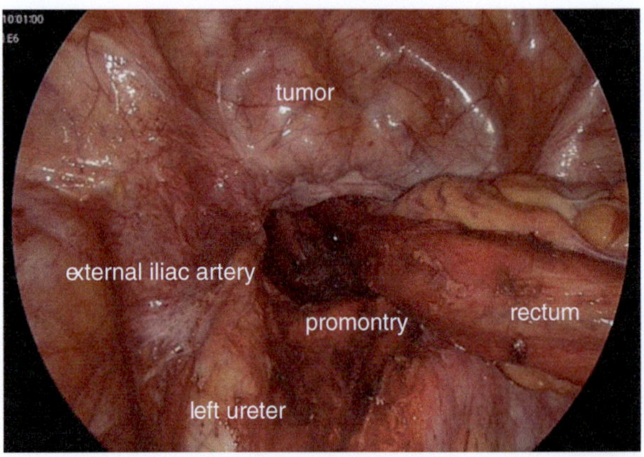

Fig. 14.2 The anatomical location of the tumor. The retroperitoneal space around the rectum was widely dissected, and the rectum was mobilized

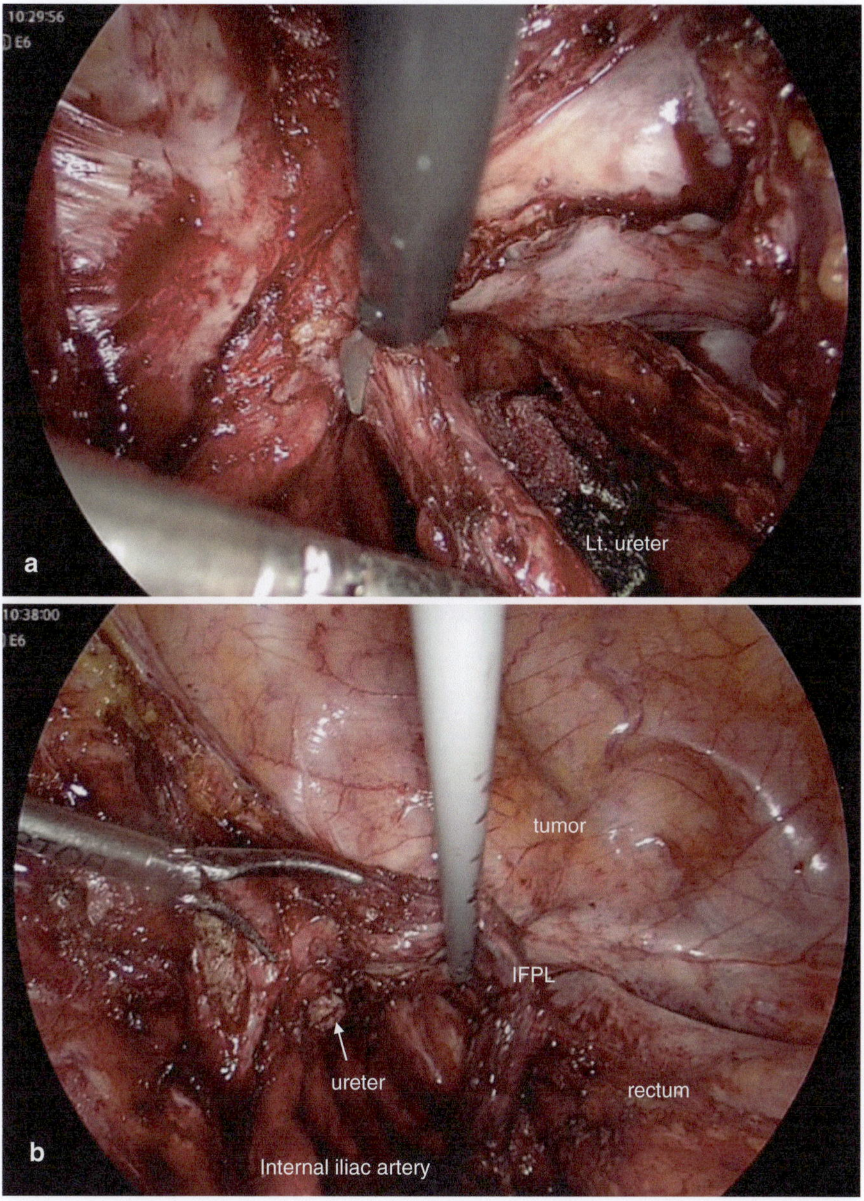

Fig. 14.3 (**a**) The transection of the left ureter. (**b**) After the transection of the ureter. *IFPL* infundibulopelvic ligament

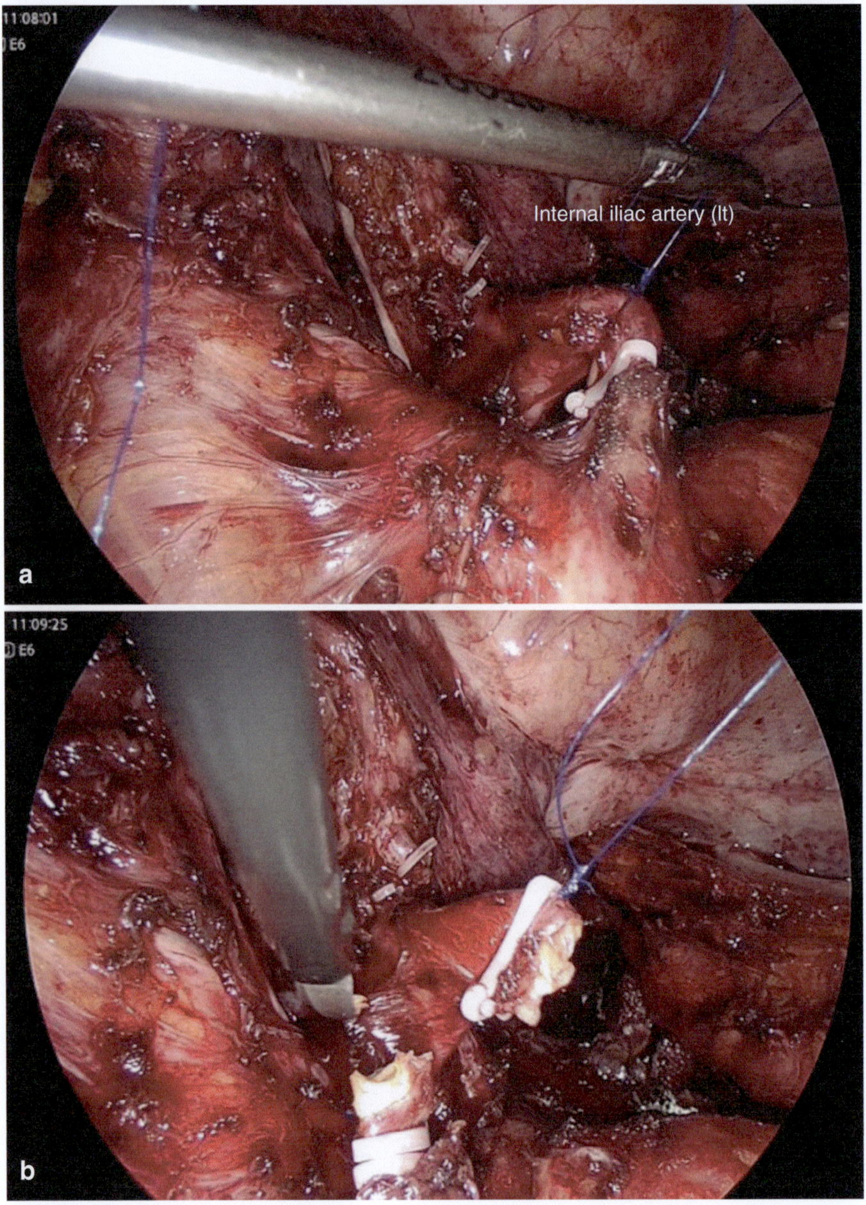

Fig. 14.4 (**a**) Hemoclips placed on the internal iliac artery. (**b**) The transection of the internal iliac artery

artery was transected with 10 mm hemoclips (Fig. 14.4). After transection of the left internal iliac artery, its branches to the pelvic sidewall (e.g., the superior gluteal artery) were clipped and transected. (The central segment of this artery must be transected before transection of the peripheral branches, whereas the peripheral branches of the internal iliac vein must be transected before transection of the central segment.) The tumor extended to the inferior piriform foramen, so the

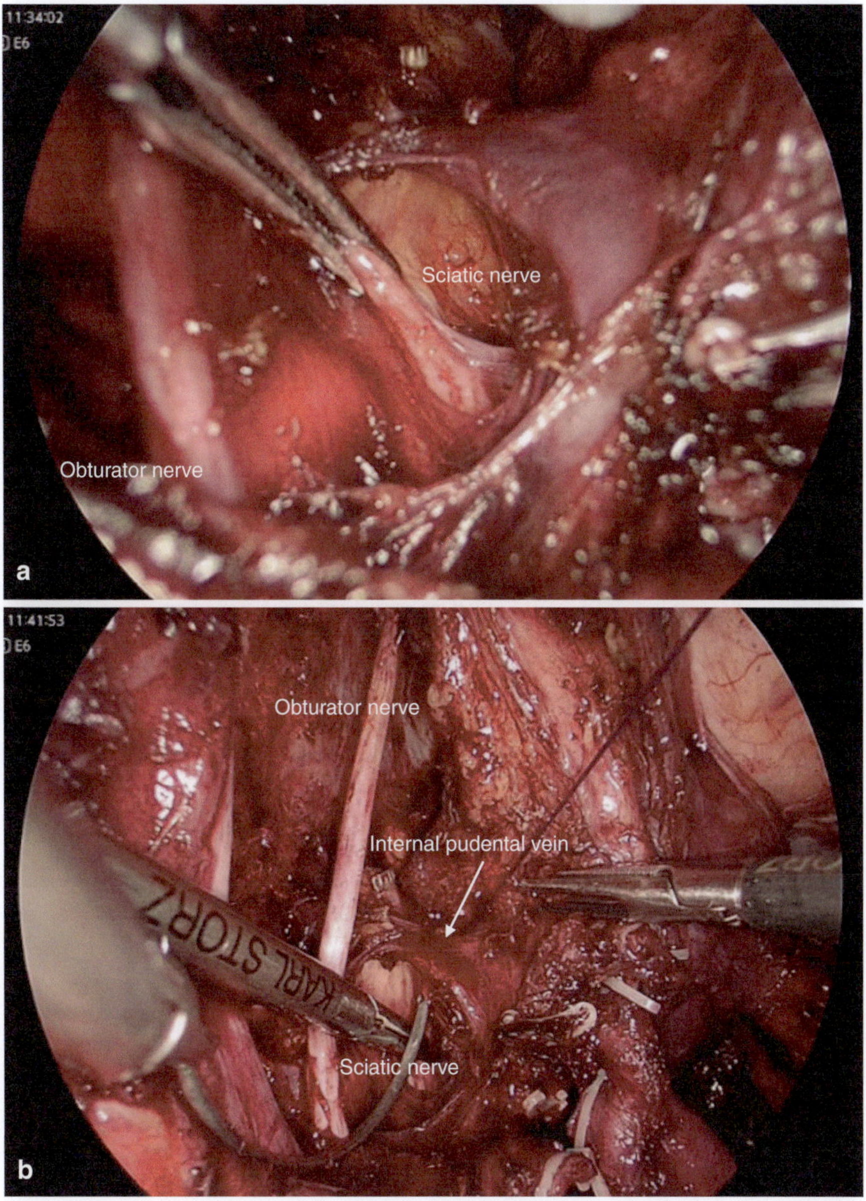

Fig. 14.5 (**a**) Sciatic nerve (lt). (**b**) The ligation of the lt. internal pudendal vein

dissection was continued to the inferior piriform foramen, where the sciatic nerve was identified (Fig. 14.5a). During pelvic exenteration, two structures must be preserved: the external iliac artery and the sciatic nerve. The sciatic nerve is very close to the cardinal ligament, and gynecologic malignancy often involves this nerve. Thus, it is very important to identify the sciatic nerve during pelvic exenteration. After isolation of the sciatic nerve, the internal pudendal vessels were ligated and transected at the inferior piriform foramen. The close proximity between the sciatic nerve and internal pudendal vessels at the internal pudendal foramen is seen in Fig. 14.5b. After transection of the internal pudendal vein (a peripheral vein), the internal iliac vein (a central vein) was safely transected (Fig. 14.6). At this stage, the tumor was detached from the pelvic sidewall (Fig. 14.7).

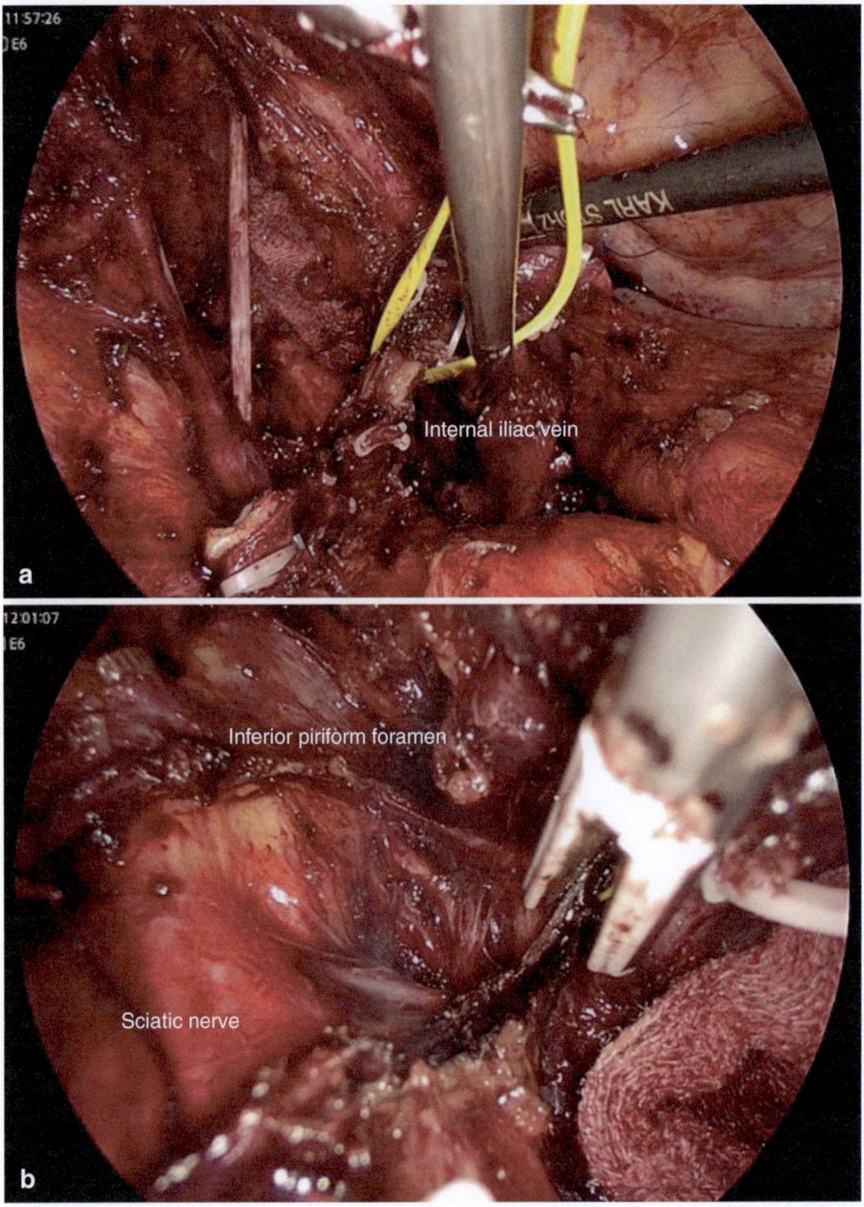

Fig. 14.6 The transection of the internal iliac vein. (**a**) Isolation of the internal iliac vein. (**b**) Transection of the internal iliac vein

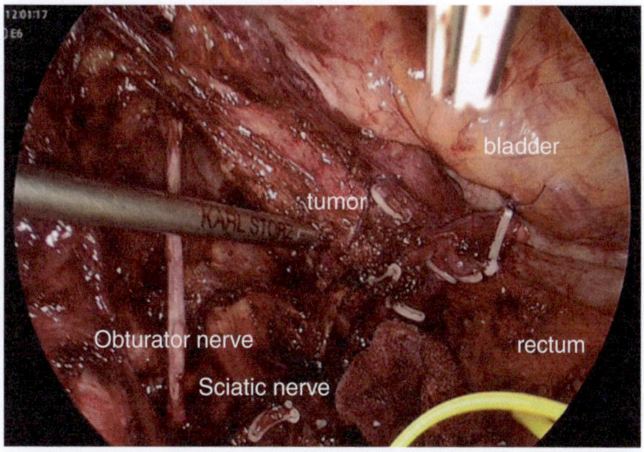

Fig. 14.7 The tumor was detached from the pelvic sidewall

Development of the Prevesical Space (Fig. 14.8)
The prevesical space, which is an avascular area, was dissected and developed widely. The bladder was then detached from the pubic bone, and the urethra was easily identified. The adipose tissue was dissected around the urethra, and the dorsal vein complex was exposed. The dorsal vein complex was ligated and transected at the level of the levator ani muscle. (The dorsal vein complex is not as well developed in females as it is in males, and it can be transected without ligation when a vessel sealing device is used.) Note that after the bladder is detached from the pubic bone, a good operative view is very difficult to obtain, so detaching the bladder should be the final procedural step.

Transection of the Vagina and the Surgical Specimen
After the urethra was transected, the vagina was transected at the same level (Fig. 14.9).

The final intraoperative view is shown in Fig. 14.10. It is important to understand the anatomical position of the sciatic nerve, which is a key anatomical structure in the performance of pelvic exenteration. The surgical specimen is shown in Fig. 14.11. Complete R0 resection was achieved without complications.

(For surgical creation of an ileal conduit, please refer to a urology textbook.)

14.5.2 Infralevator Pelvic Exenteration plus Vulvectomy for a Rectal Carcinoma with Pagetoid Spread

14.5.2.1 Case
The patient presented with intractable itching and erythema in the perineal region. Multiple skin biopsies revealed Paget's disease, which had infiltrated the urethra, vagina, vulva, and anal canal. In addition, rectal cancer was detected by colonofiberscopy, so rectal carcinoma with pagetoid spread was diagnosed, and infralevator total pelvic exenteration and vulvectomy were performed.

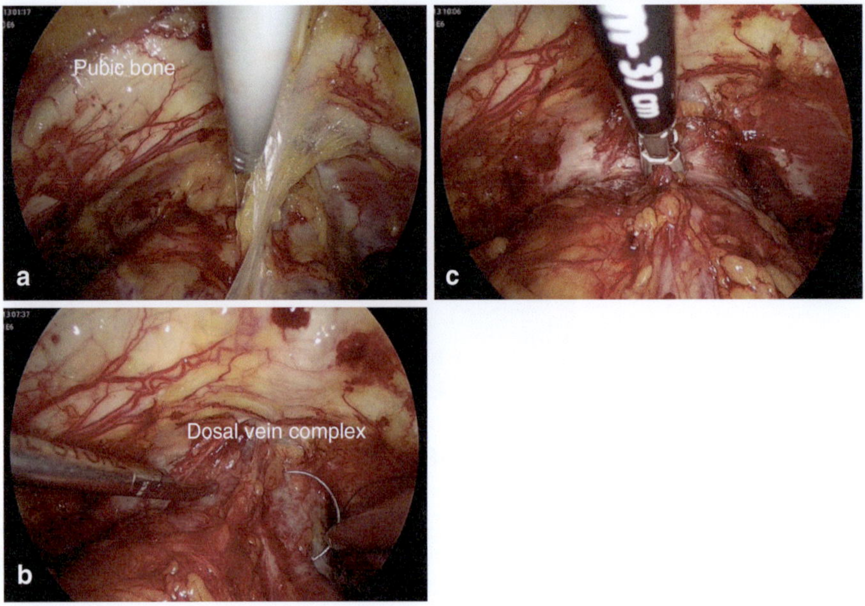

Fig. 14.8 Dissection of the prevesical space. (**a**) Exposure of the urethra. (**b**) Ligation of the dorsal vein complex. (**c**) Transection of the urethra

14.5.2.2 Operative Procedure

Dissection down to the levator ani muscle was similar to that described above. The subsequent steps were as follows:

Dissection of the Ischiorectal Fossa (Fig. 14.12)

Because the tumor had not invaded the levator ani muscle, dissection included the ischiorectal fossa which was reached by excision of the pubococcygeal muscle. This is considered the best way because, of the levator ani muscles, the pubococcygeal muscle is most easily identified due to its anatomical location. In this case, the ischiorectal fossa was developed by transection of the pubococcygeal muscle. The ischiorectal fossa is a fat-filled space, so, it is very easy to dissect and expand this space with a vessel sealing device. Dissecting and developing this space as extensively as possible laparoscopically are essential to safe and smooth performance of infralevator exenteration with vulvectomy.

Perineal Approach (Vulvectomy) (Fig. 14.13)

After laparoscopic development of the ischiorectal fossa, an incision was placed in the vulva in accordance with the preoperative skin mapping, and the underlying tissue was dissected in line with the laparoscopic incision. The ischiorectal fossa was easily reached in this manner. (If dissection of the ischiorectal fossa is inadequate,

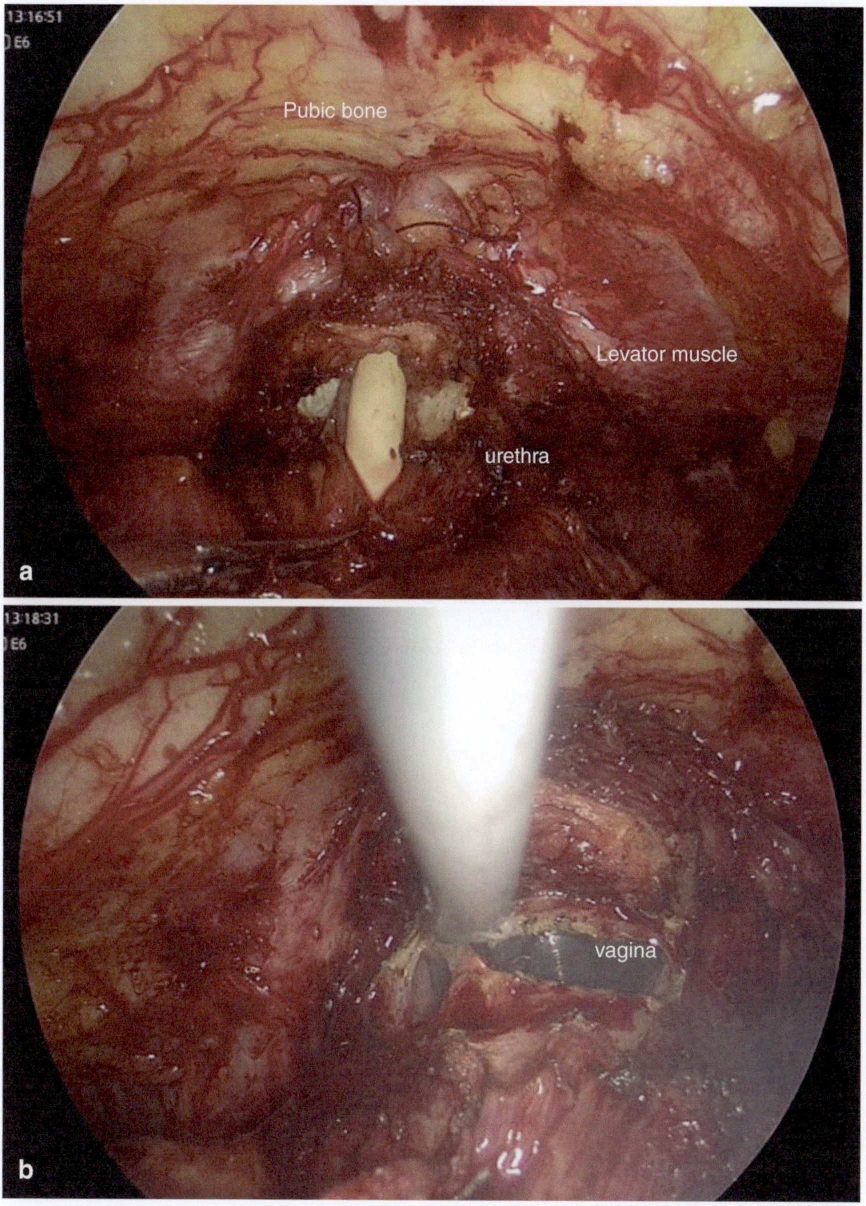

Fig. 14.9 (**a**) Transection of the urethra at the level of levator ani muscle. (**b**) Transection of the vagina

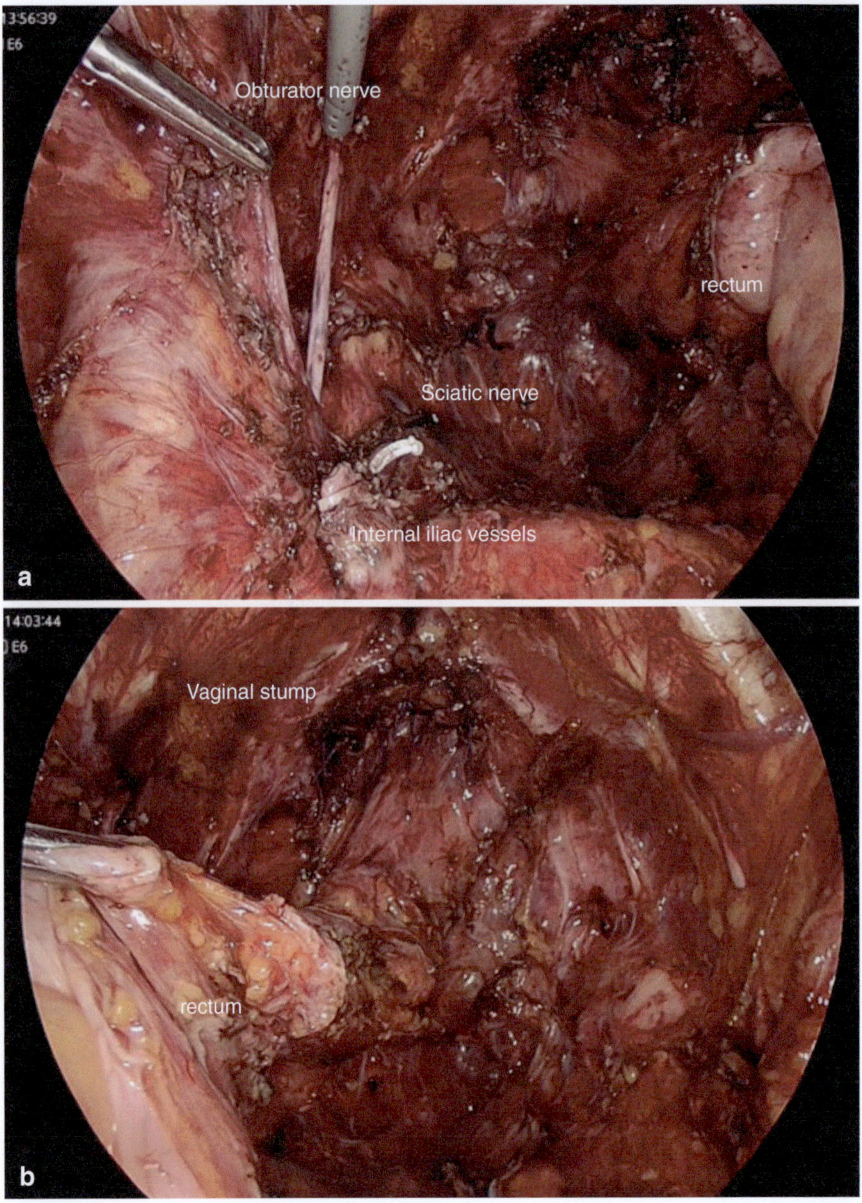

Fig. 14.10 Final intraoperative view. (**a**) Left pelvic sidewall. (**b**) Right pelvic sidewall

reaching the space by perineal approach is very difficult and time-consuming.) The surgical specimens were extracted via the vulvar incision. R0 en bloc resection of the pelvic organs was achieved.

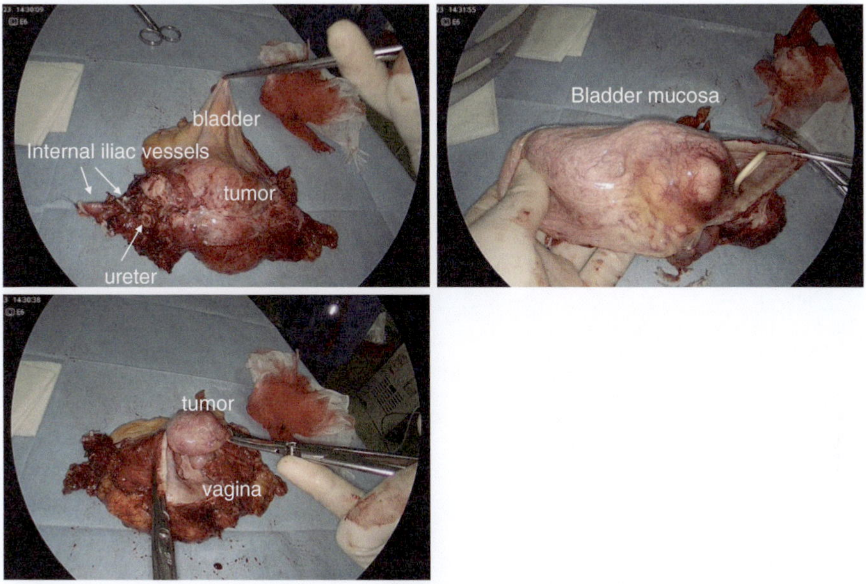

Fig. 14.11 Surgical specimen. R0 resection could be achieved

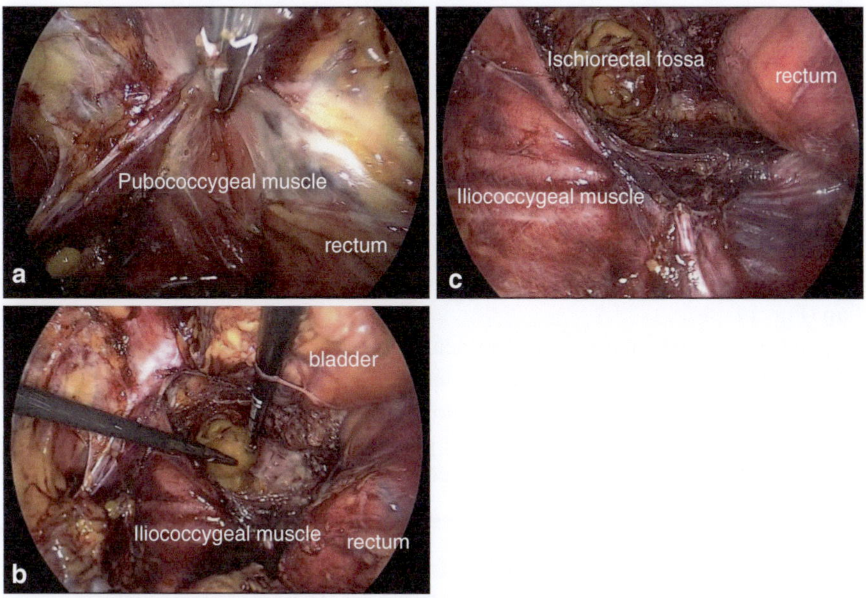

Fig. 14.12 Ischiorectal fossa. (**a**) Transection of the pubococcygeal muscle. (**b** and **c**) The development of the ischiorectal fossa

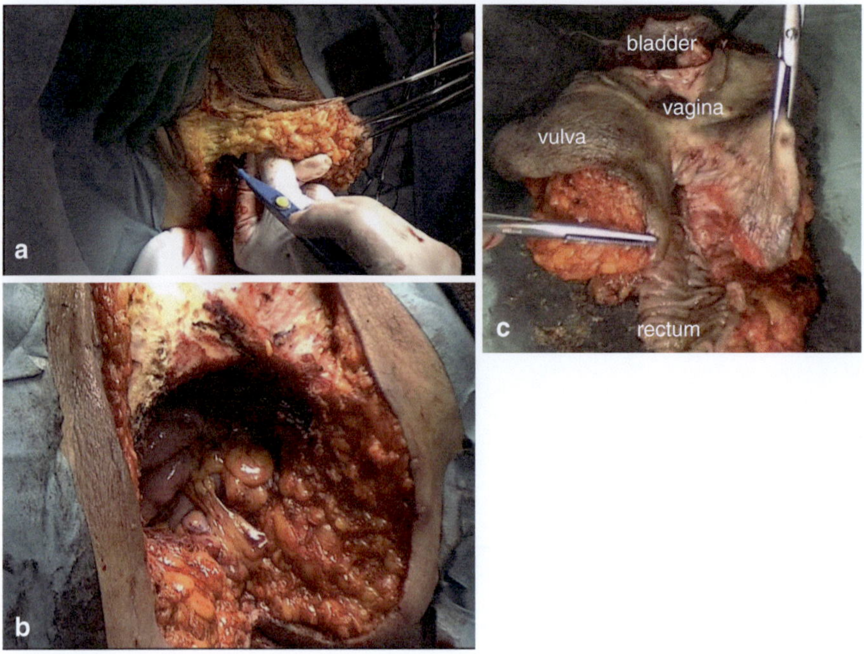

Fig. 14.13 Vulvectomy. (**a**) Incision of the vulva. (**b**) Vulvectomy. (**c**) Surgical specimen

Perineal Reconstruction (Fig. 14.14)
Perineal reconstruction was performed with a gracilis muscle flap. The gracilis muscle was harvested from its bed via a medial femoral skin incision (Fig. 14.14a), the flap was brought into the pelvis, and the developed ischiorectal fossa was filled with this flap (Fig. 14.14b). The dead space can lead to pelvic abscess and intractable infection, so the gracilis muscle flap is quite important. A femoral skin flap was brought into the perineal region through an adequately large subcutaneous tunnel made between the perineum and thigh, and the skin defect was covered by the skin flap (Fig. 14.14c).

(Radical vulvectomy requires perineal reconstruction. There are various techniques; please refer to a plastic surgery textbook.)

In cases of recurrent cervical carcinoma, the pelvic exenteration procedure is more complicated due to the presence of previously irradiated tissue.

The case below is that of a recurrent cervical carcinoma.

14.5.3 Total Laparoscopic Pelvic Exenteration for a Laterally Recurrent Cervical Carcinoma and Vesicovaginal Fistula that Developed After CCRT

14.5.3.1 Case (This case report is cited from reference [15])

The patient had a stage IVA cervical carcinoma. The tumor, which measured 10 cm upon MRI, involved the bladder and right ureter, and it caused right hydronephrosis

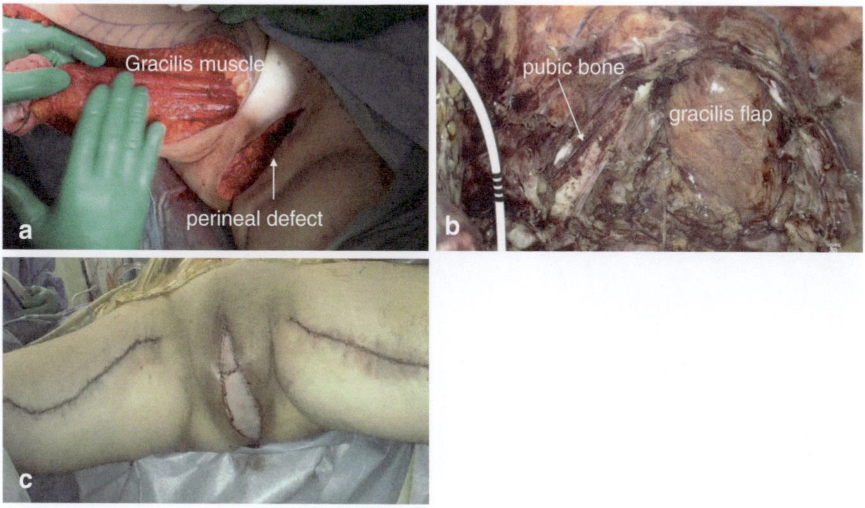

Fig. 14.14 (**a**) Harvest of the gracilis muscle; (**b**) The ischiorectal fossa is fulfilled by the gracilis flap; (**c**) Skin reconstruction

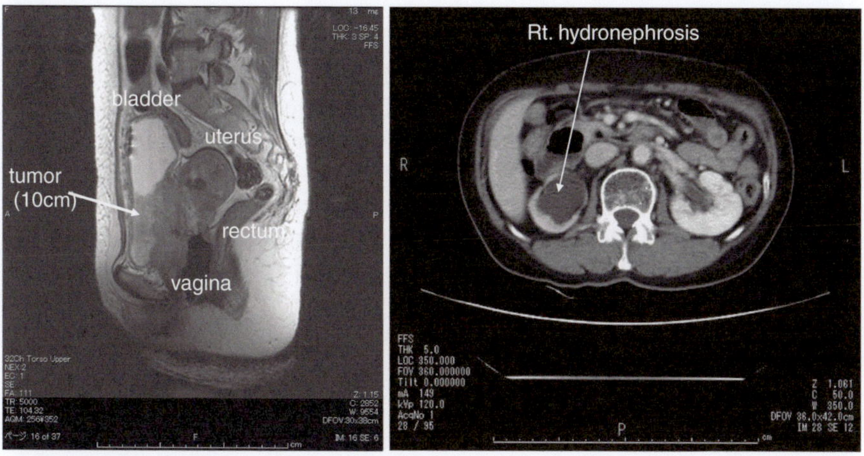

Fig. 14.15 MRI before CCRT. The tumor which measured 10 cm on a MRI involved the bladder and the right ureter, causing right hydronephrosis

(Fig. 14.15). Treatment with platinum-based CCRT was successful, and no residual tumor was detected upon completion of the CCRT. Approximately 7 months after completion of the CCRT, a recurrent tumor at the right pelvic sidewall and a vesicovaginal fistula were detected (Fig. 14.16). The tumor involved the right ureter and bladder and was attached to the rectum. The patient's right renal function was lost. A left nephrostomy tube was placed, but steady leakage of urine from the vagina continued, severely affecting the patient's quality of life. No other recurrent tumor was detected.

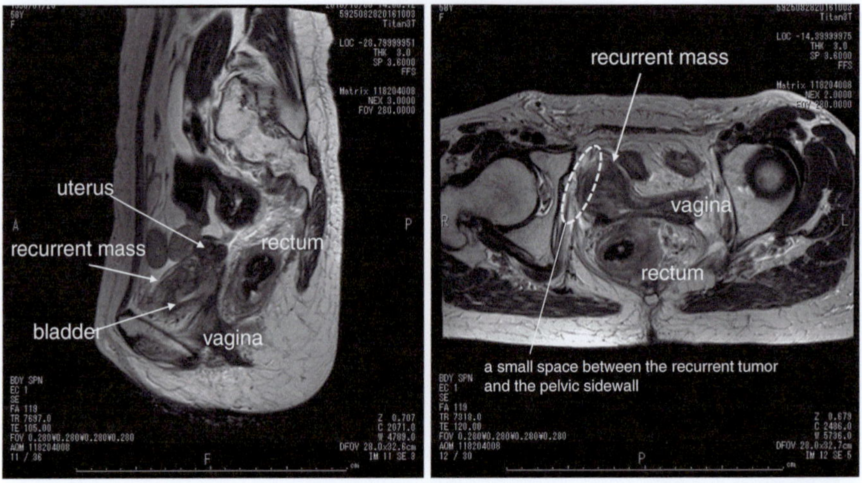

Fig. 14.16 Recurrent cervical carcinoma (MR images). Seven months after completion of the CCRT, a recurrent mass at the right pelvic sidewall and a vesicovaginal fistula were detected. The mass involved the right ureter and bladder and was attached to the rectum. The patient's right renal function was lost. At this point, a left nephrostomy tube was placed; however, steady leakage of urine from the vagina continued, severely affecting the patient's quality of life

Treatment options for patients with recurrent disease after platinum-based CCRT are limited. Chemotherapy with bevacizumab is now the standard treatment for such patients, but this treatment is associated with fistula formation, so a bevacizumab regimen was not appropriate for our patient. Resection with a completely negative margin offers the most promise, but R0 resection was judged to be difficult in this case because, as noted above, pelvic examination revealed that the tumor was fixed to the pelvic sidewall. It has been reported that complete surgical resection with negative margins can be achieved in about a third of patients with a lateralized, previously irradiated, recurrent "unresectable" cervical cancer. MRI in our case revealed a small space between the recurrent tumor and the pelvic sidewall, so laparoscopic surgery was decided upon.

14.5.3.2 Operative Procedure

Dissection and Mobilization of the Rectum

No distinct adhesion was detected around the uterus, but the uterus was completely fixed to the pelvis (Fig. 14.17a). The retroperitoneal space around the rectum was widely dissected, and the rectum was mobilized. The avascular space between the mesorectal fascia and the presacral fascia was dissected and developed. This space, in comparison to the prevesical space, was not affected by the previous irradiation. The inferior hypogastric nerves and pelvic nerve plexus were identified during the

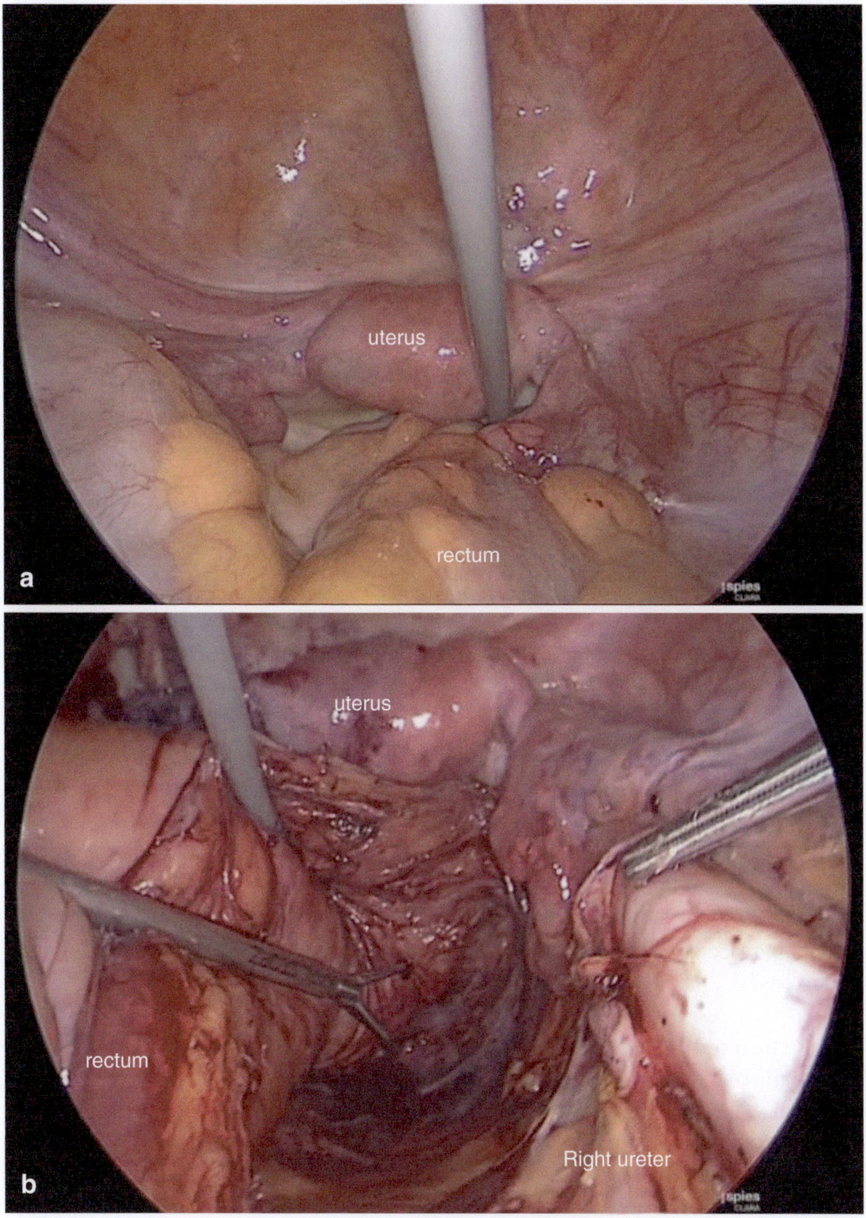

Fig. 14.17 Intraoperative view. (**a**) Preoperative view. (**b**) Dissection of the pararectal space

dissection, and they were transected completely. Dissection proceeded down to the levator ani muscle, while the assistant lifted the rectum with forceps (Fig. 14.17b).

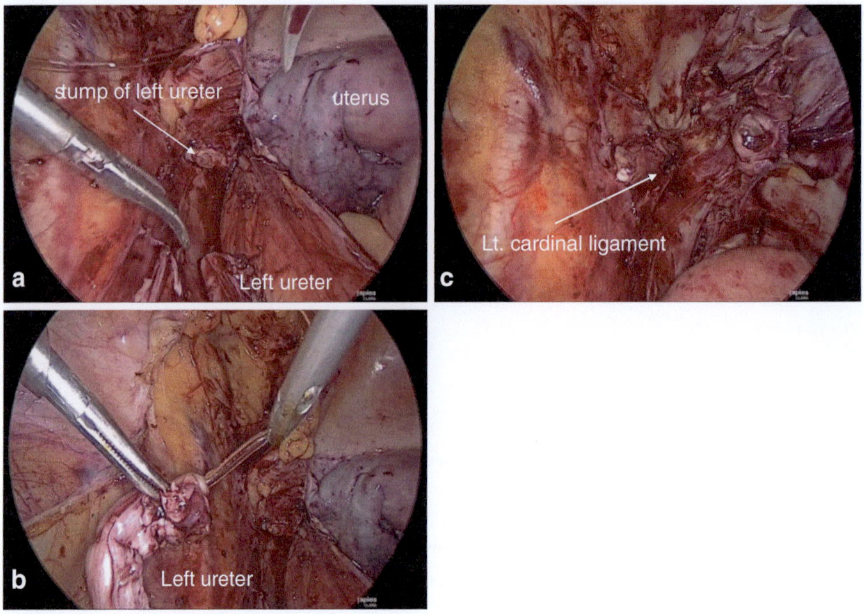

Fig. 14.18 Intraoperative view. (**a**) Transection of the lt. ureter. (**b**) Temporary urinary stent. (**c**) Exposure of the cardinal ligament

Transection of the Left Ureter (Fig. 14.18)
The left ureter was identified, and the left pararectal space was dissected. Severe fibrosis was found, especially around the left ureter, and this was most likely due to the previous CCRT. The fibrosis prevented dissection of the left ureter from the left cardinal ligament; therefore, the left ureter was transected, and a temporary ureteral stent was placed to secure left renal function during the operation. The left paravesical and pararectal spaces were dissected and opened until the left cardinal ligament was exposed.

Transection of the Left Cardinal Ligament (Fig. 14.19)
Severe fibrosis was found around the left cardinal ligament, and the left cardinal ligament was transected completely (en bloc resection) so that the left levator ani muscle could be reached. (In cases of laparoscopic radical hysterectomy, we expose the components [artery, vein, and nerve] of the cardinal ligament and transect them one by one. However, in a previously irradiated field, en bloc resection is safer because of the resulting severe fibrosis.) The right pararectal and retrorectal spaces were then dissected, and the right cardinal ligament was transected completely so that the pelvic floor could be reached, as on the left side. Right nephroureterectomy was performed because the right renal function was considered unrecoverable.

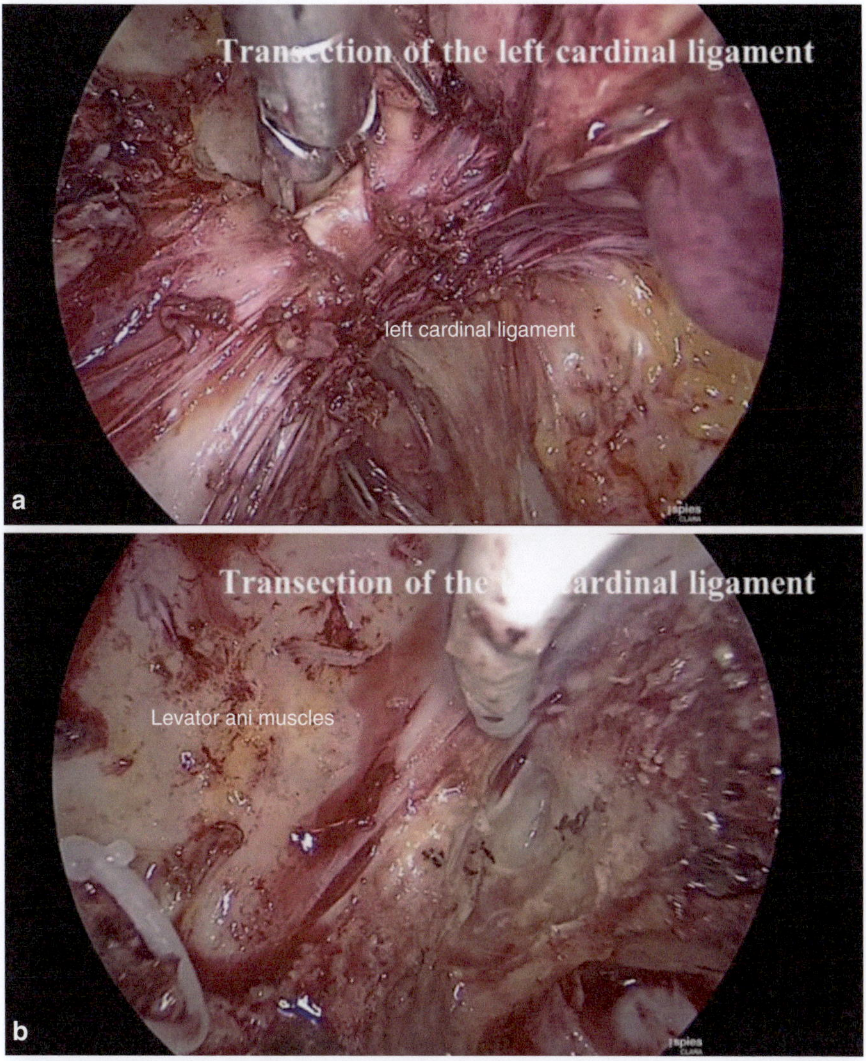

Fig. 14.19 Transection of the left cardinal ligament. (**a**) Exposure of the left cardinal ligament. (**b**) Transection of the left cardinal ligament down to the levator ani muscle

Dissection of the Prevesical Space (Fig. 14.20)

The prevesical space was dissected and developed. The recurrent mass was found to be firmly attached to the pubic bone, but the attachment was a fibrotic adhesion, most likely due to the previous CCRT. There was no direct tumor invasion of the pelvic sidewall. Therefore, complete dissection of this attachment without tumor spillage was possible. (For hemostasis when bleeding occurs in the pubic bone area, the soft coagulation mode is quite effective.)

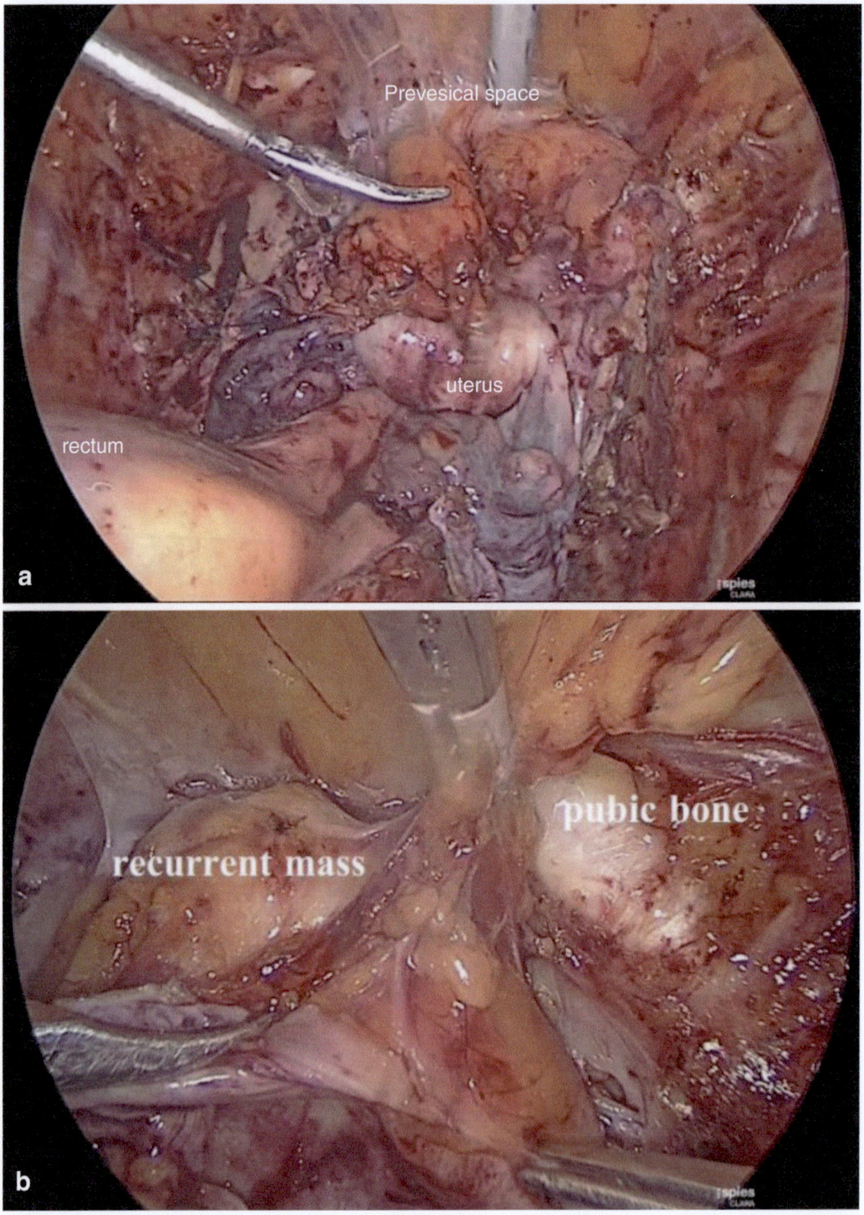

Fig. 14.20 Dissection of the prevesical space. (**a**) Opening of the prevesical space. (**b**) Detachment of the recurrent tumor from the pubic bone

Transection of the Rectum

Because the recurrent tumor was attached to the rectum, total pelvic exenteration was decided upon to ensure R0 resection. At this stage, the rectum was already mobilized, so the rectum was transected quite easily with a laparoscopic stapling device.

(For transection of the rectum, please refer to another chapter.) After the rectum was transected, the pubococcygeal muscle was partially transected, and the ischio-anal fossa was dissected and developed widely. (For a detailed description, please refer to the previous section, **Infralevator Pelvic Exenteration plus Vulvectomy for a Rectal Carcinoma with Pagetoid Spread**.)

Perineal Approach (Fig. 14.21)
The pelvic cavity was approached perineally, and this allowed for the pelvic exenteration. A surgical incision was placed in the vulva, in line with the laparoscopic

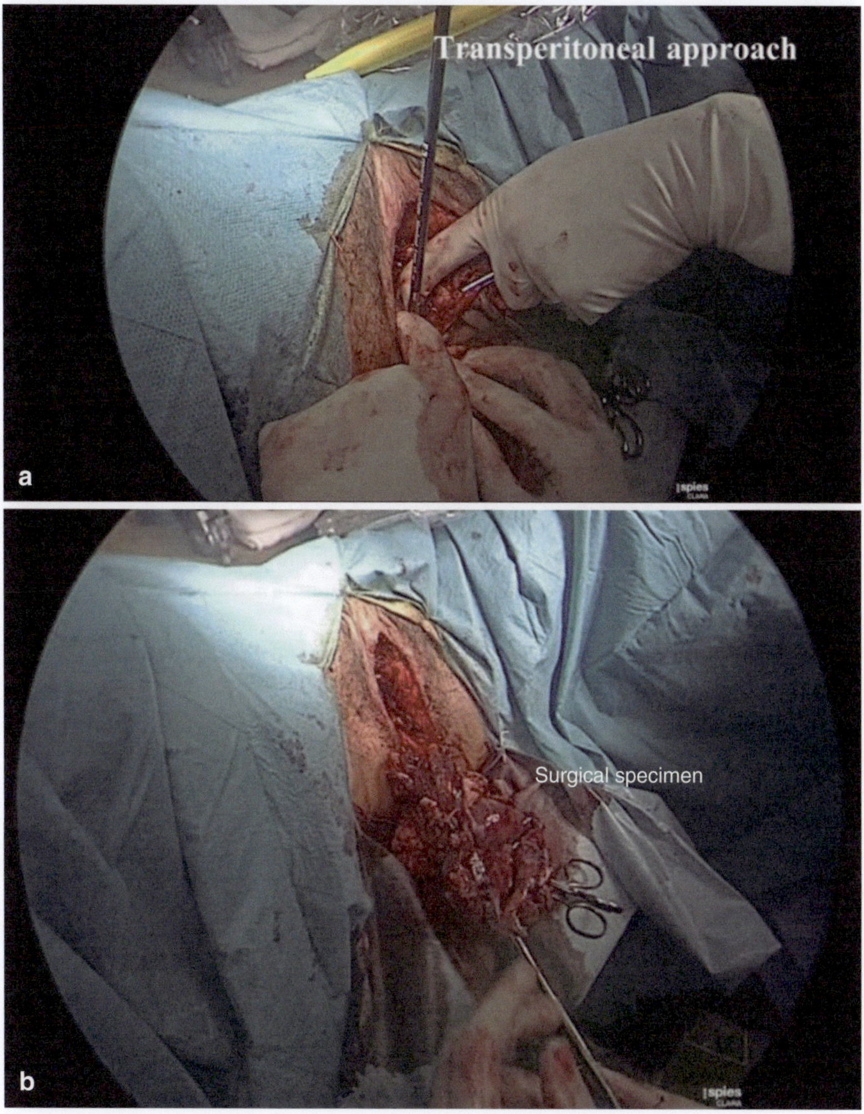

Fig. 14.21 Perineal approach. (**a**) Vulval incision. The underlying tissue was detached so that the ischiorectal fossa could be reached. (**b**) Extraction of the surgical specimen

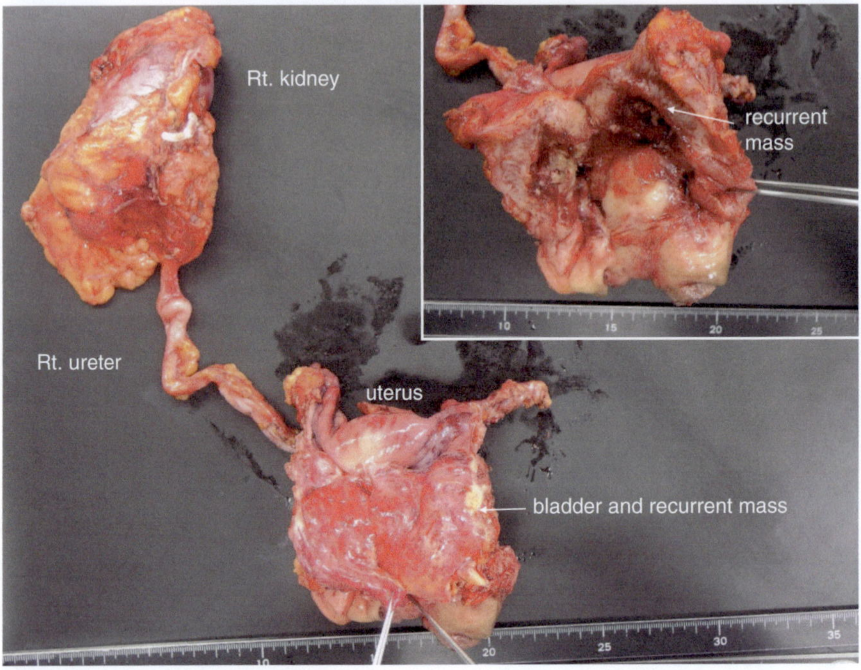

Fig. 14.22 Surgical specimen

incision, and the underlying tissue was detached so that the ischiorectal fossa could be reached. The surgical specimens were extracted via the vulvar incision. R0 en bloc resection of the pelvic organs was achieved. The recurrent tumor had fully penetrated the bladder, creating a huge vesicovaginal fistula. Upon pathologic examination of the surgical specimens, all surgical margins were found to be cancer free (Fig. 14.22).

The total laparoscopic right nephroureterectomy and pelvic exenteration were performed safely. The total operation time was 566 min. The blood loss volume was 250 mL, and there was no need for transfusion.

There were no postoperative complications, and the patient was discharged on postoperative day 14. There has been no sign of recurrence during the 18 months that have passed since the surgery.

14.6 Future Prospect

Pelvic exenteration is usually indicated in cases of recurrent cervical carcinoma only when the recurrence is central. Patients with lateral pelvic recurrence are usually abandoned because the resectability rate is low, and 5-year survival rates are close to zero when a resection margin is positive [16]. Höckel et al. described laterally extended endopelvic resection (LEER), which includes lateral extension of the surgical excision, moving toward the medial aspect of the lumbosacral plexus, piriform muscle, internal obturator muscle, and acetabulum [17]. They reported 5-year survival and overall survival rates of 62% and 55%, respectively, for 100 patients who were treated by LEER and followed up for a median time of 30 months. However, there were two procedure-related deaths, and the morbidity rate was 70% [18].

As noted above, Jurado et al. reported that about a third of patients with laterally recurrent previously irradiated cervical carcinoma classified as unresectable may ultimately undergo complete resection. They reported that when resection was complete (R0), there was no difference in 10-year survival between patients with central and those with lateral recurrence [11].

Based on these reports, we conclude that previously irradiated recurrent cervical carcinoma at pelvic sidewall is not contraindication of surgery. However, incomplete resection is more harmful than observation, so the indication for this surgery (LEER) is very important. Höckel et al. reported the following selection criteria: tumor diameter <5 cm, a disease-free interval of at least 5 months after the completion of CCRT, and a disease-free greater sciatic foramen [18]. Thus, not every recurrence that extends to the pelvic sidewall is eligible for LEER.

In cases of recurrent previously irradiated cervical carcinoma, fibrosis around the recurrent mass can obscure the tumor border, and it is thus sometimes very difficult to determine by preoperative imaging whether the recurrent mass is resectable.

Abdominal MR images of two laterally recurrent cervical carcinomas are shown in Fig. 14.23. Whether the tumor has invaded the sciatic nerve is unclear on these images. In cases in which tumor invasion of the sciatic cannot be identified upon MRI or CT, limb pain is a very important clue to tumor resectability. The Case A patient had right lower limb pain, and the Case B patient did not. In fact, in the Case A patient, denervation atrophy of the right gluteus medius is seen (A-2), which is the result of the tumor invasion of the sciatic nerve. In this case, LEER was ruled out, whereas in Case B, R0 resection was achieved by LEER (Fig. 14.24).

We performed laparoscopic LEER in three patients with a laterally recurrent previously irradiated cervical carcinoma. In all three cases, R0 resection was achieved. The morbidity rate was 33%, and the mortality rate was 0%. The survival impact of LEER is unclear, however, because of the short follow-up periods and small number of patients in whom we have performed the procedure.

The prognosis of laterally recurrent previously irradiated cervical carcinoma is currently poor, and surgery is contraindicated in such cases. However, we believe that laparoscopic LEER will become the treatment of choice for patients with this type of recurrence. The next step to determining the selection criteria and discussing the technical feasibility and oncologic outcome of LEER for laterally recurrent previously irradiated cervical carcinoma will be further data collection.

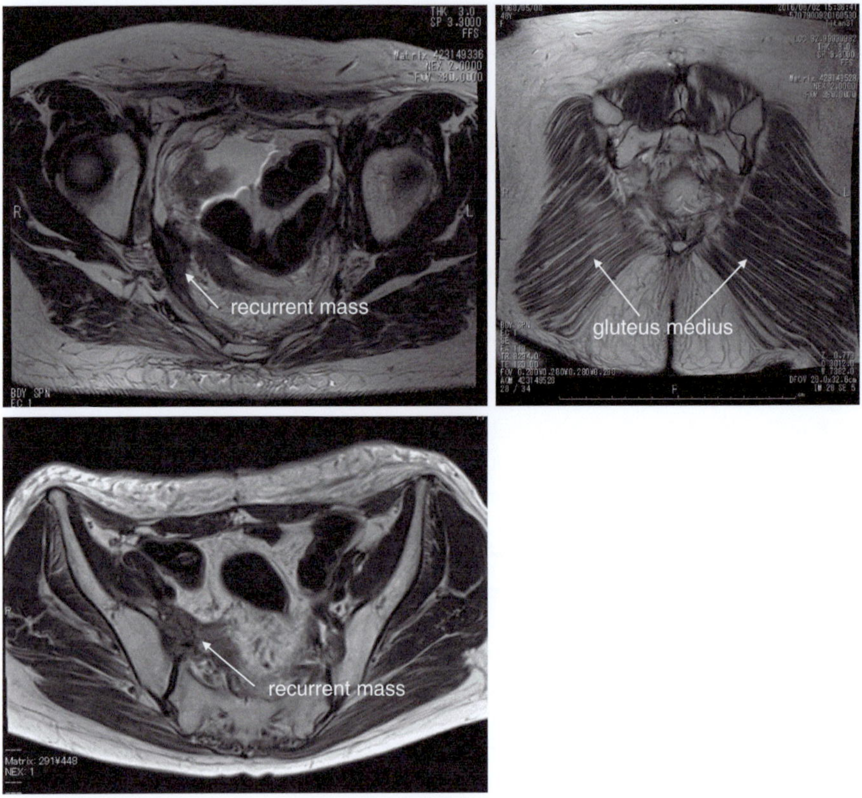

Fig. 14.23 The difficulty of evaluation of extent of the recurrent tumor

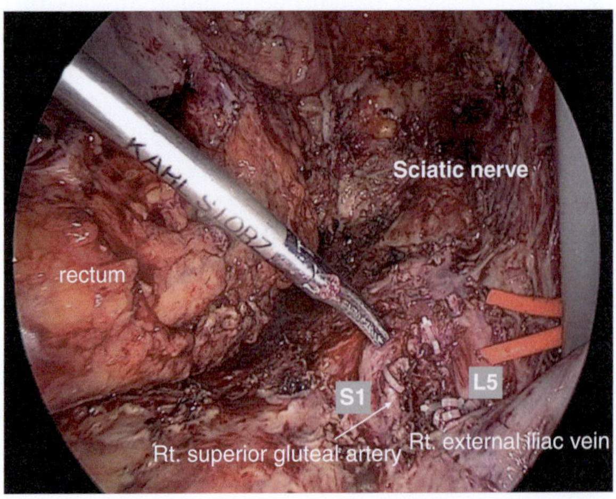

Fig. 14.24 The final operation view (Case B). R0 resection could be achieved

References

1. Peiretti M, Zapardiel I, Zanagnolo V, Landoni F, Morrow CP, Maggioni A. Management of recurrent cervical cancer: a review of the literature. Surg Oncol. 2012;21(2):e59–66.
2. Marnitz S, Köhler C, Müller M, Behrens K, Hasenbein K, Schneider A. Indications for primary and secondary exenterations in patients with cervical cancer. Gynecol Oncol. 2006;103(3):1023–30.
3. Sardain H, Lavoue V, Redpath M, Bertheuil N, Foucher F, Levêque J. Curative pelvic exenteration for recurrent cervical carcinoma in the era of concurrent chemotherapy and radiation therapy. A systematic review. Eur J Surg Oncol. 2015;41(8):975–85.
4. Berek JS, Howe C, Lagasse LD, Hacker NF. Pelvic exenteration for recurrent gynecologic malignancy: survival and morbidity analysis of the 45-year experience at UCLA. Gynecol Oncol. 2005;99(1):153–9.
5. Brunschwig A. The surgical treatment of cancer of the cervix uteri; a radical operation for cancer of the cervix. Bull N Y Acad Med. 1948;24(10):672–83.
6. Magrina JF. Types of pelvic exenterations: a reappraisal. Gynecol Oncol. 1990;37(3):363–6.
7. Magrina JF, Stanhope CR, Weaver AL. Pelvic exenterations: supralevator, infralevator, and with vulvectomy. Gynecol Oncol. 1997;64(1):130–5.
8. Iavazzo C, Vorgias G, Akrivos T. Laparoscopic pelvic exenteration: a new option in the surgical treatment of locally advanced and recurrent cervical carcinoma. Bratisl Lek Listy. 2008;109(10):467–9.
9. Rockall AG, Ghosh S, Alexander-Sefre F, Babar S, Younis MT, Naz S, Jacobs IJ, Reznek RH. Can MRI rule out bladder and rectal invasion in cervical cancer to help select patients for limited EUA? Gynecol Oncol. 2006;101(2):244–9.
10. Forner DM, Meyer A, Lampe B. Preoperative assessment of complete tumour resection by magnetic resonance imaging in patients undergoing pelvic exenteration. Eur J Obstet Gynecol Reprod Biol. 2010;148(2):182–5.
11. Jurado M, Alcázar JL, Martinez-Monge R. Resectability rates of previously irradiated recurrent cervical cancer (PIRCC) treated with pelvic exenteration: is still the clinical involvement of the pelvis wall a real contraindication? A twenty-year experience. Gynecol Oncol. 2010;116(1):38–43.
12. Unger JB, Ivy JJ, Connor P, Charrier A, Ramaswamy MR, Ampil FL, Monsour RP. Detection of recurrent cervical cancer by whole-body FDG PET scan in asymptomatic and symptomatic women. Gynecol Oncol. 2004;94(1):212–6.
13. Husain A, Akhurst T, Larson S, Alektiar K, Barakat RR, Chi DS. A prospective study of the accuracy of 18Fluorodeoxyglucose positron emission tomography (18FDG PET) in identifying sites of metastasis prior to pelvic exenteration. Gynecol Oncol. 2007;106(1):177–80.
14. Chu Y, Zheng A, Wang F, Lin W, Yang X, Han L, Chen Y, Bai L. Diagnostic value of 18F-FDG-PET or PET-CT in recurrent cervical cancer: a systematic review and meta-analysis. Nucl Med Commun. 2014;35(2):144–50.
15. Kanao H, Aoki Y, Hisa T, Takeshima N. Total laparoscopic pelvic exenteration for a laterally recurrent cervical carcinoma with a vesicovaginal fistula that developed after concurrent chemoradiotherapy. Gynecol Oncol. 2017;146(2):438–9.
16. Höckel M, Sclenger K, Hamm H, Knapstein PG, Hohenfellner R, Rösler HP. Five-year experience with combined operative and radiotherapeutic treatment of recurrent gynecologic tumors infiltrating the pelvic wall. Cancer. 1996;77(9):1918–33.
17. Höckel M. Laterally extended endopelvic resection. Novel surgical treatment of locally recurrent cervical carcinoma involving the pelvic side wall. Gynecol Oncol. 2003;91(2):369–77.
18. Höckel M. Laterally extended endopelvic resection (LEER)—principles and practice. Gynecol Oncol. 2008;111(2 Suppl):S13–7.

Sentinel Node Navigation Surgery

15

Hitoshi Niikura

Abstract

Cervical cancer patients with stage IA1 disease with lympho-vascular involvement, IA2 or IB1 disease, or squamous, adenocarcinoma, or adenosquamous histology require a sentinel lymph node navigation surgery (SNNS) via sentinel lymph node biopsy. Bilateral detection rates are high in tumors smaller than 2 cm, and such tumors are the most favorable for SNNS. Utilization of this technique increases the detection rate of lymph node micrometastasis by identification of the target node outside the usual field dissected using formal systematic lymphadenectomy and/or by ultrastaging and has the potential to decrease morbidity associated with standard lymphadenectomy, particularly lymphedema. Sentinel lymph node mapping utilizing both radioisotope and blue dye is the most effective. In more recent years, indocyanine green has emerged as an equally useful tracer compared to the traditional dual tracer technique. Indocyanine green may be particularly useful during laparoscopic or robotic surgery. In order to decide whether or not to omit systematic lymphadenectomy intraoperatively, convenient strategies for intraoperative micrometastatic diagnosis, such as cytokeratin 19 mRNA detection, need to be established.

Keywords

Cervical cancer · Sentinel lymph node · Navigation surgery · Micrometastasis CK19

H. Niikura (✉)
Department of Obstetrics and Gynecology,
National Hospital Organization Sendai Medical Center,
Sendai, Japan
e-mail: niikura@med.tohoku.ac.jp

M. Mikami (ed.), *Surgery for Gynecologic Cancer*, Comprehensive Gynecology and Obstetrics, https://doi.org/10.1007/978-981-13-1519-0_15

15.1 History

The concept behind sentinel lymph node detection is that the SLN is the first site to harbor metastases and that no systemic metastases will be present in cases without SLN metastases. This concept was reported initially in patients with penile cancer by Cabanas [1] and then applied and developed for malignant melanoma and breast cancer. Currently, SLN biopsy is standardized in melanoma [2] and breast cancer [3].

Radical hysterectomy with pelvic lymphadenectomy is performed routinely to treat early-stage cervical cancer. However, the procedure is frequently associated with complications including lymphocele, lymphedema, and urologic disorders. Furthermore, the incidence of lymph node metastasis in patients with clinical stage IB cervical carcinoma is approximately 15–20% [4, 5], suggesting that lymphadenectomy may be unnecessary in most of these early-stage cancers. To avoid systematic lymphadenectomy and minimize postoperative complications, the SLN concept has been applied to the treatment of cervical cancer. SLN biopsy for patients with cervical cancer was first reported by Echt et al. in 1995 [6] using blue dye (lymphazurin) only. This concept has also been investigated in Japan [7–9].

SLN biopsy techniques in cervical cancer have been developed in recent years, and many studies from single institutions have been reported. In a review of 842 patients in whom SLN mapping was performed, 1 study reported a 97% detection rate and 92% sensitivity when a combined method (both radioactive tracer and blue tracer) was employed [10]. These results are not inferior to those of breast cancer. Moreover, multicenter studies have reported that SLN detection is fully reliable when SLNs are detected bilaterally [11, 12].

In several systematic reviews, sentinel lymph node mapping utilizing both radioisotope (RI) and blue dye is feasible and effective [13]. As for radioisotopes, albumin nanocolloids are commonly utilized in Europe, antimonalis in Australia, and sulfur colloids in the United States. In Japan, ^{99m}Tc-phytate has been utilized for sentinel node detection at many institutes [6–8]. In more recent years, it has been understood that indocyanine green (ICG) is an equally useful tracer compared to the double tracer method with RI and blue dye [14]. ICG may be a more useful tracer during laparoscopic or robotic surgery.

15.2 Principle and Indication

The SLN is the first site of lymphatic flow from the primary tumor site, and SLN biopsy is indicated in patients with tumor limited to the uterine cervix and with no clinically evident distant metastases. In general, cervical cancer patients with stage IA1 disease with lympho-vascular involvement, IA2 or IB1 disease, or squamous, adenocarcinoma, or adenosquamous histology require a sentinel lymph node navigation surgery (SNNS) via sentinel lymph node biopsy. SLN detection rate is low, and the false-negative rate is high in patients with bulky (>4 cm) tumors. On the other hand, in cases with tumors smaller than 2 cm, bilateral detection rate is high; such tumors are ideal for SNNS [11, 12]. Previous cervical conization should not be considered a contraindication to SNNS [13].

The number of detected SLNs is 2–3 in most pelvic cavities [6]. Intraoperative frozen section analysis can be performed, and the decision to proceed to formal lymphadenectomy can be made intraoperatively.

The benefit of SLN biopsy seems to be its ability to identify a target node outside the usual field of formal, complete pelvic lymphadenectomy (e.g., presacral and para-aortic areas). In an analysis of 3012 SLNs, SLN basins were identified along the common iliac vessels (6.6%), the lower para-aortic region (2%), the presacral region (1.26%), and the inguinal chain (0.07%) [15].

Moreover, even if the SLN detection site is a common location for metastases, the lymph node micrometastases detection rate increases through ultrastaging. Ultrastaging is performed by stepwise serial sectioning at 0.1–0.2 mm intervals and immunostaining for antigens including pancytokeratin. In our studies, lymph node metastases were detected in approximately 30% of patients who underwent SNNS, and five cases had micrometastases (between 0.2 and 2 mm); two cases had isolated tumor cells (ITCs) (smaller than 0.2 mm) [16]. Another study demonstrated that lymph node metastasis was detected in 14 of 81 SNNS cases (17%) and 15 of 218 systematic lymphadenectomy cases (7%) [17].

The clinical significance of micrometastasis is not established in cervical cancer. A retrospective multicenter study demonstrated that overall survival was significantly reduced in patients with macrometastasis and micrometastasis, but the presence of ITCs was not associated with significant risk in patients who underwent SLN biopsy followed by ultrastaging. Micrometastasis identified by SLN biopsy and ultrastaging may be a significant prognostic factor [18].

There was no significant difference in recurrence rate between SNNS with intraoperative diagnosis and surgery with complete, formal lymphadenectomy [17]. No pelvic recurrence could be detected in the SNNS group evaluated with intraoperative, 2 mm interval frozen sections [16]. Intraoperative diagnosis of frozen section may be feasible at 2 mm intervals parallel to the short axis of the dissected node. In adenocarcinoma cases, it is important to distinguish between endosalpingiosis and a metastatic adenocarcinoma lesion.

The number of young women with cervical cancer has increased in recent years, and survivors must live with treatment-associated sequelae for long periods of time if treated at an early age. To that end, prevention of lymphedema is important in cervical cancer patients. In breast cancer, the rate of postoperative complications including lymphedema has been reported to significantly decrease in patients who undergo sentinel lymphadenectomy alone [19]. A significant difference in the incidence of lymphedema between the SNNS group and the systematic lymphadenectomy group was recognized in our study [16]. In cervical cancer patients, omitting formal lymphadenectomy may lead to a similar decrease in leg lymphedema as seen in the upper extremities after surgery in breast cancer patients.

15.3 Technique

15.3.1 Lymphoscintigraphy with ^{99m}-Technetium and Single-Photon Emission Computed Tomography/Computed Tomography (SPECT/CT)

On the day before surgery, lymphoscintigraphy is performed with injection of 0.4 mL of fluid containing 90 MBq ^{99m}Tc-phytate (DRL, Tokyo, Japan) into the cervix at the 3, 6, 9, and 12 o'clock positions (0.1 mL per injection site). This procedure is carried out in the Nuclear Medicine Department. No anesthesia is needed during this procedure. Dynamic lymphoscintigraphy lasts for approximately 30 min to 1 h. In most cases, sentinel lymph nodes are identified as hot spots within several minutes of injection. The first lymphoscintigram is taken at this time, and the second lymphoscintigram is taken the next morning, just before the patient enters the operating room (Fig. 15.1). The SLNs can be detected at the second scintigram in some but not all cases.

In the cases where SLNs can be detected as visualized hot spots by scintigram, SPECT/CT is added (Fig. 15.2). SLNs sometimes exist deep in the pelvic cavity in cervical cancer patients. SPECT/CT is useful for easy detection of such SLNs during surgery.

15.3.2 Intraoperative Lymphatic Mapping and Sentinel Lymph Node Identification

After the abdominal cavity is opened (or all trocars are inserted in laparoscopic or robotic surgery), 4.0 mL of blue dye (patent blue violet: SIGMA Co. St. Louis, MO)

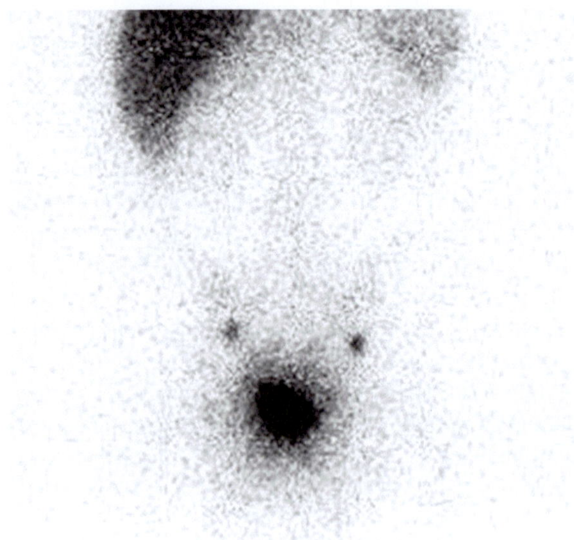

Fig. 15.1 Preoperative lymphoscintigram. Two hot nodes are visible in the pelvic area

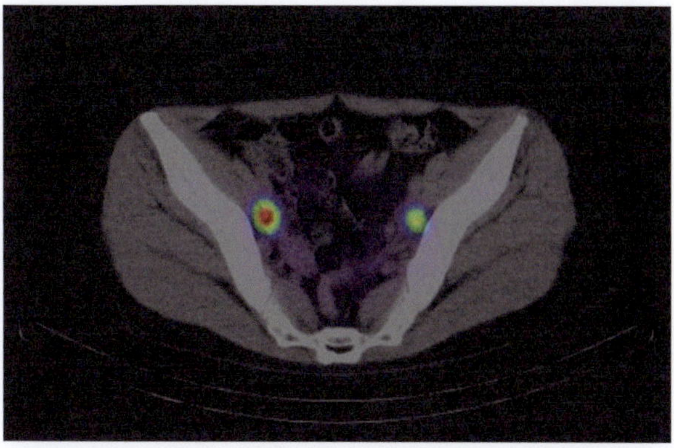

Fig. 15.2 Bilateral obturator lymph nodes are visualized in SPECT/CT

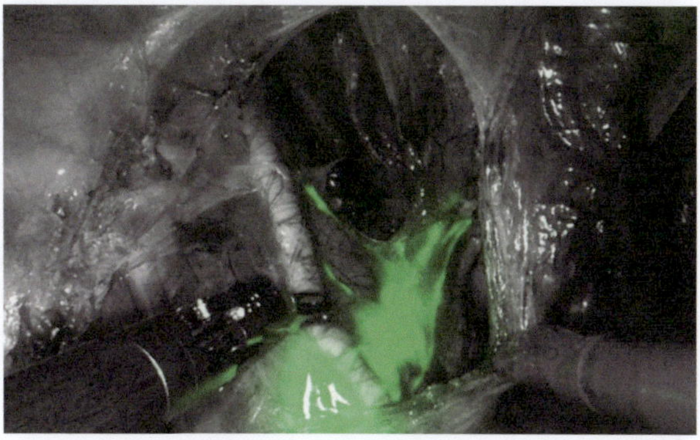

Fig. 15.3 External iliac and obturator sentinel lymph nodes are detected utilizing indocyanine green

is injected into the cervix in four quadrants (1.0 mL per injection site) as the RI solution. In our institution, photodynamic dye (ICG; Daiichi Sankyo, Tokyo) is injected into the cervix as ICG disperses more quickly than other kinds of tracer. ICG is injected at the 8 and 10 o'clock positions, and SLN biopsy is performed in the right pelvic cavity. Next, a left side SLN biopsy is performed after injecting at the 2 and 4 o'clock positions. Injecting the tracer is facilitated by moving the uterus manually from the abdominal cavity. Before SLN biopsy is attempted, the retroperitoneal cavity (paravesical space and pararectal space) should be opened, and radioactive and/or blue lymph nodes located using a gamma-detecting probe and by inspection. The gamma-detecting probe for laparoscopy is inserted into the 12 mm port (assistant port in robotic surgery) in laparoscopic surgery. The procedure to trace dye or photodynamic dye by inspection is useful in cases in which it is difficult to detect SLNs by scintigram (Fig. 15.3). In patients with SLNs in unusual sites (e.g., sacral or para-aortic nodes), it is necessary to remove all involved tissue. Radical hysterectomy requires examination of the tissue around the deep uterine veins, in order that parametrial lymph nodes are removed. In SNNS, lymph nodes around the deep uterine veins must be surveyed by a gamma-detecting probe and by inspection. If parametrial SLNs are detected, those nodes are removed and submitted for intraoperative pathological diagnosis in a similar way.

In SLN biopsy, the iliac vessels and obturator nerve are not exposed completely, so anatomical knowledge is more important than formal lymphadenectomy. Special attention is required to not injure nerves or vessels. It is important that clinically suspicious and enlarged nodes should be removed regardless of SLN detection and that systematic lymphadenectomy should be performed in at least not detected side of hemipelvis if SLN mapping is not successful [20].

When the gamma-detecting probe registers counts more than tenfold above background radiation levels, the node is considered radioactive. All radioactive and blue nodes are considered SLNs. All surgically removed lymph nodes are reexamined with the gamma-detecting probe ex vivo.

After lymphadenectomy or SLN biopsy during SNNS is performed, the pelvic cavity is scanned with the probe to confirm that no radioactive tissues remain.

After SLN biopsy, radical or semiradical hysterectomy is performed routinely (see Chap. 7 or 8).

Even if lymph node metastases are identified intraoperatively by pathological examination of frozen sections, the scheduled radical hysterectomy is not abandoned, and formal lymphadenectomy is performed. In cases with metastases limited to the SLN or in cases with micrometastasis (or ITCs), the role of hysterectomy and formal lymphadenectomy is not clear at present. Moreover, in such cases, adjuvant therapy with chemotherapy may be adequate and decrease the side effects by radiation.

15.3.3 Pathological Examination

Frozen section analysis of detected SLNs is performed intraoperatively. Each SLN is examined utilizing stepwise sectioning at 2 mm intervals parallel to the short axis of the node and examined with hematoxylin and eosin (H&E) staining. The remaining tissue is formalin-fixed and embedded in paraffin for routine histological analysis. Formal lymphadenectomy is omitted in patients with no SLN metastases in SNNS. In cases with SLN mapping only, all surgically removed non-SLNs are examined histopathologically using routine H&E staining. One section from each lymph node is divided at the maximal diameter in non-SLNs. After SLNs are reexamined and diagnosed as negative for metastasis by routine H&E staining postoperatively, the blocks are cut at 0.1 mm intervals, and slides are immunostained with an antibody directed against cytokeratin (AE1/AE3, DAKO, Japan), expression of which is a characteristic of metastatic cancer cells. It is recommended to measure and record the size of metastasis for deciding adjuvant therapy, but the significance of ITCs (defined as metastases measuring $\leq$0.2 mm) and micrometastases (defined as tumors ranging from 0.2 to 2 mm) is not clear. Most of them lead to adjuvant therapy in current practice.

15.4 Morbidity

Anaphylactic reaction to tracers (patent blue, Tc-colloidal albumin, etc.) has been reported, but we have not experienced a single such reaction in several hundreds of cases with SLN detection using patent blue and ^{99m}Tc-phytate.

The morbidity of radical or semiradical hysterectomy is present in surgeries using SNNS (see Chaps. 7 or 8), but the rate of lymphedema decreases [16].

15.5 Future and Prospect

SLN biopsy is indicated for patients with stage IA1–IB1 cervical cancer, and its feasibility and utility for more advanced-stage patients have been reported [21]. SLN detection procedure needs to be completed in all operable cases as an adjunct treatment, and the difference in the prognostic value between metastases limited to SLN and that extended to non-SLN beyond SLN needs to be clarified. The biological malignant potential may be different between cases with multiple metastases limited to sentinel nodes and those with metastases to non-sentinel nodes, and the therapeutic strategy will be modified considering the individual metastatic pattern.

In breast carcinoma, cases with micrometastases or less do not need formal axillary lymphadenectomy. In cervical cancer patients with micrometastases or ITCs, formal lymphadenectomy may be not necessary based on previous studies [22]. Further studies are needed to clarify the need for formal lymphadenectomy in such cervical cancer cases.

Previous studies have demonstrated that the detection rate of lymph node metastasis by SNNS increased compared with conventional methods as confirmed by formal lymphadenectomy and routine pathological examinations. These data have been confirmed by not only intraoperative but also postoperative ultrastaging. On the other hand, the evaluation of intraoperative pathological diagnosis is not consistent among previous reports. Examination of SLN by stepwise sectioning at 2 mm intervals parallel to the short axis of the node is time-consuming but feasible compared with examination of only a single level on frozen sections. The sensitivity of lymph node metastasis detection by single-level evaluation of frozen sections intraoperatively was reported to be low (20.7%) [23]. While the detection rate of lymph node metastasis has improved by increasing the number of frozen sections examined, the workload of pathologists has also increased. Other convenient strategies for intraoperative diagnosis, such as mRNA expression analysis and one-step nucleic acid amplification techniques, need to be established. Micrometastases or larger metastases in cervical cancer patients may be identified by evaluation of cytokeratin 19 mRNA expression [24].

SLN biopsy in cervical cancer cases is performed at very few institutions in Japan. Feasibility studies performed at a single institute are necessary even if the number of patients is limited, and the utility of SLN biopsy should be established in more institutions prior to performing multicenter prospective validation studies.

It is necessary for gynecological oncologists to have experience with at least ten cases of sentinel lymph node mapping with backup systematic lymphadenectomy using a double tracer, not single tracer, method (RI with dye or RI with ICG) and to understand the precise diffusion pattern of pelvic SLNs.

Ultrastaging and intraoperative diagnosis using frozen sections are necessary in the future. Therefore, cooperation with histopathologists is important. The feasibility of pathological diagnosis should also be evaluated in individual institutions.

If the utility of SNNS for cervical cancer in Japan can be confirmed by multicenter studies involving gynecologists who have acquired adequate experience with SLN biopsy, SNNS will provide significant clinical benefit for patients with cervical cancer.

References

1. Cabanas RM. An approach for the treatment of penile carcinoma. Cancer. 1977;39:456–66.
2. Lyman GH, Giuliano MR, Somerfield MR, Benson AB III, Bodurka DC, Burstein HJ, et al. American Society of Clinical Oncology guideline recommendations for sentinel lymph node biopsy in early-stage breast cancer. J Clin Oncol. 2005;23:7703–20.
3. Morton DJ, Thompson JF, Cochran AJ, Mozzillo N, Elashoff R, Essner R, et al. N Engl J Med. 2006;355:1307–17.
4. Delgado G, Bundy BN, Fowler WC Jr, Stehman FB, Sevin B, Creasman WTA, et al. A prospective surgical pathological study of stage I squamous carcinoma of the cervix: a Gynecologic Oncology Group Study. Gynecol Oncol. 1989;35:314–20.
5. Henriksen E. Distribution of metastases in stage I carcinoma of the cervix. Am J Obstet Gynecol. 1960;80:919–32.
6. Echt ML, Finan MA, Hoffman MS, Kline RC, Roberts WS, Fiorica JV. Detection of sentinel lymph nodes with lymphazurin in cervical, uterine, and vulvar malignancies. South Med J. 1999;92:204–8.
7. Niikura H, Okamura C, Akahira J, Takano T, Ito K, Okamura K, et al. Sentinel lymph node detection in early cervical cancer with combination 99mTc phytate and patent blue. Gynecol Oncol. 2004;94:528–32.
8. Yamashita T, Katayama H, Kato Y, Nishiwaki K, Hayashi H, Miyokawa N, et al. Management of pelvic lymph nodes by sentinel node navigation surgery in the treatment of invasive cervical cancer. Int J Gynecol Cancer. 2009;19:1113–8.
9. Ogawa S, Kobayashi H, Amada S, Yahata H, Sonoda K, Abe K, et al. Sentinel node detection with (99m)Tc phytate alone is satisfactory for cervical cancer patients undergoing radical hysterectomy and pelvic lymphadenectomy. Int J Clin Oncol. 2010;15:52–8.
10. van de Lande J, Davelaar EM, von Mensdorff-Pouilly S, Hoekstra OS, van Baal MW, Brölmann HA, et al. Sentinel lymph node detection in early stage uterine cervix carcinoma: A systematic review. Gynecol Oncol. 2007;106:604–13.
11. Altgassen C, Hertel H, Brandstadt A, Köhler C, Dürst M, Schneider A, et al. Multicenter validation study of the sentinel lymph node concept in cervical cancer: AGO Study Group. J Clin Oncol. 2008;26:2943–51.
12. Lecuru F, Mathevet P, Querleu D, Leblanc E, Morice P, Daraï E, et al. Bilateral negative sentinel nodes accurately predict absence of lymph node metastasis in early cervical cancer: results of the SENTICOL study. J Clin Oncol. 2011;29:1686–91.
13. Kadkhodayan S, Hasanzadeh M, Treglia G, Azad A, Yousefi Z, Zarifmahmoudi L, et al. Sentinel node biopsy for lymph nodal staging of uterine cervix cancer: a systematic review and meta-analysis of the pertinent literature. Eur J Surg Oncol. 2015;41:1–20.

14. Jewell EL, Huang JJ, Abu-Rustum NR, Gardner GJ, Brown CL, Sonoda Y, et al. Detection of sentinel lymph nodes in minimally invasive surgery using indocyanine green and near-infrared fluorescence imaging for uterine and cervical malignancies. Gynecol Oncol. 2014;133:274–7.
15. Ouldamer L, Marret H, Acker O, Barillot I, Body G. Unusual localizations of sentinel lymph nodes in early stage cervical cancer. A review. Surg Oncol. 2012;21:e153–7. https://doi.org/10.1016/j.suronc.2012.04.003. Epub 2012 May 16
16. Niikura H, Okamoto S, Otsuki T, Yoshinaga K, Utsunomiya H, Nagase S, et al. Prospective study of sentinel lymph node biopsy without further pelvic lymphadenectomy in patients with sentinel lymph node-negative cervical cancer. Int J Gynecol Cancer. 2012;22:1244–50.
17. Gortzak-Uzan L, Jimenez W, Nofech-Mozes S, Ismiil N, Khalifa MA, Dubé V, et al. Sentinel lymph node biopsy vs. pelvic lymphadenectomy in early stage cervical cancer: is it time to change the gold standard? Gynecol Oncol. 2010;116:28–32.
18. Cibula D, Abu-Rustum NR, Dusek L, Zikán M, Zaal A, Sevcik L, et al. Prognostic significance of low volume sentinel lymph node disease in early-stage cervical cancer. Gynecol Oncol. 2012;124:496–501.
19. McLaughlin SA, Wright MJ, Morris KT, Giron GL, Sampson MR, Brockway JP, et al. Prevalence of lymphedema in women with breast cancer 5 years after sentinel lymph node biopsy or axillary dissection: objective measurements. J Clin Oncol. 2008;26:5213–9.
20. Cervical Cancer Guideline (Version 1. 2017). NCCN Clinical Practice Guidelines in Oncology http://www.nccn.org/professionals/physician_gls/PDF/cervical.pdf
21. Chereau E, Feron JG, Ballester M, Coutant C, Bezu C, Rouzier R, et al. Contribution of pelvic and para-aortic lymphadenectomy with sentinel node biopsy in patients with IB2-IIB cervical cancer. Br J Cancer. 2012;106:39–44.
22. Okamoto S, Niikura H, Yoshinaga K, Nagase S, Takano T, Ito K, et al. Detection of micrometastases in cervical cancer with a system that evaluates both sentinel and nonsentinel lymph nodes. Int J Gynecol Cancer. 2009;19:708–11.
23. Bats AS, Buénerd A, Querleu D, Leblanc E, Daraï E, Morice P, et al. Diagnostic value of intraoperative examination of sentinel lymph node in early cervical cancer: prospective, multicenter study. Gynecol Oncol. 2011;123:230–5.
24. Okamoto S, Niikura H, Nakabayashi K, Hiyama K, Matoda M, Takeshima N, et al. Detection of sentinel lymph node metastases in cervical cancer; assessment of KRT19 mRNA in the one-step nucleic acid amplification(OSNA) method. Gynecol Oncol. 2013;130:530–6.

16 Outline of Surgery (Refer to Hysterectomy in Section of Cervical Cancer)

Yukiharu Todo

Abstract

Surgery is usually the principal treatment for endometrial cancer and includes hysterectomy, often along with salpingo-oophorectomy and lymph node dissection. Acquisition of pelvic washing samples is preferable. In some cases, the omentum is removed and/or peritoneal biopsies are obtained. If the cancer has spread throughout the pelvis and abdomen, as much cancer as possible should be removed.

Keywords

Ovarian preservation · Peritoneal washing cytology · Omentectomy · Debulking surgery

16.1 History

Endometrial cancer is the most common malignancy of the female genital tract in the United States, with an estimated 61,380 new cases reported in 2017 [1]. The annual number of deaths increased from 6000 in 1997 [2] to 10,920 in 2017 [1]. However, the International Federation of Gynecology and Obstetrics (FIGO) annual report demonstrated that the survival rates of patients with endometrial cancer have continued to increase during recent decades [3]. This trend applies to all cases, including stage IIIC. Meanwhile, surgical staging has become a principal step in the treatment of endometrial cancer. This concept includes appropriate use of adjuvant therapy to improve the prognosis for patients at high risk of recurrence.

Y. Todo (✉)
Division of Gynecologic Oncology, National Hospital Organization,
Hokkaido Cancer Center, Sapporo, Japan
e-mail: yukiharu@sap-cc.go.jp

M. Mikami (ed.), *Surgery for Gynecologic Cancer*, Comprehensive Gynecology and Obstetrics, https://doi.org/10.1007/978-981-13-1519-0_16

16.2 Principles and Indications

Potential procedures required for surgical staging include hysterectomy, bilateral salpingo-oophorectomy, lymph node dissection, peritoneal washing cytology, omentectomy, and peritoneal biopsy. Hysterectomy and bilateral salpingo-oophorectomy are the cornerstone procedures for surgical staging, and additional procedures are implemented when a patient is presumed to be at high risk of recurrence or to have a poor prognosis. Ovarian preservation is considered based on the patient's age. Whether extensive surgery including lymph node dissection should be performed depends largely on the extent and aggressiveness of the disease. Assessment of myometrial invasion when determining the extent of disease is of great importance in patients with endometrial cancer presumed to be confined to the uterine corpus.

16.2.1 Hysterectomy

The standard hysterectomy procedure for stage I endometrial cancer is considered to be extrafascial hysterectomy (Piver-Rutledge class I). One prospective randomized study showed no difference in the 5-year overall and disease-free survival rates between modified radical hysterectomy and extrafascial hysterectomy (overall survival, 92.2% vs. 88.9%, $P = 0.34$; disease-free survival, 89.7% vs. 87.7%, $P = 0.72$) [4]. However, modified radical hysterectomy (Piver-Rutledge class II) is another option. In one retrospective study, the 5-year disease-free survival rate in the modified radical hysterectomy group was higher than that in the extrafascial hysterectomy group, although the difference was not statistically significant (96.0% vs. 88.2%, $P = 0.24$) [5]. In contrast, the standard hysterectomy procedure for stage II endometrial cancer is considered to be modified radical hysterectomy or radical hysterectomy. Implementation of radical hysterectomy for patients with cervical involvement is permitted in some cases because it is difficult to distinguish endometrial carcinoma with cervical involvement from cervical adenocarcinoma.

16.2.2 Salpingo-oophorectomy

The reported rate of ovarian metastasis is 5% to 10% in patients with endometrial cancer presumed to be confined to the uterus [6–10] and 13% in patients with clinical stage I through III cancer [11], which cannot be clinically ignored (Table 16.1). Therefore, this procedure is recommended for postmenopausal patients. However, removing both ovaries will cause premenopausal patients to go into menopause. The quality of life of women of reproductive age is affected by surgical castration. Early surgical menopause is associated with an increased risk of future cardiovascular disease and osteoporosis [12, 13]. In 2009, a retrospective study of data from the Surveillance, Epidemiology, and End Results (SEER) program showed that ovary-sparing surgery in women aged ≤45 years with stage I endometrial cancer was not

Table 16.1 A literature review of ovarian metastasis and ovary-sparing surgery in endometrial cancer

Author	Year of publication	*N*	Outcome
Ovarian metastasis in endometrial cancer			
Boronow [6]	1984	222	OVM 7.2% in clinical stage I (not available for information on non-endometrioid histological variant)
Creasman [7]	1987	621	OVM 5.5% in clinical stage I (not available for information on non-endometrioid histological variant)
Boente [8]	1993	202	OVM 6.9% in clinical stage II (6.9% for non-endometrioid histological variant)
Takeshima [9]	1998	439	OVM 5.0% in clinical stage I (0% for non-endometrioid histological variant)
Creasman [10]	1999	148	OVM 8.9% in clinical stage II (not available for information on non-endometrioid histological variant)
Sakuragi [11]	2000	240	OVM 12.9% in clinical stages I–III (5.4% for non-endometrioid histological variant)
Ovary-sparing surgery for reproductive women with endometrial cancer			
Wright [14]	2009	402	DSS, HR 0.58 (95% CI = 0.14–2.44); OS, HR 0.68 (95% CI = 0.34–1.35)
Koskas [15]	2012	184	No difference in DSS/OS between castration and ovary-sparing surgery
Lee [16]	2013	176	RFS, HR 0.73 (95% CI = 0.29–1.81); OS, HR 1.33 (95% CI = 0.43–4.09)

OVM ovarian metastasis, *DSS* disease-specific survival, *RFS* recurrence-free survival, *OS* overall survival

associated with an increase in cancer-related mortality [14]. Similar results were confirmed in other studies [15, 16]. Ovarian preservation can be one option for pre-menopausal women with early-stage endometrial cancer. Notably, however, synchronous ovarian malignancies are significantly associated with endometrial cancer in premenopausal women aged ≤45 years [17, 18].

16.2.3 Peritoneal Washing Cytology

One reliable systematic review revealed a positive peritoneal cytology rate of 11% in patients with endometrial cancer [19]. Positive peritoneal cytology is associated with an increased incidence of extrauterine disease, but it is not consistently linked to other high-risk factors such as deep myometrial invasion, lymphovascular space invasion, or lymph node metastasis. Several studies have confirmed that positive peritoneal cytology is not an independent prognostic factor in patients with endometrial cancer confined to the uterus [20–25] (Table 16.2). Consequently, peritoneal cytology findings were disregarded in the 2008 FIGO surgical staging protocol; however, conflicting results were present in the literature [26–31] (Table 16.2). Therefore, Mariani et al. [32] stated that the continued collection of peritoneal cytology may provide useful information when making postoperative treatment

Table 16.2 A literature review of positive peritoneal cytology in endometrial cancer

Author	Year of publication	*N*	Study population	Overall incidence (%)	Treatment		Impact of positive PC on prognosis (multivariate analysis result)
					LND	Adjuvant TX	
Positive PC: not an independent prognostic factor							
Hirai [20]	1989	235	All surgical stage	18.7%	100%	NA	NA
Ebina [21]	1997	114	All surgical stage	35.1%	100%	NA	NA
Takeshima [22]	2001	534	All surgical stage	22.3%	100%	22%*	NA
Mariani [23]	2002	51	FIGO stage IIIA (1988)	NA	71%	86%†	NA
Kasamatsu [24]	2003	280	Surgical stage I	17.1%	61%	1%‡	aHR 0.83 (95% CI = 0.2–2.9), RFS, adjusting factors: age, grade, myometrial invasion, cervical involvement
Tebeu [25]	2004	311	Surgical stage I	10.6%	2%	52%‡	aHR 0.74 (95% CI = 0.2–2.3), DSS, adjusting factors: age, stage, grade, myometrial invasion, RT
Positive PC: an adverse prognostic factor							
Turner [26]	1989	567	Surgical stage I	4.9%	24%	82%‡	Coefficient 1.53 $p = 0.0037$, OS, adjusting factors: stage, grade, myometrial invasion
Lurain [27]	1991	230	Clinical stage I	16.5%	65%	NA	NA
Kashimura [28]	1997	303	All surgical stage	14.5%	NA	NA	NA
Obermair [29]	2001	369	Surgical stage I	3.5%	51%	NA	NA
Saga [30]	2006	307	Surgical stage I	10.4%	100%	NA	aHR 4.7 (95% CI = 1.1–12.5), DSS, adjusting factors: age, grade, myometrial invasion, cervical involvement, LVSI
Havrilesky [31]	2007	524	Surgical stages I–IIIA	NA	100%	24%‡	aHR 1.7 (95%CI = 1.02–2.66), OS, adjusting factors:age, race, ovarian/serosal involvement, histology, LND, RT
Shiozaki [33]	2014	265	Surgical stage I	10.2%	59%	51%§	aHR4.3 (95% CI = 1.5–12.0), PFS, adjusting factors: age, histology, myometrial invasion, LVSI, LND, CT
Milgrom [34]	2013	196	Surgical stage III	NA	92%	93%ǁ	aHR 2.9 (95% CI = 1.6–5.1), DSS, adjusting factors: age, histology, myometrial invasion, LVSI, LND, RT, CT
Garg [35]	2013	14,704	Surgical stages I and II	3.3%	92%	30%‡	aHR 4.6 (95% CI = 3.8–5.7), DSS, adjusting factors: age, race, histology, grade, LND, RT

aHR adjusted hazard risk, *CI* confidence interval, *CT* chemotherapy, *DSS* disease-specific survival, *LND* lymph node dissection, *LVSI* lymphovascular space invasion, *NA* not available, *OS* overall survival, *PC* peritoneal cytology, *PFS* progression-free survival, *RFS* recurrence-free survival, *RT* radiation therapy, *TX* treatment; *RT 7% and CT15%; †RT84% and CT 2%; ‡RT, #RT30% and CT2%; §RT1% and CT50%; ǁRT 23%, CT23% and concurrent chemoradiation 47%

decisions or planning future research. Indeed, several researchers subsequently reported the prognostic significance of positive peritoneal washings [33–35] (Table 16.2). In particular, a 2013 study of the SEER database showed the prognostic significance of positive peritoneal cytology in 14,704 patients with early-stage endometrial cancer. However, there is no definitive consensus on the prognostic significance of positive peritoneal cytology when the disease is confined to the uterus. According to pooled data, the recurrence rate in patients with positive peritoneal cytology as the only manifestation of extrauterine extension was 4.1%, but 37.1% of the relevant patients received adjuvant treatment [19]. This high rate of adjuvant treatment confounds the results in terms of predicting the risk of recurrence when these patients are not treated.

16.2.4 Omentectomy

The reported rate of omental metastasis ranges from 0.5% to 8.3% in patients with endometrial cancer presumed to be confined to the uterine corpus [36–43] (Table 16.3). A recent systematic review suggested that microscopic omental metastases were not negligible in patients with clinical stage I endometrial cancer and that selective omentectomy was recommended for patients at high risk of omental metastasis [44]. Omental metastasis was associated with deep myometrial invasion, type II corpus cancer, adnexal involvement, and lymph node metastasis. In particular, the rate of omental metastasis increased to 43–45% in patients with positive peritoneal cytology [37, 40]. Although whether omentectomy itself has therapeutic significance remains unclear, it is possible that the diagnosis of

Table 16.3 A literature review of omental metastasis in endometrial cancer

Author	Year of publication	Patient number	Background and study design	Omental metastasis (%)
Chen [36]	1991	84	Clinical stage I, 19% for serous/clear histological variant, prospective design	8.3%
Saygili [37]	2001	97	Clinical stage I, 12% for serous/clear histological variant, retrospective design	6.2%
Dilek [38]	2006	51	Clinical stage I, 100% for endometrioid histology, retrospective design	5.9%
Fujiwara [39]	2008	134	Clinical stage I, 100% for endometrioid histology, prospective design	3.0%
Metindir [40]	2008	65	Clinical stage I, 100% for endometrioid histology, retrospective design	6.2%
Ozdal [41]	2013	189	Clinical stage I and more, 100% for endometrioid histology, retrospective design	0.5%
Ulker [42]	2014	322	Clinical stage I and more, 100% for endometrioid histology, retrospective design	3.4%
Sasaki [43]	2014	98	Clinical stage I and more, 33% for non-endometrioid histology, retrospective design	9.2%

omental metastasis indirectly contributes to an improved prognosis in certain groups of patients. Omentectomy followed by intraoperative rapid peritoneal cytology might be proposed as part of the surgical management of endometrial cancer.

16.2.5 Lymph Node Dissection

Establishment of a patient's nodal status is necessary to determine the stage of endometrial cancer. The most accurate method with which to detect lymph node metastasis is systematic removal of the regional lymph nodes and pathological inspection of those nodes. Another method is lymph node palpation only or selective removal of only enlarged nodes. However, systematic lymphadenectomy is significantly associated with increased postoperative complications. Lymph node dissection must therefore be tailored to maximize the therapeutic effect of surgery and minimize its invasiveness and adverse effects. Regional lymph nodes in endometrial cancer are classified into pelvic lymph nodes (PLNs) and para-aortic lymph nodes (PANs). PANs are widely known as regional lymph nodes in endometrial cancer through sentinel mapping [45, 46] and surgicopathologic studies [7, 47–70]. PLN metastases are identified in 14.4% of patients with endometrial cancer who have undergone surgical removal and pathological examination of the PLNs + PANs (Table 16.4). The rates vary with the depth of myometrial invasion and histological findings as follows: negligible in cases of no myoinvasion, negligible in cases of small (<2 cm) tumors with superficial myoinvasion and type I histology, 5% in cases of superficial myoinvasion and type I histology, 15% in cases of superficial myoinvasion and type II histology, and 40% in cases of deep myoinvasion and type II histology. PAN metastases are identified in 9.7% of patients with endometrial cancer who have undergone surgical removal and pathological examination of the PLNs + PANs (Table 16.4). While PAN metastasis is detected in only 2.7% of patients without PLN metastasis, it is detected in 51.4% of those with PLN metastasis (Table 16.4). In addition, occult PAN micrometastasis is detected in 73.0% of patients with stage IIIC1 disease [71].

16.3 Preoperative Evaluation

The surgical stage should be based on the patient's physical status, age, body mass index, comorbidities, disease extent, and disease aggressiveness. The extent of the disease, including the presence of myometrial invasion, cervical involvement, adnexal metastasis, lymph node metastasis, and distant metastasis, can be assessed by imaging modalities. The use of magnetic resonance imaging is recommended to assess myometrial invasion and cervical involvement, and computed tomography is preferable for assessing lymph node metastasis and distant metastasis. The aggressiveness of the disease can be assessed by microscopic examination of preoperative specimens obtained from endometrial curettage.

Table 16.4 Lymphatic spread pattern in endometrial cancer

Author	Year	*N*	FIGO stage III/IV (%)	NE histology (%)	Number[a] of PLNs removed	Number[a] of PANs removed	*A* PLN−/PAN−	*B* PLN−/PAN+	*C* PLN+/PAN−	*D* PLN+/PAN+	*C* + *D*/*N* (%)	*B* + *D*/*N* (%)	*B*/*A* + *B* (%)	*D*/*C* + *D* (%)
Median (mean) number of PAN removed: <10														
Larson [47]	1993	50	28%	0%	13	5	40	0	2	8	20.0%	16.0%	0.0%	80.0%
Fanning [48]	1996	60	8%	0%	21	7	55	0	5	0	8.3%	0.0%	0.0%	0.0%
Yokoyama [49]	1997	63	13%	3%	14	6	45	4	6	8	22.2%	19.0%	8.2%	57.1%
Lee [50]	2009	349	NA	0%	(22.8)	(9.5)	277	7	26	39	18.6%	13.2%	2.5%	60.0%
Abu-Rustum [51]	2009	847	NA	NA	16	5	722	12	52	61	13.3%	8.6%	1.6%	54.0%
Chiang [52]	2011	171	22%	6%	17	5	154	2	12	3	8.8%	2.9%	1.3%	20.0%
Solmaz [53]	2015	516	NA	0%	22	8.5	449	4	37	26	12.2%	5.8%	0.9%	41.3%
Subtotal		2056					1742	29	140	145	13.9%	8.5%	1.6%	50.9%
Median (mean) number of PAN removed: not available														
Chen [54]	1983	74	NA	11%	NA	NA	63	3	3	5	10.8%	10.8%	4.5%	62.5%
Creasman [7]	1987	621	22%	4%	NA	NA	551	12	36	22	9.3%	5.5%	2.1%	37.9%
Ayhan [55]	1995	209	NA	NA	NA	NA	173	6	17	13	14.4%	9.1%	3.4%	43.3%
Hirahatake [56]	1997	200	42%	4%	NA	NA	158	2	24	16	20.0%	9.0%	1.3%	40.0%
Milam [57]	2012	582	11%	0%	NA	NA	520	12	31	19	8.6%	5.3%	2.3%	38.0%
Sueoka [58]	2014	502	17%	18%	NA	NA	422	15	27	38	12.9%	10.6%	3.4%	58.5%
Mahdi [59]	2014	91	NA	NA	NA	NA	56	6	18	11	31.9%	18.7%	9.7%	37.9%
Subtotal		2279					1943	56	156	124	12.3%	7.9%	2.8%	44.3%
Median (mean) number of PAN removed: >10														
Onda [60]	1997	173	24%	1%	(37.9)	(28.7)	143	2	10	18	16.2%	11.6%	1.4%	64.3%
Matsumoto [61]	2002	106	NA	5%	(36.8)	(30.5)	79	2	7	18	23.6%	18.9%	2.5%	72.0%
Mariani [62]	2008	281	NA	NA	35	17	218	10	24	29	18.9%	13.9%	4.4%	54.7%
Fujimoto [63]	2009	355	25%	0%	42	19	306	7	20	22	11.8%	8.2%	2.2%	52.4%

(continued)

Table 16.4 (continued)

Author	Year	*N*	FIGO stage III/IV (%)	NE histology (%)	Number[a] of PLNs removed	Number[a] of PANs removed	*A* PLN−/PAN−	*B* PLN−/PAN+	*C* PLN+/PAN−	*D* PLN+/PAN+	*C* + *D*/*N* (%)	*B* + *D*/*N* (%)	*B*/*A* + *B* (%)	*D*/*C* + *D* (%)
Dogan [64]	2011	161	21%	21%	(49.5)	(19.0)	143	2	11	5	9.9%	4.3%	1.4%	31.3%
Odagiri [65]	2014	266	NA	17%	62.5	20	224	7	16	19	13.2%	9.8%	3.0%	54.3%
Altay [66]	2014	173	NA	27%	26	12	135	7	12	19	17.9%	15.0%	4.9%	61.3%
Tomisato [67]	2014	260	46%	17%	50	22	169	9	34	48	31.5%	21.9%	5.1%	58.5%
Fotopoulou [68]	2015	128	15%	24%	29	21.5	101	4	8	15	18.0%	14.8%	3.8%	65.2%
Sautua [69]	2015	90	NA	NA	(11.9)	(10.7)	77	6	3	4	7.8%	11.1%	7.2%	57.1%
Alay [70]	2015	204	26%	23%	(44.1)	(24.9)	160	8	17	19	17.6%	13.2%	4.8%	52.8%
Subtotal		2197					1755	64	162	216	17.2%	12.7%	3.5%	57.1%
Total		6532					5440	149	458	485	14.4%	9.7%	2.7%	51.4%

[a]Median (mean); *FIGO* International Federation of Gynecology and Obstetrics; *NA* not available; *NE* non-endometrioid; *PLN* pelvic lymph node; *PAN* para-aortic lymph node

16.4 Technique

The patient is placed in either the supine or dorsal lithotomy position depending on the surgical approach. If the lithotomy position is used, extra caution is required during positioning to ensure that no pressure points are created or hyperextension of joints occurs. The risk of nerve injury is higher in this position. The abdominopelvic cavity should be explored to identify any ascites and peritoneal dissemination. Any free peritoneal fluid should be sent for cytology. If no free fluid is present, peritoneal washings for cytologic examination should be obtained by irrigating the pelvis with warm saline. If no evidence of peritoneal dissemination is found, peritoneal biopsies can be performed for type II endometrial cancer. The omentum should be carefully inspected. The infracolic omentum might be removed in patients with type II endometrial cancer. If any suspicious area is present between the stomach and transverse colon, then the entire gastrocolic omentum should be removed. Hysterectomy and lymphadenectomy are discussed in detail in Chaps. 6, 7, 8 and 18, respectively. All regional lymph nodes are not removed in every patient, and the actual extent of lymphadenectomy depends on the disease status and patient's characteristics including age, body mass index, and complications. Consensus regarding this issue has not been reached.

Lymphatic spread of endometrial cancer may occur by three routes. The first route is from the fundus toward the adnexa and infundibulopelvic ligaments to the PANs. The second route is from the lower and middle thirds of the uterus in the base of the broad ligaments toward the lateral pelvic wall. The third route is along the round ligaments to the circumflex iliac nodes to the distal external iliac nodes.

16.5 Morbidity

Surgical morbidity rates in patients with endometrial cancer vary depending on the surgical approach (laparotomy vs. minimally invasive surgery), procedure (with vs. without lymphadenectomy and extent thereof), and patient characteristics (age, obesity, and comorbidities). Laparotomy and lymphadenectomy are significantly associated with increased complications compared with minimally invasive surgery performed by experienced surgeons and hysterectomy alone. Intraoperative organ injuries include intestinal, bladder, ureteral, vascular, and neurologic injuries. Perioperative and postoperative complications include reoperation, postoperative hemorrhage, ileus, wound separation, surgical site infection, and venous thromboembolism. Wound complications are significantly associated with obesity and diabetes mellitus. Lower extremity lymphedema and lymphocele formation are lymphadenectomy-related complications. Surgery-associated morbidity in patients with endometrial cancer is significantly higher in women aged >80 years, even after medical comorbidities have been considered [72].

16.6 Surgical Treatment of Advanced Disease

Most patients with endometrial cancer are diagnosed at an early stage, but 3% to 13% of all patients have stage IV disease at the time of diagnosis. Previous studies of advanced disease have suggested that optimal cytoreduction may be beneficial [73–78]. Chi et al. [73] showed a survival benefit of surgical cytoreduction for patients with stage IV cancer by dividing patients into three groups: optimal cytoreduction, in which the largest residual tumor is ≤2 cm; suboptimal cytoreduction, in which the largest residual tumor is >2 cm; and unresectable disease. The median survival periods in the three groups were 31, 12, and 3 months, respectively ($P < 0.01$). Bristow et al. [74] showed a survival benefit of optimal cytoreduction for patients with stage IVb cancer by dividing patients into two groups: optimal cytoreduction, in which the largest residual tumor was ≤1 cm, and suboptimal cytoreduction, in which the largest residual tumor was >1 cm. The median survival periods in these groups were 34 and 11 months, respectively ($P = 0.0001$). Ueda et al. [76] concluded that optimal cytoreduction (residual tumor of <2 cm) is associated with improved survival of patients with stage IVb disease with extra-abdominal metastasis. The median survival periods for these groups were 57 and 6 months, respectively ($P = 0.016$). In other studies, optimal cytoreduction showed a survival benefit for patients with advanced uterine serous papillary carcinoma [77, 78].

References

1. Siegel RL, Miller KD, Jemal A. Cancer statistics, 2017. CA Cancer J Clin. 2017;67:7–30.
2. Parker SL, Tong T, Bolden S, Wingo PA. Cancer statistics, 1997. CA Cancer J Clin. 1997;47:5–27.
3. Creasman WT, Odicino F, Maisonneuve P, Quinn MA, Beller U, Benedet JL, Heintz AP, Ngan HY, Pecorelli S. Carcinoma of the corpus uteri FIGO 26th annual report on the results of treatment in gynecological cancer. Int J Gynaecol Obstet. 2006;95:S105–43.
4. Signorelli M, Lissoni AA, Cormio G, Katsaros D, Pellegrino A, Selvaggi L, Ghezzi F, Scambia G, Zola P, Grassi R, Milani R, Giannice R, Caspani G, Mangioni C, Floriani I, Rulli E, Fossati R. Modified radical hysterectomy versus extrafascial hysterectomy in the treatment of stage I endometrial cancer: results from the ILIADE randomized study. Ann Surg Oncol. 2009;16:3431–41.
5. Han CH, Lee KH, Lee HN, Kim CJ, Park TC, Park JS. Does the type of hysterectomy affect the prognosis in clinical stage I endometrial cancer? J Obstet Gynecol Res. 2010;36:581–7.
6. Boronow RC, Morrow CP, Creasman WT, Disaia PJ, Silverberg SG, Miller A, Blessing JA. Surgical staging in endometrial cancer: clinical-pathologic findings of a prospective study. Obstet Gynecol. 1984;63:825–32.
7. Creasman WT, Morrow CP, Bundy BN, Homesley HD, Graham JE, Heller PB. Surgical pathologic spread patterns of endometrial cancer. A Gynecologic Oncology Group Study. Cancer. 1987;60:2035–41.
8. Boente MP, Yordan EL Jr, McIntosh DG, Grendys EC Jr, Orandi YA, Davies S, Beck D, Graham JE Jr, Miller A, Marshall R, et al. Prognostic factors and long-term survival in endometrial adenocarcinoma with cervical involvement. Gynecol Oncol. 1993;51:316–22.
9. Takeshima N, Hirai Y, Yano K, Tanaka N, Yamauchi K, Hasumi K. Ovarian metastasis in endometrial carcinoma. Gynecol Oncol. 1998;70:183–7.

10. Creasman WT, DeGeest K, DiSaia PJ, Zaino RJ. Significance of true surgical pathologic staging: a Gynecologic Oncology Group Study. Am J Obstet Gynecol. 1999;181:31–4.
11. Sakuragi N, Hareyama H, Todo Y, Yamada H, Yamamoto R, Fujino T, Sagawa T, Fujimoto S. Prognostic significance of serous and clear cell adenocarcinoma in surgically staged endometrial carcinoma. Acta Obstet Gynecol Scand. 2000;79:311–6.
12. Michelesen TM, Pripp AH, Tonstad S, Trope CG, Dorum A. Metabolic syndrome after risk-reducing salpingo-oophorectomy in women at high risk for hereditary breast ovarian cancer: a controlled observational study. Eur J Cancer. 2009;45:82–9.
13. Dorum A, Tonstad S, Liavaag AH, Michelesen TM, Hildrum B, Dahl AA. Bilateral oophorectomy before 50 years of age is significantly associated with the metabolic syndrome and Framingham risk score: a controlled, population-based study (HUNT-2). Gynecol Oncol. 2008;109:377–83.
14. Wright JD, Buck AM, Shah M, Burke WM, Schiff PB, Herzog TJ. Safety of ovarian preservation in premenopausal women with endometrial cancer. J Clin Oncol. 2009;27:1214–9.
15. Koskas M, Bendifallah S, Luton D, Daraï E, Rouzier R. Safety of uterine and/or ovarian preservation in young women with grade 1 intramucous endometrial adenocarcinoma: a comparison of survival according to the extent of surgery. Fertil Steril. 2012;98:1229–35.
16. Lee TS, Lee JY, Kim JW, Oh S, Seong SJ, Lee JM, Kim TJ, Cho CH, Kim SM, Park CY. Outcomes of ovarian preservation in a cohort of premenopausal women with early-stage endometrial cancer: a Korean Gynecologic Oncology Group study. Gynecol Oncol. 2013;131:289–93.
17. Evans-Metcalf ER, Brooks SE, Reale FR, Baker SP. Profile of women 45 years of age and younger with endometrial cancer. Obstet Gynecol. 1998;91:349–54.
18. Gitsch G, Hanzal E, Jensen D, Hacker NF. Endometrial cancer in premenopausal women 45 years and younger. Obstet Gynecol. 1995;85:504–8.
19. Wethington SL, Barrena Medel NI, Wright JD, Herzog TJ. Prognostic significance and treatment implications of positive peritoneal cytology in endometrial adenocarcinoma: Unraveling a mystery. Gynecol Oncol. 2009;115:18–25.
20. Hirai Y, Fujimoto I, Yamauchi K, Hasumi K, Masubuchi K, Sano Y. Peritoneal fluid cytology and prognosis in patients with endometrial carcinoma. Obstet Gynecol. 1989;73:335–8.
21. Ebina Y, Hareyama H, Sakuragh N, Yamamoto R, Furuya M, Sogame M, Fujino T, Makinoda S, Fujimoto S. Peritoneal cytology and its prognostic value in endometrial carcinoma. Int Surg. 1997;82:244–8.
22. Takeshima N, Nishida H, Tabata T, Hirai Y, Hasumi K. Positive peritoneal cytology in endometrial cancer: enhancement of other prognostic indicators. Gynecol Oncol. 2001;82:470–3.
23. Mariani A, Webb MJ, Keeney GL, Aletti G, Podratz KC. Assessment of prognostic factors in stage IIIA endometrial cancer. Gynecol Oncol. 2002;86:38–44.
24. Kasamatsu T, Onda T, Katsumata N, Sawada M, Yamada T, Tsunematsu R, Ohmi K, Sasajima Y, Matsuno Y. Prognostic significance of positive peritoneal cytology in endometrial carcinoma confined to the uterus. Br J Cancer. 2003;88:245–50.
25. Tebeu PM, Popowski Y, Verkooijen HM, Bouchardy C, Ludicke F, Usel M, Major AL. Positive peritoneal cytology in early-stage endometrial cancer does not influence prognosis. Br J Cancer. 2004;91:720–4.
26. Turner DA, Gershenson DM, Atkinson N, Sneige N, Wharton AT. The prognostic significance of peritoneal cytology for stage I endometrial cancer. Obstet Gynecol. 1989;74:775–80.
27. Lurain JR, Rice BL, Rademaker AW, Poggensee LE, Schink JC, Miller DS. Prognostic factors associated with recurrence in clinical stage I adenocarcinoma of the endometrium. Obstet Gynecol. 1991;78:63–9.
28. Kashimura M, Sugihara K, Toki N, Matsuura Y, Kawagoe T, Kamura T, Kaku T, Tsuruchi N, Nakashima H, Sakai H. The significance of peritoneal cytology in uterine cervix and endometrial cancer. Gynecol Oncol. 1997;67:285–90.
29. Obermair A, Geramou M, Tripcony L, Nicklin JL, Perrin L, Crandon AJ. Peritoneal cytology: impact on disease-free survival in clinical stage I endometrioid adenocarcinoma of the uterus. Cancer Lett. 2001;164:105–10.

30. Saga Y, Imai M, Jobo T, Kuramoto H, Takahashi K, Konno R, Ohwada M, Suzuki M. Is peritoneal cytology a prognostic factor of endometrial cancer confined to the uterus? Gynecol Oncol. 2006;103:277–80.
31. Havrilesky LJ, Cragun JM, Calingaert B, Alvarez Secord A, Valea FA, Clarke-Pearson DL, Berchuck A, Soper JT. The prognostic significance of positive peritoneal cytology and adnexal/serosal metastasis in stage IIIA endometrial cancer. Gynecol Oncol. 2007;104:401–5.
32. Mariani A, Dowdy SC, Podratz KC. New surgical staging of endometrial cancer: 20 years later. Int J Gynaecol Obstet. 2009;105:110–1.
33. Shiozaki T, Tabata T, Yamada T, Yamamoto Y, Yamawaki T, Ikeda T. Does positive peritoneal cytology not affect the prognosis for stage I uterine endometrial cancer?: the remaining controversy and review of the literature. Int J Gynecol Cancer. 2014;24:549–55.
34. Milgrom SA, Kollmeier MA, Abu-Rustum NR, Makker V, Gardner GJ, Barakat RR, Alektiar KM. Positive peritoneal cytology is highly predictive of prognosis and relapse patterns in stage III (FIGO 2009) endometrial cancer. Gynecol Oncol. 2013;130:49–53.
35. Garg G, Gao F, Wright JD, Hagemann AR, Mutch DG, Powell MA. Positive peritoneal cytology is an independent risk-factor in early stage endometrial cancer. Gynecol Oncol. 2013;128:77–82.
36. Chen SS, Spiegel G. Stage I endometrial carcinoma. Role of omental biopsy and omentectomy. J Reprod Med. 1991;36:627–9.
37. Saygili U, Kavaz S, Altunyurt S, Uslu T, Koyuncuoglu M, Erten O. Omentectomy, peritoneal biopsy and appendectomy in patients with clinical stage I endometrial carcinoma. Int J Gynecol Cancer. 2001;11:471–4.
38. Dilek S, Dilek U, Dede M, Deveci MS, Yenen MC. The role of omentectomy and appendectomy during the surgical staging of clinical stage I endometrial cancer. Int J Gynecol Cancer. 2006;16:795–8.
39. Fujiwara H, Saga Y, Takahashi K, Ohwada M, Enomoto A, Konno R, Tanaka A, Suzuki M. Omental metastases in clinical stage I endometrioid adenocarcinoma. Int J Gynecol Cancer. 2008;18:165–7.
40. Metindir J, Dilek GB. The role of omentectomy during the surgical staging in patients with clinical stage I endometrioid adenocarcinoma. J Cancer Res Clin Oncol. 2008;134:1067–70.
41. Ozdal B, Unlu BS, Yalcin HR, Tapisiz OL, Energin H, Besli M, Gungor T. Role of omentectomy and appendectomy in surgical staging of endometrioid endometrial cancer. Eur J Gynaecol Oncol. 2013;34:322–4.
42. Ulker V, Tunca A, Numanoglu C, Akbayir O, Akyol A, Erim A, Ongut C. Should omentectomy be a part of surgical staging in patients with endometrioid adenocarcinoma of the uterine corpus? Gynecol Obstet Investig. 2014;77:58–63.
43. Sakai K, Yamagami W, Susumu N, Nomura H, Kataoka F, Banno K, Tsuda H, Aoki D. Pathological factors associated with omental metastases in endometrial cancer. Eur J Gynaecol Oncol. 2015;36:397–401.
44. Joo WD, Schwartz PE, Rutherford TJ, Seong SJ, Ku J, Park H, Jung SG, Choi MC, Lee C. Microscopic omental metastasis in clinical stage I endometrial cancer: a meta-analysis. Ann Surg Oncol. 2015;22:3695–700.
45. Burke TW, Levenback C, Tornos C, Morris M, Wharton JT, Gershenson DM. Intraabdominal lymphatic mapping to direct selective pelvic and para-aortic lymphadenectomy in women with high-risk endometrial cancer: results of a pilot study. Gynecol Oncol. 1996;62:169–73.
46. Niikura H, Okamura C, Utsunomiya H, Yoshinaga K, Akahira J, Ito K, Yaegashi N. Sentinel lymph node detection in patients with endometrial cancer. Gynecol Oncol. 2004;92:669–74.
47. Larson DM, Johnson KK. Pelvic and para-aortic lymphadenectomy for surgical staging of high-risk endometrioid adenocarcinoma of the endometrium. Gynecol Oncol. 1993;51:345–8.
48. Fanning J, Nanavati PJ, Hilgers RD. Surgical staging and high dose rate brachytherapy for endometrial cancer: limiting external radiotherapy to node-positive tumors. Obstet Gynecol. 1996;87:1041–4.
49. Yokoyama Y, Maruyama H, Sato S, Saito Y. Indispensability of pelvic and paraaortic lymphadenectomy in endometrial cancers. Gynecol Oncol. 1997;64:411–7.

50. Lee KB, Ki KD, Lee JM, Lee JK, Kim JW, Cho CH, et al. The risk of lymph node metastasis based on myometrial invasion and tumor grade in endometrioid uterine cancers: a multicenter, retrospective Korean study. Ann Surg Oncol. 2009;16:2882–7.
51. Abu-Rustum NR, Khoury-Collado F, Pandit-Taskar N, Soslow RA, Dao F, Sonoda Y, et al. Sentinel lymph node mapping for grade 1 endometrial cancer: is it the answer to the surgical staging dilemma? Gynecol Oncol. 2009;113:163–9.
52. Chiang AJ, Yu KJ, Chao KC, Teng NN. The incidence of isolated para-aortic nodal metastasis in completely staged endometrial cancer patients. Gynecol Oncol. 2011;121:122–5.
53. Solmaz U, Mat E, Dereli ML, Turan V, Tosun G, Dogan A, et al. Lymphovascular space invasion and positive pelvic lymph nodes are independent risk factors for para-aortic nodal metastasis in endometrioid endometrial cancer. Eur J Obstet Gynecol Reprod Biol. 2015;186:63–7.
54. Chen SS, Lee L. Retroperitoneal lymph node metastases in Stage I carcinoma of the endometrium: correlation with risk factors. Gynecol Oncol. 1983;16:319–25.
55. Ayhan A, Tuncer ZS, Tuncer R, Yüce K, Küçükali T. Tumor status of lymph nodes in early endometrial cancer in relation to lymph node size. Eur J Obstet Gynecol Reprod Biol. 1995;60:61–3.
56. Hirahatake K, Hareyama H, Sakuragi N, Nishiya M, Makinoda S, Fujimoto S. A clinical and pathologic study on para-aortic lymph node metastasis in endometrial carcinoma. J Surg Oncol. 1997;65:82–7.
57. Milam MR, Java J, Walker JL, Metzinger DS, Parker LP, Coleman RL. Gynecologic Oncology Group. Nodal metastasis risk in endometrioid endometrial cancer. Obstet Gynecol. 2012;119:286–92.
58. Sueoka K, Umayahara K, Abe A, Usami T, Yamamoto A, Nomura H, et al. Prognosis for endometrial cancer patients treated with systematic pelvic and para-aortic lymphadenectomy followed by platinum-based chemotherapy. Int J Gynecol Cancer. 2015;25:81–6.
59. Mahdi H, Jernigan A, Nutter B, Michener C, Rose PG. Lymph node metastasis and pattern of recurrence in clinically early stage endometrial cancer with positive lymphovascular space invasion. J Gynecol Oncol. 2015;26:208–13.
60. Onda T, Yoshikawa H, Mizutani K, Mishima M, Yokota H, Nagano H, et al. Treatment of node-positive endometrial cancer with complete node dissection, chemotherapy and radiation therapy. Br J Cancer. 1997;75:1836–41.
61. Matsumoto K, Yoshikawa H, Yasugi T, Onda T, Nakagawa S, Yamada M, et al. Distinct lymphatic spread of endometrial carcinoma in comparison with cervical and ovarian carcinomas. Cancer Lett. 2002;180:83–9.
62. Mariani A, Dowdy SC, Cliby WA, Gostout BS, Jones MB, Wilson TO, et al. Prospective assessment of lymphatic dissemination in endometrial cancer: a paradigm shift in surgical staging. Gynecol Oncol. 2008;109:11–8.
63. Fujimoto T, Nanjyo H, Fukuda J, Nakamura A, Mizunuma H, Yaegashi N, et al. Endometrioid uterine cancer: histopathological risk factors of local and distant recurrence. Gynecol Oncol. 2009;112:342–7.
64. Dogan NU, Gungor T, Karsli F, Ozgu E, Besli M. To what extent should para-aortic lymphadenectomy be carried out for surgically staged endometrial cancer? Int J Gynecol Cancer. 2012;22:607–10.
65. Odagiri T, Watari H, Kato T, Mitamura T, Hosaka M, Sudo S, et al. Distribution of lymph node metastasis sites in endometrial cancer undergoing systematic pelvic and para-aortic lymphadenectomy: a proposal of optimal lymphadenectomy for future clinical trials. Ann Surg Oncol. 2014;21:2755–61.
66. Altay A, Toptas T, Dogan S, Simsek T, Pestereli E. Analysis of Metastatic Regional Lymph Node Locations and Predictors of Para-aortic Lymph Node Involvement in Endometrial Cancer Patients at Risk for Lymphatic Dissemination. Int J Gynecol Cancer. 2015;25:657–64.
67. Tomisato S, Yamagami W, Susumu N, Kuwahata M, Takigawa A, Nomura H, et al. Clinicopathological study on para-aortic lymph node metastasis without pelvic lymph node metastasis in endometrial cancer. J Obstet Gynaecol Res. 2014;40:1733–9.

68. Fotopoulou C, El-Balat A, du Bois A, Sehouli J, Harter P, Muallem MZ, et al. Systematic pelvic and paraaortic lymphadenectomy in early high-risk or advanced endometrial cancer. Arch Gynecol Obstet. 2015;292:1321–7.
69. Sautua RR, Goiri K, Calle MA, Marin IJ, Artola AL. Incidence of nodal metastasis and isolated aortic metastases in patients with surgically staged endometrioid endometrial cancer. Int J Gynecol Cancer. 2015;25:875–8.
70. Alay I, Turan T, Ureyen I, Karalok A, Tasci T, Ozfuttu A, et al. Lymphadenectomy should be performed up to the renal vein in patients with intermediate-high risk endometrial cancer. Pathol Oncol Res. 2015;21:803–10.
71. Todo Y, Suzuki Y, Azuma M, et al. Ultrastaging of para-aortic lymph nodes in stage IIIC1 endometrial cancer. Gynecol Oncol. 2012;127:532–7.
72. Wright JD, Lewin SN, Barrena Medel NI, Sun X, Burke WM, Deutsch I, Herzog TJ. Morbidity and mortality of surgery for endometrial cancer in the oldest old. Am J Obstet Gynecol. 2011;205:66.e1–8.
73. Chi DS, Welshinger M, Venkatraman ES, Barakat RR. The role of surgical cytoreduction in Stage IV endometrial carcinoma. Gynecol Oncol. 1997;67:56–60.
74. Bristow RE, Zerbe MJ, Rosenshein NB, Grumbine FC, Montz FJ. Stage IVB endometrial carcinoma: the role of cytoreductive surgery and determinants of survival. Gynecol Oncol. 2000;78:85–91.
75. Ayhan A, Taskiran C, Celik C, Yuce K, Kucukali T. The influence of cytoreductive surgery on survival and morbidity in stage IVB endometrial cancer. Int J Gynecol Cancer. 2002;12:448–53.
76. Ueda Y, Enomoto T, Miyatake T, Egawa-Takata T, Ugaki H, Yoshino K, Fujita M, Kimura T. Endometrial carcinoma with extra-abdominal metastasis: improved prognosis following cytoreductive surgery. Ann Surg Oncol. 2010;17:1111–7.
77. Memarzadeh S, Holschneider CH, Bristow RE, Jones NL, Fu YS, Karlan BY, Berek JS, Farias-Eisner R. FIGO stage III and IV uterine papillary serous carcinoma: impact of residual disease on survival. Int J Gynecol Cancer. 2002;12:454–8.
78. Thomas MB, Mariani A, Cliby WA, Keeney GL, Podratz KC, Dowdy SC. Role of cytoreduction in stage III and IV uterine papillary serous carcinoma. Gynecol Oncol. 2007;107:190–3.

Retroperitoneal Lymph Node Dissection 17

Yukiharu Todo

Abstract

The regional lymph nodes in patients with endometrial cancer are usually categorized into pelvic lymph nodes and para-aortic lymph nodes. Thus, lymph node dissection in patients with endometrial cancer includes a wide variety of surgical procedures. Although the consensus is that pelvic lymphadenectomy is not necessary for patients with low-risk endometrial cancer, it is possible that combined pelvic and para-aortic lymphadenectomy is useful for patients with intermediate- and high-risk endometrial cancer. Another important aspect of lymphadenectomy is the risk of lymphedema of the lower extremities. Leg edema is the most frequent complication of lymphadenectomy. Therefore, lymphadenectomy must be tailored to maximize the therapeutic effect of surgery and minimize its invasiveness and adverse effects. Two strategies may be used: (1) removal of lymph nodes most likely to harbor disease with preservation of lymph nodes unlikely to be affected and (2) performance of full lymphadenectomy only in patients who can potentially benefit from this procedure with preservation of the lymph nodes most closely associated with the incidence of lymphedema.

Keywords

Para-aortic lymphadenectomy · Circumflex iliac nodes · Lymphedema · Inferior mesenteric artery · Renal vein

Y. Todo (✉)
Division of Gynecologic Oncology, National Hospital Organization, Hokkaido Cancer Center, Sapporo, Japan
e-mail: yukiharu@sap-cc.go.jp

M. Mikami (ed.), *Surgery for Gynecologic Cancer*, Comprehensive Gynecology and Obstetrics, https://doi.org/10.1007/978-981-13-1519-0_17

17.1 History

Before 2008, all studies regarding the role of lymphadenectomy in patients with endometrial cancer were retrospective. Some studies supported a survival benefit of lymphadenectomy [1–8], while others did not [9–12]. The regional lymph nodes in patients with endometrial cancer are usually categorized into pelvic lymph nodes (PLNs) and para-aortic lymph nodes (PANs). Although PANs are widely known as regional lymph nodes in patients with endometrial cancer, para-aortic lymphadenectomy had not been well valued. Mariani et al. [8] focused on the PANs and showed a potential survival benefit of para-aortic lymphadenectomy in patients with endometrial cancer. They reported that removal of five or more PANs is associated with improved survival of high-risk patients.

In 2008, Benedetti-Panici et al. [13] conducted the first randomized controlled trial to assess the therapeutic effect of lymphadenectomy. A Study in the Treatment of Endometrial Cancer (ASTEC), the second randomized controlled trial of the therapeutic role of lymphadenectomy, was performed in 2009 [14]. Because both randomized controlled trials showed negative effects of lymphadenectomy on prognosis, many gynecologists have declared at conferences that standard surgery for endometrial cancer should not include lymphadenectomy. Conversely, this idea has also been criticized. The problem most often criticized is that para-aortic lymphadenectomy is performed at the discretion of the attending physician, and only a small number of patients undergo para-aortic lymphadenectomy in previous randomized studies.

In 2010, the significance of lymphadenectomy was revaluated in a retrospective observational study from Japan. The survival effect of para-aortic lymphadenectomy (SEPAL) study showed no survival benefit of combined pelvic and para-aortic lymphadenectomy over pelvic lymphadenectomy alone for low-risk patients but showed a significant survival benefit of the implementation of para-aortic lymphadenectomy in addition to pelvic lymphadenectomy for intermediate- and high-risk patients [15]. In that study, the combination of pelvic and para-aortic lymphadenectomy resulted in a 10.6% increase in the 5-year overall survival rate compared with pelvic lymphadenectomy alone in intermediate- and high-risk patients. In addition, para-aortic lymphadenectomy improved survival independent of the efficacy of adjuvant treatment.

17.2 Principles and Indications

17.2.1 Regional Lymph Nodes in Endometrial Cancer

Figure 17.1 shows the locations of the regional lymph node sites defined below. PLNs are classified into nine sites: circumflex iliac nodes to distal external iliac nodes (CINDEINs), external iliac nodes (EINs), circumflex iliac nodes to distal obturator nodes (CINDONs), interiliac nodes (IINs), obturator nodes (ONs), para-uterine artery nodes (PUNs), cardinal ligament nodes (CLNs), sacral nodes (SNs),

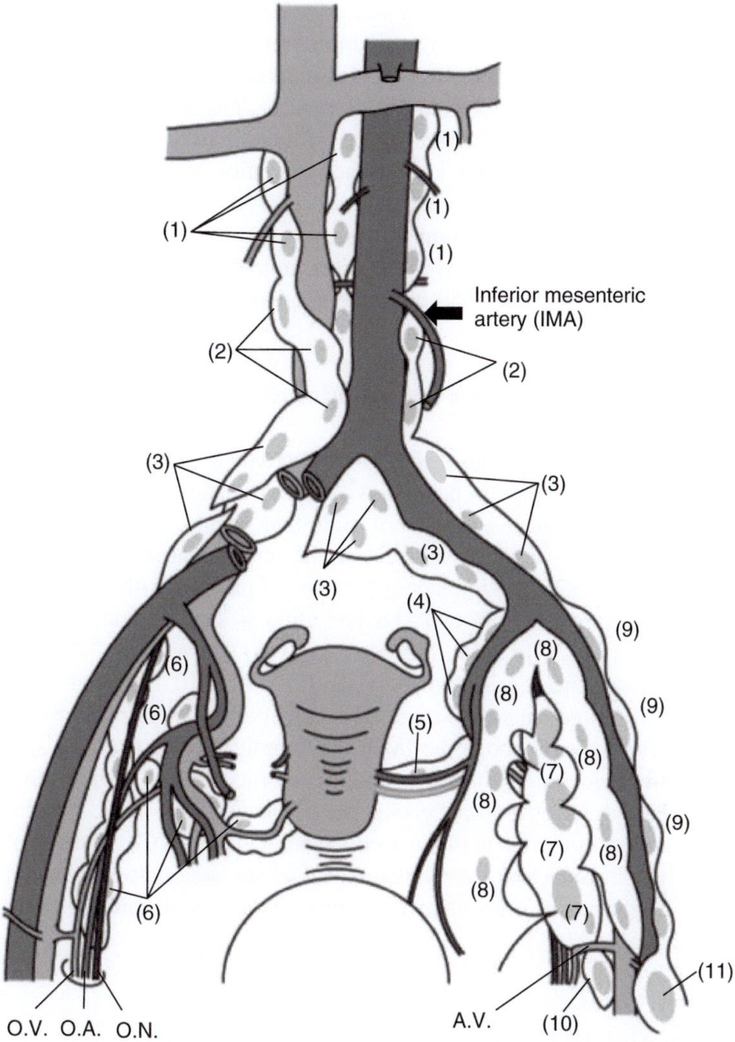

Fig. 17.1 Grouping and nomenclature of retroperitoneal lymph nodes. Para-aortic nodes: (*1*) the area above the inferior mesenteric artery (326b1), (*2*) the area below the inferior mesenteric artery (326b2), Pelvic nodes: (*3*) common iliac nodes, (*4*) sacral nodes, (*5*) para-uterine artery nodes, (*6*) cardinal ligament nodes, (*7*) obturator nodes, (*8*) internal iliac nodes, (*9*) external iliac nodes, (*10*) circumflex iliac nodes distal to the obtrator nodes, (*11*) circumflex iliac nodes distal to the external iliac nodes. *AV* anonymous vein, *OA* obturator artery, *ON* obturator nerve, *OV* obturator vein

and common iliac nodes (CINs). The definitions of each site are as follows. The EINs are located outside a lateral iliac artery and below the level of the bifurcation of the common iliac artery. The CINDEINs are the most distal EINs. The IINs are located on the anterior side of a medial iliac artery below the level of the bifurcation of the common iliac artery, between both iliac arteries. The ONs are located on the anterior side of an obturator nerve and under the IINs. The CINDONs are the most distal ONs, being located below an anonymous vein. The PUNs are located along the uterine artery or uterine vein. The CLNs are located on the posterior side of an obturator nerve and are often called the deep ONs. The SNs are located inside a medial iliac artery and below the level of the bifurcation of the common iliac artery. The CINs are located between the level of the bifurcation of the common iliac artery and the level of the bifurcation of the aorta. Conversely, the PANs are located between the level of the bifurcation of the aorta and the level of the renal veins. Namely, the PANs are all nodes from the precaval and laterocaval, interaortocaval, and preaortic and lateroaortic areas up to the renal veins.

17.2.2 Extent of Para-aortic Lymphadenectomy

Although the addition of para-aortic lymphadenectomy to pelvic lymphadenectomy might have a survival benefit in patients with intermediate- and high-risk endometrial cancer, this situation is actually not quite that simple. The PANs are usually categorized into the areas above and below the inferior mesenteric artery (IMA) (Fig. 17.1). Some sentinel node mapping studies of patients with endometrial cancer showed that more than half of PANs identified as sentinel nodes were located above the IMA [16, 17]. In 2008, Mariani et al. [18] showed that 77% of patients with PAN metastasis harbor disease above the IMA. In 2010, Fotopoulou et al. [19] showed that 54% of patients with stage IIIC cancer and 70% of patients with PAN metastasis harbor disease above the IMA. They indicated the need for systematic lymphadenectomy including the pelvic and para-aortic areas up to the renal vessels. In the SEPAL study, almost all patients in the pelvic and para-aortic lymphadenectomy group underwent removal of the section above the IMA. Combined pelvic and para-aortic lymphadenectomy without removal of the area between the IMA and renal veins might be insufficient to improve survival for patients with high-risk endometrial cancer.

17.2.3 Decision of the Need for Lymphadenectomy

The Mayo Clinic initiated a paradigm for surgical management of endometrial cancer. According to the Mayo algorithm, women with endometrial cancer are divided into a high-risk group (at risk for nodal metastasis) and low-risk group (not at risk for nodal metastasis). Full lymphadenectomy is performed in the high-risk group, and lymphadenectomy is no longer necessary for the low-risk group (defined as grade 1–2 endometrioid histology, depth of invasion of ≤50%, and tumor size of ≤2 cm; any grade endometrioid histology, no myometrial invasion, and any tumor size) [20]. This algorithm has been recognized as a cornerstone in decision-making regarding implementation of lymph node dissection because it warrants a sufficiently low (negligible) false-negative rate (undertreatment rate) in this situation. Some other risk-stratification models can also reportedly be applied in clinical

Table 17.1 Risk-stratification models for predicting lymph node metastasis in endometrial cancer

Model	Author	Low-risk (NOT at-risk) criteria	NOT at-risk population (%)	FNR* (%)	FPR** (%)
Mayo criteria	Mariani [20]	(1) Endometrioid G1/G2, myoinvasion <50%, tumor diameter <2 cm; (2) endometrioid any grade, myoinvasion 0%, any tumor diameter	21–40%†	0–2.3%††	88–94%†††
Helsinki model	Tuomi [21, 22]	Endometrioid, 0 risk score point (1 point for thrombocytosis, 2 points for grade 3, 2 points for tumor diameter ≥ 3 cm, 3 points for CA125 ≥ 35 U/mL)	38%§	0%§§	85%§§§
Milwaukee model	Cox Bauer [23]	Endometrioid, tumor diameter ≤ 5 cm, myoinvasion ≤33%	39–51%‖	0–2.0%¶	84–85%¶¶
Hokkaido Japan model	Todo [24, 25]	Endometrioid G1/G2, small volume index (<36), low CA125 (<70 U/mL for patients <50 years of age and <28 U/mL for patients ≥50 years of age)	54%‡	3.1–3.3%‡‡	72–74%‡‡‡
Korean model	Kang [26, 27]	Endometrioid, myoinvasion <50%, CA125 < 35 U/mL, no extrauterine disease	51–53%∫	1.6–1.9%∬	76%$
Modified ESMO criteria	Bendifallah [28]	(1) Endometrioid G1/G2, myoinvasion <50%; (2) endometrioid G1/G2, myoinvasion ≥50%, no lymphovascular space invasion (LVSI); (3) endometrioid G3, myoinvasion <50%, no LVSI	61%	7.6%	67%
Modified Mayo criteria	Vargas [29]	(1) Endometrioid G1, myoinvasion <50%, any tumor diameter; (2) endometrioid G2, myoinvasion <50%, tumor diameter < 3 cm; (3) endometrioid G3, myoinvasion 0%, any tumor diameter	Not available	Not available	Not available

**FNR* false-negative rate (positive lymph node metastasis rate in NOT at-risk population); ***FPR* false-positive rate (negative lymph node metastasis rate in at-risk population); † 21% [29], 29% [22], 32% [31], 40% [30]; †† 0% [20], 0.8% [30], 1.4% [29], 2.3% [22]; ††† 88% [22], 89% [31], 94% [29]; § 38% [22]; §§ 0% [22]; §§§ 85% [22]; ‖39% [23], 51% [22]; ¶ 0% [23], 2.0% [22]; ¶¶ 84% [22], 85% [23]; ‡ 54% [24], 54% [25]; ‡‡ 3.1% [25], 3.3% [24]; ‡‡‡ 72% [24], 74% [25]; ∫51% [27], 53% [26]; ∬1.6% [26], 1.9% [27]; $ 76% [27]

practice (Table 17.1) [20–30]. These models might be divided into three types. The Mayo criteria, the Helsinki model [21, 22], and the Milwaukee model [23] are examples of the first type of model, which provides an excellent false-negative rate by reducing the low-risk population to a minimum limit. However, some researchers have recently criticized this type of model because of its high false-positive rate (overtreatment rate) [31]. The model by Todo et al. [24, 25], the Korean Gynecologic Oncology Group criteria [26, 27], and the modified Mayo criteria [29] are examples of the second type of model, which can reduce false positives while controlling false negatives by expanding the low-risk population. The third type of model might not be practical because an incorporated factor is not available before hysterectomy. The modification of the European Society of Medical Oncology criteria incorporates lymphovascular space invasion, but information on lymphovascular space invasion is not available before hysterectomy and is difficult to confirm intraoperatively [28]. Generally, these models keep false negatives to a minimum limit but cause false positives; i.e., lymphadenectomies are frequently performed in patients with no lymph node metastasis. Sentinel lymph node mapping is expected to dramatically reduce false positives while controlling false negatives, thus offering a trade-off between systematic lymphadenectomy and no dissection in early-stage endometrial cancer.

17.3 Preoperative Evaluation

The risk of lymph node metastasis is highly associated with myometrial invasion, tumor size, and histological grade/variant. The use of magnetic resonance imaging (MRI) is recommended for assessment of myometrial invasion and tumor size. The histological grade/variant can be assessed by microscopic examination based on preoperative specimens obtained from endometrial curettage. The surgical stage should be also based on the patient's physical status, age, body mass index, and comorbidities. Obesity is an established risk factor for developing endometrial cancer and is common among patients with endometrial cancer. Therefore, obesity is an important issue when treating endometrial cancer. Obesity is reportedly associated with a well-differentiated histological grade, a younger age, or a FIGO stage of I, all of which are associated with favorable survival outcomes; nevertheless, obesity has never been shown to be associated with a survival advantage in patients with endometrial cancer [32–38]. It is possible that the paradoxical findings are resulted from insufficient surgical staging [39].

17.4 Technique

17.4.1 PLN Dissection

There are two priority tasks in terms of pelvic lymphadenectomy: development of the pararectal space and development of the paravesical space. The landmarks for development of the pararectal space are the ureter and the interiliac (hypogastric) artery. The inlet into the pararectal space is located between the ureter and interiliac artery. After the ureter has been identified, it is retracted medially to identify the interiliac artery. The pararectal space can then be bluntly developed, retracting the rectum medially. On the other hand, the landmark for development of the paravesical space is the umbilical ligament. The inlet into the paravesical space is present between the umbilical ligament and external iliac vein. After the umbilical ligament has been identified, it is retracted medially to identify the external iliac vein. The paravesical space can then be bluntly developed. Surgical retractor fixation systems are available for stable development of these spaces (Fig. 17.2).

The dissection begins with the EINs, but the CINDEINs might be spared to prevent postoperative lower extremity lymphedema (Fig. 17.3). The EINs can be detached from the external iliac artery and psoas muscle. The genitofemoral nerve should be spared during dissection. The IINs can be dissected from the external iliac vein and the nodal package consisting of the ONs. The ONs may be accessed from a lateral approach. After the external iliac vein has been medially mobilized, the obturator nodal package can be detached from the psoas muscle (Fig. 17.4). It may

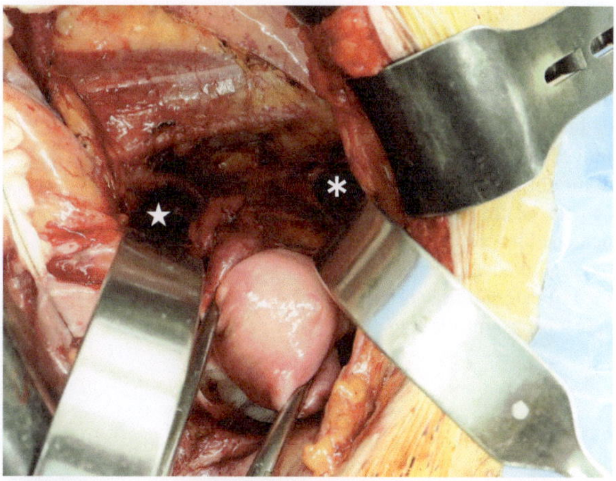

Fig. 17.2 The left pararectal (★) and the left paravesical (*) spaces are stably developed using a surgical retractor fixation system. The uterus is medially retracted with fine serrations forceps

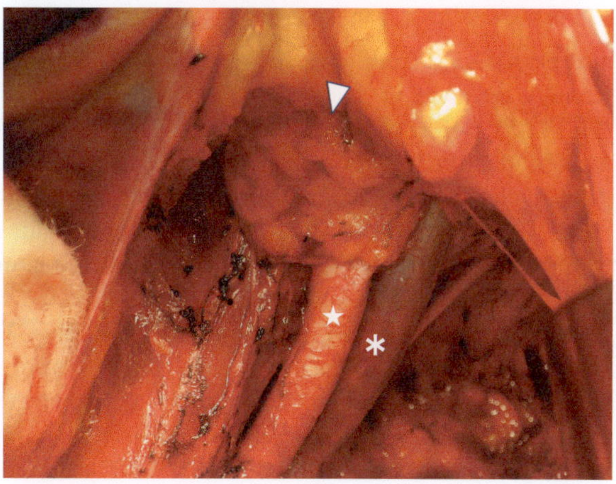

Fig. 17.3 The left EINs are removed, while the left CINDEIN (arrowhead) is spared. (★ left external iliac artery, * left external iliac vein)

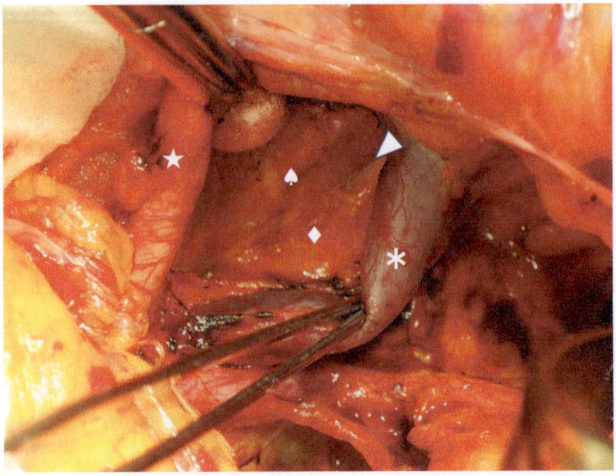

Fig. 17.4 Lateral approach for left ON dissection. The arrowhead indicates the boundary between the left obturator nodal package (♦) and the left psoas muscle (♠) (★ left external iliac artery, * left external iliac vein)

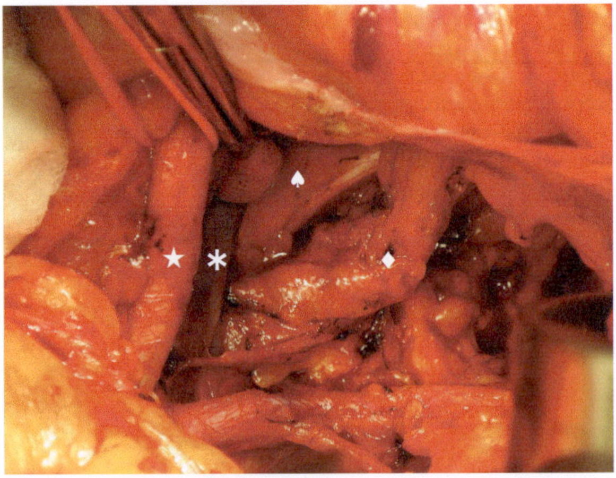

Fig. 17.5 Medial approach for left ON dissection. While the external iliac vein (*) is moved laterally, the left obturator nodal package (♦) can be completely detached from the left external iliac vein (*) (★ left external iliac artery, ♠ left psoas muscle)

also be accessed from a medial approach. While the external iliac vein is moved laterally, the nodal package can be completely detached from the external iliac vein (Fig. 17.5). Before the caudal limit of the nodal package is cut, the obturator nerve must be identified (Fig. 17.6). Pushing the obturator nerve in a dorsal direction with gentle counterattraction of the caudal limit of the package in a ventral direction may enable the package to be dissected from the obturator nerve. The CLNs are found below the ONs (Fig. 17.7), but they may be spared in most cases.

The CINs may be classified into three parts: the superficial (Fig. 17.8), deep (Fig. 17.9), and medial (Fig. 17.8 and 17.10) CINs. The superficial CINs receive lymphatic vessels from the superficial lymphatic trunks along the ventral aspect of the external iliac vessels. The superficial CINs may be dissected in a state connected from the PANs. The deep lateral CINs receive the lymphatic vessels from the deep lymphatic trunks, which consist of the ONs and CLNs. When the external iliac

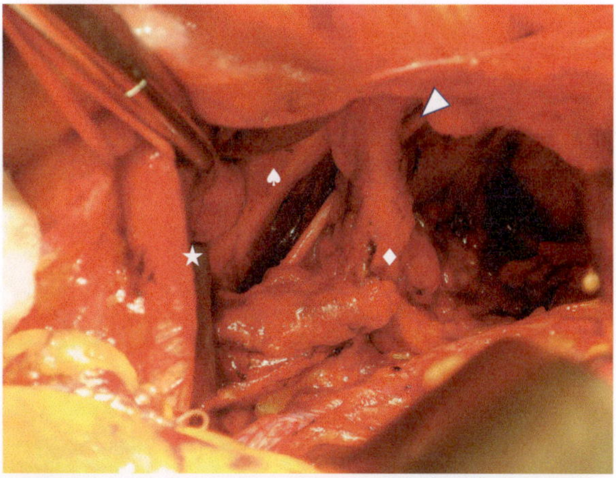

Fig. 17.6 Identification of the left obturator nerve (arrowhead) (★ left external iliac vessels, ◆ left obturator nodal package, ♠ left psoas muscle)

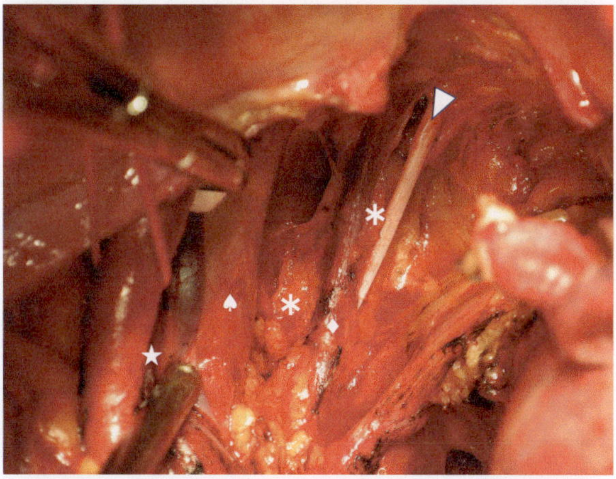

Fig. 17.7 Left cardinal lymph nodes (*) are seen below the left obturator nerve (arrowhead) (★ left external iliac vessels, ◆ left obturator vein, ♠ left psoas muscle)

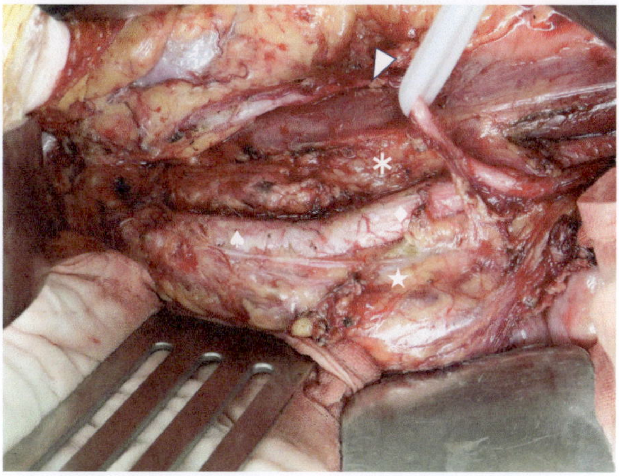

Fig. 17.8 Left superficial (*) CINs are located along the external side of the left common iliac artery (◆). Left medial (★) CINs are seen along the medial side of the left common iliac artery. The left ureter (arrowhead) is laterally retracted with a Penrose drain (♠ aorta)

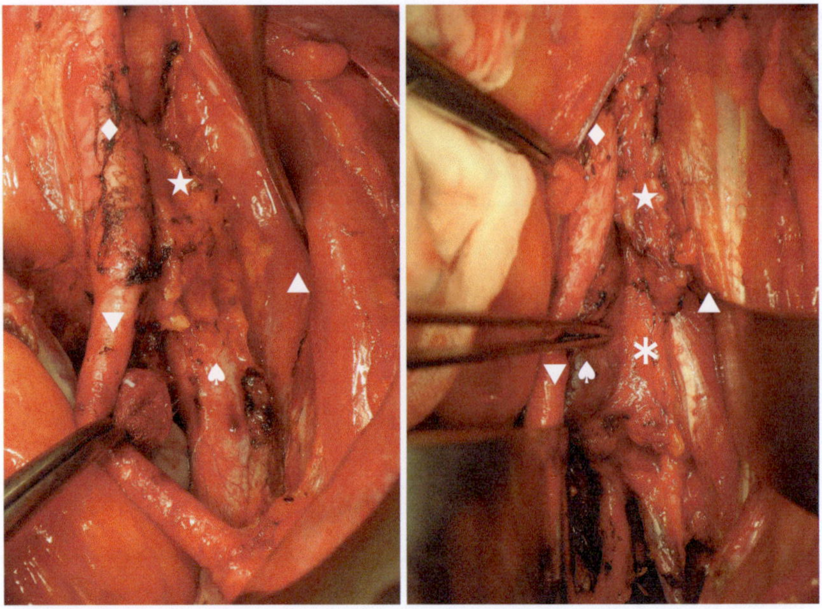

Fig. 17.9 Working space for dissection of the deep lateral CIN (★) before (left) and after (right) medial retraction of the external iliac vein (♠). The deep lateral CINs directly receive lymphatic vessels from the ONs (*) (◆ left common iliac artery, ▲ left psoas muscle, ▼ left external iliac artery)

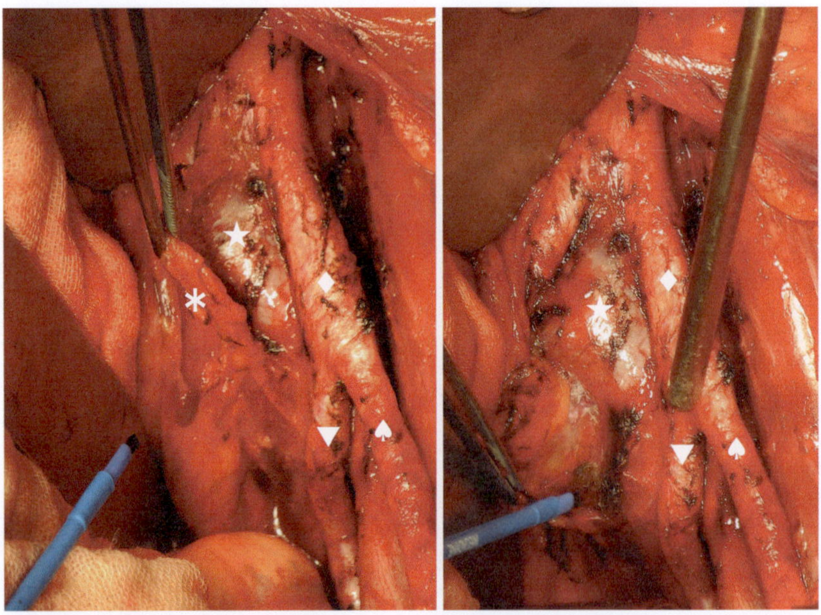

Fig. 17.10 Aortic bifurcation before (left) and after (right) dissection of the medial CIN (*) (★ left common iliac vein, ◆ left common iliac artery, ▼ left internal iliac artery, ♠ left external iliac vein)

vessels are moved medially, the deep lateral CINs can be completely dissected from the psoas muscle, obturator nerve, and common iliac vein (Fig. 17.9). The medial CINs receive the other lymphatic vessels from the deep lymphatic trunks consisting of the SNs. The SNs receive lymphatic vessels from the ONs and CLNs, and they may be dissected from the interiliac vessels. Special caution is needed to avoid injury to the interiliac vein.

17.4.2 PAN Dissection

First, the small intestine is isolated in a specimen bag and then flipped over outside the body in a direction opposite the operative field. When working on the left side, the peritoneum outside the descending colon is incised along the paracolic gutter and over the left kidney toward the splenic flexure (Fig. 17.11). To facilitate development of the working space, the mesentery must be detached from the anterior leaf of the renal fascia (Gerota's fascia). The fusion fascia of the two layers of mesentery (Toldt's fusion fascia) might serve as a landmark for the detachment process (Fig. 17.12). The descending colon is retracted medially, and this fusion fascia is

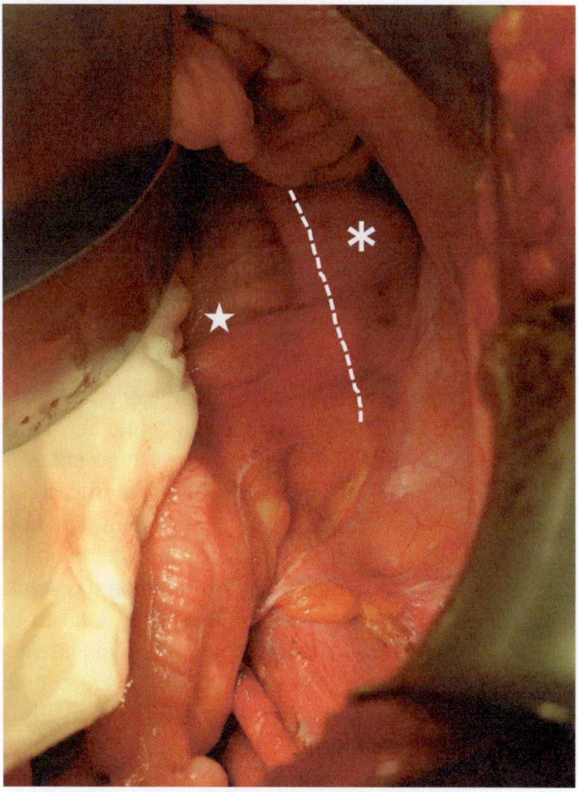

Fig. 17.11 Incision line (broken line) for development of the working space for left para-aortic lymph node dissection (★ descending colon, * left kidney)

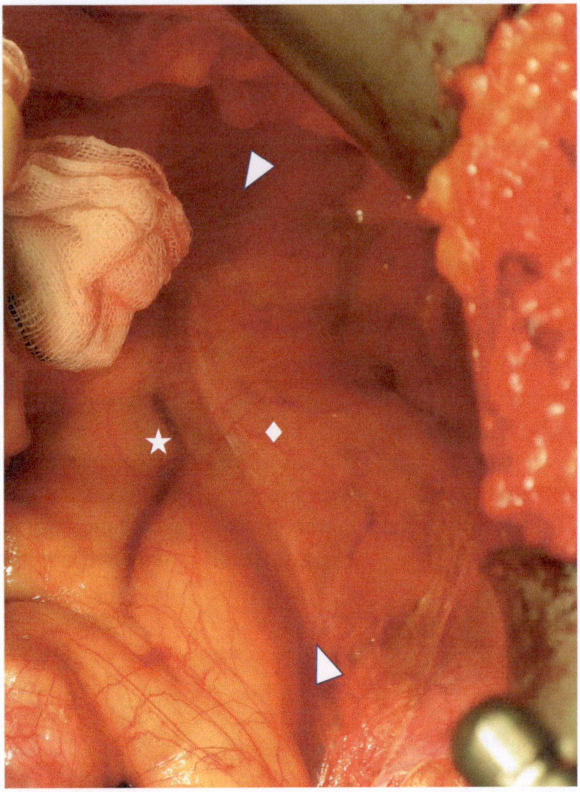

Fig. 17.12 Boundary (arrowhead) between the mesentery (★) and Gerota's fascia (♦)

detached from Gerota's fascia. As the separation proceeds, the left renal vein and its branch, which the left ovarian vein joins, are identified (Fig. 17.13). The fascia on the renal vein and ovarian vessels, which extends through the same surface as Gerota's fascia, may be dissected. The left ovarian artery may also be cut and ligated. The left ovarian vessels are then completely detached from the left ureter. Next, the left ovarian vein is cut and ligated. The descending colon and mesentery are retracted medially and cephalad, while the left ureter is retracted laterally (Fig. 17.14). Surgical retractor fixation systems are available for stable development of the working space (Fig. 17.15). The preaortic and lateroaortic lymph nodes are then dissected up to the level of the renal vein. The left para-aortic lymphatic tissue bundle can be separated from the aorta and then mobilized from the medial to lateral direction. When the incision is performed on the ventral surface of the aorta in the first step of this separation, particular care is taken to avoid injury in its branch, which the IMA joins. Although the upper hypogastric plexus is sometimes injured in this step, such injury does not lead to severe complications. Using an Allis forceps and monopolar scissors, this lymphatic bundle is elevated, and the lumbar vessels are then usually found on the anterior surface of the lumbar spine. While sparing these vessels as much as possible, the relevant lymphatic bundle is horizontally

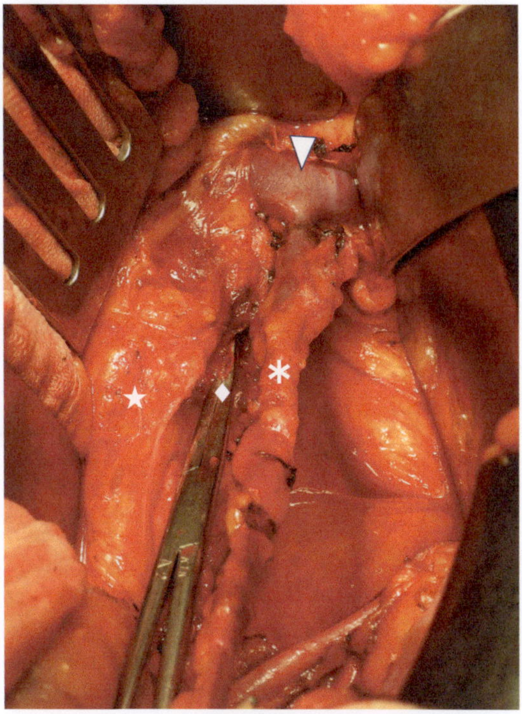

Fig. 17.13 Identification of the left renal vein (arrowhead) and its branch, which the left ovarian vein (*) joins. The left ovarian artery was cut and ligated by a Kelly clamp (◆) (★ aorta)

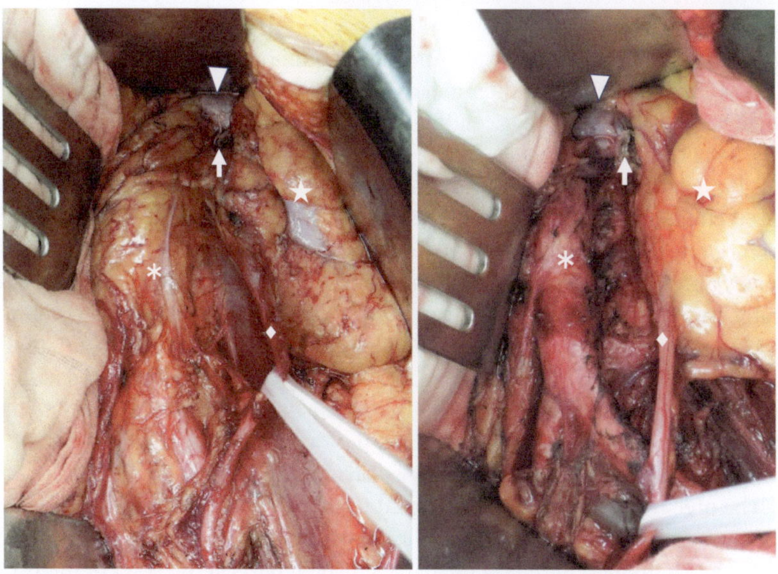

Fig. 17.14 Working space for the left para-aortic area before (left) and after (right) para-aortic lymphadenectomy. The left renal vein (arrowhead) and its branch (arrow), which the left ovarian vein joins, are identified at the upper limit (★ left kidney, * aorta, ◆ left ureter)

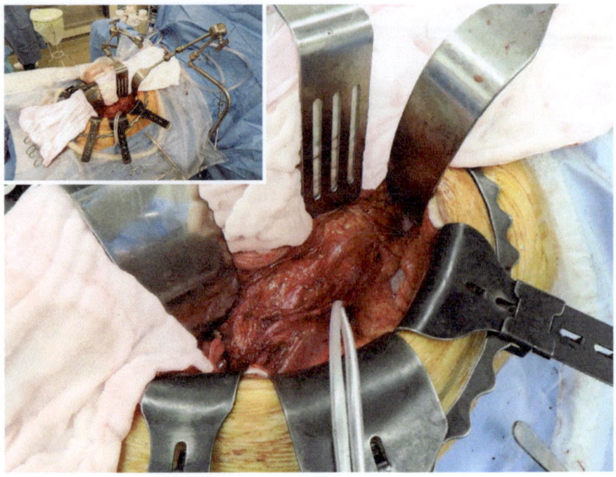

Fig. 17.15 The working space for left para-aortic lymph node dissection is stably developed using a surgical retractor fixation system. The left ureter is laterally retracted with a Penrose drain

separated from the aorta and vertically separated from the spine. The lymphatic bundle may also be divided into its cephalad and caudal parts at the level of the IMA. After continuing the separation up to the left renal vein, the upper end of the lymphatic bundle is ligated, and this bundle is finally resected. During this ligation procedure, particular care is taken to avoid injury to the communicating branches between the upper end of the lymphatic bundle and the hemiazygos vein. The upper end of the left PANs might be carefully divided into a few parts, and then each part may be separately ligated.

When working on the right side, the peritoneum outside the ascending colon is incised along the paracolic gutter and over the right kidney toward the level of the duodenum (Fig. 17.16). The ascending colon is retracted medially, and the mesentery is detached from Gerota's fascia. As the separation proceeds, the vena cava and its branch, which the right ovarian vein joins, are identified, and the right renal vein is then identified. After the right ovarian vessels are completely detached from the right ureter, the ovarian vessels are cut and ligated. The ascending colon and mesentery are retracted medially and cephalad, while the right ureter is retracted laterally. Surgical retractor fixation systems are available for stable development of the working space. The right-sided lymphatic flow consists of a route along the inferior vena cava (IVC) and another route crossing over the IVC caudad and along the aorta cephalad (Fig. 17.17). These lymphatic tissues may be divided along the ventral surface of the IVC to differentiate the two above-mentioned bundles. The precaval and laterocaval lymphatic tissues are dissected up to the level of the renal vein. The precaval bundle can be separated from the superior hypogastric plexus on the ventral surface of the aorta and then mobilized from medial to lateral. This bundle may be divided into its cephalad and caudal parts at the level of the IMA. A few small veins from the caudal part are usually found inserting into the ventral

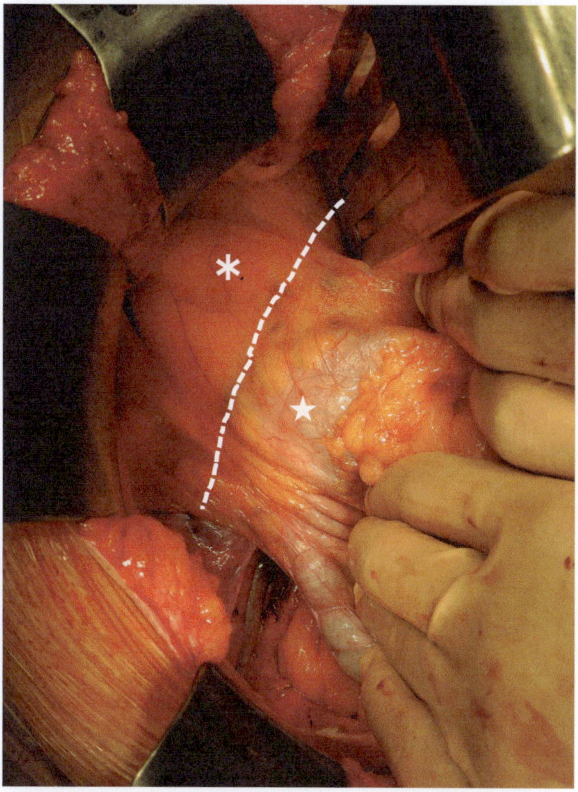

Fig. 17.16 Incision line (broken line) for development of the working space for right para-aortic lymph node dissection (★ ascending colon, * right kidney)

surface of the IVC. Particular care is taken to identify and ligate these veins. The caudal part is easily dissected after successful performance of this step. The cephalad part is vertically separated from the interaortocaval lymph nodes and then dissected after ligation of its upper end. The laterocaval lymphatic bundle can be separated from the IVC while sparing lumbar vessels. The lymph node dissection is carried cephalad to the desired level, usually near the insertion of the right ovarian vein into the IVC.

Finally, the lymphatic tissues residing between the great vessels are separately dissected at the level of the IMA. Two Tupfel gazes are available for stable development of the working space (Fig. 17.18). One Tupfel pushes aside the IVC laterally, and the other pushes aside the aorta in the opposite direction. Using an Allis forceps and monopolar scissors, the interaortocaval lymphatic tissues are elevated and separated from the great vessels. The lumbar vessels are usually found crossing the anterior surface of the lumbar spine. The caudal part of the interaortocaval lymphatic tissues is dissected while sparing the lumbar vessels, and the cephalad part is then dissected after ligation of its upper end.

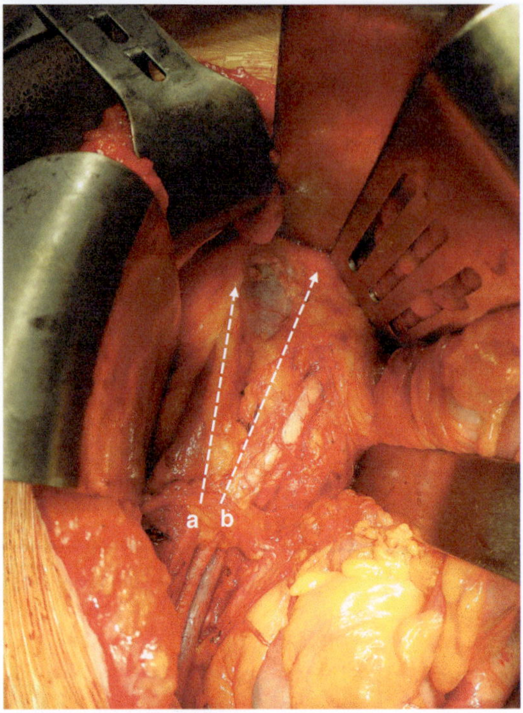

Fig. 17.17 The right-sided lymphatic flow consists of a route along the inferior vena cava (**a**) and another route crossing over the IVC caudad and along the aorta cephalad (**b**)

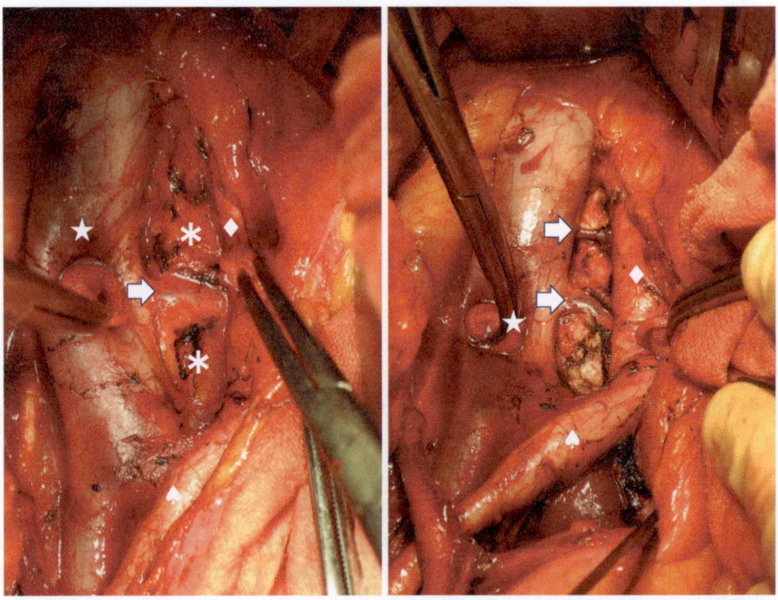

Fig. 17.18 Interaortocaval space before (left) and after (right) dissection of the interaortocaval lymph nodes (*). Lumbar vessels (arrow) are seen crossing the anterior surface of the lumbar spine (★ inferior vena cava, ♦ aorta, ♠ right common iliac artery)

17.5 Morbidity

17.5.1 Lower Extremity Lymphedema

Lower extremity lymphedema is the most common complication after lymphadenectomy [40, 41]. Postoperative leg edema is a serious complication and a chronic disease that lasts a lifetime in most patients. Previous reports describe a wide range of incidences (1.2–50.0%) of postoperative lower extremity lymphedema in patients with endometrial cancer [42–45]; this wide variation might be due to the difference in the total number of resected lymph nodes and diagnostic methods for lymphedema. Two strategies for minimizing the incidence of postoperative lower extremity lymphedema are (1) removal of the lymph nodes most likely to harbor disease with preservation of the lymph nodes unlikely to be affected and (2) performance of full lymphadenectomy with preservation of the lymph nodes most closely associated with the development of lymphedema. Sentinel lymph node mapping, fully described in another chapter, is the core technique in the first strategy, while CINDEIN-sparing lymphadenectomy is the core technique in the second strategy. Recent studies have shown that removal of the CINDEINs increases leg edema after lymphadenectomy [44, 46, 47]. As described in Chap. 17, lymphatic spread of endometrial cancer may occur by three routes. However, the third route (along the round ligaments to the CINDEINs) is a minor route in terms of metastasis [17, 48, 49]. Todo et al. [49] showed that high-risk histology results (grade 3 endometrioid cancer or non-endometrioid cancer) and pelvic node metastasis were independent risk factors for CINDEIN metastasis. Removal of the CINDEINs can be eliminated without anxiety in patients with low-risk endometrial cancer.

17.5.2 Lymphoceles

Lymphoceles are a common complication after lymphadenectomy and may be the cause of severe morbidity [50, 51]. Symptomatic lymphoceles compress adjacent structures and cause lymphedema, deep vein thrombosis, or inflammation. Two strategies for minimizing the incidence of lymphoceles are to leave the peritoneum open after surgery and to ensure proper timing of retroperitoneal drainage tube placement. The rationale for leaving the peritoneum open is that lymph moving from the retroperitoneal cavity to the peritoneal cavity is reabsorbed into the peritoneum or omentum. One prospective randomized trial that assessed the clinical significance of nonclosure of the peritoneum showed that the incidence of lymphoceles in the "closure" group was significantly higher than that in the "nonclosure" group (52% vs. 23%, $P < 0.05$) [52]. In other recent studies, however, the placement of drainage tubes resulted in a higher risk of symptomatic lymphocele formation. A recent Cochrane review reported that drainage tube placement is associated with a higher risk of symptomatic lymphocyst formation when the peritoneum is left open [53]. Lymphocele formation is probably caused by the drainage tube, which may act as a foreign body. If external stimulation by the drainage tube induces adhesion between the mesenterium/intestinal tract and a retroperitoneum-deficient region, the abovementioned rationale for preventing lymphocele formation in the peritoneal nonclosure method would not apply. From this point of view, a preventative agent for postsurgical adhesion might help to reduce the incidence of lymphocele formation.

17.5.3 Complications with or Without Para-aortic Lymphadenectomy

Whether para-aortic lymphadenectomy itself increases perioperative complications has been a matter of debate. One retrospective analysis in which morbidity rates were compared with versus without para-aortic lymphadenectomy showed that para-aortic lymphadenectomy was not associated with increased rates of lower extremity lymphedema, lymphoceles, severe ileus, postoperative thrombosis, or intraoperative organ injury [41]. The study showed a significant increase in postoperative ileus secondary to the addition of para-aortic lymphadenectomy, but no significant difference in severe ileus with or without para-aortic lymphadenectomy (1.4% vs. 0.7%, $P = 0.58$). Postoperative ileus after para-aortic lymphadenectomy occurs with a relatively high incidence rate but is manageable [41, 54]. Para-aortic lymphadenectomy might be a safe operative procedure when performed by experienced surgeons in tertiary centers.

References

1. Kilgore LC, Partridge EE, Alvarez RD, Austin JM, Shingleton HM, Noojin F 3rd, Conner W. Adenocarcinoma of the endometrium: survival comparisons of patients with and without pelvic node sampling. Gynecol Oncol. 1995;56:29–33.
2. Trimble EL, Kosary C, Park RC. Lymph node sampling and survival in endometrial cancer. Gynecol Oncol. 1998;71:340–3.
3. Fanning J. Long-term survival of intermediate risk endometrial cancer (stageIG3, IC, II) treated with full lymphadenectomy and brachytherapy without teletherapy. Gynecol Oncol. 2001;82:371–4.
4. Cragun JM, Havrilesky LJ, Calingaert B, Synan I, Secord AA, Soper JT, et al. Retrospective analysis of selective lymphadenectomy in apparent early-stage endometrial cancer. J Clin Oncol. 2005;23:3668–75.
5. Lutman CV, Havrilesky LJ, Cragun JM, Secord AA, Calingaert B, Berchuck A, et al. Pelvic lymph node count is an important prognostic variable for FIGO stage I and II endometrial carcinoma with high-risk histology. Gynecol Oncol. 2006;102:92–7.
6. Chan JK, Wu H, Cheung MK, Shin JY, Osann K, Kapp DS. The outcome of 27,063 women with unstaged endometrioid uterine cancer. Gynecol Oncol. 2007;106:282–8.
7. Abu-Rustum NR, Iasonos A, Zhou Q, Oke E, Soslow RA, Alektiar KM, et al. Is there a therapeutic impact to regional lymphadenectomy in the surgical treatment of endometrial carcinoma? Am J Obstet Gynecol. 2008;198(457):E1–5.
8. Mariani A, Webb MJ, Galli L, Podratz KC. Potential therapeutic role of para-aortic lymphadenectomy in node-positive endometrial cancer. Gynecol Oncol. 2000;76:348–56.

9. Candiani GB, Belloni C, Maggi R, Colombo G, Frigoli A, Carinelli SG. Evaluation of different surgical approaches in the treatment of endometrial cancer at FIGO stage I. Gynecol Oncol. 1990;37:6–8.
10. Bar-Am A, Ron IG, Kuperminc M, Gal I, Jaffa A, Kovner F, Wigler N, et al. The role of routine pelvic lymph node sampling in patients with stage I endometrial carcinoma: second thoughts. Acta Obstet Gynecol Scand. 1998;77:347–50.
11. Sartori E, Gaddicci A, Landoni F, Lissoni A, Maggino T, Zola P, et al. Clinical behavior of 203 stage II endometrial cancer cases: the impact of primary surgical approach and of adjuvant radiation therapy. Int J Gynecol Cancer. 2001;11:430–7.
12. Hidaka T, Kato K, Yonezawa R, Shima T, Nakashima A, Nagira K, et al. Omission of lymphadenectomy is possible for low-risk corpus cancer. Eur J Surg Oncol. 2007;33:86–90.
13. Benedetti-Panici P, Basile S, Maneschi F, et al. Systematic pelvic lymphadenectomy vs no lymphadenectomy in early-stage endometrial carcinoma: randomized clinical trial. J Natl Cancer Inst. 2008;100:1707–16.
14. ASTEC Study Group. Efficacy of systematic pelvic lymphadenectomy in endometrial cancer (MRC ASTEC trial): a randomized study. Lancet. 2009;373:125–36.
15. Todo Y, Kato H, Kaneuchi M, Watari H, Takeda M, Sakuragi N. Survival Effect of Para-aortic Lymphadenectomy in Endometrial Cancer (SEPAL Study): a retrospective cohort analysis. Lancet. 2010;375:1165–72.
16. Burke TW, Levenback C, Tornos C, Morris M, Wharton JT, Gershenson DM. Intraabdominal lymphatic mapping to direct selective pelvic and para-aortic lymphadenectomy in woman with high-risk endometrial cancer: results of a pilot study. Gynecol Oncol. 1996;62:169–73.
17. Niikura H, Okamura C, Utsunomiya H, Yoshinaga K, Akahira J, Ito K, Yaegashi N. Sentinel lymph node detection in patients with endometrial cancer. Gynecol Oncol. 2004;92:669–74.
18. Mariani A, Dowdy SC, Cliby WA, Gostout BS, Jones MB, Wilson TO, Podratz KC. Prospective assessment of lymphatic dissemination in endometrial cancer: a paradigm shift in surgical staging. Gynecol Oncol. 2008;109:11–8.
19. Fotopoulou C, Savvatis K, Kraetschell R, Schefold JC, Lichtenegger W, Sehouli J. Systematic pelvic and aortic lymphadenectomy in intermediate and high-risk endometrial cancer: lymph-node mapping and identification of predictive factors for lymph-node status. Eur J Obstet Gynecol Reprod Biol. 2010;149:199–203.
20. Mariani A, Webb MJ, Keeney GL, Hoddock MG, Calori G, Podratz KC. Low-risk corpus cancer: is lymphadenectomy or radiotherapy necessary? Am J Obstet Gynecol. 2000;182:1506–19.
21. Tuomi T, Pasanen A, Luomaranta A, Leminen A, Bützow R, Loukovaara M. Risk-stratification of endometrial carcinomas revisited: a combined preoperative and intraoperative scoring system for a reliable prediction of an advanced disease. Gynecol Oncol. 2015;137:23–7.
22. Tuomi T, Pasanen A, Leminen A, Bützow R, Loukovaara M. Prediction of lymphatic dissemination in endometrioid endometrial cancer: comparison of three risk-stratification models in a single-institution cohort. Gynecol Oncol. 2017;144:510–4.
23. Cox Bauer CM, Greer DM, Kram JJF, Kamelle SA. Tumor diameter as a predictor of lymphatic dissemination in endometrioid endometrial cancer. Gynecol Oncol. 2016;141:199–205.
24. Todo Y, Okamoto K, Hayashi M, Minobe S, Nomura E, Hareyama H, et al. A validation study of a scoring system to estimate the risk of lymph node metastasis for patients with endometrial carcinoma for tailoring the indication of lymphadenectomy. Gynecol Oncol. 2007;104:623–8.
25. Todo Y, Choi HJ, Kang S, Kim JWMD, Nam JH, Watari H, Tamakoshi A, Sakuragi N. Clinical significance of tumor volume in endometrial cancer: a Japan-Korea cooperative study. Gynecol Oncol. 2013;131:294–8.
26. Kang S, Kang WD, Chung HH, Jeong DH, Seo SS, Lee JM, et al. Preoperative identification of a low-risk group for lymph node metastasis in endometrial cancer: a Korean gynecologic oncology group study. J Clin Oncol. 2012;30:1329–34.
27. Kang S, Todo Y, Odagiri T, Mitamura T, Watari H, Kim JW, Nam JH, Sakuragi N. A low-risk group for lymph node metastasis is accurately identified by Korean gynecologic oncology group criteria in two Japanese cohorts with endometrial cancer. Gynecol Oncol. 2013;129:33–7.

28. Bendifallah S, Canlorbe G, Raimond E, Hudry D, Coutant C, Graesslin O, Touboul C, Huguet F, Cortez A, Daraï E, Ballester M. A clue towards improving the European Society of Medical Oncology risk group classification in apparent early stage endometrial cancer? Impact of lymphovascular space invasion. Br J Cancer. 2014;110:2640–6.
29. Vargas R, Rauh-Hain JA, Clemmer J, Clark RM, Goodman A, Growdon WB, Schorge JO, Del Carmen MG, Horowitz NS, Boruta DM 2nd. Tumor size, depth of invasion, and histologic grade as prognostic factors of lymph node involvement in endometrial cancer: a SEER analysis. Gynecol Oncol. 2014;133:216–20.
30. Milam MR, Java J, Walker JL, Metzinger DS, Parker LP, Coleman RL. Nodal metastasis risk in endometrioid endometrial cancer. Obstet Gynecol. 2012;119:286–92.
31. Lefringhouse JR, Elder JW, Baldwin LA, Miller RW, DeSimone CP, van Nagell JR Jr, Samoyoa LM, West DS, Dressler EV, Liu M, Ueland FR. Prospective validation of an intraoperative algorithm to guide surgical staging in early endometrial cancer. Gynecol Oncol. 2017;145:50–4.
32. Crosbie EJ, Roberts C, Qian W, et al. Body mass index does not influence post-treatment survival in early stage endometrial cancer: results from the MRC ASTEC trial. Eur J Cancer. 2012;48:853–64.
33. Arem H, Park Y, Pelser C, et al. Prediagnosis body mass index, physical activity, and mortality in endometrial cancer patients. J Natl Cancer Inst. 2013;105:342–9.
34. von Gruenigen VE, Tian C, Frasure H, et al. Treatment effects, disease recurrence, and survival in obese women with early endometrial carcinoma: a Gynecologic Oncology Group study. Cancer. 2006;107:2786–91.
35. Mauland KK, Trovik J, Wik E, et al. High BMI is significantly associated with positive progesterone receptor status and clinico-pathological markers for non-aggressive disease in endometrial cancer. Br J Cancer. 2011;104:921–6.
36. Chia VM, Newcomb PA, Trentham-Dietz A, et al. Obesity, diabetes, and other factors in relation to survival after endometrial cancer diagnosis. Int J Gynecol Cancer. 2007;17:441–6.
37. Calle EE, Rodriguez C, Walker-Thurmond K, et al. Overweight, obesity, and mortality from cancer in a prospectively studied cohort of U.S. adults. N Engl J Med. 2003;348:1625–38.
38. Modesitt SC, Tian C, Kryscio R, et al. Gynecologic Oncology Group. Impact of body mass index on treatment outcomes in endometrial cancer patients receiving doxorubicin and cisplatin: a Gynecologic Oncology Group study. Gynecol Oncol. 2007;105:59–65.
39. Todo Y, Okamoto K, Minobe S, Kato H. Clinical significance of surgical staging for obese women with endometrial cancer: a retrospective analysis in a Japanese cohort. Jpn J Clin Oncol. 2014;44:903–9.
40. Kodama J, Seki N, Ojima Y, Nakamura K, Hongo A, Hiramatsu Y. Risk factors for early and late postoperative complications of patients with endometrial cancer. Eur J Obstet Gynecol Reprod Biol. 2006;124:222–6.
41. Konno Y, Todo Y, Minobe S, Kato H, Okamoto K, Sudu S, Takeda M, Watari H, Kaneuchi M, Sakuragi N. A retrospective analysis of postoperative complications with or without para-aortic lymphadenectomy in endometrial cancer. Int J Gynecol Cancer. 2011;21:385–90.
42. Abu-Rustum NR, Alekitar K, Iasonos A, Lev G, Sonoda Y, Aghajanian C, Chi DS, Barakat RR. The incidence of symptomatic lower-extremity lymphedema following treatment of uterine corpus malignancies: a 12-year experience at Memorial Sloan-Kettering Cancer Center. Gynecol Oncol. 2006;103:714–8.
43. Tada H, Teramukai S, Fukushima M, Sasaki H. Risk factors for lower limb lymphedema after lymph node dissection in patients with ovarian and uterine carcinoma. BMC Cancer. 2009;9:47.
44. Todo Y, Yamamoto R, Minobe S, Suzuki Y, Takeshi U, Nakatani M, Aoyagi Y, Ohba Y, Okamoto K, Kato H. Risk factors for postoperative lower-extremity lymphedema in endometrial cancer survivors who had treatment including lymphadenectomy. Gynecol Oncol. 2010;119:60–4.

45. Tanaka T, Ohki N, Kojima A, Maeno Y, Miyahara Y, Sudo T, et al. Radiotherapy negates the effect of retroperitoneal nonclosure for prevention of lymphedema of the legs following pelvic lymphadenectomy for gynecological malignancies: an analysis from a questionnaire survey. Int J Gynecol Cancer. 2007;17:460–4.
46. Abu-Rustum NR, Barakat RR. Observations on the role of circumflex iliac node resection and the etiology of lower extremity lymphedema following pelvic lymphadenectomy for gynecologic malignancy. Gynecol Oncol. 2007;106:4–5.
47. Hareyama H, Ito K, Hada K, Uchida A, Hayakashi Y, Hirayama E, Oikawa M, Okuyama K. Reduction/prevention of lower extremity lymphedema after pelvic and para-aortic lymphadenectomy for patients with gynecologic malignancies. Ann Surg Oncol. 2012;19:268–73.
48. Matsumoto K, Yoshikawa H, Yasugi T, Onda T, Nakagawa S, Yamada M, Kawana K, Minaguchi T, Oda K, Hasumi Y, Taketani Y. Distinct lymphatic spread of endometrial carcinoma in comparison with cervical and ovarian carcinomas. Cancer Lett. 2002;180:83–9.
49. Todo Y, Kato H, Okamoto K, Minobe S, Suzuki Y, Ohba Y, Takeda M, Watari H, Kaneuchi M, Sakuragi N. Incidence of metastasis in circumflex iliac nodes distal to the external iliac nodes in intermediate- and high-risk endometrial cancer. Gynecol Oncol. 2011;122:55–8.
50. Weinberger V, Cibula D, Zikan M. Lymphocele: prevalence and management in gynecological malignancies. Expert Rev Anticancer Ther. 2014;14:307–17.
51. Zikan M, Fischerova D, Pinkavova I, Slama J, Weinberger V, Dusek L, Cibula D. A prospective study examining the incidence of asymptomatic and symptomatic lymphoceles following lymphadenectomy in patients with gynecological cancer. Gynecol Oncol. 2015;137:291–8.
52. Suzuki M, Ohwada M, Sato I. Pelvic lymphocysts following retroperitoneal lymphadenectomy: retroperitoneal partial "no-closure" for ovarian and endometrial cancers. J Surg Oncol. 1998;68:149–52.
53. Charoenkwan K, Kietpeerakool C. Retroperitoneal drainage versus no drainage after pelvic lymphadenectomy for the prevention of lymphocyst formation in patients with gynaecological malignancies. Cochrane Database Syst Rev. 2014;6:CD007387.
54. Fujita K, Nagano T, Suzuki A, Sakakibara A, Takahashi S, Hirano T, Okagaki A, Ban C. Incidence of postoperative ileus after para-aortic lymph node dissection in patients with malignant gynecologic tumors. Int J Clin Oncol. 2005;10:187–90.

18 Laparoscopic Surgery for Endometrial Cancer

Yoshito Terai

Abstract

Endometrial cancer is one of the most common of gynecological malignancies among women worldwide. Most cancers are detected early in the course of the disease, and this has resulted in improved survival rates. Within this population, reducing the surgical morbidity rate is of considerable importance for the survival and quality of life of the patient. Over the past two decades, laparoscopic surgery has been incorporated into gynecological oncology, with this approach now being used in the treatment of endometrial cancer to reduce surgical morbidity. In this section, we demonstrated about the preoperative evaluation of the laparoscopic surgery, the techniques of the laparoscopic surgery including pelvic and para-aortic lymphadenectomy, and the morbidity of the laparoscopic surgery compared with laparotomic surgery for the patients with endometrial cancer. In the previous randomized clinical studies and our institution data, we indicated that laparoscopic surgery tended to be longer in each study compared with open surgical operation. On the other hand, intraoperative blood loss tended to be significantly less in laparoscopic surgery compared with that in laparotomy. In addition, the hospital stay was significantly shortened by laparoscopic surgery in all of the studies. Moreover, we discuss that the correspondence to the intermediate-risk or advanced uterine endometrial cancer. We concluded that laparoscopic surgery is a curative surgery equivalent to that of conventional laparotomic surgery, and it is very important for gynecologic oncologic surgeons to perform laparoscopic surgery which results in less blood loss, fewer complications, quicker recovery, and less invasiveness for patients with early-stage endometrial cancer.

Y. Terai (✉)
Department of Obstetrics and Gynecology,
Kobe University Graduate School of Medicine, Kobe, Japan
e-mail: yterai@med.kobe-u.ac.jp

M. Mikami (ed.), *Surgery for Gynecologic Cancer*, Comprehensive Gynecology and Obstetrics, https://doi.org/10.1007/978-981-13-1519-0_18

Keywords
Laparoscopic surgery · Endometrial cancer · Para-aortic lymphadenectomy · Pelvic lymphadenectomy

18.1 Introduction

Endometrial cancer is one of the most common of gynecological malignancies among women worldwide. Most cancers are detected early in the course of the disease, and this has resulted in improved survival rates. Within this population, reducing the surgical morbidity rate is of considerable importance for the survival and quality of life of the patient.

The standard surgical procedure for early endometrial cancer for many decades has been total abdominal hysterectomy (TAH) and bilateral salpingo-oophorectomy (BSO) with or without bilateral pelvic/para-aortic lymph node dissection. Lymphadenectomy is part of the staging of endometrial carcinoma, and its therapeutic value is a subject of ongoing debate [1].

Over the past two decades, laparoscopic surgery has been incorporated into gynecological oncology, with this approach now being used in the treatment of endometrial cancer to reduce surgical morbidity. Recently, the Gynecologic Oncology Group LAP2 protocol randomized over 2600 women with endometrial cancer to compare laparotomy versus laparoscopy, and it reported fewer postoperative moderate or severe adverse events, shorter hospital stays, less pain, earlier resumption of normal activities, and improved quality of life in the laparoscopy cohort [2].

18.2 History

The first laparoscopically assisted vaginal hysterectomy for stage I endometrial cancer was reported by Childers and colleagues in 1992 [3]. Subsequently, Childers also reported about the laparoscopic lymphadenectomy of pelvic and para-aortic lymph nodes for staging endometrial cancer [4].

18.3 Principle and Indication

Uterine endometrial carcinoma has been on an increasing trend in recent years. 71.1% of carcinomas at stage I are confined to the uterus, and 77.4% of carcinomas at stage I are stage 1A which is muscle invasion less than 1/2 according to the FIGO staging system. As described above, in cases of uterine body cancer, most are primary cancers, and, therefore, surgical therapy, which is the main treatment, becomes an important factor for the curability of the tumor. In laparoscopic surgery for uterine endometrial cancer, six RCTs (randomized control trials) have been reported (Table 18.1) [2, 5–9]. Although two cases were included at stage II, the rate of stage I endometrial cancer was 74.5–87.7% in these studies.

Table 18.1 A six-study randomized control comparison between laparoscopy vs. open surgery for endometrial cancer

Author		Procedure	Operation time (min)	Blood loss (mL)	Conversion rate (%)	Hospital stay
Tozzi (2005)	Laparoscopy (63)	LAVH		241.3*	1.4	7.8**
	Open (59)			586.1*		11.4**
Malzoni (2009)	Laparoscopy (81)	TLH	136**	50**	0	2.1**
	Open (78)		123**	145**		5.1**
Zullo (2009)	Laparoscopy (40)	LAVH	196.7	173.9	12.5	3.0**
	Open (38)		135.3	282.5		6.9**
Walker (2012) LAP2 study	Laparoscopy (1696)	LAVH, TLH, Robotic	204**		25.8	3**
	Open (920)		130**			4**
Janda (2010) LACE study	Laparoscopy (190)	TLH	138**		5.1	62%; less than 2 days**
	Open (142)		109**			97%; more than 2 days**
Mourits (2010)	Laparoscopy (185)	TLH	115**	100**	10.8	3**
	Open (94)		71**	200**		5**

$^{*}p < 0.05$

$^{**}p < 0.01$

In the six RCT studies, laparoscopic surgery tended to be longer in each study compared with open surgical operation. On the other hand, intraoperative blood loss tended to be significantly less in laparoscopic surgery compared with that in laparotomy. In addition, the hospital stay was significantly shortened by laparoscopic surgery in all of the studies.

Regarding the perioperative complications, ureteral injury was 1–5% in laparoscopic surgery compared to 0–2.6% in laparotomic surgery. Also, bowel injury and vascular injury showed no significant difference between laparoscopic procedure and laparotomy. Postoperative complications in laparoscopic surgery showed a significantly lower rate compared with that in laparotomy. The LAP2 study also showed that laparoscopic surgery significantly reduced the incidence of postoperative ileus, thus indicating the superiority of the technique.

18.4 Preoperative Evaluation

Before reviewing the laparoscopic procedure, it is important to understand some general concepts about laparoscopy. A laparoscopic approach is contraindicated in any patient whose uterus is too large to be removed intact through the vagina and also in medically compromised patients for whom a laparoscopic approach might not be safe. Patient characteristics, including a history of prior surgery and body weight, are also important considerations. Attempting laparoscopy in patients with prior surgery is acceptable; however, conversion may be necessary if adhesions are too dense and exposure is compromised. Moreover, the size of the uterus is an important factor since, for oncologic procedures, the organ must be removed intact. In our previous report, total laparoscopic hysterectomy can be performed successfully in most patients whose uterus is no larger than 10 cm at its greatest transverse diameter [10]. The preoperative total length of myoma nodules determined by MRI is also a useful preoperative indicator of uterine weight.

An increasing body mass index and its associated thickening of the subcutaneous tissue have been shown to increase the risk of perioperative complications and conversion to laparotomy [11]. Obesity is not a contraindication to laparoscopy, as many series have reported successful surgeries in the obese population [11–13]. In the study of 1266 cases in Italy, the transfusion rate, postoperative complication occurrence rate, and postoperative hospital stay period in laparoscopic surgery were significantly lower than those in laparotomic surgery. Although the number of lymph nodes removed during laparoscopic surgery was not different from that in laparotomic surgery, there was no difference in laparoscopic surgery when the patient's BMI was 40 or more. Moreover, the number of lymph nodes removed was significantly fewer in the laparotomic surgery group than in the laparoscopic surgery group. It should be noted, however, that the rate of lymphadenectomy in highly obese patients with a BMI exceeding 40 mg/m^2 tended to be significantly lower, and the conversion rate from laparoscopic surgery to laparotomic surgery was also significantly higher than in patients with a BMI under 40 mg/m^2 [13]. In the subanalysis of obesity cases in the LAP2 study, the rate of well-differentiated-type endometrial adenocarcinoma tended to be higher in stage IA obese patients, lymph node metastasis was also significantly lower, and the risk of recurrence tended to be lower than in nonobese patients [12].

There is a definite learning curve for laparoscopic procedures, and the risk of complications changes according to the skills of the operator. As it is a well-known fact that obese patients are at a higher risk of perioperative complications in general surgery than nonobese patients, it is necessary to perform laparoscopic surgery with special attention paid to complications that may arise in each particular case. We highly recommend that surgeons convert to laparotomy without hesitation at the onset of any intraoperative complication or difficulties in proceeding with laparoscopy.

18.5 Technique

We insert the first trocar using the open Hasson technique. Then, four accessory trocars without intrauterine manipulation for laparoscopic endometrial cancer surgery are placed in the Trendelenburg position. A 12 mm balloon trocar (Auto Suture Blunt Tip Trocar, Tyco), used for a 30 degree 10 mm laparoscope, is briefly inserted under direct visualization (open laparoscopy) through an intraumbilical incision of 1.5 cm. Three lateral 5 mm trocars are then inserted (left and right lower abdominal quadrant and left under the costal arch) for the ancillary instruments, and one 12 mm trocar is placed midline suprapubically for further manipulations and the extraction of lymph nodes (Fig. 18.1). Exploration of the peritoneal surface of the abdominal

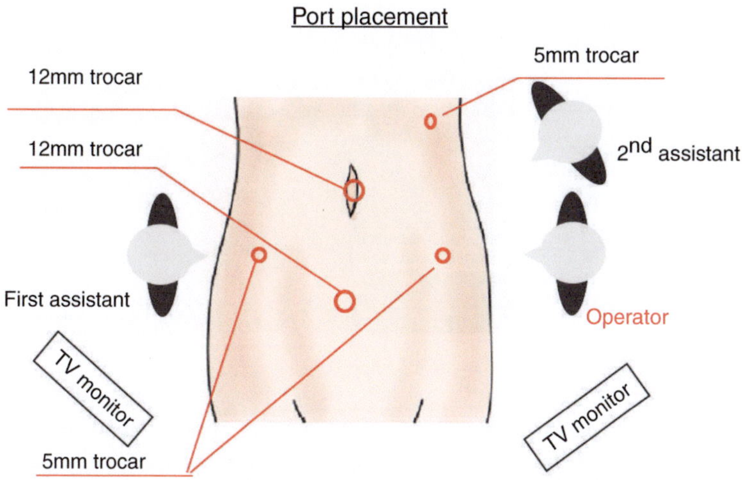

Fig. 18.1 Trocar placement of laparoscopic surgery for endometrial cancer

and pelvic cavities from the diaphragm to the pelvic cul-de-sac is carried out, and pelvic peritoneal cytology is obtained. A total laparoscopic hysterectomy with bilateral salpingo-oophorectomy is then performed. The uterus is retracted using 5 mm grasping forceps that were inserted into the left under the costal arch, as the use of a uterine manipulator during laparoscopic hysterectomy for endometrial cancer is a concern about the possible increased incidence of positive peritoneal cytology and cancer cell spillage potential. After collecting peritoneal fluid or washings for cytological examination, the round and broad ligaments are coagulated and transected by an Enseal® (Ethicon Endo-Surgery Inc., OH, USA), LigaSure Maryland® (Medtronic Inc., MN, USA), or bipolar coagulation device. After clamping the uterine artery lateral to the ureters and opening the ureteral tunnels, the ureters are unroofed and rolled laterally. The bilateral infundibulopelvic ligaments are then coagulated and transected by an Enseal® or LigaSure Maryland® sealing device. The vesicouterine and uterosacral ligaments are also transected. After the bilateral paracolpium are ligated by 1-0 PDS, the vaginal cuff (10–20 mm) and the corresponding paracolpos are resected. A circumferential colpotomy is performed on the rim of the Vagi-Pipe® (Hakko Co., Japan) with monopolar scissors. After removal of the uterus or adnexa, or both, through the vagina, the vaginal cuff is closed laparoscopically with running absorbable sutures. The uterus is then submitted for frozen histologic section.

A pelvic lymphadenectomy is performed for all patients with endometrial cancer, excluding those with grade 1 tumors who had no muscle invasion, as was noted in previous studies [5]. If the intraoperative frozen section assessment of the uterus is reported to have muscle invasion of grades 1 and 2 in more than half of the tissue or grade 3 and other subtypes, a para-aortic lymphadenectomy is performed.

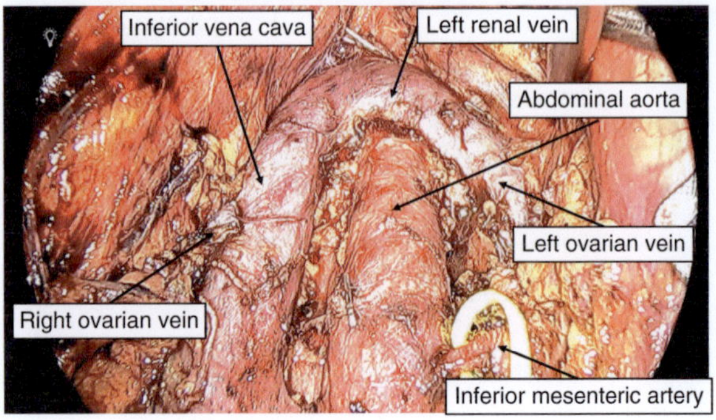

Fig. 18.2 Operating field of laparoscopic systematic para-aortic lymphadenectomy for endometrial cancer. The left renal vein which is the cranial border of dissection is exposed. The vena cava and the anterior aspect of the aorta are cleared. The superficial intercavoaortic nodes were also removed

A laparoscopic pelvic lymphadenectomy involves dissection of the common, external, and internal iliac lymph nodes and obturator nodes. Next, a para-aortic lymphadenectomy is performed. The aortic nodes are removed up to the left renal vein. The posterior peritoneum is incised by a diagonal cut to the peritoneum which goes along the route of the mesentery from the cecum to the Treitz's ligament. The peritoneum is then cleaved and retracted laterally to the right (or left) side of the patient in order to create a "wall" between the operative field and the bowel loops (Fig. 18.2). The inferior mesenteric artery and left ureter are routinely identified and divided to prove ample access to the upper side of the left aortic nodes. The retroperitoneal space is gently opened, and the anterior aspects of the aorta and of the vena cava are identified up to the left renal vein. When we develop the retroperitoneal field, we usually use the vessel clips to secure hemostasis and lymphostasis. Both ovarian arteries are divided and occluded by vessel clips, either an Enseal® or LigaSure Maryland® sealing device. The left lateroaortic and the precaval, interaorticocaval, and laterocaval nodal areas are removed separately.

The operation is completed with a final laparoscopic inspection to check for hemostasis.

18.6 Morbidity

Among the six RCTs, four studies showed that the recurrence rate for laparoscopic surgery was 8.1–20% and 8.5–18.4% for laparotomic surgery. The number of pelvic lymph nodes was also reported in the 6 RCTs, with 11.5– 23.5 nodes removed by laparoscopic surgery and 10.7– 22.2 nodes removed by laparotomy. These data indicated that laparoscopic pelvic lymph node dissection is equivalent to that of laparotomy. In addition, the recurrence rate in the pelvis was 1.3–5.0%, which is equivalent to the 1.0–15.8% recurrence in laparotomy operations. In 2012, a prognostic analysis of the LAP2 large study was announced [14]. The mean follow-up period was 59.3 (38–62.9) months, the 3 year recurrence rate was 11.4%, there was no significant difference from the 10.2% in laparotomy operations, and the estimated 5-year survival rate was 89.8%, which is not different from the rate in

Table 18.2 Comparison of results of laparoscopic and abdominal operations at Osaka Medical College

	Laparoscopic group ($n = 39$)	Laparotomic group ($n = 93$)	P value
Median (SD) duration of surgery (min)	321.1 ± 65.9	262.6 ± 75.0	<0.0001
Median (SD) EBL (mL)	42.9 ± 76.3	236.8 ± 186.6	<0.0001
No. of transfusion patients	0 (Autologous 1)	2 (Autologous 7)	0.46
Length of uterus (cm)	10.3 ± 11.6	8.5 ± 2.0	0.14
Length of cervical cuff (SD) (mm)	12.0 ± 4.1	5.5 ± 6.6	<0.0001
Median (SD) number of lymph nodes removed	32.3 ± 13.1	28.0 ± 11.9	0.15
Conversion to laparotomy	0	—	—

laparotomy procedures. However, the follow-up period in these studies which was 38.5–78 (2–96) months is short, and NCCN guidelines mention that there needs to be a long-term prognostic observation in cases of laparoscopic surgery.

In our institution, we have released the first report of laparoscopic surgery for 39 Japanese patients with endometrial cancer compared with the laparotomy (Table 18.2) [15]. Patients in the laparoscopic group had longer operations compared with those in the laparotomic surgery group (median, 321.1 ± 65.9 vs. 262.6 ± 75.0 min, $p < 0.0001$). The estimated blood loss in the laparoscopic group was significantly lower than that in the laparotomic group (42.9 ± 76.3 vs. 236.8 ± 186.6, $p < 0.0001$). Nine patients received blood transfusions, including seven autologous blood transfusions in the laparotomic group; however, only one patient received an autologous blood transfusion in the laparoscopic group. There were no patients who were initially approached via laparoscopy who required conversion to laparotomy. The uterine diameter was 10.3 ± 11.6 cm in the laparoscopic group and 8.5 ± 2.0 cm in the laparotomic group ($p = 0.14$). The median length of vagina removed was 12.0 ± 4.1 mm in the laparoscopic group and was 5.5 ± 6.6 mm in the laparotomic group ($p < 0.0001$). Pelvic lymphadenectomy was performed in 61.5% of the laparoscopic patients ($n = 24$). In the laparotomic group, pelvic lymphadenectomy was performed in 67.8% of patients ($n = 63$). The mean number of pelvic nodes removed was 32.3 ± 13.1 in the laparoscopic group and 28.0 ± 11.9 in the laparotomic group. There were no significant differences between the two groups ($p = 0.15$). The mean lowest postsurgical hemoglobin (Hgb) level was 11.3 ± 1.7 g/dL in the laparoscopic group and 10.9 ± 1.1 g/dL in the laparotomic group, which was significantly different between the groups ($p = 0.01$). The mean highest postsurgical C-reactive protein (CRP) level was also significantly different between the laparoscopic group and the laparotomic group (3.77 ± 2.7 mg/dL vs. 7.3 ± 4.3 mg/dL, $p < 0.0001$). Patients who underwent laparoscopic surgery had less intense postoperative pain (assessed by the duration time of analgesics used) than patients in the laparotomic group (1.1 days vs. 2.4 days; $p < 0.0001$). The mean time to the first passage of flatus was 1.6 ± 0.6 days in the laparoscopic group and 1.3 ± 0.7 days in the laparotomic group ($p = 0.11$). The mean time to tolerance of a regular diet was 6.0 ± 1.4 days in the laparotomic group and 6.6 ± 3.0 days in the laparotomic group ($p = 0.27$). There were no patients who developed any intraoperative complications, such as ureteric injury or major vessel injury, in either of the two groups. No major perioperative complications, such as suture failure in the vaginal wound, infection, ileus, or thrombosis, occurred in the laparoscopic group; however, 14 patients (14.3%) had postoperative complications in the laparotomic group. One patient had postoperative ileus, 2 patients had lymph cysts, and 11 patients had wound dehiscence. The postoperative hospital stay in the laparoscopic group was 9.3 ± 2.5 days and was significantly shorter than that in the laparotomic group (14.6 ± 12.6 days, $p = 0.009$). Three patients in the laparoscopic group and 14 patients in the laparotomic group received adjuvant chemotherapy. After the median follow-up of 17.3 months (range 1–27 months) in the laparoscopic group and 37.8 months (range 6–74 months) in the laparotomic group, there were no recurrent patients in either of the two groups.

18.7 Correspondence to Para-aortic Lymph Node Dissection and Advanced Endometrial Cancer

Para-aortic lymphadenectomy is a major surgical procedure for patients with gynecologic cancer. This technique has improved their prognosis [1–6] and has facilitated correct staging [7–9] among patients with endometrial cancer. Para-aortic lymph node metastasis was reported to be 1% in the low risk of recurrence group, 11.9% in the intermediate-risk group, and 23.8% in the high-risk group, and patients with retroperitoneal lymph node metastasis are classified as stage IIIC [10]. In the six RCT studies, the effective rate of para-aortic lymph node dissection was 10–95.8%, and the number of excised lymph nodes was 7–12.3. Among cases suspected of preoperative stage I, it is also true that there are some cases that should undergo curative surgery including para-aortic lymph node dissection in this way. Todo et al. reported that systematic lymphadenectomy, including para-aortic lymphadenectomy, has therapeutic significance for patients at intermediate/high risk of recurrence, such as those with deeply invasive lesions, high-grade histology, and tumors of serous carcinoma, clear cell carcinoma, or carcinosarcoma [11]. According to the National Comprehensive Cancer Network, para-aortic nodal evaluation from the inframesenteric and infrarenal regions may also be utilized for staging of select high-risk tumors, such as deeply invasive lesions, high-grade histology, and tumors of serous carcinoma, clear cell carcinoma, or carcinosarcoma in patients undergoing primary surgical management of endometrioid uterine cancer [12]. There have been several studies demonstrating the feasibility of laparoscopic surgery for patients with endometrial cancer. In these studies, laparoscopic surgery involved less intraoperative blood loss and a shorter hospital stay compared with laparotomic surgery [16–21]. The GOG LAP2 study, which was a multicenter randomized trial comparing the treatment of endometrial cancer performed by laparoscopy versus laparotomy, demonstrated not only the short-term feasibility of laparoscopy but also its non-inferiority with regard to the long-term prognosis compared with laparotomy.

We also reported the feasibility of laparoscopic para-aortic systematic lymph node dissection for Japanese patients with clinical stage I endometrial cancer of intermediate/high risk of recurrence, such as those with deeply invasive lesions, high-grade histology, and tumors of serous carcinoma, clear cell carcinoma, or carcinosarcoma endometrial cancer (Table 18.3) (Fig. 18.2) [16]. Comparison between the laparoscopic para-aortic lymph node dissection group (54 cases) and the laparotomic surgery group (99 cases) at the same facility showed no significant difference between the two groups at the time of operation. Moreover, the laparoscopic group had less

Table 18.3 Comparison of para-aortic lymphadenectomy between laparoscopy and laparotomy

	Laparoscopy *n* = 54	Laparotomy *n* = 99	*P* value
Age[a], year-old	57.9 ± 11.0	58.0 ± 10.3	0.9
BMI[a]	22.8 ± 3.4	22.4 ± 4.3	0.6
Median (SD) duration of surgery (min)[a]	483 ± 102	481 ± 106	0.9
Median (SD) estimated blood loss[a] (mL)	143 ± 253	988 ± 694	<0.01
No. of patients of transfusion (%)	2 (3.7)	10 (10.0)	0.1
Median (SD) number of pelvic lymph node[a]	31.8 ± 10.1	39.9 ± 15.9	<0.01
Median (SD) number of para-aortic lymph node[a]	26.2 ± 10.9	31.1 ± 13.2	0.02
Minimum level of Hb[a] (SD) (g/dL)	10.4 ± 1.1	9.9 ± 1.4	0.02
Maximum level of CRP[a] (SD) (mg/dL)	6.3 ± 3.8	10.2 ± 4.9	<0.01
No. of patients with intraoperative complications	3	8	0.7
Vessel injury	2	6	0.6
Ureter injury	0	1	0.5
Nerve injury	0	1	0.5
Compartment syndrome	1	0	0.1
No. of patients with postoperative complications			
Urinary tract infection	0	1	0.5
Pelvic cellulitis	0	1	0.5
Venous thrombosis	0	3	0.2
Pulmonary embolus	0	3	0.2
Bowel obstruction	0	0	
Urinary fistula	0	0	
Ileus	0	10	0.02
Wound infection	2	3	0.7
Lymphocyst	2	1	0.2
Chyle or lymphorrhea	10	7	0.02
Lymphedema	2	13	0.07
Median (SD) time (days) to hospital stay[a]	8.4 ± 5.7	16.1 ± 8.0	<0.01
Follow-up[b], day (quantile)	364 (110–681)	693 (267–1222)	0.01
Recurrence (%)	4 (7.4)	15 (14.3)	0.2

BMI body mass index, *Hb* hemoglobin, *CRP* C-reactive protein
[a]Based on an ANOVA (mean ± SD)
[b]Median (+interquartile ranges)

intraoperative blood loss than the laparotomic group (143 ± 253 vs. 988 ± 694 mL, $p < 0.01$). Naturally, the rate of blood transfusion was lower in the laparoscopic group than in the laparotomic group (3.7% vs. 10.0%, $p = 0.1$). The number of resected pelvic lymph nodes was less in the laparoscopic group than in the laparotomic group (31.8 ± 10.1 vs. 39.9 ± 15.9, $p < 0.01$), and the number of resected para-aortic lymph nodes was also less in the laparoscopic group than in the laparotomic group (26.2 ± 10.9 vs. 31.1 ± 13.2, $p = 0.02$). The postoperative minimum level of hemoglobin was higher in the laparoscopic group than in the laparotomic group (10.4 ± 1.1 g/dL vs. 9.9 ± 1.4 g/dL, $p = 0.02$). In contrast, the postoperative maximum level of C-reactive protein (CRP) was lower in the laparoscopic group than in the laparotomic group (6.3 ± 3.8 mg/dL vs. 10.2 ± 4.9 mg/dL, $p < 0.01$). There was no difference in the intraoperative complications between the two groups, and intestinal obstruction due to postoperative complications was not significantly generated in the laparoscopic group and was significantly lower. Hospital stay, as well, was significantly shorter in the laparoscopic group, and the rate of intraoperative complications was not significantly different between the groups (5.6% vs. 8.1%, $p = 0.7$). Two vessel injuries and one compartment syndrome occurred in the laparoscopic group, and six vessel injuries (one ureter injury and one obturator nerve injury) occurred in the laparotomic group. The two patients with vessel injuries in the laparoscopic group were converted to laparotomy for hemostasis, and the conversion rate of laparoscopic group was 3.7%. Postoperatively, there was one urinary tract infection, one case of pelvic cellulitis, three cases of venous thrombosis, and three cases of pulmonary embolus in the laparotomic group. No complications described above occurred in the laparoscopic group. Bowel obstruction and urinary fistula did not occur in either group. While no cases of ileus occurred in the laparoscopic group, ten occurred in the laparotomic group. There were two wound infections in the laparoscopic group and three in the laparotomic group. There were two cases of lymphocyst in the laparoscopic group and one in the laparotomic group. The rate of chyle or lymphorrhea was higher in the laparoscopic group than in the laparotomic group (18.5% vs. 7.1%, $p = 0.02$). These symptoms were spontaneously resolved in a few days with observation and basic support. The rate of lymphedema was lower in the laparoscopic group than in the laparotomic group (3.7% vs. 13.1%, $p = 0.07$). The laparoscopic group tended to have a shorter hospital stay than the laparotomic group (8.4 ± 5.7 days vs. 16.1 ± 8.0 days, $p < 0.01$). The medium (quantile) duration of follow-up was 364 (110–681) days in the laparoscopic group and 693 (267–1222) days in the laparotomic group. The recurrence rate was not significantly different between the groups in the period above (7.4% vs. 14.3%, $p = 0.2$). We conclude that laparoscopic para-aortic lymphadenectomy was safe and feasible compared with laparotomy, although a longer follow-up will be needed before long-term survival can be evaluated accurately.

Regarding laparoscopic surgery for stage II endometrial cancer, six RCT studies have included 6–15% of stage II endometrial cancer. In the results of these studies, laparoscopic surgery for stage II endometrial cancer is likely to be applied.

Can we perform laparoscopic surgery for stage IV advanced endometrial cancer, especially when peritoneal dissemination or intestinal infiltration is suspected?

Unfortunately, there is no prospective study between the laparoscopic surgery and laparotomy for advanced endometrial cancer. Correspondence to stage IV endometrial cancer is considered to be similar to surgery for advanced ovarian cancer with disseminated lesions. However, there are few reports on laparoscopic surgery for the same disease. In a retrospective study, Nezhat reported that the optimal laparoscopic surgery for tumors less than 0.5 cm in size can be done in 88.2% of cases, and the amount of blood loss, as well as recurrence rate, is less than that in laparotomy operations [17]. There is insufficient evidence that laparoscopic surgery is considered an effective and safe procedure for patients with stage IV advanced endometrial cancer, as six RCT studies only included 0–2% in stage IV endometrial cancer. The LAP2 study indicated that metastatic lesions increased the rate of conversion to open surgery. In other words, laparoscopic surgery for advanced endometrial cancer in which the lesion is spreading outside the uterus is not currently recommended in general clinical treatment.

18.8 Future Prospect

Since laparoscopic surgery is a curative surgery equivalent to that of conventional laparotomic surgery, it is very important for gynecologic oncologic surgeons to perform laparoscopic surgery which results in less blood loss, fewer complications, quicker recovery, and less invasiveness for patients with endometrial cancer. In the future, we believe that laparoscopic surgery, compared with conventional laparotomic surgery, for patients with either advanced stage or recurrent endometrial cancer will be performed widely, as laparoscopic surgery has the advantage of being a more precise surgery with an enlarged visual view.

References

1. Blake P, et al. Adjuvant external beam radiotherapy in the treatment of endometrial cancer (MRC ASTEC and NCIC CTG EN.5 randomised trials): pooled trial results, systematic review, and meta-analysis. Lancet. 2009;373(9658):137–46.
2. Walker JL, et al. Laparoscopy compared with laparotomy for comprehensive surgical staging of uterine cancer: Gynecologic Oncology Group Study LAP2. J Clin Oncol. 2009;27(32):5331–6.
3. Childers JM, Surwit EA. Combined laparoscopic and vaginal surgery for the management of two cases of stage I endometrial cancer. Gynecol Oncol. 1992;45(1):46–51.
4. Childers JM, et al. Laparoscopically assisted surgical staging (LASS) of endometrial cancer. Gynecol Oncol. 1993;51(1):33–8.
5. Janda M, et al. Quality of life after total laparoscopic hysterectomy versus total abdominal hysterectomy for stage I endometrial cancer (LACE): a randomised trial. Lancet Oncol. 2010;11(8):772–80.
6. Malzoni M, et al. Total laparoscopic hysterectomy versus abdominal hysterectomy with lymphadenectomy for early-stage endometrial cancer: a prospective randomized study. Gynecol Oncol. 2009;112(1):126–33.
7. Mourits MJ, et al. Safety of laparoscopy versus laparotomy in early-stage endometrial cancer: a randomised trial. Lancet Oncol. 2010;11(8):763–71.

8. Tozzi R, et al. Laparoscopy versus laparotomy in endometrial cancer: first analysis of survival of a randomized prospective study. J Minim Invasive Gynecol. 2005;12(2):130–6.
9. Zullo F, et al. Laparoscopic surgery vs laparotomy for early stage endometrial cancer: long-term data of a randomized controlled trial. Am J Obstet Gynecol. 2009;200(3):296.e1–9.
10. Hatta K, et al. Preoperative assessment by magnetic resonance imaging is useful for planning the treatment of an enlarged uterus by total laparoscopic hysterectomy. J Obstet Gynaecol Res. 2013;39(4):814–9.
11. Bouwman F, et al. The impact of BMI on surgical complications and outcomes in endometrial cancer surgery--an institutional study and systematic review of the literature. Gynecol Oncol. 2015;139(2):369–76.
12. Gunderson CC, et al. The impact of obesity on surgical staging, complications, and survival with uterine cancer: a Gynecologic Oncology Group LAP2 ancillary data study. Gynecol Oncol. 2014;133(1):23–7.
13. Uccella S, et al. Impact of obesity on surgical treatment for endometrial cancer: a multicenter study comparing laparoscopy vs open surgery, with propensity-matched analysis. J Minim Invasive Gynecol. 2016;23(1):53–61.
14. Walker JL, et al. Recurrence and survival after random assignment to laparoscopy versus laparotomy for comprehensive surgical staging of uterine cancer: Gynecologic Oncology Group LAP2 Study. J Clin Oncol. 2012;30(7):695–700.
15. Terai Y, et al. Total laparoscopic modified radical hysterectomy with lymphadenectomy for endometrial cancer compared with laparotomy. J Obstet Gynaecol Res. 2014;40(2):570–5.
16. Tanaka T, et al. Comparison between laparoscopy and laparotomy in systematic para-aortic lymphadenectomy for patients with endometrial cancer: a retrospective multicenter study. J Gynecol Surg. 2017;33(3):105–10.
17. Nezhat FR, et al. The safety and efficacy of laparoscopic surgical staging and debulking of apparent advanced stage ovarian, fallopian tube, and primary peritoneal cancers. JSLS. 2010;14(2):155–68.

Sentinel Node Navigation Surgery for Endometrial Cancer

19

Nobuyuki Susumu, Wataru Yamagami, Fumio Kataoka, Takuro Hirano, Takeshi Makabe, Kensuke Sakai, Tatsuyuki Chiyoda, Hiroyuki Nomura, Akira Hirasawa, and Daisuke Aoki

Abstract

To date, the results of the clinical trial of sentinel node navigation surgery (SNNS) for endometrial cancer are not reported, and SNNS should be not yet performed as a clinical practice. SNNS is thought to be performed as a clinical trial in the institutions with enough experiences of SN mapping. Regarding the methods of the tracer injection and tracer detection, the diagnostic accuracy of metastasis, the clinical significance of ITC, or micrometastasis, the oncologic significance of solitary metastasis-positive sentinel lymph node (SN) in para-aortic basin, the usefulness of SN biopsy using surgical robots with fluorescence imaging system for detecting ICG, accumulations of clinical trials, and the data analysis in many facilities are needed so that SNNS comes to be safely performed as a clinical practice. Furthermore, the standardization of the diagnosing method for the pathological search for SN and the establishment of the molecular biologic laboratory procedure are necessary, too. However, we think SNNS will emerge as a promising, elegant solution to the ongoing discussion regarding lymphadenectomy in the initial surgical management of endometrial cancer in order to prevent many patients from receiving oversurgery, in order to properly

N. Susumu (✉)
Department of Gynecologic Center, International University of Health and Welfare Mita Hospital, Minato-ku, Tokyo, Japan

Department of Obstetrics and Gynecology, Keio University School of Medicine, Shinjuku-ku, Tokyo, Japan
e-mail: susumu35@iuhw.ac.jp

W. Yamagami · F. Kataoka · T. Hirano · T. Makabe · K. Sakai · T. Chiyoda · H. Nomura
A. Hirasawa · D. Aoki
Department of Obstetrics and Gynecology, Keio University School of Medicine, Shinjuku-ku, Tokyo, Japan

M. Mikami (ed.), *Surgery for Gynecologic Cancer*, Comprehensive Gynecology and Obstetrics, https://doi.org/10.1007/978-981-13-1519-0_19

select patients who need to receive lymphadenectomy, and in order to definitely evaluate the risk of recurrence by using ultra-staging or biological diagnosing method in the near future.

Keywords
Endometrial cancer · Sentinel node navigation surgery · Sentinel node mapping · Minimally invasive surgery · ICG

19.1 Principle and History

Sentinel lymph node (SN) is defined as a lymph node which receives lymphatic flow directly from tumors. From SNs, lymphatic fluid flows into many lymph nodes. Therefore, SNs may have first metastasis among regional lymph nodes. Non-SN metastasis might occur from SN with metastasis. In principle, no direct metastasis occurs from tumor to non-SN. Concerning lymphatic metastasis, metastatic tumor cells should harbor in the SN(s) (first SN), and direct metastasis from tumor to non-SNs cannot be recognized. Requirements for SN detection method are high detection rate, high sensitivity, high specificity, and high negative predictive value (NPV). One of the aims of SN navigation surgery (SNNS) is a reduced surgery-associated morbidity, such as lymphedema, injury of artery or vein, and increased blood loss, without influencing oncologic outcomes.

In the gynecologic field, the concept of SN dissection was first developed in vulvar cancer and next in cervical cancer as a tool to select patients most suitable for surgical management. In vulvar cancer, clinical trials for verifying the omission of systemic lymphadenectomy have been reported [1], and in cervical cancer, the result of validation study in many facilities came to be reported [2]. As for endometrial cancer, papers for SN biopsy have gradually increased in number after the article of Burke et al. [3] in 1996, and the interest increases about SN biopsy with an argument of the significance of lymph node dissection in endometrial cancer. A prospective multicenter study in France [4] was reported in 2011, and the NCCN Clinical Practice Guidelines in Oncology for Uterine Neoplasms (Version 1.2018) [5] state that prospective and retrospective studies demonstrate that compared to systemic lymphadenectomy, SLN mapping with ultra-staging may increase the detection of lymph node metastasis with low false-negative rates in women with apparent uterine-confined disease. The NCCN Guidelines also mention that the role of SN mapping in endometrial cancer is under evaluation; however, it states that "Previously, a full standard lymphadenectomy was recommended for all patients; however, a more selective and tailored lymphadenectomy approach that may include the SLN algorithm is now recommended by the NCCN Panel to avoid systematic overtreatment." And "SLN mapping can be considered as an alternative to full lymphadenectomy in the setting of apparent uterine-confined disease." Recommendation strength is category 2A. In the ESMO-ESGO-ESTRO guideline

[6], ultra-staging of the SNs is referred to detect micrometastases otherwise undiagnosed by conventional histology, even in patients considered at low risk, on the basis of grade and depth myometrial invasion. It also states that SN dissection is still experimental, but large series suggest its feasibility and SN dissection increase the detection of lymph nodes with small metastases and isolated tumor cells; however, the importance of these findings is unclear (level of evidence, IV; strength of recommendation, D). The guideline concludes that SN dissection may be useful in the management of endometrial cancers, although evidence is accumulating. Recently, the Society of Gynecologic Oncology's (SGO) Clinical Practice Committee and SN Working Group reviewed the current literature and reported a review and literature-based recommendations for the inclusion of SN assessment in the treatment of patients with endometrial cancer [7].

In Japan, Japan Society of Gynecologic Oncology (JSGO) published "Treatment guideline for endometrial cancer version 2013," and now JSGO is revising a new version. Regarding SN, at present, there is no definite evidence enough for omitting retroperitoneal lymph node dissection based on SN sampling. SNNS should be performed as a clinical study. And recommendation grade is C2; however, in the next version, it might be written that pathological diagnosis of SN may be taken into account in order to improve the accuracy of diagnosis of tumor spread, if it would be performed by a well-trained team under the circumstances with good cooperation of pathologists. And recommendation grade might become C1.

Unfortunately, SNNS has not been yet reported in endometrial cancer. Therefore, in this chapter, some evidences regarding SN mapping in endometrial cancer are introduced in order. In the fields of surgery for endometrial cancer, a new attempt of "precision" or "personalized" surgery has already been made for reducing morbidity associated with comprehensive lymphadenectomy and for improving diagnostic accuracy of lymph node metastasis and moreover for improving prognosis after surgery.

19.2 Indication for SN mapping

In principle, SN mapping can be considered for the surgical staging of apparent uterine-confined malignancy when there is no metastasis demonstrated by imaging studies or no obvious extrauterine disease at exploration; however, there is a movement of the adaptation expansion. Historically, SN mapping was controversial in patients with high-risk histology (e.g., serous carcinoma, clear cell carcinoma, carcinosarcoma). The NCCN Guidelines Version 1.2018 [5] stated that SN mapping in patients with high-risk histologies (i.e., grade 3, serous, clear cell, carcinosarcoma) has been reported with promising results as a potential alternative to complete lymphadenectomy [8, 9]. The main contraindication for SN mapping is uterine sarcoma. However, this guideline sequentially emphasizes that SN mapping should be done in institutions with expertise in this procedure.

19.3 Preoperative Evaluation

SN mapping can be considered for the surgical staging of apparent uterine-confined malignancy when there is no metastasis demonstrated by imaging studies or no obvious extrauterine disease at exploration [5]. For preoperative evaluation, MRI, CT, or PET-CT is applied. MRI is useful for checking myometrial invasion, cervical invasion, or adnexal metastasis [10]. On the other hand, CT or PET/CT is useful for diagnosing metastasis and peritoneal dissemination. According to a systematic review and meta-analysis for the diagnostic performances of 18F-FDG-PET or PET/CT in detecting pelvic and/or para-aortic lymph node metastasis [11], sensitivity and specificity of FDG-PET or PET/CT scans in the detection of pelvic and/or para-aortic metastasis were 63% and 95%, respectively. The high positive likelihood value confirms the reliability of a positive FDG-PET or PET/CT to detect pelvic and/or para-aortic lymph node metastasis in patients with untreated endometrial cancer. However, the efficacy of PET-CT for detecting lymph node metastasis has the limitation relating to the size of metastasis in lymph node and the region of metastatic lymph node [12]. In metastatic lymph nodes with a short-axis diameter of 4 mm or less, between 5 and 9 mm, and 10 mm or greater, PET had a detection sensitivity of 16.7%, 66.7%, and 93.3%, respectively [13]. The sensitivities for the interiliac and parametrial regions were very low, compared with obturator, interiliac, parametrial, and common iliac lymph nodes [12].

Preoperative pathological diagnosis is also important for presuming the risk of lymph node metastasis of endometrial cancer. Pathological diagnosis can usually be made by an office endometrial biopsy; however, office endometrial biopsies have a false-negative rate of about 10% [5]. In order to fully examine the endometrium, patients must be followed up by a fractional dilation and curettage (D and C) under anesthesia.

19.4 Technique of SN Mapping and SNNS

19.4.1 Selection of Tracers and Injection Sites

Historically, blue dyes, 99m-Technetium, or a combination of the two tracers has been used for SN mapping in endometrial cancer patients. In this chapter, the selection and injection sites of tracers employed in some validating studies in relatively small number patients are introduced, and the results of SN detection are also shown.

Ansari et al. [14] comprehensively reviewed the available reports on SN biopsy of endometrial cancer in 2013. Overall, 35 studies had enough information for false-negative rate evaluation and 51 studies for detection rate evaluation (2071 patients overall). Pooled detection rate was 77.8% (95% confidence interval [CI] 73.5–81.5%), and pooled sensitivity was 89% (95% CI 83–93%). Cervical injection, as well as using both blue dye and radiotracer, results in higher detection rate and sensitivity. New techniques such as fluorescent dye injection and robotic-assisted surgery showed high detection rate and sensitivity. They concluded that using both blue dye and radiotracer and cervical injection of the mapping material can optimize the sensitivity and detection rate of this technique.

Recently, one of the green dyes, indocyanine green (ICG), has been widely used with near-infrared fluorescence imaging using specific instruments. ICG, as a tracer, has been recently introduced in this setting. Ruscito et al. [15] reviewed 6 studies including 538 patients. Compared with blue dyes, ICG SN mapping had higher overall (odds ratio [OR] 0.27; 95% CI 0.15–0.50; $p < 0.0001$) and bilateral detection rates (OR 0.27; 95% CI 0.19–0.40; $p < 0.00001$). No difference was found between ICG and 99m-Technetium, although these results are based on data of a single series. No difference in overall and bilateral detection rates was found between ICG and the combination of blue dyes and 99m-Technetium. The pooled analysis of false-negative rate data showed no difference in false-negative rates between tracers. They concluded that ICG SN mapping seems to be equivalent to the combination of blue dyes and 99m-Technetium in terms of overall and bilateral detection rates. Its safety profile and ease of use may favor its employment respect to conventional tracers.

Regarding the tracer injection sites, Delpech et al. [16] reviewed papers concerning correlations between SN distribution and tracer injection sites, such as cervical injection, subendometrial injection under hysteroscopy, and subserosal injection at operation. When tracers were injected at the cervix, the sites of detected SNs were confined only to the pelvic region, whereas, when tracers were injected to the corpus either subendometrially or subserosally, SNs are detected also at the para-aortic region. Kataoka et al. [17] showed as much as 80% detection rate of SNs in the para-aortic region by injecting RI subendometrially and by injecting dye subserosally into the corpus.

By using radioisotope and dye, Niikura et al. [18] detected SNs in 82% cases by injecting RI into the corpus submucosally under hysteroscopy and injecting dye into the corpus subserosally in 2004. SNs were distributed in the pelvic region and also in the para-aortic region. SN localization was 10% only in the pelvic region, 25% only in the para-aortic region, and 65% in both pelvic and para-aortic regions. Namely, 90% of cases revealed to have SNs in the para-aortic region. And 40% of metastatic LNs were localized in the para-aortic region. The average number of detected SNs was 3.7 (range: 1–9). In 2013, they also evaluated the most effective combination of injected tracer types and injection sites in order to detect SNs in early endometrial cancer [19]. They examined 100 consecutive patients with endometrial cancer by either RI injection into the endometrium during hysteroscopy (55 cases) or direct RI injection into the uterine cervix (45 cases). SN detection rate was highest (96%) by cervical RI injection; however, no SN was detected in the para-aortic area. Para-aortic SNs were detected only by hysteroscopic RI injection (56%). All cases with pelvic lymph node metastases were detected by pelvic SN biopsy. Isolated positive para-aortic lymph nodes were detected in three patients. Bilateral SN detection rate was high (96%) by cervical RI injection combined with dye. They concluded that RI injection into the uterine cervix is highly sensitive in the detection of SN metastasis in early-stage endometrial cancer. It is a useful and safe modality when combined with blue dye injection into the uterine body.

In 2015, Kataoka et al. [17] evaluated the detection rate and diagnostic accuracy of SN mapping using hysteroscopic subendometrial injection of 99m-Technetium-labeled phytate and subserosal ICG injection in patients with endometrial cancer. They prospectively evaluated 57 endometrial cancer patients undergoing SN mapping using RI method combined with dye method. As for 32 cases, both (RI + dye) methods were used, and 23 cases were performed only in dye method. At least one SN was detected in 100%, and the average number of detected SNs was 6.0 in RI + dye method. Sensitivity and NPV were 100% and 100%, respectively. From the results of SN mapping, 62.8% of SNs were present in the pelvic and 37.1% in para-aortic lymph nodes (PAN). A total of 56.3% of lymph nodes with metastasis were present in the pelvic and 43.8% in PAN, and the distribution has no difference with SN mapping results ($p = 0.602$). Among 13 cases with metastatic SNs, 76.9% of cases showed metastasis in PAN. They concluded that their SN mapping procedure revealed high detection rate, sensitivity, and NPV and also indicated the importance of the SN exploration in PAN basin. The same study group [20] also assessed tracers for SN mapping in endometrial cancer patients, comparing the dye and near-infrared fluorescence imaging to clarify a suitable method. They enrolled 92 patients and performed three methods using either dye or fluorescence solutions in conjunction with a RI method. In the dye method, they injected ICG in the uterine subserosa, visually identifying SNs as stained green. In the fluorescence method, a dilute ICG solution (0.5 mg, fluorescence A or 0.25 mg, fluorescence B, each per 10 mL of solvent) was injected and the SN identified by the HyperEye Medical System. The SN detection rates were 100%, 100%, and 96% using dye and fluorescence A or B solution, respectively. Pelvic SNs were detected by the three methods in 98%, 100%, and 96% of cases and para-aortic SNs in 65%, 88%, and 74%, respectively. Fluorescence A solution was somewhat better than dye in detecting para-aortic SNs, although not significantly ($p = 0.07$). The sensitivity and NPV for detecting SNs with metastases with the dye method were 92% and 98% compared with 100% and 100%, respectively, for both fluorescence solutions. On these data, although both dye and fluorescence methods performed well, no method perfectly identified para-aortic SNs. The concomitant use of the RI method is required to detect para-aortic SNs.

Tanaka et al. [21] also evaluated the feasibility and detection rates of SN biopsy in patients with endometrial cancer and explored some clinicopathologic factors that might affect SN detection. They enrolled 211 patients for SN mapping using 3 kinds of tracers including 99m-Technetium, indigo carmine, and ICG. The detection rates of the SN biopsy using 99m-Technetium, indigo carmine, and ICG were 77.9%, 17.0%, and 73.4%, respectively. The detection rate was lower in elderly patients (≥60 years) (67.9% vs. 89.2%, $p < 0.01$), patients with >50% myometrial invasion (68.3% vs. 85.2%, $p < 0.01$), patients with high-grade tumors (69.5% vs. 84.9%, $p < 0.01$), and patients who underwent laparotomy (71.2% vs. 84.9%, $p < 0.01$). There were no significant differences in body mass index. The sensitivity was not significantly different in any factor. However, the false-negative rate was higher in patients with >50% myometrial invasion (11.5% vs. 1.2%, $p < 0.01$) and high-grade tumors (13.3% vs. 0.8%, $p < 0.01$) and who underwent laparotomy (12.2% vs. 0.4%, $p < 0.01$). They concluded that patients who underwent laparoscopy with <50% myometrial invasion and low-grade tumors not only have higher detection rates but also have lower false-negative rates. These patients may avoid systemic lymphadenectomy according to the status of the SN biopsy.

Some meta-analysis papers are available regarding SN detection in endometrial cancer. In 2015, Cormier et al. [22] conducted a PubMed search and included all original research of endometrial cancer patients having undergone SN procedure with an $n > 30$. Data collected included injection technique; unilateral, bilateral, and para-aortic detection rates; and ultra-staging results. They identified 17 eligible studies. Injection sites were categorized into cervical versus corporeal. Overall detection rates ranged from 60% to 100%; studies with $n > 100$ all had overall detection rates of >80%. Bilateral detection rates were higher with a combination of two injection agents. Para-aortic mapping was most frequent after corporeal injection techniques (39%) and was higher after deep vs. standard cervical injection (17% vs. 2%). The proportion of metastatic lymph nodes diagnosed through ultra-staging was high (around 40%), and ultra-staging of SN upstaged approximately in 5% of patients. Retrospectively applying a surgical algorithm revealed a sensitivity of 95%, a NPV of 99%, and a false-negative rate of 5%. They concluded that results of SN research for endometrial cancer are promising. In 2016, Bodurtha Smith et al. [23] conducted a systematic review to evaluate the diagnostic accuracy and clinical impact of SN mapping in the management of endometrial cancer. They identified 55 eligible studies, which included 4915 women. The overall detection rate of SN mapping was 81% (95% CI, 77–84%) with a 50% (95% CI, 44–56%) bilateral pelvic node detection rate and 17% (95% CI, 11–23%) para-aortic detection rate. There was no difference in detection rates by patient body mass index or tumor histology and grade. The use of ICG increased the bilateral detection rate compared with blue dye. Additionally, cervical injection increased the bilateral SN detection rate but decreased the para-aortic detection rate compared with alternative injection techniques. The sensitivity of SN mapping to detect metastases was 96% (95% CI, 91–98%). Compared with women staged with complete lymphadenectomy, women staged with SN mapping were more likely to receive adjuvant treatment. They concluded that SN mapping is feasible and accurately predicts nodal status in women with endometrial cancer. This data favors the use of cervical injection techniques with ICG.

Several lymphatic pathways directly reach even to the para-aortic region. Reginal lymph node is rather wide than those of cervical cancer and vulvar cancer. This is one of the reasons for the delay of SN study in endometrial cancer. However, those cases with para-aortic lymph node metastasis and without pelvic lymph node metastasis are reported to be rare; most of the papers regarding SN mapping referred solely to the pelvic SN. In NCCN Clinical Practice Guidelines in Oncology for Uterine Neoplasms Version 1.2018 [5], the combination method using both superficial (1–3 mm) injection and deep (1–2 cm) injection into the cervix is useful in delivering dye to the main layers of lymphatic channel origins in the cervix and corpus. Main uterine lymphatic trunks commonly cross over the umbilical ligament and flow to the most common location of pelvic SNs, which are located medial to the external iliac region and ventral to the hypogastric region, and also located in the superior (cranial) part of obturator lymph nodes. The guideline also referred to the less common pathway of injected dye, which does not cross over the umbilical ligament and runs toward cranial direction along with the mesoureter and reaches to less common SNs locations, such as presacral region.

Regarding the training curve in detecting SNs, Khoury-Collado et al. [24] examined how many cases are needed to achieve >90% SN detection. They included 115 patients with endometrial cancer. The cervix was the only site of injection in 82 cases (71%), while a combined cervical and fundal injection was performed in 33 cases (29%). Overall, SN detection was achieved in 98 (85%) cases. In the initial 27 months of the study, a SN was identified in 50 of 64 cases (78%), with two false-negative cases. In the subsequent 15 months, successful mapping was achieved in 48 of 51 cases (94%) with no false-negative cases. When examining an individual provider's performance, after the first 30 cases, the rate of successful mapping significantly increased from 77% to 94% ($p = 0.033$). They concluded that high SN detection rates can be achieved in women with uterine cancer, and increasing surgical volume (30 cases) is associated with significantly increased detection rates.

19.4.2 Results of Detected SNs

In this chapter, two prospective multicenter cohort studies will be referred and discussed.

A prospective, multicenter cohort study (SENTI-ENDO study) [4] was first reported to assess the detection rate and diagnostic accuracy of the SN procedure in predicting the pathological pelvic node status in patients with early-stage endometrial cancer in 2011. Eligibility is stage I/II endometrial cancer. All lymph nodes were histopathologically examined, and SNs were serial sectioned and examined by immunochemistry. The primary endpoint was the estimation of the NPV of SN biopsy per hemipelvis. One hundred thirty-three patients were enrolled at nine centers in France. Pelvic SNs were assessed by cervical dual injection (with technetium and patent blue) and systematic pelvic node dissection. SN detection rate was 89% (111/125), and 19 of 111 (17%) had pelvic lymph node metastases. Five of 111 patients (5%) had an associated SN in the para-aortic area. Considering the patient as the unit of analysis, NPV was 100% and sensitivity 100%. Three patients had false-negative results (two had metastatic nodes in the contralateral pelvic area and one in the para-aortic area), giving an NPV of 97% and sensitivity of 84%. All three of these patients had type 2 endometrial cancer. The authors concluded that SNNS by the use of cervical dual labeling could be an alternative to systematic lymphadenectomy in patients with low-risk and intermediate-risk endometrial cancer. However, further study is needed for protocol standardization and for validating prognosis of patients with SN mapping.

In 2017, Rossi et al. [25] reported the results of a multicenter, prospective, cohort study (FIRES trial) comparing SN biopsy to lymphadenectomy for endometrial cancer staging for patients with clinical stage 1. In the FIRES multicenter, prospective, cohort study, patients with clinical stage 1 endometrial cancer of all histologies and grades undergoing robotic staging were eligible for study inclusion. Patients received a standardized cervical injection of ICG and SN mapping followed by pelvic lymphadenectomy with or without para-aortic lymphadenectomy. Negative SNs (by hematoxylin and eosin staining on sections) were ultra-staged with immunohistochemistry for cytokeratin. The primary endpoint was sensitivity of the SN-based detection of metastatic disease. They enrolled 340 patients, and 196 (58%) patients received para-aortic lymphadenectomy as well as pelvic lymphadenectomy. Two hundred ninety-three (86%) patients had successful mapping of at least one SN. Forty-one (12%) patients had positive nodes, 36 of whom had at least one mapped SN. Nodal metastases were identified in the SNs of 35 (97%) of these 36 patients, yielding a sensitivity to detect node-positive disease of 97.2% and a NPV of 99.6%. They detected SNs also in 23% of cases in the para-aortic region. Isolated para-aortic SN was detected in three cases (<1%). They concluded that SNs identified with ICG have a high degree of diagnostic accuracy in detecting endometrial cancer metastases and can safely replace lymphadenectomy in the staging of endometrial cancer.

19.4.3 Pathologic Diagnosis and Molecular Biological Diagnosis of SNs

Metastasis is classified into three categories according to the maximum diameter of metastasis. Metastasis with a maximum diameter greater than 2 mm is called macrometastasis and 0.2–2.0 mm a micrometastasis, and metastasis with a diameter less than 0.2 mm is called isolated tumor cells (ITCs). Recent data suggest the potential significance and impact of SN ultra-staging (i.e., serial sectioning and immunohistochemistry) to improve the accuracy of detecting micrometastases.

Niikura et al. [26] reported that SNs detected by immunostaining with step-serial sectioning had micrometastases more frequently than non-SNs. Easy detection of micrometastases by immunostaining is only possible when the SNs are evaluated with step-serial section combined by cytokeratin immunostaining. They examined consecutive patients undergoing laparotomy (total abdominal hysterectomy, bilateral salpingo-oophorectomy, total pelvic lymphadenectomy, and para-aortic lymphadenectomy to the level of renal veins) with SN biopsy for endometrial cancer. All surgically removed lymph nodes, including SNs, were examined histopathologically by immunohistochemistry staining with an anti-cytokeratin antibody (AE1/AE3) combined with step-serial sectioning at 200–500 micrometer intervals. Four of 74 SNs (5%) obtained from 20 patients had micrometastases or ITCs. In contrast, only 4 of the 1350 non-SNs obtained from 20 patients (0.3%) had detectable micrometastases. They concluded that easy detection of micrometastases by immunostaining is only possible with step-serial sectioning of the SNs.

Holloway et al. [27] compared the performance of SN mapping with staging lymphadenectomy versus staging lymphadenectomy alone for the detection of metastasis and the use of adjuvant therapies in patients with endometrial cancer. They examined patients with apparent early-stage endometrial cancer ($n = 780$) who underwent robotic-assisted hysterectomy with pelvic ± aortic lymphadenectomy and they compared pelvic ± aortic lymphadenectomy ($n = 661$) with SN-mapped cases with pelvic ± aortic lymphadenectomy ($n = 119$). Isosulfan blue and ICG with near-infrared imaging were used for SN mapping. SNs were processed in blocks and H&E slides were evaluated. The H&E negative blocks were further microsectioned 50 μm apart to get three H&E slides and one immunohistochemistry slide using anti-cytokeratin AE1/AE3. Non-SNs were examined only by routine H&E. The mapped group had more LN metastasis detected (30.3% vs. 14.7%, $p < 0.001$), more stage IIIC (30.2% vs. 14.5%, $p < 0.001$), and more GOG high-risk cases (32.8% vs. 21.8%, $p = 0.013$) and received more chemotherapy + radiation (28.6% vs. 16.3%, $p < 0.003$). The SN was the only metastasis in 18 (50%) mapped cases with positive nodes. The SN false-negative rate was 1/36 (2.8%). Micrometastases or ITCs were identified in 22/35 (62.9%) SN metastases. Multivariate analysis demonstrated that SN mapping imparted a significant effect on the detection of metastatic disease. The performance of SN mapping with staging lymphadenectomy increased the detection of lymph node metastasis and was associated with more use of adjuvant therapies.

In the SENTI-ENDO study by Ballester et al. [4], immunohistochemistry and serial sectioning detected metastases undiagnosed by conventional histology in 9 of 111 (8%) patients with detected SNs, representing 9 of the 19 patients (47%) with metastases. SN biopsy upstaged 10% of patients with low-risk and 15% of those with intermediate-risk endometrial cancer. This study suggests that SN biopsy could provide important data to tailor adjuvant therapy.

Kim et al. [28] reported that SN mapping with pathologic ultra-staging in endometrial cancer detects additional low-volume metastases (4.5%) that would otherwise go undetected with routine evaluations, and they also found that lymphovascular invasion was frequently recognized in those cases with low-volume metastases. Ultra-stage detected metastases more commonly in the cases with some evidence of myometrial invasion. In contrast to tumors with no myoinvasion, in which ultra-stage-detected nodal metastases were only found in 0.8% of cases, patients with any myoinvasion had approximately 7–8% low-volume, ultra-stage-detected nodal metastases in SNs. This is the largest single-institution study to date with standardized specialized pathology review reporting the incidence of low-volume, ultra-stage-detected metastases in SNs during the surgical staging of endometrial cancer. They described the incidence of low-volume ultra-stage-detected metastases in SNs identified at surgical staging for endometrial cancer and they correlated it with depth of myoinvasion and tumor grade. They reviewed 508 patients who underwent primary surgery for endometrial cancer with successful mapping of at least one SN. All patients underwent a cervical injection for mapping. The SN ultra-staging protocol involved cutting an additional two adjacent 5-μm sections at each of two levels, 50-μm apart, from each paraffin block lacking metastatic carcinoma on routine hematoxylin and eosin (H&E) staining. At each level, one slide was stained with H&E and with IHC using anti-cytokeratin AE1/AE3. Micrometastases and ITCs were classified as low-volume ultra-stage-detected metastases if pathologic ultra-staging was the only method allowing detection of such nodal disease. 64 (12.6%) of the 508 patients had positive nodes: routine H&E detected 35 patients (6.9%), ultra-staging detected an additional 23 patients (4.5%) who would have otherwise been missed (4 micrometastases and 19 ITCs), and 6 patients (1.2%) had metastatic disease in their non-SNs. The incidence rates of low-volume ultra-stage-detected nodal metastases in patients with grades 1, 2, and 3 tumors were 3.8%, 3.4%, and 6.9%, respectively. The frequency rates of low-volume ultra-stage-detected metastases in patients with a depth of myoinvasion of 0, less than 50%, and 50% or more were 0.8%, 8.0%, and 7.4%, respectively. Lymphovascular invasion was present in 20 (87%) of the cases containing low-volume ultra-stage-detected metastases in the lymph nodes. They proposed that the pathologic ultra-staging of SNs should be incorporated in endometrial cancer with any degree of myoinvasion.

In the field of diagnosis of SN metastasis, an epoch-making diagnostic method, a one-step nucleic acid amplification (OSNA) assay, was introduced. Nagai et al. [29] examined if an OSNA assay might improve lymph node (LN) metastasis identification for patients with endometrial cancer. Using quantitative reverse transcription polymerase chain reaction (qRT-PCR), an optimal mRNA marker was selected, and its expression was compared between histopathologically positive and negative LNs using an OSNA assay. They also investigated whether an OSNA assay could detect LN metastases with sensitivity and specificity equivalent to the 2-mm-interval histopathology method. Cytokeratin 19 (CK19) was selected as a useful mRNA marker for the OSNA assay. When the cutoff value was set at 250 copies, an OSNA assay using CK19 mRNA had a sensitivity of 93.3%, a specificity of 99.5%, and a concordance rate of 99.1%. For performance evaluations using SNs (120 histopathologically negative LNs and 17 histopathologically positive LNs from 35 patients), a OSNA assay using CK19 mRNA had a sensitivity of 82.4%, a specificity of 99.2%, a positive predictive value of 93.3%, and a concordance rate of 97.1%. Thus, an OSNA assay using CK19 mRNA provided results equivalent to those with the 2-mm-interval histopathology method. They demonstrated that an OSNA assay using CK19 mRNA was applicable for detecting LN metastases. A combined analysis using an OSNA assay and SNs may improve individualized treatments according to LN metastatic status. The OSNA assay also showed high sensitivity and specificity in another report. López-Ruiz et al. [30] enrolled 94 SNs from 34 patients with endometrial cancer. Using the breast cancer cutoff value for detecting lymph node metastasis (OSNA criteria for breast cancer, >250 copies of CK19/μL), the sensitivity of the OSNA assay was 100%; specificity was 87.6%; diagnostic accuracy was 88.3%. In two SNs from the same patient, histopathological examination revealed the presence of benign epithelial inclusions that were CK19 positive; both SNs yielded a positive result in the OSNA assay (true/false positive). All remaining nine histologically negative/OSNA-positive SNs were classified as micrometastasis (+)

by the OSNA assay. The OSNA assay shows high sensitivity and specificity, which suggests its utility as a novel tool for the molecular detection of SN metastasis.

19.4.4 Algorithm of SNNS

Barlin et al. [31] examined the effectiveness of their algorithm in detecting metastatic endometrial cancer while minimizing the need for complete lymphadenectomy. They reviewed 498 patients who received SN mapping in a single institution, and they applied retrospectively their algorithm to all patients. The surgical algorithm is as follows: (1) peritoneal and serosal evaluation and washings; (2) retroperitoneal evaluation including excision of all mapped SNs with ultra-staging and suspicious nodes regardless of mapping; and (3) if there is no mapping on a hemipelvis, a side-specific pelvic, common iliac, and interiliac lymph node dissection is performed. Para-aortic lymph node dissection is performed at the attendings' discretion. At least one LN was removed in 95% of cases (474/498); at least one SN was identified in 81% (401/498). SN correctly diagnosed 40/47 patients with nodal metastases who had at least one SN mapped, resulting in a 15% false-negative rate. After applying the algorithm, the false-negative rate dropped to 2%. Only one patient, whose LN spread would not have been caught by the algorithm, had an isolated positive right para-aortic LN with a negative ipsilateral SN and pelvic lymph node dissection. After limiting their analysis to patients with at least ten LNs removed, the endometrial cancer SN algorithm still performed well, with a sensitivity of 96.9%, NPV of 99.5%, and false-negative rate of 3.1%. They concluded that satisfactory SN mapping requires adherence to a surgical SN algorithm and goes beyond just the removal of blue SNs. Removal of any suspicious node along with side-specific lymphadenectomy for failed mapping is an integral part of this algorithm. Further validation of the false-negative rate of this algorithm is necessary. NCCN Clinical Practice Guidelines Version 1.2018 [5] cited this algorithm and recommended as category 2A.

19.5 Morbidity

There are few reports referring to the morbidity in the SN mapping. A prospective multicenter study, SENTI-ENDO [4] with 133 patients enrolled, revealed no complication after injection of technetium colloid, and no anaphylactic reactions after patent blue injection. No surgical complication was reported during SN biopsy, including procedures that involved conversion to open surgery. On the other hand, in the FIRES trial [25], 33 (9%) of 356 patients had an adverse event, and 22 of these patients had a serious adverse event. The most common grade 3 or 4 adverse events or serious adverse events were postoperative neurological changes, such as peripheral nerve injuries, or central nervous symptoms, such as syncope or vertigo (4 patients); postoperative respiratory distress or failure (4 patients); postoperative nausea and vomiting (3 patients); and bowel injury (3 patients). They reported one serious adverse event related to the study intervention: a ureteral injury incurred during SN dissection. The surgeon reported difficulty visualizing the ureter in the retroperitoneum during activation of the near-infrared imaging modality when bleeding was encountered. The ureter received a thermal injury that was immediately recognized. The ureter was stented and the patient did not sustain long-term adverse sequelae.

Geppert et al. [32] compared the rate of lymphatic complications in women with endometrial cancer undergoing SN biopsy versus a full pelvic and infrarenal para-aortic lymphadenectomy. This prospective study included 188 patients with endometrial cancer planned for robotic surgery. ICG was used to identify SNs. In low-risk patients, the lymphadenectomy was restricted to the removal of SNs, whereas in high-risk patients also a full lymphadenectomy was performed. The bilateral detection rate of SNs was 96% after cervical tracer injection. No intraoperative complication was associated with the SN biopsy per se. Compared with hysterectomy alone, the additional average operative time for the removal of SNs was 33 min whereas 91 min was saved compared with a full pelvic and para-aortic lymphadenectomy. SN biopsy alone resulted in a lower incidence of leg lymphedema than infrarenal para-aortic and pelvic lymphadenectomy (1.3% vs. 18.1%, $p = 0.0003$).

19.6 Future Prospect

There remain some problems in SN mapping or SNNS for endometrial cancer, such as the standard tracer selection, the standard tracer injection sites for detecting SNs in the para-aortic basin, the standard method of pathological diagnosis or biological diagnosis of SNs, the clinical significance of ITCs or micrometastases, the oncologic significance of solitary metastasis-positive SN in the para-aortic basin, the usefulness of SN biopsy using surgical robots with fluorescence imaging system for detecting ICG, and so on. Recently, a few articles regarding these problems were announced.

Ultra-staging of SNs with serial sectioning and immunohistochemistry in endometrial cancer with any degree of myoinvasion is useful for detecting low-volume metastases that would otherwise go undetected with routine evaluations. However, the oncologic significance of low-volume nodal metastases requires long-term follow-up [27] or, if possible, a randomized prospective study comparing the prognosis of those patients with early-stage endometrial cancer with micrometastases or ITCs with or without adjuvant chemotherapy.

St Clair et al. [33] characterized treatment patterns and oncologic outcomes in 844 patients with low-volume lymph node metastasis (ITCs and micrometastases [MM]) discovered during SN mapping for endometrial cancer. The median number of lymph nodes resected was six (range 0–60), and the median number of SNs was two (range 0–15). Overall, 753 (89.2%) patients were node-negative, 23 (2.7%) had ITCs only, 21 (2.5%) had MM only, and 47 (5.6%) had macrometastasis. Adjuvant chemotherapy was administered to 106 (14%) of 753 node-negative patients, 19 (83%) of 23 patients with ITCs, 17 (81%) of 21 patients with MM, and 42 (89%) of 47 with macrometastasis. The median follow-up was 26 months (range 0–108).

Three-year recurrence-free survival was as follows: node-negative patients, 90%; ITCs only, 86%; MM only, 86%; and macrometastasis, 71% [$p < 0.001$]. Patients with ITCs and MM frequently received adjuvant chemotherapy and had improved oncologic outcomes in comparison to those with macrometastasis to the lymph nodes. Further prospective study is needed to determine optimal post-resection management in patients with ITCs or MM alone.

In the Fluorescence Imaging for Robotic Endometrial Sentinel lymph node biopsy (FIRES) trial [25], da Vinci Si or Xi surgical robots (Intuitive Surgery, Sunnyvale, CA, USA) were used in all patients. This study using ICG for tracers injected into the cervix revealed 23% as a detecting rate of SNs in the para-aortic basin. This detecting rate is higher than those of other studies with cervical injection of tracers, and the high detecting rate is next to those of studies with corporal (subendometrial or subserosal) injection methods [17, 19]. This might be derived from the usefulness of the fluorescence detecting system of robots or from robotic surgery itself. SN biopsy with this robotic system might solve the problem of the difficulties in detecting SNs in the para-aortic basin even by injecting tracers into the cervix.

How et al. [34] reviewed 472 patients with endometrial cancer who underwent either SN mapping (SN cohort) or systematic lymphadenectomy (LND cohort) from sequential, non-overlapping historical time points and compared the possible impact of SN mapping on the location of disease recurrence between the two cohorts. No significant difference in overall recurrence-free survival (RFS) could be identified between the cohorts at 48 months (HR 0.74, 95% CI 0.43–1.28, $p = 0.29$). However, the SN cohort had improved the pelvic sidewall RFS compared to the LND cohort (HR 0.32, 95% CI 0.14–0.74, $p = 0.007$). The pelvic sidewall recurrences accounted for 30% of recurrences in the SN cohort (8 out of 26 recurrences) compared to 71.4% in the LND cohort (20 out of 28 recurrences). They concluded that SN mapping may enable more efficient detection of the LNs at greatest risk of metastasis and help to guide adjuvant therapy according to the pathologic results using ultra-staging, which in turn seems to decrease the risk of pelvic sidewall recurrences. SN mapping in addition to complete lymphadenectomy appears to be beneficial compared to complete lymphadenectomy alone; however, it is not known whether SN mapping on its own is superior to lymphadenectomy in terms of outcomes of RFS or overall survival.

Daraï et al. [35] reported the long-term follow-up results of the SENTI-ENDO study [4].

Patients with stages I–II endometrial cancer underwent pelvic SN biopsy after cervical dual injection (technetium and patent blue) and systematic pelvic node dissection. The secondary endpoint is the long-term recurrence-free survival (RFS) and the impact of the SN procedure on adjuvant therapies. The median follow-up was 50 months (range 3–77 months). Eighteen of the 125 patients (14.4%) experienced a recurrence. The 50-month RFS was 84.7% with no difference between patients with and without detected SN ($p = 0.09$). Among patients with detected SN (111), no difference in RFS was observed between those with and without positive SN ($p = 0.5$). In the whole population, adjuvant therapy was performed in low-, intermediate-, and high-risk groups in 31 of 64 patients (48.4%), 28 of 37 patients (75.7%), and 14 of

17 patients (82.3%), respectively ($p = 0.0001$). For the 111 patients with detected SN, EBRT was performed in 27 of the 89 with negative SN and in 11 of the 14 with positive SN ($p = 0.001$). Chemotherapy was performed more frequently in patients with positive SN (6/12, 50%) than in patients with negative SN (7/56, 12.5%) ($p = 0.009$). Their data support the impact of SN biopsy on surgical management and indications for adjuvant therapies. Further studies are required to assess the clinical impact of the SN biopsy in early-stage endometrial cancer.

Plante et al. [36] evaluated the outcome and the role of adjuvant treatment in the management of patients with endometrial cancer and ITCs identified by SN mapping. They enrolled 519 patients undergoing hysterectomy, salpingo-oophorectomy, lymphadenectomy, and SN mapping for endometrial cancer in a single institute. Data was prospectively collected. Overall, 85 patients (16.4%) were found to have SN metastases of which 43 (51%) were macrometastasis, 11 (13%) micrometastasis (MM), and 31 (36%) ITC. Eleven (35%) of patients with ITCs received adjuvant chemotherapy ± whole pelvic radiation therapy (WPRT), 10 (32%) received WPRT, and 10 (32%) received either no adjuvant treatment or vault brachytherapy (VBT) only. ITC patients received significantly less chemotherapy ($p = 0.0001$) and WPRT ($p = 0.007$) compared to patients with macrometastasis. Remarkably, the authors did not consider ITC as node positive. With a median follow-up of 29 months (range 0–67), the PFS at 3 years for the ITC patients was 95.5%, similar to node-negative (87.6%) and micrometastasis patients (85.5%) but statistically better than patients with macrometastasis (58.5%) ($p = 0.0012$). Only 1/31 patient with ITC recurred (IB, 7 cm carcinosarcoma) despite adjuvant treatments. None of the ITC patients with endometrioid histology recurred (0/28). Patients with endometrial cancer found to have SN ITCs have an excellent outcome. The use of adjuvant treatment should be tailored to uterine factors and histology and not solely based on the presence of ITCs. Patients with ITCs and otherwise low-risk uterine disease probably received little benefit from additional treatments. More studies are needed to confirm their results.

As mentioned above, there remain some difficult problems in SN mapping; however, we think SNNS will emerge as a promising, elegant solution to the ongoing discussion regarding lymphadenectomy in the initial surgical management of endometrial cancer in order to prevent most patients from receiving overtreatment, in order to select patients who need to receive lymphadenectomy, and in order to definitely evaluate the risk of recurrence by using ultra-staging or biological diagnosing method in the near future.

References

1. Van der Zee AG, Oonk MH, De Hullu JA, Ansink AC, Vergote I, Verheijen RH, et al. Sentinel node dissection is safe in the treatment of early-stage vulvar cancer. J Clin Oncol. 2008;26(6):884–9. https://doi.org/10.1200/JCO.2007.14.0566.
2. Altgassen C, Hertel H, Brandstädt A, Köhler C, Dürst M, Schneider A, AGO Study Group. Multicenter validation study of the sentinel lymph node concept in cervical cancer: AGO Study Group. J Clin Oncol. 2008;26(18):2943–51. https://doi.org/10.1200/JCO.2007.13.8933.

3. Burke TW, Levenback C, Tornos C, Morris M, Wharton JT, Gershenson DM. Intraabdominal lymphatic mapping to direct selective pelvic and paraaortic lymphadenectomy in women with high-risk endometrial cancer: results of a pilot study. Gynecol Oncol. 1996;62(2):169–73.
4. Ballester M, Dubernard G, Lécuru F, Heitz D, Mathevet P, Marret H, et al. Detection rate and diagnostic accuracy of sentinel-node biopsy in early stage endometrial cancer: a prospective multicentre study (SENTI-ENDO). Lancet Oncol. 2011;12(5):469–76. https://doi.org/10.1016/S1470-2045(11)70070-5.
5. NCCN Clinical Practice Guidelines in Oncology (NCCN Guidelines®) Uterine Neoplasms. Version 1.2018—October 13, 2017. NCCN.org. https://www.nccn.org/professionals/physician_gls/pdf/uterine.pdf. Accessed 25 Feb 2018.
6. Colombo N, Creutzberg C, Amant F, Bosse T, González-Martín A, Ledermann J, et al.; ESMO-ESGO-ESTRO Endometrial Consensus Conference Working Group. ESMO-ESGO-ESTRO Consensus Conference on Endometrial Cancer: Diagnosis, Treatment and Follow-up. Int J Gynecol Cancer. 2016;26(1):2–30. https://doi.org/10.1097/IGC.0000000000000609.
7. Holloway RW, Abu-Rustum NR, Backes FJ, Boggess JF, Gotlieb WH, Jeffrey Lowery W, et al. Sentinel lymph node mapping and staging in endometrial cancer: A Society of Gynecologic Oncology literature review with consensus recommendations. Gynecol Oncol. 2017;146(2):405–15. https://doi.org/10.1016/j.ygyno.2017.05.027.
8. Soliman PT, Westin SN, Dioun S, Sun CC, Euscher E, Munsell MF, et al. A prospective validation study of sentinel lymph node mapping for high-risk endometrial cancer. Gynecol Oncol. 2017;146(2):234–9. https://doi.org/10.1016/j.ygyno.2017.05.016.
9. Schiavone MB, Zivanovic O, Zhou Q, Leitao MM Jr, Levine DA, Soslow RA, et al. Survival of patients with uterine carcinosarcoma undergoing sentinel lymph node mapping. Ann Surg Oncol. 2016;23(1):196–202. https://doi.org/10.1245/s10434-015-4612-2.
10. Antonsen SL, Jensen LN, Loft A, Berthelsen AK, Costa J, Tabor A, et al. MRI, PET/CT and ultrasound in the preoperative staging of endometrial cancer—a multicenter prospective comparative study. Gynecol Oncol. 2013;128(2):300–8. https://doi.org/10.1016/j.ygyno.2012.11.025.
11. Chang MC, Chen JH, Liang JA, Yang KT, Cheng KY, Kao CH. 18F-FDG PET or PET/CT for detection of metastatic lymph nodes in patients with endometrial cancer: a systematic review and meta-analysis. Eur J Radiol. 2012;81(11):3511–7. https://doi.org/10.1016/j.ejrad.2012.01.024.
12. Nogami Y, Banno K, Irie H, Iida M, Kisu I, Masugi Y, et al. The efficacy of preoperative positron emission tomography-computed tomography (PET-CT) for detection of lymph node metastasis in cervical and endometrial cancer: clinical and pathological factors influencing it. Jpn J Clin Oncol. 2015;45(1):26–34. https://doi.org/10.1093/jjco/hyu161.
13. Kitajima K, Murakami K, Yamasaki E, Fukasawa I, Inaba N, Kaji Y, et al. Accuracy of 18F-FDG PET/CT in detecting pelvic and paraaortic lymph node metastasis in patients with endometrial cancer. AJR Am J Roentgenol. 2008;190(6):1652–8. https://doi.org/10.2214/AJR.07.3372.
14. Ansari M, Rad MA, Hassanzadeh M, Gholami H, Yousefi Z, Dabbagh VR, et al. Sentinel node biopsy in endometrial cancer: systematic review and meta-analysis of the literature. Eur J Gynaecol Oncol. 2013;34(5):387–401.
15. Ruscito I, Gasparri ML, Braicu EI, Bellati F, Raio L, Sehouli J, et al. Sentinel node mapping in cervical and endometrial cancer: indocyanine green versus other conventional dyes-a meta-analysis. Ann Surg Oncol. 2016;23(11):3749–56. https://doi.org/10.1245/s10434-016-5236-x.
16. Delpech Y, Coutant C, Darai E, Barranger E. Sentinel lymph node evaluation in endometrial cancer and the importance of micrometastases. Surg Oncol. 2008;17:237–45. https://doi.org/10.1016/j.suronc.2008.04.001.
17. Kataoka F, Susumu N, Yamagami W, Kuwahata M, Takigawa A, Nomura H, et al. The importance of para-aortic lymph nodes in sentinel lymph node mapping for endometrial cancer by using hysteroscopic radio-isotope tracer injection combined with subserosal dye injection: Prospective study. Gynecol Oncol. 2016;140(3):400–4. https://doi.org/10.1016/j.ygyno.2015.12.023.

18. Niikura H, Okamura C, Utsunomiya H, Yoshinaga K, Akahira J, Ito K, et al. Sentinel lymph node detection in patients with endometrial cancer. Gynecol Oncol. 2004;92:669–74.
19. Niikura H, Kaiho-Sakuma M, Tokunaga H, Toyoshima M, Utsunomiya H, Nagase S, et al. Tracer injection sites and combinations for sentinel lymph node detection in patients with endometrial cancer. Gynecol Oncol. 2013;131(2):299–303. https://doi.org/10.1016/j.ygyno.2013.08.018.
20. Yamagami W, Susumu N, Kataoka F, Makabe T, Sakai K, Ninomiya T, et al. A comparison of dye versus fluorescence methods for sentinel lymph node mapping in endometrial cancer. Int J Gynecol Cancer. 2017;27(7):1517–24. https://doi.org/10.1097/IGC.0000000000000997.
21. Tanaka T, Terai Y, Fujiwara S, Tanaka Y, Sasaki H, Tsunetoh S, et al. The detection of sentinel lymph nodes in laparoscopic surgery can eliminate systemic lymphadenectomy for patients with early stage endometrial cancer. Int J Clin Oncol. 2018;23(2):305–13. https://doi.org/10.1007/s10147-017-1196-9.
22. Cormier B, Rozenholc AT, Gotlieb W, Plante M, Giede C, Communities of Practice (CoP) Group of Society of Gynecologic Oncology of Canada (GOC). Sentinel lymph node procedure in endometrial cancer: A systematic review and proposal for standardization of future research. Gynecol Oncol. 2015;138(2):478–85. https://doi.org/10.1016/j.ygyno.2015.05.039.
23. Bodurtha Smith AJ, Fader AN, Tanner EJ. Sentinel lymph node assessment in endometrial cancer: a systematic review and meta-analysis. Am J Obstet Gynecol. 2017;216(5):459–476.e10. https://doi.org/10.1016/j.ajog.2016.11.1033.
24. Khoury-Collado F, Glaser GE, Zivanovic O, Sonoda Y, Levine DA, Chi DS, et al. Improving sentinel lymph node detection rates in endometrial cancer: how many cases are needed? Gynecol Oncol. 2009;115(3):453–5. https://doi.org/10.1016/j.ygyno.2009.08.026.
25. Rossi EC, Kowalski LD, Scalici J, Cantrell L, Schuler K, Hanna RK, et al. A comparison of sentinel lymph node biopsy to lymphadenectomy for endometrial cancer staging (FIRES trial): a multicentre, prospective, cohort study. Lancet Oncol. 2017;18(3):384–92. https://doi.org/10.1016/S1470-2045(17)30068-2.
26. Niikura H, Okamoto S, Yoshinaga K, Nagase S, Takano T, Ito K, et al. Detection of micrometastases in the sentinel lymph nodes of patients with endometrial cancer. Gynecol Oncol. 2007;105(3):683–6.
27. Holloway RW, Gupta S, Stavitzski NM, Zhu X, Takimoto EL, Gubbi A, et al. Sentinel lymph node mapping with staging lymphadenectomy for patients with endometrial cancer increases the detection of metastasis. Gynecol Oncol. 2016;141(2):206–10. https://doi.org/10.1016/j.ygyno.2016.02.018.
28. Kim CH, Soslow RA, Park KJ, Barber EL, Khoury-Collado F, Barlin JN, et al. Pathologic ultrastaging improves micrometastasis detection in sentinel lymph nodes during endometrial cancer staging. Int J Gynecol Cancer. 2013;23:964–70.
29. Nagai T, Niikura H, Okamoto S, Nakabayashi K, Matoda M, Utsunomiya H, et al. A new diagnostic method for rapid detection of lymph node metastases using a one-step nucleic acid amplification (OSNA) assay in endometrial cancer. Ann Surg Oncol. 2015;22(3):980–6. https://doi.org/10.1245/s10434-014-4038-2.
30. López-Ruiz ME, Diestro MD, Yébenes L, Berjón A, Díaz de la Noval B, Mendiola M, et al. One-step nucleic acid amplification (OSNA) for the detection of sentinel lymph node metastasis in endometrial cancer. Gynecol Oncol. 2016;143(1):54–9. https://doi.org/10.1016/j.ygyno.2016.07.106.
31. Barlin JN, Khoury-Collado F, Kim CH, Leitao MM Jr, Chi DS, Sonoda Y, et al. The importance of applying a sentinel lymph node mapping algorithm in endometrial cancer staging: beyond removal of blue nodes. Gynecol Oncol. 2012;125(3):531–5. https://doi.org/10.1016/j.ygyno.2012.02.021.
32. Geppert B, Lönnerfors C, Bollino M, Persson J. Sentinel lymph node biopsy in endometrial cancer-Feasibility, safety and lymphatic complications. Gynecol Oncol. 2018;148(3):491–8. https://doi.org/10.1016/j.ygyno.2017.12.017.

33. St Clair CM, Eriksson AG, Ducie JA, Jewell EL, Alektiar KM, Hensley ML, et al. Low-volume lymph node metastasis discovered during sentinel lymph node mapping for endometrial carcinoma. Ann Surg Oncol. 2016;23(5):1653–9. https://doi.org/10.1245/s10434-015-5040-z.
34. How J, Gauthier C, Abitbol J, Lau S, Salvador S, Gotlieb R, et al. Impact of sentinel lymph node mapping on recurrence patterns in endometrial cancer. Gynecol Oncol. 2017;144(3):503–9. https://doi.org/10.1016/j.ygyno.2017.01.013.
35. Daraï E, Dubernard G, Bats AS, Heitz D, Mathevet P, Marret H, et al. Sentinel node biopsy for the management of early stage endometrial cancer: long-term results of the SENTI-ENDO study. Gynecol Oncol. 2015;136(1):54–9. https://doi.org/10.1016/j.ygyno.2014.09.011.
36. Plante M, Stanleigh J, Renaud MC, Sebastianelli A, Grondin K, Grégoire J. Isolated tumor cells identified by sentinel lymph node mapping in endometrial cancer: does adjuvant treatment matter? Gynecol Oncol. 2017;146(2):240–6. https://doi.org/10.1016/j.ygyno.2017.05.024.

Outline of Surgical Treatments

20

Katsutoshi Oda, Kazunori Nagasaka, Mayuyo Mori-Uchino, Takahide Arimoto, Yoko Matsumoto, Yutaka Osuga, and Tomoyuki Fujii

Abstract

Surgery is among the most important therapeutic and diagnostic modalities in ovarian cancer. In general, staging laparotomy is needed even for early-stage patients, while primary debulking surgery or interval debulking surgery is indicated mainly for patients with advanced ovarian cancer. Because more than 10% of cases of early-stage ovarian cancer have lymph node involvement, lymph node dissection is included in staging laparotomy. Secondary debulking surgery can be a treatment option for recurrent cases, particularly those in which tumors are expected to be completely resected. Fertility-sparing surgery and minimally invasive surgery have gained much attention recently. The increasing rate of risk-reducing salpingo-oophorectomy for hereditary breast and ovarian carcinomas indicates the importance of prevention against ovarian cancer.

Keywords

Staging laparotomy · Primary debulking surgery · Interval debulking surgery Secondary debulking surgery · Fertility-sparing surgery

20.1 Introduction

Ovarian cancer is the leading cause of death among all gynecologic malignancies. Its prognosis is associated with surgical outcomes, particularly the size of residual tumors [1–3]. Surgical outcome is generally classified according to the size of the

K. Oda (✉) · K. Nagasaka · M. Mori-Uchino · T. Arimoto · Y. Matsumoto · Y. Osuga · T. Fujii
Department of Obstetrics and Gynecology, Graduate School of Medicine, The University of Tokyo, Tokyo, Japan
e-mail: katsutoshi-tky@umin.ac.jp

M. Mikami (ed.), *Surgery for Gynecologic Cancer*, Comprehensive Gynecology and Obstetrics, https://doi.org/10.1007/978-981-13-1519-0_20

maximum residual tumor. No residual macroscopic disease (R0) is considered as complete resection, regardless of positivity of the peritoneal cytology. Otherwise, it is classified according to the largest diameter of the macroscopic residual tumors. Cytoreduction with small residual tumor burden of 1–10 mm is optimal debulking, whereas cytoreduction with any residual tumors larger than 10 mm is suboptimal debulking. In advanced ovarian cancers, the prognosis is significantly favorable in patients with complete resection [4]. Optimal debulking by primary debulking surgery (PDS) is an alternative goal of the surgery; however, its impact on prognosis is limited compared with complete resection [4]. To improve the surgical resectability, interval debulking surgery (IDS) between cycles of chemotherapy has been used [5–7]. Complete resection was also shown to be the most significant prognostic factor in patients receiving IDS [8]. Therefore, complete resection is the desired surgical treatment for advance ovarian carcinomas. Fertility-sparing surgery should be considered in patients when the staging is early (mainly IA and possibly a part of IC) and the tumors are completely resectable under appropriate staging surgery [9]. However, the criteria for fertility-sparing surgery have not been established yet. The usefulness of minimally invasive surgery (MIS), such as laparoscopic surgery, is still controversial [10]. However, inspection laparoscopy before neoadjuvant chemotherapy may be an option for accurate diagnosis of the histological subtypes and evaluation of peritoneal dissemination. Here, we review the surgical modalities for epithelial ovarian cancer.

20.2 History

The importance of primary cytoreduction in ovarian cancer was initially described in 1934 and has been widely reported to date [11–13]. Intensive surgical management has been the standard strategy for advanced ovarian cancers, regardless of the chemotherapeutic regimen [14–16]. The high incidence of lymph node metastasis (pelvic and/or para-aortic) in advanced ovarian cancer has been also broadly reported [17–19]. The significance of systematic lymphadenectomy is supported by the findings that the prognosis of ovarian cancer upstaged to stage III after lymphadenectomy was similar to that of stage I/II patients [20]. However, the therapeutic effect of systematic lymphadenectomy is still under debate, particularly for advanced ovarian cancer. Recently, a large randomized trial for advanced ovarian cancer patients who received macroscopic complete resection strongly suggested that systematic pelvic and para-aortic lymphadenectomy (LION, lymphadenectomy in ovarian neoplasms) did not improve the prognosis of patients with (pre- and intra-operatively) clinically negative lymph nodes compared with the other group without lymphadenectomy [21]. Therefore, the optimal technique for primary surgical management is yet to be established.

"Second-look" surgery was widely performed for abdominal malignancies, including ovarian cancer since the 1940s [22–24]. Until the 1980s, multidisciplinary treatment for advanced ovarian cancer often includes whole-abdomen irradiation as well as chemotherapy [25, 26]. Sequential therapy included primary surgery, chemotherapy, second-look exploratory laparotomy, and whole-abdomen irradiation [25]. "Second-look" surgery was mainly diagnostic and occasionally therapeutic. It was indicated to (a) assess disease with the intent of stopping therapy, (b) evaluate recurrent or persistent disease, and (c) determine the need for further tumor resection following chemotherapy [27]. For diagnosis, "second-look" laparoscopy was introduced around the 1980s [28]. "Second-look surgery" often included both inspection and debulking surgery (interval and secondary). Currently, diagnostic "second-look surgery" is not routinely performed. Although IDS for patients with suboptimal PDS or neoadjuvant chemotherapy has already been performed for several decades, the prognostic significance of IDS remains controversial and needs more evaluation. No randomized controlled trials for secondary debulking surgery (SDS) have been performed; however, complete cytoreduction via SDS has been reported to be of prognostic importance for recurrent ovarian cancer [29–33]. In any case, debulking surgery has since been considered as one of the treatment options for advanced and recurrent ovarian cancer.

20.3 Staging Laparotomy

Staging laparotomy is a surgery that includes procedures necessary for the determination of tumor stage. The standard surgical procedure includes bilateral salpingo-oophorectomy, hysterectomy, and greater omentectomy as well as peritoneal cytology, peritoneal biopsies, and retroperitoneal (pelvic and para-aortic) lymphadenectomy (or biopsy) (Table 20.1). The extent of dissection for para-aortic lymph nodes is generally up to the level of the left renal vessel.

More than 10% of apparent stage I (pT1M0) disease has pelvic and/or para-aortic lymph node involvement [19, 34–36], indicating the importance of lymphadenectomy for diagnosis and treatment. The incidence of lymph node metastasis in stage I/II (pT1/2M0) was the highest in grade 3 tumors (20.0%) and the serous subtype (23.3%) [36]. In a retrospective study of 6686 patients with clinical stage I ovarian cancer, lymphadenectomy was significantly associated with improved 5-year disease-specific survival (87.0% vs. 92.6%, $P < 0.001$) [37]. In a randomized trial in patients with macroscopically intrapelvic ovarian cancer, the risks for progression were lower in the systematic lymphadenectomy arm than the node

Table 20.1 Staging laparotomy for ovarian cancer

Total abdominal hysterectomy, bilateral salpingo-oophorectomy, infracolic omentectomy, and excision of masses when prudent
Lymphadenectomy (or biopsy) of pelvic and para-aortic nodes
Peritoneal cytology (ascites or peritoneal washing)
Biopsy of peritoneum of vesicouterine excavation, Douglas' pouch, right and left pelvic sidewalls, and right and left paracolic gutters
Biopsy or cytology from undersurface of right hemidiaphragm
Biopsy of all suspicious lesions
Careful inspection and palpation of all peritoneal surfaces

sampling arm, although the difference was not statistically significant [38]. The incidence of para-aortic node metastasis is as high as that of pelvic node metastasis. In a retrospective study of 116 patients with stage IIIC or IV epithelial ovarian cancer who underwent systematic bilateral pelvic and aortic lymphadenectomy, 78% of patients had pelvic nodal metastases, whereas 84% had aortic lymph node metastases. A total of 59% of patients had both pelvic and aortic node metastasis [39]. Among the pelvic and/or aortic node-positive patients, the incidence of metastases to the aortic lymph nodes was high in both the level above the inferior mesenteric artery (79%) and below the inferior mesenteric artery (71%) [19]. Therefore, systematic dissection of lymph nodes should include both pelvic and para-aortic regions (up to the level of the renal vessel).

Greater omentectomy has been included as a part of staging laparotomy for ovarian cancer since the 1960s [40], with the omentum as a frequent site of metastasis. Occult omental metastases in otherwise early disease indicated the necessity of omentectomy for accurate staging and possible therapeutic benefit [41]. Microscopic disease in the omentum has been reported in 5–10% of cases of early-stage epithelial ovarian cancer [13, 42, 43]. Therefore, infracolic omentectomy should be performed even in cases without macroscopic dissemination.

Multiple biopsies of the peritoneum are important for accurate staging in ovarian cancer. Careful inspection of the abdominal cavity is necessary. In patients who are suspected to have peritoneal dissemination, biopsy and cytology of the peritoneum, such as vesicouterine excavation, Douglas' pouch, right and left pelvic sidewalls, right and left paracolic gutters, and right hemidiaphragm, are recommended.

20.4 Primary Debulking Surgery and Interval Debulking Surgery for Advanced Ovarian Cancer

The prognosis of advanced ovarian cancer (FIGO stages III to IV) is poor, with a median overall survival (OS) of less than 25 months and a 5-year survival rate of 20% [44]. PDS to achieve no residual diseases (R0) followed by platinum-based chemotherapy is the standard treatment for advanced ovarian cancer [45, 46]. Despite the accumulated evidence supporting the clinical significance of PDS, whether the good outcome depends on the background of patients' functional status and surgical tolerability or the surgical quality of professional gynecologic oncologists remains debated [47, 48]. PDS sometimes induces perioperative complications, particularly in advanced cases with massive ascites and high tumor load.

To evaluate an alternative treatment strategy for advanced patients, two large clinical trials have been conducted. The European Organization for Research and Treatment of Cancer (EORTC) Gynecologic Group conducted a large phase III study (EORTC 55971) and suggested that neoadjuvant chemotherapy (NAC) followed by IDS (NAC therapy [NACT]) has a comparable survival rate as that of PDS followed by adjuvant chemotherapy among those with stages IIIC and IV ovarian cancer [5]. The study reported no significant difference in progression-free survival

(PFS) or OS between the two treatment arms, concluding that NACT was not inferior to, and was possibly safer than, PDS. The other study was a phase II/III randomized controlled trial (CHORUS) conducted by the Medical Research Council Clinical Trials Unit in the United Kingdom. It has showed results consistent with those of EORTC 55971, strengthening the evidence for NACT as a non-inferior treatment modality in terms of survival rate and a decrease in surgical morbidity and mortality owing to less invasiveness compared with PDS [49].

Furthermore, a phase III, non-inferiority trial (JCOG0602) has recently analyzed the prognostic impact comparing PDS and NACT followed by IDS [50]. In the study, they have referred to two earlier studies; EORTC 55971 and CHORUS included a certain number of patients whose main bulk tumors were resected as diagnostic procedures before treatment in NACT arm. Therefore, the less invasiveness of NACT needs further validation. In this context, the JCOG0602 study has clearly demonstrated differences in treatment invasiveness comparing PDS and NACT by not adding diagnostic laparotomy or laparoscopy before the treatment. The JCOG0602 study showed noteworthy evidence for less invasiveness of NACT considering the frequencies of adverse events during the perioperative management [50]. In addition, the other phase III randomized clinical trial, SCORPION trial (NCT01461850), has also shown a more favorable perioperative morbidity as well as quality of life in the NACT arm than in the PDS arm [51]. The international Trial on Radical Upfront Surgery in Advanced Ovarian Cancer (TRUST) investigating OS after PDS or NACT is ongoing and aims to resolve optimal timing of IDS [52]. However, evidence for the benefit of NACT is still limited, if the cases in which appropriate maximum debulking at IDS is hard to perform even after NACT are considered. In addition, a high risk of platinum-resistant recurrence has been suggested in patients who underwent NACT [53, 54]. Hence, the clinicopathological factors that may influence poor prognosis should be investigated during IDS to understand the true benefit of NACT. In a retrospective study, positive peritoneal cytology at IDS with no residual tumors was suggested to be the most important prognostic factor for PFS [55]. The normalization of CA125 before IDS was reported to be a good predictor to receive appropriate IDS during NACT [54]. Collectively, NACT may prolong the survival of those with poor prognosis if the therapeutic effect of chemotherapy can be improved. For instance, the addition of bevacizumab to conventional platinum-based chemotherapy prolongs PFS [56], although the clinical benefit of the addition of bevacizumab for NACT has limited evidence for the outcome of IDS [57]. Recently, maintenance chemotherapy with olaparib has been shown to induce long OS for platinum-sensitive recurrent cases with *BRCA*-mutant ovarian cancer [58]. These novel chemotherapies may be effective for a certain number of suitable cases when it can be performed as NACT, as shown in previous studies of NACT with a combination of paclitaxel and carboplatin chemotherapy. Novel adjuvant chemotherapies may also improve the prognosis of patients with advanced ovarian cancer whose tumors are optimally debulked via PDS or IDS.

Collectively, NACT may become a novel alternative standard strategy, although up-front cytoreductive surgery is still important for advanced ovarian cancer. Further studies of NACT with specific molecular-targeted drugs are warranted to improve the prognosis of advanced ovarian cancer.

20.5 Secondary Debulking Surgery

SDS may have a therapeutic benefit for patients with recurrent ovarian cancer who have poor prognosis. Although no randomized controlled trials have been performed, the prognosis of patients who received complete cytoreduction via SDS has been favorable [32, 59]. Disease-free interval (DFI) is an essential factor to appropriately select patients for SDS. DFI with >6 m is often among the selection criteria for SDS [30, 59]. Although optimal surgery with residual tumors smaller than 1 cm is associated with favorable prognosis [60–62], a meta-analysis suggested that complete resection alone was the only predictor of favorable prognosis [32]. Predictive factors for complete resection via SDS include recurrence of stage I/II, complete resection via the previous PDS, good PS, an amount of ascites <500 mL, solitary tumor, and tumor size smaller than 10 cm in diameter [30, 60, 63–65]. Suitable criteria for SDS should be established.

20.6 Fertility-Sparing Surgery and Minimally Invasive Surgery

Patients with ovarian tumors with suspected malignant potential (such as endometrioma sized over 10 cm and tumors with solid and papillary component) are recommended to undergo surgical resection [66], mainly via open laparotomy and after appropriate surgical staging. Intraoperative assessment of ovarian tumors using frozen sections is useful for managing tumors, with a reported accuracy of 91–97%. However, the accuracy of frozen section biopsy for epithelial borderline malignant tumors, particularly mucinous tumors, decreases to 65–84% (sensitivity, 44–87%; specificity, 64–98%) with a tendency of underdiagnosis rather than overdiagnosis [67–71]. Re-laparotomy is recommended for cases whose final diagnosis was corrected after initial surgery. Approximately 16–31% of patients who underwent re-laparotomy were upstaged after staging laparotomy [41, 72]. Fertility-preserving procedure may be considered for patients with stage I ovarian cancer (mainly stage IA and grade 1/2) [73]. In such cases, treatment options must be discussed thoroughly before surgery as both the surgical staging and the completion of surgery are important prognostic factors. Patients who did not undergo staging laparotomy had high rate of recurrence [74–76]. However, fertility preservation has become a major issue in patients with ovarian cancer because late childbearing is much more common now. A prospective study is warranted to expand the indications in which fertility-sparing surgery followed by adjuvant chemotherapy is acceptable [77].

MIS for gynecologic malignancies is a recent medical advancement. The number of MIS, such as laparoscopic and robotically assisted surgery, for endometrial and cervical cancer is increasing [78, 79]. Although laparoscopic cytoreduction may be technically applied even for advanced ovarian neoplasms [80], a higher frequency of intraoperative rupture or metastasis to port site than laparotomy is reported [81, 82], implying the risk of laparoscopic cytoreduction. Although laparoscopic surgery may be performed by a well-trained and experienced gynecologic oncologist for patients with early ovarian cancer, with similar survival outcomes, less blood loss, and shorter hospitalization [83–85], further studies are needed to standardize laparoscopic surgery as an alternative option. Laparoscopic surgery can be useful particularly for ovarian neoplasms to evaluate whether maximum cytoreduction can be achieved in patients with advanced ovarian cancer [86]. Patients with advanced ovarian cancer are often in poor general condition, which may make standard cytoreductive surgery too invasive. As tumor samples may be helpful for predicting tumor biology, drug sensitivity, ovarian cancer prognosis, and treatment planning, MIS may be widely used for patients with unresectable ovarian cancer who will undergo neoadjuvant chemotherapy. No high-quality randomized control studies comparing laparoscopy and laparotomy for ovarian cancer have been performed [87]. Further accumulation of data and evidence is warranted to apply MIS for ovarian cancer.

20.7 Future Perspectives

Both tumor debulking and accurate diagnosis through surgery are essential for ovarian cancer as the prognosis of advanced ovarian cancer is poor even after molecular-targeted drugs and/or improvement of chemotherapy regimen. Although the surgical strategy depends on the tumor extent, drug sensitivity and/or drug availability may influence the indication of the surgeries. For instance, PARP inhibitors are effective for recurrent ovarian cancers with *BRCA1/BRCA2* mutations, and the European Medicines Agency has approved olaparib for patients with recurrent ovarian cancer with either somatic or germline *BRCA* mutations in 2014 [88], indicating that the tumor specimen needs to receive accurate companion diagnostic. Molecular-based tumor biology using genome-wide analysis is associated with ovarian cancer prognosis [89–91]. Therefore, NACT without any tumor sampling prior to chemotherapy may prevent appropriate drug selection, particularly of the molecular-targeted drugs.

Ovarian cancer prevention should also be considered. The fimbria is considered the origin of high-grade ovarian cancer (at least in part), and risk-reducing salpingo-oophorectomy is now recommended to women with germline *BRCA1/BRCA2* mutations, and even the use of risk-reducing salpingectomy is currently under debate [92, 93]. Precision medicine should be advocated in ovarian cancer, along with the improvement of drug treatment and preventive care.

Acknowledgments This work was financially supported by a research program of the Project for Cancer Research and Therapeutic Evolution (P-CREATE) (to K Oda) from the Japan Agency for Medical Research and Development (AMED). We thank Editage for their English editing service (www.editage.com).

Conflict of Interest Disclosure Statement The authors have no competing interests to disclose.

References

1. Winter WE 3rd, Maxwell GL, Tian C, Sundborg MJ, Rose GS, Rose PG, et al. Tumor residual after surgical cytoreduction in prediction of clinical outcome in stage IV epithelial ovarian cancer: a Gynecologic Oncology Group Study. J Clin Oncol. 2008;26:83–9.
2. Winter WE 3rd, Maxwell GL, Tian C, Carlson JW, Ozols RF, Rose PG, et al. Prognostic factors for stage III epithelial ovarian cancer: a Gynecologic Oncology Group Study. J Clin Oncol. 2007;25(24):3621–7.
3. Chi DS, Eisenhauer EL, Lang J, Huh J, Haddad L, Abu-Rustum NR, et al. What is the optimal goal of primary cytoreductive surgery for bulky stage IIIC epithelial ovarian carcinoma (EOC)? Gynecol Oncol. 2006;103:559–64.
4. du Bois A, Reuss A, Pujade-Lauraine E, Harter P, Ray-Coquard I, Pfisterer J. Role of surgical outcome as prognostic factor in advanced epithelial ovarian cancer: a combined exploratory analysis of 3 prospectively randomized phase 3 multicenter trials: by the Arbeitsgemeinschaft Gynaekologische Onkologie Studiengruppe Ovarialkarzinom (AGO-OVAR) and the Groupe d'Investigateurs Nationaux Pour les Etudes des Cancers de l'Ovaire (GINECO). Cancer. 2009;115:1234–44.
5. Vergote I, Trope CG, Amant F, Kristensen GB, Ehlen T, Johnson N, et al. Neoadjuvant chemotherapy or primary surgery in stage IIIC or IV ovarian cancer. N Engl J Med. 2010;363:943–53.
6. Tangjitgamol S, Manusirivithaya S, Laopaiboon M, Lumbiganon P, Bryant A. Interval debulking surgery for advanced epithelial ovarian cancer. Cochrane Database Syst Rev. 2016;2016:CD006014.
7. Makar AP, Trope CG, Tummers P, Denys H, Vandecasteele K. Advanced ovarian cancer: primary or interval debulking? Five categories of patients in view of the results of randomized trials and tumor biology: primary debulking surgery and interval debulking surgery for advanced ovarian cancer. Oncologist. 2016;21:745–54.
8. Vermeulen CKM, Tadesse W, Timmermans M, Kruitwagen RFPM, Walsh T. Only complete tumour resection after neoadjuvant chemotherapy offers benefit over suboptimal debulking in advanced ovarian cancer. Eur J Obstet Gynecol Reprod Biol. 2017;219:100–5.
9. Bentivegna E, Gouy S, Maulard A, Pautier P, Leary A, Colombo N, et al. Fertility-sparing surgery in epithelial ovarian cancer: a systematic review of oncological issues. Ann Oncol. 2016;27:1994–2004.
10. Fagotti A, Perelli F, Pedone L, Scambia G. Current recommendations for minimally invasive surgical staging in ovarian cancer. Curr Treat Options in Oncol. 2016;17:3.
11. Griffiths CT, Parker LM, Fuller AF Jr. Role of cytoreductive surgical treatment in the management of advanced ovarian cancer. Cancer Treat Rep. 1979;63:235–40.
12. Buchsbaum HJ, Lifshitz S. Staging and surgical evaluation of ovarian cancer. Semin Oncol. 1984;11:227–37.
13. Hoskins WJ. Epithelial ovarian carcinoma: principles of primary surgery. Gynecol Oncol. 1994;55:S91–6.
14. Bristow RE. Surgical standards in the management of ovarian cancer. Curr Opin Oncol. 2000;12:474–80.
15. Mutch DG. Surgical management of ovarian cancer. Semin Oncol. 2002;29:3–8.
16. Carnino F, Fuda G, Ciccone G, Iskra L, Guercio E, Dadone D, et al. Significance of lymph node sampling in epithelial carcinoma of the ovary. Gynecol Oncol. 1997;65:467–72.
17. Burghardt E, Pickel H, Stettner H. Management of advanced ovarian cancer. Eur J Gynaecol Oncol. 1984;5:155–9.
18. Onda T, Yoshikawa H, Yokota H, Yasugi T, Taketani Y. Assessment of metastases to aortic and pelvic lymph nodes in epithelial ovarian carcinoma. A proposal for essential sites for lymph node biopsy. Cancer. 1996;78:803–8.

19. Onda T, Yoshikawa H, Yasugi T, Mishima M, Nakagawa S, Yamada M, et al. Patients with ovarian carcinoma upstaged to stage III after systematic lymphadenctomy have similar survival to Stage I/II patients and superior survival to other Stage III patients. Cancer. 1998;83:1555–60.
20. Harter P, Sehouli J, Lorusso D, Reuss A, Vergote I, Marth C, et al. LION: lymphadenectomy in ovarian neoplasms—a prospective randomized AGO study group led gynecologic cancer intergroup trial. J Clin Oncol. 2017;35(15_suppl):abstr 5500.
21. Griffen WO Jr, Gilbertsen VA, Wangensteen OH. The second-look operation for abdominal malignancies, 1948–1963. Natl Cancer Inst Monogr. 1964;15:267–76.
22. Gilbertsen VA, Wangensteen OH. A summary of thirteen years' experience with the second look program. Surg Gynecol Obstet. 1962;114:438–42.
23. Santoro BT, Griffen WO Jr, Wangensteen OH. The second-look procedure in the management of ovarian malignancies and pseudomyxoma peritonei. Surgery. 1961;50:354–8.
24. Piver MS, Barlow JJ, Lee FJ, Vongtama V. Sequential therapy for advanced ovarian adenocarcinoma: operation, chemotherapy, second-look laparotomy, and radiation therapy. Am J Obstet Gynecol. 1975;122:355–7.
25. Katz ME, Schwartz PE, Kapp DS, Luikart S. Epithelial carcinoma of the ovary: current strategies. Ann Intern Med. 1981;95:98–111.
26. Stuart GC, Jeffries M, Stuart JL, Anderson RJ. The changing role of "second-look" laparotomy in the management of epithelial carcinoma of the ovary. Am J Obstet Gynecol. 1982;142:612–6.
27. Piver MS, Lele SB, Barlow JJ, Gamarra M. Second-look laparoscopy prior to proposed second-look laparotomy. Obstet Gynecol. 1980;55:571–3.
28. Eisenkop SM, Friedman RL, Wang HJ. Secondary cytoreductive surgery for recurrent ovarian cancer. A prospective study. Cancer. 1995;76:1606–14.
29. Segna RA, Dottino PR, Mandeli JP, Konsker K, Cohen CJ. Secondary cytoreduction for ovarian cancer following cisplatin therapy. J Clin Oncol. 1993;11:434–9.
30. Onda T, Yoshikawa H, Yasugi T, Yamada M, Matsumoto K, Taketani Y. Secondary cytoreductive surgery for recurrent epithelial ovarian carcinoma: proposal for patients selection. Br J Cancer. 2005;92:1026–32.
31. Al Rawahi T, Lopes AD, Bristow RE, Bryant A, Elattar A, Chattopadhyay S, et al. Surgical cytoreduction for recurrent epithelial ovarian cancer. Cochrane Database Syst Rev. 2013;2013:CD008765.
32. Bristow RE, Puri I, Chi DS. Cytoreductive surgery for recurrent ovarian cancer: a meta-analysis. Gynecol Oncol. 2009;112:265–74.
33. Takeshima N, Hirai Y, Umayahara K, Fujiwara K, Takizawa K, Hasumi K. Lymph node metastasis in ovarian cancer: difference between serous and non-serous primary tumors. Gynecol Oncol. 2005;99:427–31.
34. Cass I, Li AJ, Runowicz CD, Fields AL, Goldberg GL, Leuchter RS, et al. Pattern of lymph node metastases in clinically unilateral stage I invasive epithelial ovarian carcinomas. Gynecol Oncol. 2001;80:56–61.
35. Kleppe M, Wang T, Van Gorp T, Slangen BF, Kruse AJ, Kruitwagen RF. Lymph node metastasis in stages I and II ovarian cancer: a review. Gynecol Oncol. 2011;123:610–4.
36. Chan JK, Munro EG, Cheung MK, Husain A, Teng NN, Berek JS, et al. Association of lymphadenectomy and survival in stage I ovarian cancer patients. Obstet Gynecol. 2007;109:12–9.
37. Maggioni A, Benedetti Panici P, Dell'Anna T, Landoni F, Lissoni A, Pellegrino A, et al. Randomised study of systematic lymphadenectomy in patients with epithelial ovarian cancer macroscopically confined to the pelvis. Br J Cancer. 2006;95:699–704.
38. Pereira A, Magrina JF, Rey V, Cortes M, Magtibay PM. Pelvic and aortic lymph node metastasis in epithelial ovarian cancer. Gynecol Oncol. 2007;105:604–8.
39. Barber HR, Kwon TH. Current status of the treatment of gynecologic cancer by site: ovary. Cancer. 1976;38:610–9.
40. Arie AB, McNally L, Kapp DS, Teng NN. The omentum and omentectomy in epithelial ovarian cancer: a reappraisal: part II—The role of omentectomy in the staging and treatment of apparent early stage epithelial ovarian cancer. Gynecol Oncol. 2013;131:784–90.
41. Young RC, Decker DG, Wharton JT, Piver MS, Sindelar WF, Edwards BK, et al. Staging laparotomy in early ovarian cancer. JAMA. 1983;250:3072–6.

42. Piver MS, Barlow JJ, Lele SB. Incidence of subclinical metastasis in stage I and II ovarian carcinoma. Obstet Gynecol. 1978;52:100–4.
43. Colombo N, Peiretti M, Parma G, Lapresa M, Mancari R, Carinelli S, et al. Newly diagnosed and relapsed epithelial ovarian carcinoma: ESMO Clinical Practice Guidelines for diagnosis, treatment and follow-up. Ann Oncol. 2010;21(Suppl 5):v23–30.
44. Bristow RE, Tomacruz RS, Armstrong DK, Trimble EL, Montz FJ. Survival effect of maximal cytoreductive surgery for advanced ovarian carcinoma during the platinum era: a meta-analysis. J Clin Oncol. 2002;20:1248–59.
45. Fanfani F, Ferrandina G, Corrado G, Fagotti A, Zakut HV, Mancuso S, et al. Impact of interval debulking surgery on clinical outcome in primary unresectable FIGO stage IIIc ovarian cancer patients. Oncology. 2003;65:316–22.
46. Meigs JV. Tumors of the female pelvic organs. New York: Macmillan; 1934.
47. du Bois A, Rochon J, Pfisterer J, Hoskins WJ. Variations in institutional infrastructure, physician specialization and experience, and outcome in ovarian cancer: a systematic review. Gynecol Oncol. 2009;112:422–36.
48. Crawford SC, Vasey PA, Paul J, Hay A, Davis JA, Kaye SB. Does aggressive surgery only benefit patients with less advanced ovarian cancer? Results from an international comparison within the SCOTROC-1 Trial. J Clin Oncol. 2005;23:8802–11.
49. Kehoe S, Hook J, Nankivell M, Jayson GC, Kitchener H, Lopes T, et al. Primary chemotherapy versus primary surgery for newly diagnosed advanced ovarian cancer (CHORUS): an open-label, randomised, controlled, non-inferiority trial. Lancet. 2015;386:249–57.
50. Onda T, Satoh T, Saito T, Kasamatsu T, Nakanishi T, Nakamura K, et al. Comparison of treatment invasiveness between upfront debulking surgery versus interval debulking surgery following neoadjuvant chemotherapy for stage III/IV ovarian, tubal, and peritoneal cancers in a phase III randomised trial: Japan Clinical Oncology Group Study JCOG0602. Eur J Cancer. 2016;64:22–31.
51. Fagotti A, Ferrandina G, Vizzielli G, Fanfani F, Gallotta V, Chiantera V, et al. Phase III randomised clinical trial comparing primary surgery versus neoadjuvant chemotherapy in advanced epithelial ovarian cancer with high tumour load (SCORPION trial): final analysis of peri-operative outcome. Eur J Cancer. 2016;59:22–33.
52. Mahner S, Heitz F, Burges A, Reuss A, Kraemer B, Schmalfeldt B, et al. TRUST: trial of radical upfront surgical therapy in advanced ovarian cancer (ENGOT ov33/AGO-OVAR OP7). J Clin Oncol. 2017;35(15_suppl):abstr TPS5602.
53. Sato S, Itamochi H. Neoadjuvant chemotherapy in advanced ovarian cancer: latest results and place in therapy. Ther Adv Med Oncol. 2014;6:293–304.
54. Gill SE, McGree ME, Weaver AL, Cliby WA, Langstraat CL. Optimizing the treatment of ovarian cancer: neoadjuvant chemotherapy and interval debulking versus primary debulking surgery for epithelial ovarian cancers likely to have suboptimal resection. Gynecol Oncol. 2017;144:266–73.
55. Nagasaka K, Kawana K, Tomio K, Tsuruga T, Mori-Uchino M, Miura S, et al. Positive peritoneal cytology at interval surgery is a poor prognostic factor in patients with stage T3c advanced ovarian carcinoma: a retrospective study. J Obstet Gynaecol Res. 2015;41:755–62.
56. Burger RA, Brady MF, Bookman MA, Fleming GF, Monk BJ, Huang H, et al. Incorporation of bevacizumab in the primary treatment of ovarian cancer. N Engl J Med. 2011;365:2473–83.
57. Rouzier R, Gouy S, Selle F, Lambaudie E, Floquet A, Fourchotte V, et al. Efficacy and safety of bevacizumab-containing neoadjuvant therapy followed by interval debulking surgery in advanced ovarian cancer: results from the ANTHALYA trial. Eur J Cancer. 2017;70:133–42.
58. Ledermann JA, Harter P, Gourley C, Friedlander M, Vergote I, Rustin G, et al. Overall survival in patients with platinum-sensitive recurrent serous ovarian cancer receiving olaparib maintenance monotherapy: an updated analysis from a randomised, placebo-controlled, double-blind, phase 2 trial. Lancet Oncol. 2016;17:1579–89.
59. Chi DS, McCaughty K, Diaz JP, Huh J, Schwabenbauer S, Hummer AJ, et al. Guidelines and selection criteria for secondary cytoreductive surgery in patients with recurrent, platinum-sensitive epithelial ovarian carcinoma. Cancer. 2006;106:1933–9.

60. Zang RY, Harter P, Chi DS, Sehouli J, Jiang R, Trope CG, et al. Predictors of survival in patients with recurrent ovarian cancer undergoing secondary cytoreductive surgery based on the pooled analysis of an international collaborative cohort. Br J Cancer. 2011;105:890–6.
61. Ayhan A, Gultekin M, Taskiran C, Aksan G, Celik NY, Dursun P, et al. The role of secondary cytoreduction in the treatment of ovarian cancer: Hacettepe University experience. Am J Obstet Gynecol. 2006;194:49–56.
62. Tian WJ, Jiang R, Cheng X, Tang J, Xing Y, Zang RY. Surgery in recurrent epithelial ovarian cancer: benefits on survival for patients with residual disease of 0.1-1 cm after secondary cytoreduction. J Surg Oncol. 2010;101:244–50.
63. Zang RY, Li ZT, Tang J, Cheng X, Cai SM, Zhang ZY, et al. Secondary cytoreductive surgery for patients with relapsed epithelial ovarian carcinoma: who benefits? Cancer. 2004;100:1152–61.
64. Harter P, du Bois A, Hahmann M, Hasenburg A, Burges A, Loibl S, et al. Surgery in recurrent ovarian cancer: the Arbeitsgemeinschaft Gynaekologische Onkologie (AGO) DESKTOP OVAR trial. Ann Surg Oncol. 2006;13:1702–10.
65. Tian WJ, Chi DS, Sehouli J, Trope CG, Jiang R, Ayhan A, et al. A risk model for secondary cytoreductive surgery in recurrent ovarian cancer: an evidence-based proposal for patient selection. Ann Surg Oncol. 2012;19:597–604.
66. Tanaka YO, Okada S, Yagi T, Satoh T, Oki A, Tsunoda H, et al. MRI of endometriotic cysts in association with ovarian carcinoma. AJR Am J Roentgenol. 2010;194:355–61.
67. Ilvan S, Ramazanoglu R, Ulker Akyildiz E, Calay Z, Bese T, Oruc N. The accuracy of frozen section (intraoperative consultation) in the diagnosis of ovarian masses. Gynecol Oncol. 2005;97:395–9.
68. Stewart CJ, Brennan BA, Hammond IG, Leung YC, McCartney AJ. Intraoperative assessment of ovarian tumors: a 5-year review with assessment of discrepant diagnostic cases. Int J Gynecol Pathol. 2006;25:216–22.
69. Rakhshan A, Zham H, Kazempour M. Accuracy of frozen section diagnosis in ovarian masses: experience at a tertiary oncology center. Arch Gynecol Obstet. 2009;280:223–8.
70. Akrivos N, Thomakos N, Sotiropoulou M, Rodolakis A, Antsaklis A. Intraoperative consultation in ovarian pathology. Gynecol Obstet Investig. 2010;70:193–9.
71. Morton R, Anderson L, Carter J, Pather S, Saidi SA. Intraoperative frozen section of ovarian tumors: a 6-year review of performance and potential pitfalls in an Australian Tertiary Referral Center. Int J Gynecol Cancer. 2017;27:17–21.
72. Stier EA, Barakat RR, Curtin JP, Brown CL, Jones WB, Hoskins WJ. Laparotomy to complete staging of presumed early ovarian cancer. Obstet Gynecol. 1996;87:737–40.
73. Satoh T, Hatae M, Watanabe Y, Yaegashi N, Ishiko O, Kodama S, et al. Outcomes of fertility-sparing surgery for stage I epithelial ovarian cancer: a proposal for patient selection. J Clin Oncol. 2010;28:1727–32.
74. Zanetta G, Rota S, Chiari S, Bonazzi C, Bratina G, Torri V, et al. The accuracy of staging: an important prognostic determinator in stage I ovarian carcinoma. A multivariate analysis. Ann Oncol. 1998;9:1097–101.
75. Le T, Adolph A, Krepart GV, Lotocki R, Heywood MS. The benefits of comprehensive surgical staging in the management of early-stage epithelial ovarian carcinoma. Gynecol Oncol. 2002;85:351–5.
76. Takano M, Sasaki N, Kita T, Kudoh K, Fujii K, Yoshikawa T, et al. Survival analysis of ovarian clear cell carcinoma confined to the ovary with or without comprehensive surgical staging. Oncol Rep. 2008;19:1259–64.
77. Satoh T, Yoshikawa H. Fertility-sparing surgery for early stage epithelial ovarian cancer. Jpn J Clin Oncol. 2016;46:703–10.
78. Arimoto T, Kawana K, Adachi K, Ikeda Y, Nagasaka K, Tsuruga T, et al. Minimization of curative surgery for treatment of early cervical cancer: a review. Jpn J Clin Oncol. 2015;45:611–6.
79. Rabinovich A. Minimally invasive surgery for endometrial cancer: a comprehensive review. Arch Gynecol Obstet. 2015;291:721–7.
80. Fanning J, Hojat R, Johnson J, Fenton B. Laparoscopic cytoreduction for primary advanced ovarian cancer. JSLS. 2010;14:80–2.

81. Zivanovic O, Sonoda Y, Diaz JP, Levine DA, Brown CL, Chi DS, et al. The rate of port-site metastases after 2251 laparoscopic procedures in women with underlying malignant disease. Gynecol Oncol. 2008;111:431–7.
82. Smorgick N, Barel O, Halperin R, Schneider D, Pansky M. Laparoscopic removal of adnexal cysts: is it possible to decrease inadvertent intraoperative rupture rate? Am J Obstet Gynecol. 2009;200:237.e1–3.
83. Nezhat FR, Ezzati M, Chuang L, Shamshirsaz AA, Rahaman J, Gretz H. Laparoscopic management of early ovarian and fallopian tube cancers: surgical and survival outcome. Am J Obstet Gynecol. 2009;200:83.e1–6.
84. Lee M, Kim SW, Paek J, Lee SH, Yim GW, Kim JH, et al. Comparisons of surgical outcomes, complications, and costs between laparotomy and laparoscopy in early-stage ovarian cancer. Int J Gynecol Cancer. 2011;21:251–6.
85. Ghezzi F, Malzoni M, Vizza E, Cromi A, Perone C, Corrado G, et al. Laparoscopic staging of early ovarian cancer: results of a multi-institutional cohort study. Ann Surg Oncol. 2012;19:1589–94.
86. Fagotti A, Ferrandina G, Fanfani F, Garganese G, Vizzielli G, Carone V, et al. Prospective validation of a laparoscopic predictive model for optimal cytoreduction in advanced ovarian carcinoma. Am J Obstet Gynecol. 2008;199::642.e1–6.
87. Falcetta FS, Lawrie TA, Medeiros LR, da Rosa MI, Edelweiss MI, Stein AT, et al. Laparoscopy versus laparotomy for FIGO stage I ovarian cancer. Cochrane Database Syst Rev. 2016;10:CD005344.
88. Liu JF, Matulonis UA. What is the place of PARP inhibitors in ovarian cancer treatment? Curr Oncol Rep. 2016;18:29.
89. Yang JY, Yoshihara K, Tanaka K, Hatae M, Masuzaki H, Itamochi H, et al. Predicting time to ovarian carcinoma recurrence using protein markers. J Clin Invest. 2013;123:3740–50.
90. Patch AM, Christie EL, Etemadmoghadam D, Garsed DW, George J, Fereday S, et al. Whole-genome characterization of chemoresistant ovarian cancer. Nature. 2015;521:489–94.
91. Murakami R, Matsumura N, Mandai M, Yoshihara K, Tanabe H, Nakai H, et al. Establishment of a novel histopathological classification of high-grade serous ovarian carcinoma correlated with prognostically distinct gene expression subtypes. Am J Pathol. 2016;186:1103–13.
92. Ludwig KK, Neuner J, Butler A, Geurts JL, Kong AL. Risk reduction and survival benefit of prophylactic surgery in BRCA mutation carriers, a systematic review. Am J Surg. 2016;212:660–9.
93. Long Roche KC, Abu-Rustum NR, Nourmoussavi M, Zivanovic O. Risk-reducing salpingectomy: let us be opportunistic. Cancer. 2017;123:1714–20.

Staging Laparotomy in Early Ovarian Cancer

21

Tsutomu Tabata

Abstract

If staging laparotomy is performed in the patients with early ovarian cancer, approximately 30% of them will be subject to upstaging, from stage I to stage II/III or from stage II to stage III. The standard staging laparotomy procedure for early ovarian cancer is as follows: peritoneal cytology of ascites/washings, multiple peritoneal surface biopsies, bilateral salpingo-oophorectomy, a total hysterectomy, pelvic and para-aortic lymphadenectomy, and omentectomy. Especially, the incidence of lymph node involvement is approximately 11% for stage I and 28% for stage II. The incidence of omental metastasis is approximately 10%. Histological diagnosis is also important. Serous carcinoma cases have a high frequency of lymph node metastasis, whereas mucinous and low-grade serous types have less frequency, and in patients with apparent mucinous-type stage I ovarian cancer, lymphadenectomy may be omitted. We believe that staging laparotomy will provide information to improve the treatment quality of patients with early ovarian cancer. If a patient is diagnosed as stage IA or IB, grade 1 ovarian cancer by surgical staging laparotomy, she has an excellent prognosis without chemotherapy. It can be omitted for patients with stage IA/IB, grade 1 disease confirmed by staging laparotomy. We believe that staging laparotomy will provide information to improve the survival of patients with early ovarian cancer.

Keywords

Ovarian cancer · Staging laparotomy · Lymphadenectomy · Omentectomy

T. Tabata (✉)
Department of Obstetrics and Gynecology, Tokyo Women's Medical University, Shinjuku-Ku, Tokyo, Japan
e-mail: tabatat@clin.medic.mie-u.ac.jp

M. Mikami (ed.), *Surgery for Gynecologic Cancer*, Comprehensive Gynecology and Obstetrics, https://doi.org/10.1007/978-981-13-1519-0_21

21.1 History

The International Federation of Gynecology and Obstetrics (FIGO) was established in 1954. In 1964, the committee of FIGO officially adopted clinical staging for primary ovarian carcinoma [1, 2]. The last revision of the FIGO staging classification was made in 1988 [3]. The nomenclature of "staging laparotomy" was used in these days, because ovarian cancer was recommended to be staged surgically and pathologically. In January 2014, FIGO had revised the staging of ovarian cancer [4]. Table 21.1 shows the comparison between the old and new staging classifications of FIGO. The main purpose of the staging system is to provide standard terminology that allows comparisons of patients between centers. Furthermore, the patients and tumors are assigned to the resembling group, and specific treatment is examined. It is important to create the standardization of a staging system for ovarian cancer. Especially, with regard to early ovarian cancer, a standard of staging laparotomy is needed in the world.

In the new FIGO criteria, if there is any spillage of cystic material from an ovarian tumor, it shows stage IC1. If the ovarian tumor has surface involvement or capsular rupture before surgery, it shows stage IC2. The information concerning adhesion is important. In the new FIGO criteria, if tumors that may otherwise qualify for stage I are involved with dense adhesions and dissection results in tumor rupture, these cases justify upgrading to stage II. However, it is not clear whether upstaging based on dense adhesion is warranted. A recent study suggests that it is not [5]. Any adherences to the uterus, pelvic sidewall, or adjacent pelvic structures, such as the small or large bowel, should be recorded.

If the patient has retroperitoneal lymph node involvement, she is defined as stage IIIC in the old FIGO staging criteria. However, the new staging includes a revision of stage III patients and assignment to stage IIIA1 based on spread to the retroperitoneal lymph nodes without intraperitoneal dissemination. Stage IIIA1 is further subdivided into IIIA1 (i) and IIIA1 (ii) by lymph node diameter (10 mm), even though there is no retrospective data supporting quantification of the size of metastasis in stage IIIA1 disease. Some studies reported that the patients who have the retroperitoneal lymph nodes involvement without peritoneal dissemination have a better prognosis than that of tumors with abdominal peritoneal involvement [2, 6–10].

21.2 Principle and Indication

Suspicious early-stage ovarian cancer is indicated for staging laparotomy at initial surgery. A preoperative evaluation should exclude the presence of extra peritoneal metastases. If the patient has extra peritoneal disease, staging laparotomy may not be recommended. When the patients have extra abdominal metastasis, like lung metastasis, she may be initially treated with chemotherapy.

Table 21.1 Comparison between the old FIGO Stage and new One

Stage I: Tumor confined to ovaries			
The FIGO 1988 staging		The FIGO 2014 staging	
IA	Tumor limited to one ovary, negative carcinomatous ascites, no tumor on surface, capsule intact	IA	Tumor limited to one ovary, capsule intact, no tumor on surface, negative washings
IB	Tumor involves both ovaries, otherwise like IA	IB	Tumor involves both ovaries, otherwise like IA
IC	Tumor involves one or both ovaries	IC	Tumor limited to one or both ovaries
IC(a)	Spontaneous capsule rupture	IC1	Surgical spill
IC(b)	Capsule rupture during surgery	IC2	Capsule rupture before surgery or tumor on ovarian surface
IC(1)	Positive peritoneal washing cytology	IC3	Malignant cells in the ascites or peritoneal washings
IC(2)	Positive ascites cytology		
Stage II: Tumor involves one or both ovaries with pelvic extension (below the pelvic brim) or primary peritoneal cancer			
The FIGO 1988 staging		The FIGO 2014 staging	
IIA	Extension and/or implant on the uterus and/or fallopian tubes	IIA	Extension and/or implant on the uterus and/or fallopian tubes
IB	Extension to other pelvic intraperitoneal tissues	IIB	Extension to other pelvic intraperitoneal tissues
IIC	IIA or IIB with tumor on surface, capsule rupture, or positive washings/ascites cytology		
Stage III: Tumor involves one or both ovaries with cytologically or histologically confirmed spread to the peritoneum outside the pelvis and/or metastasis to the retroperitoneal lymph nodes			
The FIGO 1988 staging		The FIGO 2014 staging	
IIIA	Microscopic metastasis beyond the pelvis	IIIA	IIIA (positive retroperitoneal lymph nodes and/or microscopic metastasis beyond the pelvis)
		IIIA1	Positive retroperitoneal lymph nodes only
		IIIA1(i)	Metastasis ≤10 mm
		IIIA1(ii)	Metastasis >10 mm
		IIIA2	Microscopic, extrapelvic (above the brim) peritoneal involvement ± positive retroperitoneal lymph nodes
IIIB	Macroscopic, extrapelvic, peritoneal metastasis ≤2 cm in greatest dimension	IIIB	Macroscopic, extrapelvic, peritoneal metastasis ≤2 cm ± positive retroperitoneal lymph nodes. Includes extension to capsule of the liver/spleen
IIIC	Macroscopic, extrapelvic, peritoneal metastasis >2 cm in greatest dimension and/or regional lymph node metastasis	IIIC	Macroscopic, extrapelvic, peritoneal metastasis >2 cm ± positive retroperitoneal lymph nodes. Includes extension to capsule of the liver/spleen

(continued)

Table 21.1 (continued)

Stage IV: Distant metastasis excluding peritoneal metastasis			
The FIGO 1988 staging		The FIGO 2014 staging	
IVA	Distant metastasis excluding peritoneal metastasis. Includes hepatic parenchymal metastasis	IVA	Pleural effusion with positive cytology
		IVB	Hepatic and/or splenic parenchymal metastasis, metastasis to extra-abdominal organs (including inguinal lymph nodes and lymph nodes outside of the abdominal cavity)

If the patient was diagnosed with early-stage ovarian cancer at initial surgery without staging surgery, i.e., only salpingo-oophorectomy, restaging surgery is recommended. The accurate stage and whether or not the patient needs to receive adjuvant chemotherapy should be decided by staging laparotomy as soon as possible.

21.3 Preoperative Evaluation

When a woman is suspected to have ovarian cancer by transvaginal ultrasonography or tumor marker, magnetic resonance imaging (MRI) should be taken. MRI may presume the histologic type of ovarian cancer. Computed tomography (CT) with contrast enhancement may be helpful in identifying the lymph node involvement. However, imaging modality is not conclusive, and if the patient has suspicious ovarian malignancy, she should be evaluated by surgery. Histological diagnosis of ovarian tumor is needed.

Before surgery, extra abdominal metastasis should be excluded. A chest X-ray may be helpful to identify a pleural effusion, and cytology of the fluid will confirm of more advanced disease. A preoperative clinical situation may require investigation of the gastrointestinal tract. Ovarian metastasis should be eliminated preoperatively.

If patients desire future childbearing, fertility preservation should be discussed before surgery. See Chap. 28.

21.4 Technique

The standard staging laparotomy procedure for early ovarian cancer is as follows: peritoneal cytology of ascites/washings, multiple peritoneal surface biopsies, bilateral salpingo-oophorectomy, a total hysterectomy, pelvic and para-aortic lymphadenectomy, and omentectomy [11–13].

In general, the abdomen should be opened through a longitudinal midline incision extending from the symphysis pubis to the umbilicus. If ascites is present in the abdominal cavity, cytologic examination should be done. If ascites is absent, the peritoneal washings with saline should be obtained. Surgeons observe visually and palpate in the abdominal cavity and investigate whether there are seeding tumors. The peritoneal surface of the liver and the diaphragm should be examined by direct observation and palpation. The surface of small bowel mesentery from the ileocecal to the ligament of Treitz should be directly observed and palpated. Furthermore, the lymph node swelling should be palpated from the pelvic area to the para-aortic area. Particularly, it is important whether the capsule of ovarian tumor is intact or not. First, the ovarian tumor should be removed by salpingo-oophorectomy. If there is adhesion of ovarian tumor to adjacent organs, care should be taken not to rupture the tumor. The ovarian tumor should be pathologically examined by frozen section during surgery. The diagnosis of ovarian cancer rests with the pathological examination, and the error rate of frozen section ranges from 5% to 15%. If the frozen examination reveals malignancy of the tumor, staging laparotomy should be recommended to the patient.

Peritoneal biopsy specimens should be obtained from the following sites: the peritoneum covering the bladder, Douglas' pouch, the peritoneal surface of paracolic gutters, and the peritoneum beneath the right hemidiaphragm. If some suspicious lesions can be seen, biopsies should be taken as pathologic specimens. Even if there is no evidence of metastasis, such biopsies are needed for staging laparotomy, as the final pathologic examination may demonstrate a metastasis of malignant disease.

The retroperitoneal spaces should be developed to perform the pelvic lymphadenectomy. First, the round ligament is cut and the peritoneum is incised along with the external iliac vessels. The para-rectal and paravesical space should be widely opened (Figs. 21.1 and 21.2). After that, pelvic lymphadenectomy will be performed. The layer between the external iliac vessels and the psoas muscle is dissected. Separate the sheath of the external and internal iliac vein (Fig. 21.3). Extract some lymph nodes and fat tissue from external iliac artery (Fig. 21.4). The external and internal lymph nodes are then gathered to the caudal side. The obturator nodes are separated from the external iliac vessels and are cut with a sealing device. The pelvic lymph nodes are gathered on the obturator nerve from both the cranial side and caudal side (Fig. 21.5). These pelvic nodes are removed from the obturator nerve and are gathered on the umbilical vessel. Then these nodes are extracted from the umbilical vessel (Fig. 21.6).

A total hysterectomy is performed [13]. The bladder is separated from the vaginal wall with an electronic device. Next thin the anterior vesicouterine ligament as soon as possible. The infundibulopelvic ligament is cut and ligated. The ureter is separated from the broad ligament. The broad ligament is cut toward to the uterosacral ligament. Incise the peritoneum of Douglas' pouch. The uterosacral ligament is divided. The parametrium is clumped and divided. Enough of the vaginal wall should be removed (Fig. 21.7). The hysterectomy is often performed before pelvic lymphadenectomy.

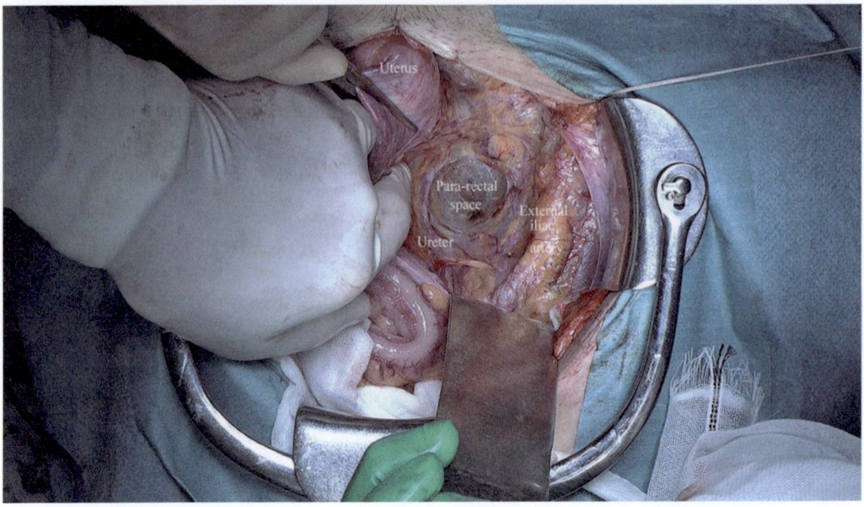

Fig. 21.1 Expansion of the para-rectal. After pulling the rectum to the opposite side from the external iliac artery can provide tension to the broad ligament, then it is possible to make a cavity between the ureter and the umbilical ligament

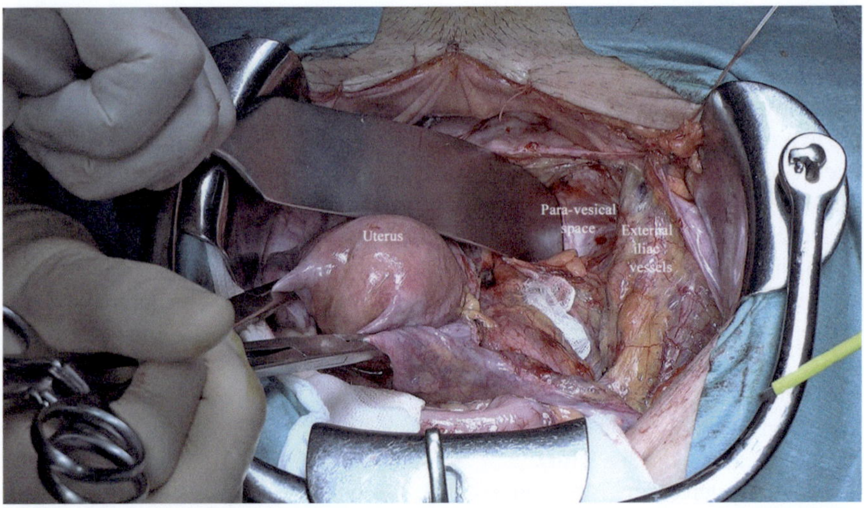

Fig. 21.2 Expansion of the paravesical space. The pelvic floor muscle can be seen. Gauze has been inserted in the para-rectal space in this photo

Ovarian cancer often has occult metastasis of para-aortic lymph nodes, and para-aortic lymphadenectomy is needed as part of staging laparotomy. An upper abdominal skin incision is added to perform a para-aortic lymphadenectomy. The para-aortic lymphadenectomy can be performed through three different approaches (Fig. 21.8). Types A and C approaches incise the peritoneum along with the paracolic gutter. In

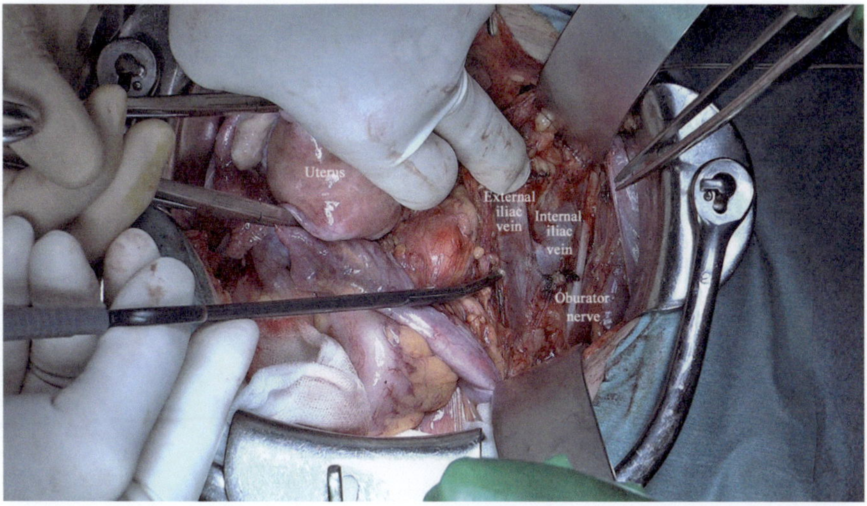

Fig. 21.3 Pelvic lymphadenectomy. Separate the sheath of the external and internal iliac vein. Bifurcation between the external iliac vein and the internal one should be cleaned. If it is possible, expose the internal iliac artery between the external iliac vein and the internal one

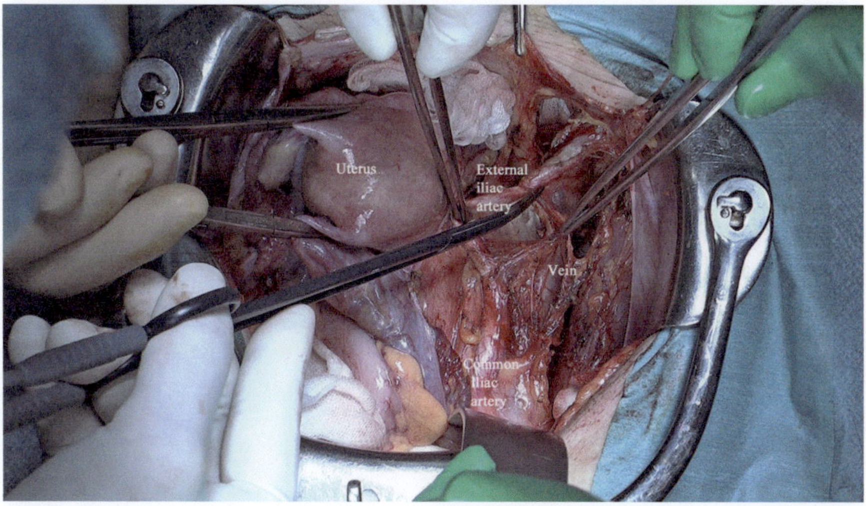

Fig. 21.4 Separate the sheath of the external iliac artery from the cranial side to the caudal side. Extract some lymph nodes and fat tissue from the external iliac artery. Lymphadenectomy means the extraction of the sheath of the vessels

type A incision, the ascending colon can be reflected over the vena cava. The most common approach is through the midline peritoneum, as line B in Fig. 21.8. An incision of the peritoneum from the cecum to the ligament of Treitz is needed. Through an incision of the peritoneum, the para-aortic lymph nodes along the aorta

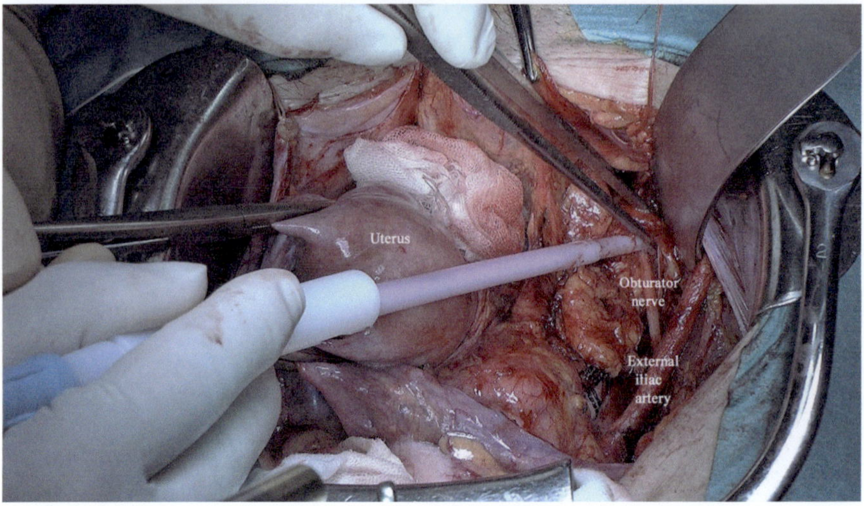

Fig. 21.5 The pelvic lymph nodes are gathered on the obturator nerve from both the cranial side and caudal side. These pelvic nodes are removed from the obturator nerve and are gathered on the umbilical vessel. Then these nodes are extracted from the umbilical vessel

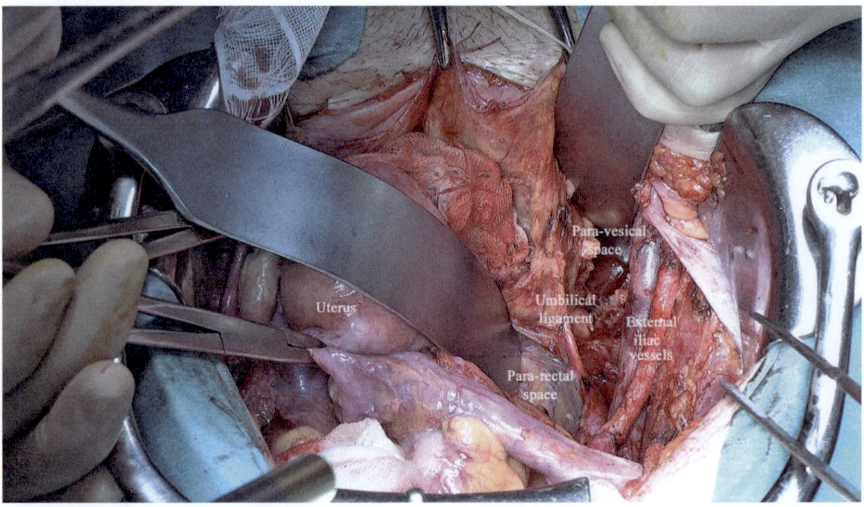

Fig. 21.6 The pelvic lymph nodes have been extracted as en bloc lymphadenectomy. Two retractors are placed into the paravesical and para-rectal space. The umbilical vessel is clearly seen

and inferior vena cava can be identified. Para-aortic lymphadenectomy should be dissected below the upper level of the renal vein (Fig. 21.9). At the same time, the common iliac lymph nodes are removed, because the appropriate surgical field can be seen.

There are three types of omentectomy: total omentectomy, subtotal omentectomy, and infracolic omentectomy. If there is no macroscopic metastasis of the

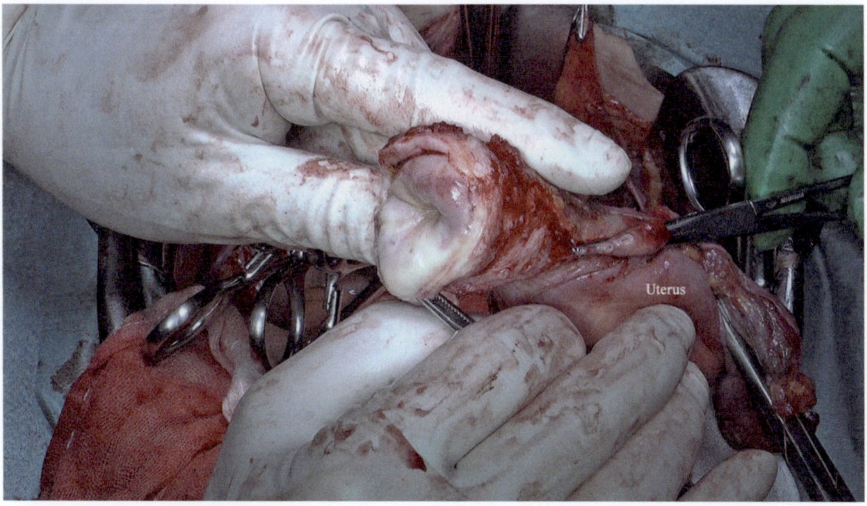

Fig. 21.7 The hysterectomy has been done. Enough vaginal cuff has been dissected

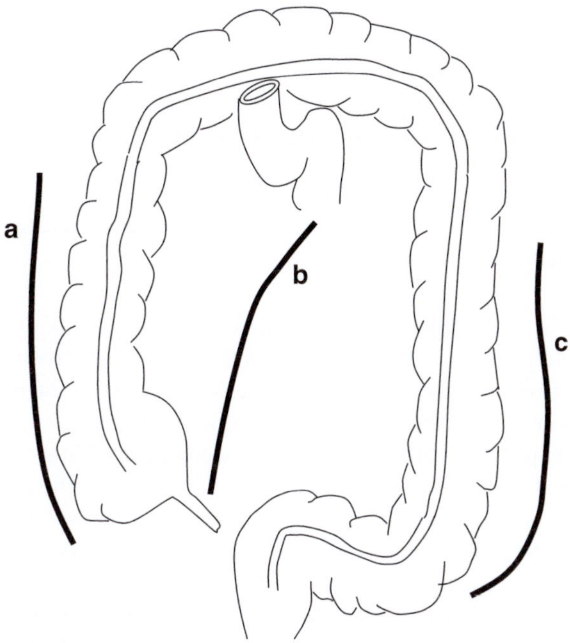

Fig. 21.8 The para-aortic lymphadenectomy can be performed through three different approaches. (**a**) Right paracolic gutter approach. (**b**) Midline approach. (**c**) Left paracolic gutter approach

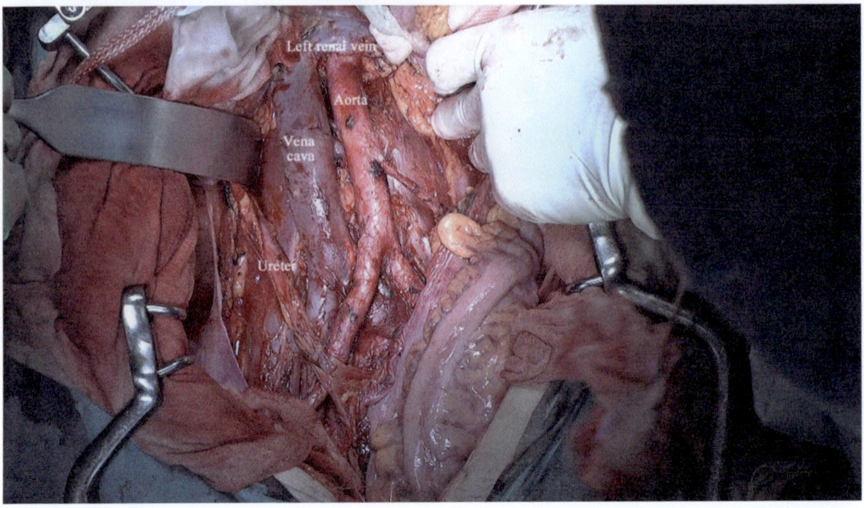

Fig. 21.9 The pelvic and para-aortic lymphadenectomy has been performed. After lymphadenectomy, we can see some running vessels clearly

omentum, an infracolic omentectomy is often performed to look for microscopic metastases that are otherwise not obvious.

Major intraoperative and postoperative complications included vessel injuries, lymphocyte, lymphedema, and pulmonary embolism [14–16]. Care should be taken for such complications.

21.5 Morbidity

Ovarian cancer is the leading cause of death among women with gynecologic cancer. Approximately 60% of patients initially present with stage III and IV disease. If the patient has been diagnosed as stage I disease by accurate staging laparotomy, more than 90% of stage I patients in Japan survive for 5 years.

The important pathologic findings have been demonstrated in the following sites: ascites, peritoneal washings, omentum, peritoneal surfaces of the paracolic gutters and diaphragm, and retroperitoneal lymph nodes. In the 1970s, some authors reported that almost half of patients with stage 1A ovarian cancer had positive cytology on peritoneal washings [17, 18]. Tumor rupture or surface involvement by tumor cells warrants a change in stage to stage IC. In multivariate analysis, capsular rupture before surgery and positive cytology means independent predictors of a worse prognosis [19, 20], but it is controversial whether rupture during surgery worsens prognosis in the absence of positive ascites or positive washings. Some authors reported that intraoperative tumor rupture portends a higher risk of disease recurrence [19, 20], whereas others did not [21–24]. However, rupture should be avoided during surgery of early ovarian cancer. If the patient has the metastasis on

Table 21.2 Lymph node metastasis in stage I/II ovarian cancer

Author	Year	Stage I	Stage II
Petru [34]	1994	9/40 (23%)	
Onda [6]	1996	7/33 (21%)	6/26 (23%)
Baiocchi [14]	1998	32/242 (13%)	
Kanazawa [7]	1999	5/44 (11%)	9/24 (38%)
Sakuragi [29]	2000	4/78 (5%)	5/16 (31%)
Suzuki [30]	2000	5/47 (11%)	
Cass [31]	2001	14/96 (15%)	
Takeshima [32]	2005	20/156 (13%)	18/37 (49%)
Desteli [33]	2010	2/33 (6%)	
Oshita [15]	2013	9/204 (4%)	14/80 (18%)
Mikami [35]	2014	11/89 (12%)	
Total		118/1062 (11%)	52/183 (28%)

Table 21.3 Lymph node metastasis in apparent stage I ovarian cancer

				Site of metastasis	
Author	Year	No. of Pts.	Positivity of LN	Pelvic	Para-aortic
Petru [34]	1994	40	9/40 (23%)	8 (20%)	2 (5%)
Onda [6]	1996	33	7/33 (21%)	6 (18%)	5 (15%)
Baiocchi [14]	1998	242	32/242 (13%)	NS[a]	NS[a]
Kanazawa [7]	1999	44	5/44 (11%)	3 (7%)	4 (9.1%)
Sakuragi [29]	2000	78	4/78 (5%)	0%	4 (5%)
Suzuki [30]	2000	47	5/47 (11%)	4 (9%)	2 (4%)
Cass [31]	2001	96	14/96 (15%)	9 (9%)	7 (7%)
Takeshima [32]	2005	156	20/156 (13%)	11 (7%)	15 (10%)
Desteli [33]	2010	33	2/33 (6%)	1 (3.0%)	1 (3.0%)
Oshita [15]	2013	204	9/204 (4%)	NS	NS
Mikami [35]	2014	89	11/89 (12%)	9 (10%)	6 (7%)
Total		1062	118/1062 (11%)	51/616 (8%)	46/616 (7%)

[a]NS: Data is not shown

the omentum, the staging reveals more than stage III disease. The incidence of omental metastasis is about 5%–12% [25–27].

The incidence of lymph node involvement is approximately 11% for stage I and 28% for stage II [6, 7, 14, 15, 28–35] (Table 21.2). Accumulated reports of lymph node metastasis in apparent stage I ovarian cancer patients are shown in Table 21.3. In these articles, the incidence of pelvic and para-aortic lymph node involvement is the same at about 8%. Furthermore, positive aortic nodes were also found in the situation of negative pelvic nodes. Systemic lymphadenectomy including both the pelvic and para-aortic area is needed.

The majority of malignant ovarian tumors are epithelial. Epithelial ovarian cancers are histologically divided into five main types: high-grade and low-grade serous, mucinous, endometrioid, and clear cell types. These tumor types have different characteristics: patterns of spread, response to chemotherapy, and prognosis. Low-grade serous carcinoma of the ovary usually contains a serous borderline component and has a good prognosis, but it will not respond to chemotherapy. Furthermore, in patients with apparent stage I epithelial ovarian cancer, the incidence of lymph node metastasis is about 10%–25% for high-grade serous type and less than 10% for endometrioid. Especially, the incidence of lymph node metastasis in low-grade serous and mucinous ovarian cancer is less than 2% [30, 32, 35, 36]. Some authors reported that the patients with mucinous ovarian cancer may be able to omit systemic lymphadenectomy [36, 37]. However, when the patient is diagnosed as mucinous carcinoma, metastatic ovarian disease from the gastrointestinal tract should be ruled out. Stage I high-grade serous ovarian cancer had the highest incidence of node metastasis (25%) [14, 30, 32]. In cases of serous tumor, the para-aortic region, particularly above the inferior mesenteric artery, is the prime site for the earliest lymph node metastasis [30, 32]. Ovarian cancers differ primarily based on histologic types.

Histologic grade is an important independent prognostic factor in patients with epithelial ovarian cancer [19]. When the tumor is limited to an ovary and the patient is diagnosed as stage I, if the histological diagnosis is grade 2 or 3, the patient will need to be treated with chemotherapy. Grade 3 tumors are more commonly seen in lymph node-positive patients [31]. In the patients with early-stage ovarian cancer who underwent comprehensive surgical staging, 16% of the patients with grade 1 lesions were upstaged, compared with 34% with grade 2 disease and 46% with grade 3 disease [27].

If the patient is diagnosed as stage IA or IB, grade 1 ovarian cancer by surgical staging, she has an excellent prognosis without chemotherapy [38–41]. Both the NCCN guideline and the Japan Society of Gynecologic Oncology guideline recommend omitting adjuvant chemotherapy for patients with stage IA/IB, grade 1 disease confirmed by staging laparotomy [42, 43]. If the surgical staging were not to be performed, occult metastasis may be present, and its stage may be recognized as less than its actual stage. As a result, the chemotherapy which should be performed as adjuvant treatment may not be carried out. Inadequate subsequent therapy may lead to an unfortunate prognosis.

There were two randomized comparative studies, EORTC-ACTION study [45, 48] and ICON 1 [46] study, conducted to evaluate the efficacy of adjuvant chemotherapy for patients with early-stage (stages I and II) ovarian cancer. In both trials, the prognosis of the patients was better in the adjuvant chemotherapy group than the observation group. Especially, in non-optimally staged patients in the EORTC-ACTION study, adjuvant chemotherapy was associated with statistically significant improvements overall and recurrence-free survival. However, the patients who underwent accurate staging did not have a benefit of adjuvant chemotherapy [44]. Furthermore, when the patients who had not performed retroperitoneal lymphadenectomy or blind biopsies did not have adjuvant chemotherapy, they had poor prognoses [47]. These results support that patients who need to have adjuvant chemotherapy should be detected by comprehensive staging laparotomy. Furthermore, Cochrane Review suggested that women with high-risk disease (stage IA/B and grade 3, stage IC) had benefited from adjuvant chemotherapy, but subgroup analyses could neither confirm nor exclude survival benefits in lower-risk disease (stage IA/IB, grade 1 or 2) or in optimally staged disease. It remains uncertain whether women with lower-risk early-stage ovarian cancer for whom performed optimally staged surgery will benefit as much from adjuvant chemotherapy as women with high-risk disease. Treatment of women with lower-risk disease should be individualized to take into account individual factors [48].

Restaging laparotomy in patients whose initial surgery was inadequate showed 16–30% incidence of upward staging reported by some authors [41, 49]. Although restaging laparotomy provides important prognostic information with minimal morbidity, they may provide little benefit to those patients already receiving chemotherapy based on the initial operative findings.

Survival is affected by the cancer stage, grade of differentiation, gross findings at surgery, and additional treatment. If staging laparotomy is performed in patients with early ovarian cancer, approximately 30% of them will be subject to upstaging, from stage I to stage II/III or from stage II to stage III. Careful surgical staging is needed in the management of stage I ovarian cancer, and accurate staging offers correct adjuvant treatment.

21.6 Future Prospect

Recently, some authors have reported about staging laparoscopy for the management of early-stage ovarian cancer. They reported that staging laparoscopy was safe and resulted in less blood loss [50–52]. However, tumor rupture during surgery is one of the most serious problems of laparoscopy. Surgeons should take care not to rupture the ovarian tumor. Regardless of whether the tumor fluid has malignant cells, if the ovarian tumor is ruptured and a spillage of tumor fluid shows, then the FIGO clinical stage will be upgraded. Surgery is necessary to remove the ovarian tumor perfectly without rupture. In the future, if staging laparoscopy can resolve the problem of rupture, staging laparoscopy in early ovarian cancer may be recommended.

It appears reasonable not to recommend adjuvant chemotherapy for patients with stage IA/IB and grade 1 lesions who have been comprehensively staged [38–43]. Patients with stage IA/IB and grade 2/3, and IC (capsule rupture during surgery) disease, who have been comprehensively staged, present a more difficult problem for receiving adjuvant chemotherapy. The Japan Gynecologic Oncology Group (JGOG) has been promoting, since 2012, the enrollment for the JGOG 3020 clinical trial: a randomized phase III clinical trial in patients with surgical stage I epithelial ovarian cancer will investigate the efficacy of adjuvant chemotherapy (Fig. 21.10). Eligible patients are determined by comprehensive staging surgery, and histological diagnoses are stage IA/IB and grade 2/3 and IC (capsule rupture during surgery). The estimated primary completion date of this study is June 2024. If the patients are diagnosed as low risk, stage IA/IB and grade 2/3, or IC (capsule rupture during surgery), such patients will be able to omit unnecessary adjuvant chemotherapy. The result of this clinical trial is expected to improve patient's QOL.

Because early ovarian cancer has the greatest opportunity for cure, optimal treatment must be taken. Therefore, patients with suspicious early ovarian cancer should have a staging laparotomy and be treated with appropriate therapy. Accurate staging is important for treatment planning and for providing an accurate prognosis.

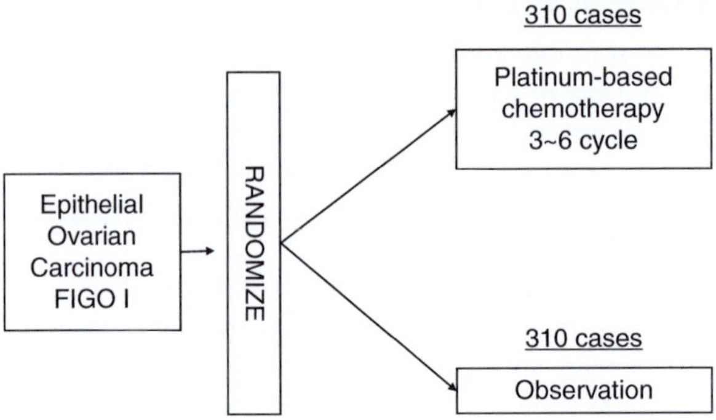

Fig. 21.10 The purpose of JGOG 3020 is to evaluate the need for platinum-based chemotherapy as adjuvant chemotherapy through comparison using overall survival for subjects diagnosed with FIGO stage I epithelial ovarian cancer after comprehensive staging surgery

References

1. Jones HW Jr. Recent advances in gynecologic cancer. J Int Fed Gynaecol Obstet. 1965;13:208.
2. Cliby WA, Aletti GD, Wilson TO, Podratz KC. Is it justified to classify patients to Stage IIIC epithelial ovarian cancer based on nodal involvement only? Gynecol Oncol. 2006;103:797–801.
3. FIGO Committee. Changes in definitions of clinical staging for carcinoma of the cervix and ovary: International Federation of Gynecology and Obstetrics. Am J Obstet Gynecol. 1987;156:263–4.
4. Prat J, FIGO Committee on Gynecologic Oncology. Staging classification for cancer of the ovary, fallopian tube, and peritoneum. Int J Gynecol Obstet. 2014;124:1–5.
5. Seidman JD, Cosin JA, Wang BG, Alsop S, Yemelyanova A, Fields A, et al. Upstaging pathologic stage I ovarian carcinoma based on dense adhesions is not warranted: a clinicopathologic study of 84 patients originally classified as FIGO stage II. Gynecol Oncol. 2010;119:250–4.
6. Onda T, Yoshikawa H, Yokota H, Yasugi T, Taketani Y. Assessment of metastases to aortic and pelvic lymph nodes in epithelial ovarian carcinoma. A proposal for essential sites for lymph node biopsy. Cancer. 1996;78:803–8.
7. Kanazawa K, Suzuki T, Tokashiki M. The validity and significance of substage IIIC by node involvement in epithelial ovarian cancer: impact of nodal metastasis on patient survival. Gynecol Oncol. 1999;73:237–41.
8. Panici PB, Maggioni A, Hacker N, Landoni F, Ackermann S, Campagnutta E, et al. Systematic aortic and pelvic lymphadenectomy versus resection of bulky nodes only in optimally debulked advanced ovarian cancer: a randomized clinical trial. J Natl Cancer Inst. 2005;97:560–6.
9. Ferrandina G, Scambia G, Legge F, Petrillo M, Salutari V. Ovarian cancer patients with "node-positive-only" Stage IIIC disease have a more favorable outcome than Stage IIIA/B. Gynecol Oncol. 2007;107:154–6.
10. Baek SJ, Park JY, Kim DY, Kim JH, Kim YM, Kim YT, et al. Stage IIIC epithelial ovarian cancer classified solely by lymph node metastasis has a more favorable prognosis than other types of stage IIIC epithelial ovarian cancer. J Gynecol Oncol. 2008;19:223–8.
11. Tabata T. Staging Laparotomy for endometrial and ovarian cancer. Osaka, Japan: Medica Corporation; 2014. p. 1–250.
12. Tabata T. Radical hysterectomy. Osaka, Japan: Medica Corporation; 2017. p. 1–214.
13. Tabata T. Total abdominal hysterectomy. Osaka, Japan: Medica Corporation; 2015. p. 1–101.

14. Baiocchi G, Raspagliesi F, Grosso G, Fontanelli R, Cobellis L, di Re E, di Re F. Early ovarian cancer: Is there a role for systematic pelvic and para-aortic lymphadenectomy? Int J Gynecol Cancer. 1998;8:103–8.
15. Oshita T, Itamochi H, Nishimura R, Numa F, Takehara K, Hiura M, et al. Clinical impact of systematic pelvic and para-aortic lymphadenectomy for pT1 and pT2 ovarian cancer: a retrospective survey by the Sankai Gynecology Study Group. Int J Clin Oncol. 2013;18:1107–13.
16. Bourne TH, Campbell S, Reynolds K, Hampson J, Bhatt L, Crayford TJ, et al. The potential role of serum CA 125 in an ultrasound-based screening program for familial ovarian cancer. Gynecol Oncol. 1994;52:379–85.
17. Keettel WC, Pixley EE, Buchsbaum HJ. Experience with peritoneal cytology in the management of gynecologic malignancies. Am J Obstet Gynecol. 1974;120:174–82.
18. Creasman WT, Rutledge F. The prognostic value of peritoneal cytology in gynecologic malignant disease. Am J Obstet Gynecol. 1971;110:773–81.
19. Vergote I, De Brabanter J, Fyles A, Bertelsen K, Einhorn N, Sevelda P, et al. Prognostic importance of degree of differentiation and cyst rupture in stage I invasive epithelial ovarian carcinoma. Lancet. 2001;357:176–82.
20. Bakkum-Gamez JN, Richardson DL, Seamon LG, Aletti GD, Powless CA, Keeney GL, et al. Influence of intraoperative capsule rupture on outcomes in stage I epithelial ovarian cancer. Obstet Gynecol. 2009;113:11–7.
21. Seidman JD, Yemelyanova AV, Khedmati F, Bidus MA, Dainty L, Boice CR, et al. Prognostic factors for stage I ovarian carcinoma. Int J Gynecol Pathol. 2010;29:1–7.
22. Chan JK, Tian C, Monk BJ, Herzog T, Kapp DS, Bell J, et al. Prognostic factors for high-risk early-stage epithelial ovarian cancer: a Gynecologic Oncology Group study. Cancer. 2008;112:2202–10.
23. Ahmed FY, Wiltshaw E, A'Hern RP, Nicol B, Shepherd J, Blake P, et al. Natural history and prognosis of untreated stage I epithelial ovarian carcinoma. J Clin Oncol. 1996;14:2968–75.
24. Obermair A, Fuller A, Lopez-Varela E, van Gorp T, Vergote I, Eaton L, et al. A new prognostic model for FIGO stage 1 epithelial ovarian cancer. Gynecol Oncol. 2007;104:607–11.
25. Knapp RC, Friedman EA. Aortic lymph node metastases in early ovarian cancer. Am J Obstet Gynecol. 1974;119:1013–7.
26. Berek JS, Hacker NF. Staging and second-look operations in ovarian cancer. In: Alberts DS, Surwit EA, editors. Ovarian cancer. Boston, MA: Martinus Nihoff; 1985. p. 109–27.
27. Young RC, Decker DG, Wharton JT, Piver S, Lindelar WF, Edwards BK, et al. Staging laparotomy in early ovarian cancer. JAMA. 1983;250:3071–6.
28. Lago V, Minig L, Fotopoulou C. Incidence of lymph node metastases in apparent early-stage low-grade epithelial ovarian cancer: a comprehensive review. Int J Gynecol Cancer. 2016;26:1407–14.
29. Sakuragi N, Yamada H, Oikawa M, Okuyama K, Fujino T, Sagawa T, Fujimoto S. Prognostic significance of lymph node metastasis and clear cell histology in ovarian carcinoma limited to the pelvis (pT1M0 and pT2M0). Gynecol Oncol. 2000;7:251–5.
30. Suzuki M, Ohwada M, Yamada T, Kohno T, Sekiguchi I, Sato I. Lymph node metastasis in stage I epithelial ovarian cancer. Gynecol Oncol. 2000;79:305–8.
31. Cass I, Li AJ, Runowicz CD, Fields AL, Goldberg GL, Leuchter RS, Lagasse LD, Karlan BY. Pattern of lymph node metastases in clinically unilateral stage I invasive epithelial ovarian carcinomas. Gynecol Oncol. 2001;80:56–61.
32. Takeshima N, Hirai Y, Umayahara K, Fujiwara K, Takizawa K, Hasumi K. Lymph node metastasis in ovarian cancer: difference between serous and non-serous primary tumors. Gynecol Oncol. 2005;99:427–31.
33. Desteli GA, Gultekin M, Usubutun A, Yuce K, Ayhan A. Lymph node metastasis in grossly apparent clinical stage Ia epithelial ovarian cancer: Hacettepe experience and review of literature. World J Surg Oncol. 2010;30:106–12.
34. Petru E, Lahousen M, Tamussino K, Pickel H, Stranzl H, Stettner H, et al. Lymphadenectomy in stage I ovarian cancer. Am J Obstet Gynecol. 1994;170:656–62.

35. Mikami M. Role of lymphadenectomy for ovarian cancer. J Gynecol Oncol. 2014;25:279–81.
36. Minig L, Heitz F, Cibula D, Bakkum-Gamez JN, Germanova A, Dowdy SC, et al. Patterns of Lymph Node Metastases in Apparent Stage I Low-Grade Epithelial Ovarian Cancer: A Multicenter Study. Ann Surg Oncol. 2017;24:2720–6.
37. Nasioudis D, Chapman-Davis E, Witkin SS, Holcomb K. Prognostic significance of lymphadenectomy and prevalence of lymph node metastasis in clinically-apparent stage I endometrioid and mucinous ovarian carcinoma. Gynecol Oncol. 2017;144:414–9.
38. Elit L, Chambers A, Fyles A, Covens A, Carey M, Fung MF. Systematic review of adjuvant care for women with Stage I ovarian carcinoma. Cancer. 2004;101:1926–35.
39. Trimbos JB, Schueler JA, van der Burg M, Hermans J, van Lent M, Heintz AP, et al. Watch and wait after careful surgical treatment and staging in well-differentiated early ovarian cancer. Cancer. 1991;67:597–602.
40. Monga M, Carmichael JA, Shelley WE, Kirk ME, Krepart GV, Jeffrey JF, et al. Surgery without adjuvant chemotherapy for early epithelial ovarian carcinoma after comprehensive surgical staging. Gynecol Oncol. 1991;43:195–7.
41. Young RC, Walton LA, Ellenberg SS, Homesley HD, Wilbanks GD, Decker DG, et al. Adjuvant therapy in stage I and stage II epithelial ovarian cancer. Results of two prospective randomized trials. N Engl J Med. 1990;322:1021–7.
42. Komiyama S, Katabuchi H, Mikami M, Nagase S, Okamoto A, Ito K, et al. Japan Society of Gynecologic Oncology guidelines 2015 for the treatment of ovarian cancer including primary peritoneal cancer and fallopian tube cancer. Int J Clin Oncol. 2016;21:435–46.
43. Ovarian cancer guideline (Ver 2. 2017). NCCN Clinical Practice Guidelines in Oncology. https://www.nccn.org/professionals/physician_gls/pdf/ovarian.pdf.
44. Trimbos JB, Vergote I, Bolis G, Vermorken JB, Mangioni C, Madronal C, et al. Impact of adjuvant chemotherapy and surgical staging in early-stage ovarian carcinoma: European Organisation for Research and Treatment of Cancer-Adjuvant ChemoTherapy in Ovarian Neoplasm trial. J Natl Cancer Inst. 2003;95:113–25.
45. Trimbos JB, Parmar M, Vergote I, Guthrie D, Bolis G, Colombo N, et al. International Collaborative Ovarian Neoplasm trial 1 and Adjuvant ChemoTherapy in Ovarian Neoplasm trial: two parallel randomized phase III trials of adjuvant chemotherapy in patients with early-stage ovarian carcinoma. J Natl Cancer Inst. 2003;95:105–12.
46. Colombo N, Guthrie D, Chiari S, Parmar M, Qian W, Swart AM, et al. International Collaborative Ovarian Neoplasm trial 1: a randomized trial of adjuvant chemotherapy in women with early-stage ovarian cancer. J Natl Cancer Inst. 2003;95:125–32.
47. Timmers PJ, Zwinderman K, Coens C, Vergote I, Trimbos JB. Lymph node sampling and taking of blind biopsies are important elements of the surgical staging of early ovarian cancer. Int J Gynecol Cancer. 2010;20:1142–7.
48. Lawrie TA, Winter-Roach BA, Heus P, Kitchener HC. Adjuvant (post-surgery) chemotherapy for early stage epithelial ovarian cancer. Cochrane Database Syst Rev. 2015;(17, 12):CD004706.
49. Stier EA, Barakat RR, Curtin JP, Brown CL, Jones WB, Hoskins WJ. Laparotomy to complete staging of presumed early ovarian cancer. Obstet Gynecol. 1996;87:737–40.
50. Park HJ, Kim DW, Yim GW, Nam EJ, Kim S, Kim YT. Staging laparoscopy for the management of early-stage ovarian cancer: a metaanalysis. Am J Obstet Gynecol. 2013;209:58.e1–8.
51. Chi DS, Abu-Rustum NR, Sonoda Y, Ivy J, Rhee E, Moore K, et al. The safety and efficacy of laparoscopic surgical staging of apparent stage I ovarian and fallopian tube cancers. Am J Obstet Gynecol. 2005;192:1614–9.
52. Koo YJ, Kim JE, Kim YH, Hahn HS, Lee IH, Kim TJ, et al. Comparison of laparoscopy and laparotomy for the management of early-stage ovarian cancer: surgical and oncological outcomes. J Gynecol Oncol. 2014;25:111–7.

Primary Debulking Surgery (Advanced)

22

Hirokuni Takano

Abstract

When performing PDS, it is desirable to achieve complete surgery. Accordingly, cases in which complete tumor resection is considered possible are selected. However, it is extremely difficult to accurately determine preoperatively whether complete resection is possible in advanced cases. As combined resection of organs other than the internal genitalia is often required to achieve complete excision for cases of advanced ovarian cancer, this means that large-scale surgical intervention is necessary. When performing such procedures, it is vital to avoid having to prematurely stop the resection despite it being incomplete. Therefore, it is optimal to be able to accurately determine whether complete resection can be performed on the basis of preoperative tests or minimally invasive procedures. The details of surgery depend on the comprehensive ability of that specific hospital. It is vital that each facility investigates what surgical procedure can be performed safely and without causing any disadvantage to the patient beforehand.

Keywords

Advanced ovarian cancer · Primary debulking surgery · Complete surgery

22.1 History

Surgical treatment for advanced ovarian cancer fundamentally involves primary debulking surgery (PDS), which aims to remove any peritoneal dissemination and metastatic lesions to the maximum extent possible. The residual tumor diameter

H. Takano (✉)
Department of Obstetrics and Gynecology, The Jikei University Kashiwa Hospital, Kashiwa, Chiba, Japan
e-mail: hirokuni@jikei.ac.jp

M. Mikami (ed.), *Surgery for Gynecologic Cancer*, Comprehensive Gynecology and Obstetrics, https://doi.org/10.1007/978-981-13-1519-0_22

correlates with prognosis. Therefore, optimal surgery is defined as PDS resulting in a maximum residual tumor diameter of <1 cm. When the maximum residual tumor diameter is ≥1 cm, it is often termed as suboptimal surgery. Performing optimal surgery improves prognosis [1–3]. If the tumor has been removed to the extent that it is no longer macroscopically visible, this is referred to as complete surgery. It has been shown that complete surgery improves prognosis significantly more than optimal surgery, in which the maximum residual tumor diameter is <1 cm [4–7]. However, in cases of advanced ovarian cancer, it is difficult to achieve complete surgery with basic procedures such as bilateral adnexectomy, hysterectomy, and omentectomy. When it is considered difficult to aim for complete surgery with PDS, another option is performing neoadjuvant chemotherapy (NAC) and then interval debulking surgery (IDS). This is referred to as NAC-IDS. In cases of advanced ovarian cancer, it has been reported that outcomes for NAC-IDS are not inferior to those achieved by performing chemotherapy after PDS (EORTC/NCICOV13 Trial [8], CHORUS Trial [9]). However, because these trials reported low-complete and optimal surgery rates and short operation times as problems, reinvestigation at a facility with a high-optimal surgery rate is required. Accordingly, the results of the ongoing TRUST (Trial on Radical Upfront Surgery in Advanced Ovarian Cancer) and SUNNY (Study of Upfront Surgery Versus Neoadjuvant Chemotherapy in Patients with Advanced Ovarian Cancer) studies are highly anticipated. In either case, it is evident that complete surgery should be the aim as far as possible when performing PDS.

22.2 Indication and Preoperative Evaluation

When performing PDS, it is desirable to achieve complete surgery. Accordingly, cases in which complete tumor resection is considered possible are selected. However, it is extremely difficult to accurately determine preoperatively whether complete resection is possible in advanced cases. It can at least be determined that complete resection is impossible according to preoperative diagnostic imaging for cases of metastasis into the mediastinal space, multiple metastases in the lungs or lung parenchyma, metastasis to large areas of lung parenchyma requiring segmentectomy, metastasis occupying the hepatic portal region, metastasis requiring resection of the pancreatic head or duodenum, and metastasis in which the course of large vessels such as the inferior vena cava is greatly altered. When the greater omentum has become lumped with the gastrointestinal tract over an extensive area and when metastasis of the tumor is noted extensively over the mesentery or gastrointestinal tract surface, complete resection is difficult. Furthermore, it is difficult to accurately diagnose such states before operating on the area. Although a method of determining whether complete resection is possible using laparoscopy has recently been reported, the surgeon usually makes the final judgment on whether resection is possible according to findings on palpation. In the future, new methods of preoperative diagnosis are expected.

22.3 Technique

The criteria for complete resection are different at each facility. When operating on cases of advanced ovarian cancer, apart from the need for a large number of gynecologist with a high level of expertise, coordination with other departments such as hepatobiliary-pancreatic surgery, gastrointestinal surgery, vascular surgery, urology, etc. is required. In addition, the cooperation of operating theater staff and anesthesiologists is required, and the cooperation of internal medicine specialists is indispensable in cases with serious internal complications. Therefore, the details of surgery depend on the comprehensive ability of that specific hospital. It is vital that each facility investigates what surgical procedure can be performed safely without causing any disadvantage to the patient beforehand.

22.3.1 If a Tumor Obstructs Douglas' Pouch

As ovarian tumors increase in size, they may invade the uterus and the neighboring sigmoid colon and rectum (Fig. 22.1). One common clinical situation is the complete obstruction of the pouch of Douglas by the tumor. In such cases, combined resection of the gastrointestinal tract and internal genitalia is performed. After separating the bladder following the necessary procedures on the round ligament and ovarian blood vessels, the rectum is separated from the anterior aspect of the sacrum, and the internal genitalia and intestinal tract are elevated together. After operating on the parametrium, the vaginal canal is resected, and the intestinal tract is resected at the necessary site to allow the combined resection of the internal genitalia and intestinal tract.

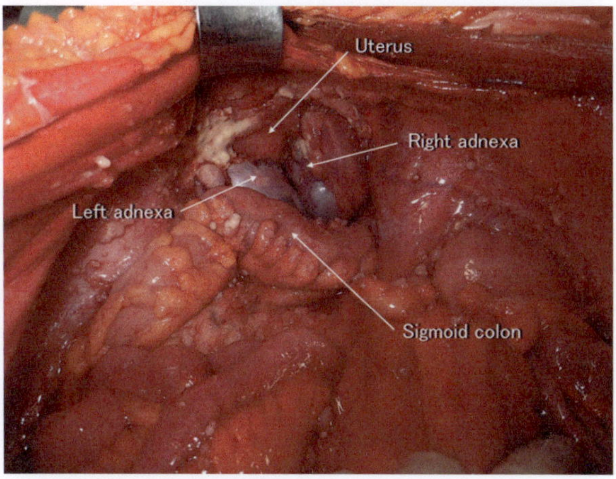

Fig. 22.1 Pelvic cavity obstructed by the tumors

22.3.2 If a Tumor Is Present in the Bladder Peritoneum

Cases in which the tumor develops in the bladder peritoneum are also common. In such cases, the retropubic space is first exposed, after which the bladder is filled with physiological saline solution to make the bladder walls taut. Then, the bladder is separated with the bladder peritoneum. If the dissection between the bladder and the bladder peritoneum reaches the uterine cervix, the bladder can be preserved without any damage in many cases.

22.3.3 If the Tumor Is Joined to the Inside of the Lesser Pelvis

Sometimes, the internal genitalia cannot be visualized at all, and the lesser pelvis actually appears to be a large tumorous mass. In such cases, surgery involving combined resection of the internal genitalia and the necessary segment of intestinal tract is planned, and a retroperitoneal approach is taken. First, the retropubic space is exposed from the posterior surface of the pubic bone, and the separation range of the retroperitoneal cavity is extended laterally, identifying the round ligament (Fig. 22.2), which is resected at its origin. The proximal side retroperitoneum is then exposed, and the ureter is separated out (Fig. 22.3). Although the ureter has often buried in the tumor, making its course difficult to identify, it can usually be identified by dissecting the retroperitoneum past the lesser pelvis until the para-aortic region. After separating out the ureter, the ovarian blood vessels are identified and resected. Next, the paravesical and pararectal spaces are exposed. If necessary, the vessels in the cardinal ligament of the uterus may also be resected after the uterine artery to avoid any unnecessary blood loss. When bladder position cannot be confirmed, the bladder is filled with physiological saline solution, as described above, to make the bladder wall taut. This makes it easier to confirm bladder position and

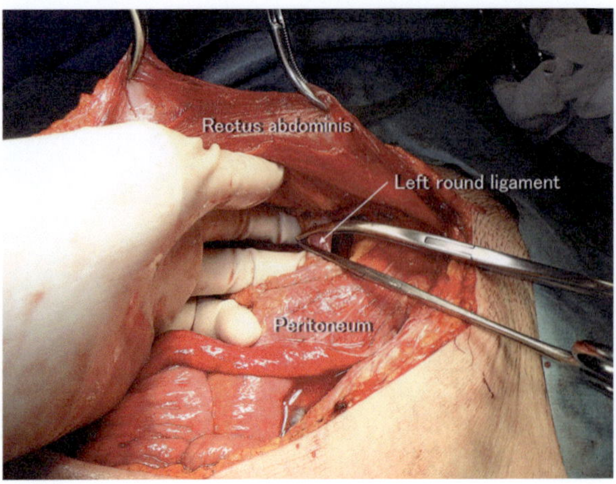

Fig. 22.2 Round ligament identified by retroperitoneal approach

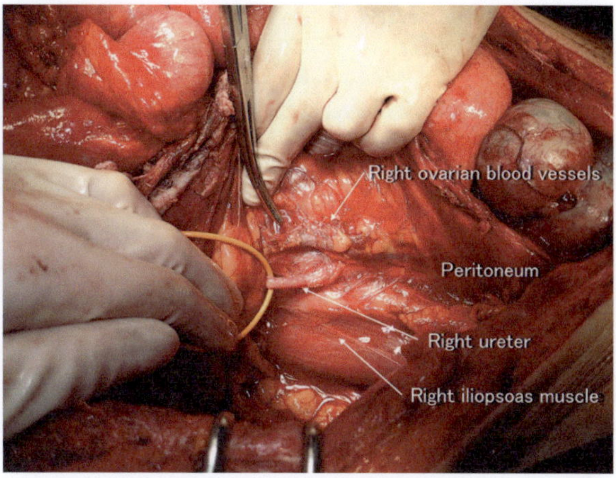

Fig. 22.3 Ureter detached by retroperitoneal approach

allows for the separation of the bladder from the uterine cervix. Next, the retroperitoneum is exposed, the rectum is separated from the anterior aspect of the sacral bone, and the rectum and internal genitalia are elevated together from the lesser pelvis. After this, the vaginal canal is resected. If palpation indicates that the vaginal fornices are not easily identifiable, a soft spatula of approximately 2-cm width is inserted from the vagina to make it easier to confirm the fornix portion. After resecting the vaginal canal, when the tumor is judged to be completely resectable, the intestinal canal is resected on the proximal and distal sides, and the tumor is extracted in one piece.

22.3.4 Diaphragmatic Lesions

The treatment of diaphragmatic lesions needs to be altered depending on their depth. Diaphragmatic stripping is performed if the lesion is confined to the diaphragmatic surface, whereas whole-thickness resection of the diaphragm is performed if the lesion is deep. For whole-thickness resection, the defect area is supplemented with Gore-Tex or a similar product. In either case, as securing clear visualization of the operative field is the most important concern, a Kent retractor or similar instrument is used to elevate the thorax so that the falciform ligament of the liver can be resected (Fig. 22.4). Once the hepatic ligaments are resected and the liver is mobilized, the left and right diaphragmatic regions can be confirmed. On the right side in particular, as metastatic tumors are often located at a deep site on the posterior surface of the liver, the visual field needs to be sufficiently secured (Figs. 22.5 and 22.6). The space between the diaphragm and the liver is sometimes partially blocked by the tumor. In such cases, if the lesion is evaluated as being on the superior surface of the liver on detailed imaging evaluations, an energy device is used for hemostasis, while the diaphragm is separated from the hepatic surface and diaphragmatic stripping is continued.

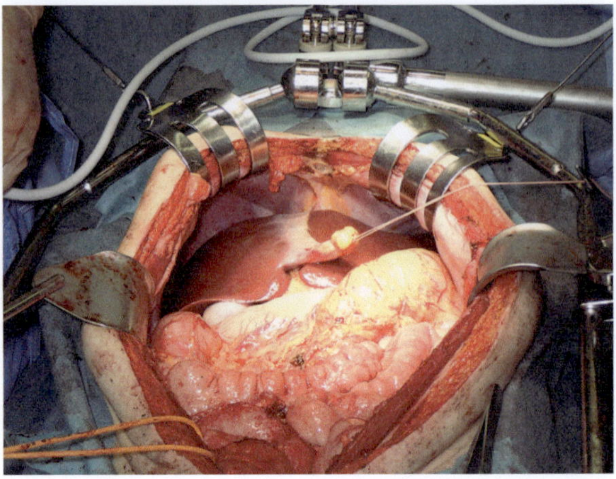

Fig. 22.4 Thorax elevated by a Kent retractor

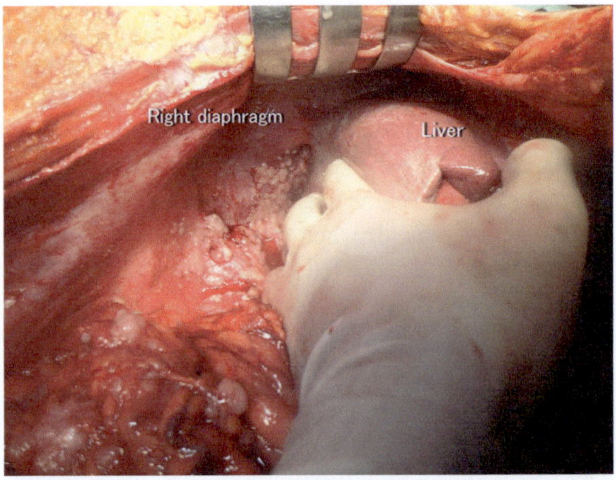

Fig. 22.5 Metastatic tumors located at a deep site on the posterior surface of the liver

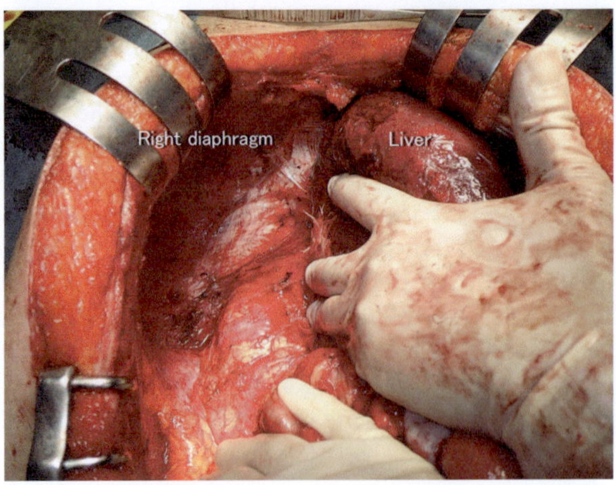

Fig. 22.6 Completely stripped diaphragm

Regardless of whether stripping or whole-thickness resection is performed, care must be taken regarding the course of the phrenic arteries and veins, which run through the diaphragm.

22.3.5 Peritoneum Lesions

When a peritoneal lesion is noted, the entire area with visible lesions is resected as a rule. Although depending on the degree of metastasis, the peritoneum might show marked hypertrophy; it is extremely rare for lesions to infiltrate up to the muscular layer of the abdominal wall, and resection is possible in most cases (Fig. 22.7). However, when resecting the peritoneum near the kidneys, care should be taken not to damage the adrenal glands. Although it is difficult to distinguish the adrenal glands by palpation, care should be taken not to manipulate them unnecessarily because they are extremely prone to bleeding. As manipulation of the adrenal glands can also cause sudden fluctuations in blood pressure, it is important to inform the anesthesiologist of this in advance when operating on this area.

22.3.6 Pancreatic Head and Duodenal Lesions

When a lesion is present in the pancreatic head or duodenum, complete resection is often impossible unless resection of the pancreatic head and duodenum is performed. Tumor resection is not to be performed for such cases because this is considered as excessive surgical invasion. Accordingly, preoperative diagnostic imaging needs to be carefully evaluated to confirm that there are no lesions in this area.

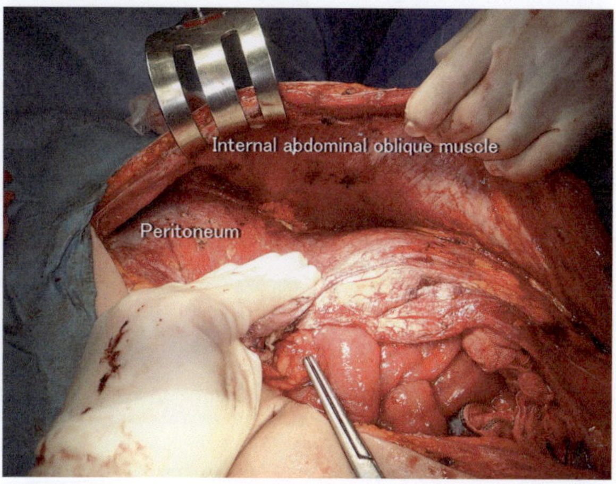

Fig. 22.7 Peritoneum stripped from fascia

22.3.7 Pancreatic Tail and Spleen

If tumor metastasis into the greater omentum is observed, metastasis into the spleen is also often noted. As the spleen is extremely prone to bleeding, splenectomy is usually performed. When a metastatic lesion is observed in the splenic hilum, it must be carefully evaluated whether there is sufficient space between the spleen and the pancreas. If the space between the tumor and the pancreatic tail is insufficient, combined splenic and pancreatic tail resection is performed.

22.3.8 Mesentery

When lesions are dispersed throughout the mesentery and are determined to be resectable, resection is performed to the maximum extent possible (Fig. 22.8). However, if the tumor is located close to the mesenteric artery, care must be taken not to damage the blood vessels as this can cause intestinal ischemia.

22.3.9 Greater Omentum

When clear metastatic lesions are observed on the greater omentum, complete omentectomy, including gastroepiploic artery ligation, is performed. If this is not the case, partial omentectomy from below the gastroepiploic artery is performed. In either case, detailed inspection is performed during omentectomy, including a detailed evaluation of whether any metastatic tumors are present in the foramen of Winslow.

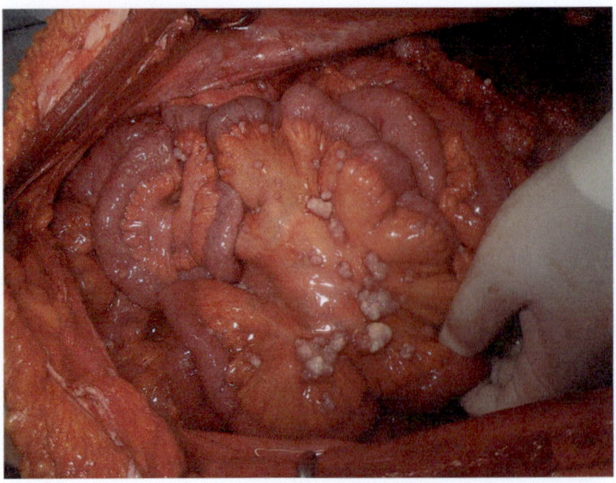

Fig. 22.8 Disseminated tumors on the mesentery

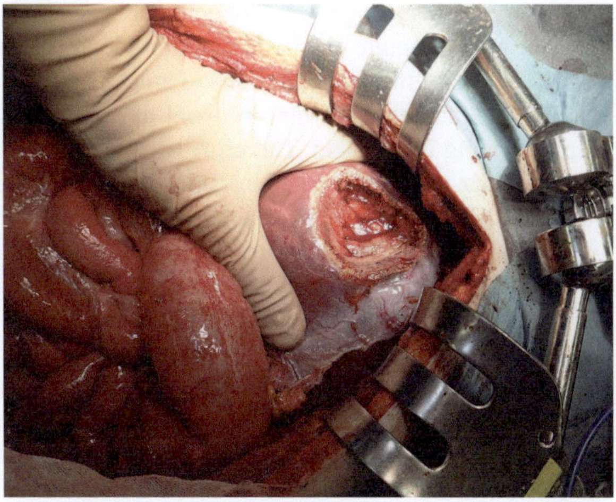

Fig. 22.9 Metastatic lesion removed by partial hepatectomy

22.3.10 Liver Parenchyma

Lesions in the hepatic parenchyma are operated on if hepatic surface resection or partial hepatectomy is possible (Fig. 22.9). Resection is not performed if segmental resection is considered necessary. During the surgery, the Pringle maneuver or similar method is used to temporarily restrict the blood flow into the liver, and resection is performed using a clamp-crushing or a power device.

22.3.11 Lymph Nodes

Even in cases of advanced ovarian cancer, systematic lymph node dissection is performed as a rule. Despite lymph node metastasis being observed, it is very rare for metastatic lymph nodes to infiltrate into the blood vessels. However, strong adhesion to the vascular wall is often observed. Such lymph nodes must be dissected carefully around veins because venous walls are much weaker than arterial walls. In particular, for the lymph nodes around the renal vein, inferior vena cava, and iliac vein, the blood vessels must be sufficiently exposed so that breakthrough bleeding can be immediately stopped while securing the necessary operative field to enable hemostasis.

22.4 Future Prospect

As combined resection of organs other than the internal genitalia is often required to achieve complete excision for cases of advanced ovarian cancer, this means that large-scale surgical intervention is necessary. Establishing specialized hospitals may contribute to raising the rate of complete operation. However, because there are many cases that require chemotherapy for a long time after surgery, it is necessary to solve problems that frequent visits to long distances are required. When performing such procedures, it is vital to avoid having to prematurely stop the resection despite it being incomplete. Therefore, it is optimal to be able to accurately determine whether complete resection can be performed on the basis of preoperative tests or minimally invasive procedures. Several reports have been reported on diagnostic accuracy of laparoscopy to diagnose unresectable disease in advanced ovarian cancer [10]. However, at the moment, there is no conclusive data that laparoscopy can diagnose the extensiveness of disease. Meanwhile, NAC-IDS may become a mainstream treatment after the results of the TRUST study and SUNNY trial are released. However, when performing surgery after chemotherapy for advanced ovarian cancer, physicians must remember that cancer tissue causes extensive fibrosis and that such surgery can often be more difficult than PDS.

References

1. Bristow RE, Tomacruz RS, Armstrong DK, Trimble EL, Montz FJ. Survival effect of maximal cytoreductive surgery for advanced ovarian carcinoma during the platinum era: a meta-analysis. J Clin Oncol. 2002;20:1248–59.
2. Eisenkop SM, Spirtos NM, Friedman RL, Lin W-CM, Pisani AL, Perticucci S. Relative influences of tumor volume before surgery and the cytoreductive outcome on survival for patients with advanced ovarian cancer: a prospective study. Gynecol Oncol. 2003;90:390–6.
3. Panici PB, Maggioni A, Hacker N, Landoni F, Ackermann S, Campagnutta E, Tamussino K, Winter R, Pellegrino A, Greggi S, Angioli R, Manci N, Scambia G, Dell'Anna T, Fossati R, Floriani I, Rossi RS, Grassi R, Favalli G, Raspagliesi F, Giannarelli D, Martella L, Mangioni C. Systematic aortic and pelvic lymphadenectomy versus resection of bulky nodes only in optimally debulked advanced ovarian cancer: a randomized clinical trial. J Natl Cancer Inst. 2005;97:560–6.
4. Chi DS, Eisenhauer EL, Lang J, Huh J, Haddad L, Abu-Rustum NR, Sonoda Y, Levine DA, Hensley M, Barakat RR. What is the optimal goal of primary cytoreductive surgery for bulky stage IIIC epithelial ovarian carcinoma (EOC)? Gynecol Oncol. 2006;103:559–64.
5. Terauchi F, Nishi H, Moritake T, Kobayashi Y, Nagashima T, Onodera T, Fujito A, Nakayama D, Isaka K. Prognostic factor on optimal debulking surgery by maximum effort for stage IIIC epithelial ovarian cancer. J Obstet Gynaecol Res. 2009;35:315–9.
6. Chi DS, Eisenhauer EL, Zivanovic O, Sonoda Y, Abu-Rustum NR, Levine DA, Guile MW, Bristow RE, Aghajanian C, Barakat RR. Improved progression-free and overall survival in advanced ovarian cancer as a result of a change in surgical paradigm. Gynecol Oncol. 2009;114:26–31.
7. du Bois A, Reuss A, Pujade-Lauraine E, Harter P, Ray-Coquard I, Pfisterer J. Role of surgical outcome as prognostic factor in advanced epithelial ovarian cancer: a combined exploratory analysis of 3 prospectively randomized phase 3 multicenter trials: by the Arbeitsgemeinschaft Gynaekologische Onkologie Studiengruppe Ovarialkarzinom (AGO-OVAR) and the Groupe d'Investigateurs Nationaux Pour les Etudes des Cancers de l'Ovaire (GINECO). Cancer. 2009;115:1234–44.
8. Vergote I, Trope CG, Amant F, Kristensen GB, Ehlen T, Johnson N, Verheijen RH, van der Burg ME, Lacave AJ, Panici PB, Kenter GG, Casado A, Mendiola C, Coens C, Verleye L, Stuart GC, Pecorelli S, Reed NS. Neoadjuvant chemotherapy or primary surgery in stage IIIC or IV ovarian cancer. N Engl J Med. 2010;363:943–53.

9. Kehoe S, Hook J, Nankivell M, Jayson GC, Kitchener H, Lopes T, Luesley D, Perren T, Bannoo S, Mascarenhas M, Dobbs S, Essapen S, Twigg J, Herod J, McCluggage G, Parmar M, Swart AM. Primary chemotherapy versus primary surgery for newly diagnosed advanced ovarian cancer (CHORUS): an open-label, randomised, controlled, non-inferiority trial. Lancet. 2015;386:249–57.
10. Rutten MJ, Leeflang MMG, Kenter GG, Mol BWJ, Buist M. Laparoscopy for diagnosing resectability of disease in patients with advanced ovarian cancer. Cochrane Database Syst Rev. 2014;2014:CD009786.

Upper Abdomen

23

Fumitoshi Terauchi

Abstract

The primary debulking surgery is performed to achieve complete debulking as the amount of residual tumor is one of the most important prognostic factors for survival of women with advanced ovarian cancer. In advanced cases, basic surgical procedures (bilateral salpingo-oophorectomy, total hysterectomy, and omentectomy) can deal with only minimal cases. And this is restrictive.

The upper abdominal disease is frequently observed in advanced cases. The reason of suboptimally debulking surgery is the presence of unresectable upper abdominal disease in advanced ovarian cancer. In other words, it means that we can get closer to complete debulking if we can extract any upper abdominal disease.

In this chapter, I describe about the surgery for some upper abdominal disease, especially diaphragmatic surgery, liver resection, splenectomy, and distal pancreatectomy.

Upper abdominal surgical technique is essential for operative treatment for advanced ovarian cancer.

For many gynecologic oncologists, it is necessary to master these techniques from now on.

Keywords

Diaphragmatic surgery · Reconstruction of diaphragm · Liver mobilization Splenectomy · Distal pancreatectomy

F. Terauchi (✉)
Department of Obstetrics and Gynecology, Tokyo Medical University, Shinjuku-ku, Tokyo, Japan
e-mail: teralfa@tokyo-med.ac.jp

M. Mikami (ed.), *Surgery for Gynecologic Cancer*, Comprehensive Gynecology and Obstetrics, https://doi.org/10.1007/978-981-13-1519-0_23

23.1 History

23.1.1 What Is the Optimal Surgery?

Prognosis of ovarian cancer is greatly affected by the diameter of residual tumor at the time of surgery. Therefore, primary debulking surgery (PDS), which removes disseminated and metastatic foci in the abdominal cavity as much as possible, is performed in advanced cases.

When residual tumors of less than 1 cm in diameter are removed in PDS, the prognosis of the case is significantly improved. Such surgery has been named as optimal surgery and has been considered as a goal of surgical treatment that should be aimed at [1, 2].

However, the analysis results of a multicenter randomized phase III study showed that prognostic indicators, both progression-free survival (PFS) and overall survival (OS), were significantly improved in only a complete surgery group, in which no residual tumors were observed. The survival rate of cases with residual tumors of less than 1 cm in diameter was almost the same level as that of cases with residual tumors of 1 cm or larger even if the group received a treatment previously considered as an optimal surgery [3]. Therefore, what is sought for surgeries of advanced ovarian cancer now is the complete surgery without residual tumors.

The plan is also similar in interval debulking surgery (IDS) conducted after the neoadjuvant chemotherapy (NAC).

The complete surgery can only be considered as an optimal surgery.

23.1.2 The Reason of Difficult to Perform the Complete Surgery

In advanced cases, basic operative procedures (bilateral salpingo-oophorectomy, total hysterectomy, and omentectomy) can deal with minimal cases. One of the reasons is that upper abdominal disease (UAD) is frequently observed in advance cases.

This is considered as a typical factor that interferes with the achievement of complete surgery.

In other words, the achievement rate of complete surgery would be improved if UAD can be surgically controlled.

This article gives an explanation about representative surgical techniques to the upper abdomen for advanced ovarian cancer.

23.2 Principle and Indication

23.2.1 Characteristic of the Upper Abdominal Disease (UAD)

Organs that specifically correspond to UAD include the right and left diaphragms, liver, stomach and lesser omentum, spleen, pancreas tail, and upper greater omentum and transverse colon. Ovarian cancer is characterized by unclear boundary between the metastatic site and healthy site due to its disseminated development.

In other words, UAD that exists with engulfing surrounding organs occurs more frequently. Therefore, this is one of UAD's characteristics that many cases require en bloc resection.

It has no standard procedures and is needed to be dealt with on an individual basis.

23.3 Does All UAD Become the Indication?

Not all UADs are suitable for surgery.

Reconstruction of the portal vein system become required especially when dissemination is observed in the hepatic portal region; therefore, exenteration is not usually applied. In addition, exenteration in PDS is also considered to be not applicable when multiple metastases are observed in the liver parenchyma. Exenteration of the pancreatic tail is applicable; however, exenteration of the pancreatic body to pancreatic head is considered to be not applicable at the current moment considering risks of the exenteration. Surgery is applicable for diaphragmatic lesion in many cases through a technique described below. However, it has no other choice other than to determine that surgery is not applicable when the lesion made progress from the dorsal midline toward a mediastinal direction because complete extraction is difficult.

Resection of UAD is often a highly invasive surgery. Therefore, preoperative evaluation of the general condition should be conducted with caution.

Especially, careful judgment of indication is required for the elderly and patients with complicating venous thromboembolism.

23.4 Preoperative Evaluation

23.4.1 Computed Tomography (CT)

Computed tomography (CT) is effective for evaluation of UADs.

However, the evaluation may be difficult depending on the metastasized organs, requiring an attention. PET/CT is a very useful examination but is affected by cancerous ascites. Therefore, the accurate evaluation for metastases is difficult.

It is difficult to conduct preoperative diagnosis of disseminated lesion of the diaphragm accurately unless the legion forms nodal mass. But when the nodal tumor is recognized at the slice between thoracic cavity and abdominal cavity in CT, full-thickness resection (described below) is often necessary (Fig. 23.1).

When ascites accumulates in large quantity, dissemination to the right diaphragm can be predicted from irregularity of the dorsal peritoneum in slices of the liver to

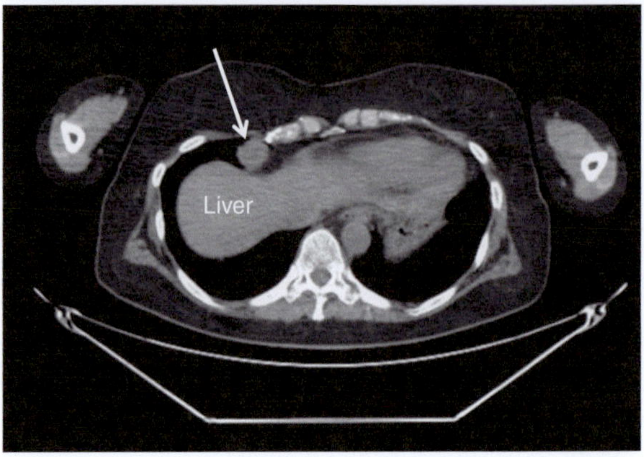

Fig. 23.1 The white arrow shows the nodal metastatic disease of the diaphragm

thoracic cavity. Accurate evaluation of the status of dissemination to surrounding organs is difficult unless findings at laparotomy are available although it is valuable for diagnosis of metastasis to the spleen.

In addition, the presence or absence of dilation of the caudal pancreatic duct shall be confirmed with CT in preparation for resection of the pancreas tail.

It is important to evaluate the extent of the lesion in preoperative image diagnosis as much as possible, but the final operative method is determined based on findings at the time of laparotomy in many cases. The algorithm to select the treatment for patients who need surgery first and who need chemotherapy first is tried by diagnostic laparoscopy [4].

Therefore, physicians must be ready so that they can deal with any individual patterns.

23.4.2 Preoperative Preparation

Resection of UAD often becomes a highly invasive surgery; hence, it is important to adequately improve the general condition prior to surgery. Especially, anemia and undernutrition need to be corrected.

When UAD is extirpated, it is desired to put a fasting period for a few days before the surgery in cases in which the necessity of combined resection and reconstruction of the digestive tract (jejunum/ileum, transverse colon, etc.) is expected.

Furthermore, when there is coexisted medical disease especially diabetes, it is important to control the condition adequately before the surgery.

It is needed to conduct ultrasonography of the veins of lower extremities when high D-dimer value was obtained in preoperative examination because venous thromboembolism, especially deep-vein thrombosis, may be accompanying.

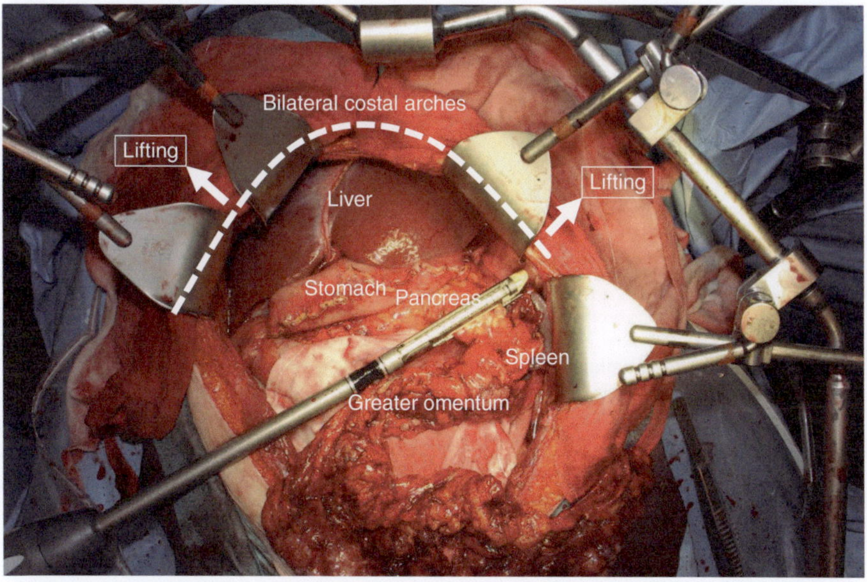

Fig. 23.2 The surgical field is expanded by lifting the bilateral costal arches up using retractors or similar devices. This is the en bloc resection of the pancreas tail, spleen and the greater omentum

23.5 Surgical Technique

23.5.1 Securement of the Surgical Field

It is extremely important to expand the surgical field sufficiently for removal of upper abdominal disease. When the expansion of surgical field is insufficient, it may hinder safe operation and becomes a factor causing an incomplete removal.

When the physicians are inexperienced in upper abdominal surgeries, they should especially pay attention to the expansion of surgical field and ensure to have sufficient surgical field.

It is basic to conduct median incision from the xiphoid process to implement upper abdominal operation. The technique can be performed more safely and unfailingly when the surgical field is expanded by lifting the bilateral costal arches up using retractors or similar devices (Fig. 23.2).

23.6 Liver Mobilization

Liver mobilization is an important technique for development. Especially, this is an essential surgical technique when diseases of the right diaphragm or liver are removed.

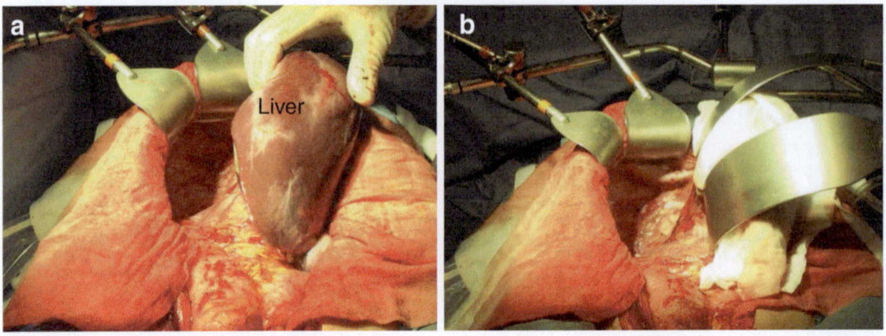

Fig. 23.3 (**a**) The liver mobilization was performed completely. The surgical field under the right side diaphragm spreads drastically by the liver mobilization. (**b**) The mobilized liver was fixed by the surgical retractor

First, liver mobilization is started with dissection of the ligamentum falciforme hepatis and right coronary ligament of liver. The dissection should not be forcedly conducted when dissemination is observed in the boundary between the diaphragm and liver.

In addition, separation of the boundary between the diaphragm and liver becomes easier by conducting separation of membrane continuing from the retroperitoneum and fascia renalis to the fascia hepatis in advance.

The procedure consists of dissection of adhesion of the transverse colon with the lower surface of the liver or gallbladder (ligamentum hepatocolicum) using an electrosurgical knife and the following dissection of the hepatorenal ligament, which is exposed to view beneath the dissected adhesion and is a membrane continuing from the retroperitoneum and fascia renalis to the fascia hepatis with an electrosurgical knife.

When the coarse membrane is dissected and separated along the periphery of the liver, the line connects with a dissection line of the right coronary ligament of the liver, which was dissected at the nearest site of the liver attachment site.

It is important to conduct this procedure cautiously and thoroughly with an attention to a group of short hepatic veins flowing into the right hepatic vein as well as the vena cava inferior. When the right margin of the vena cava inferior can be confirmed, the detachment is completed, and the liver is removed and turned from the site and fixed using surgical retractors (Fig. 23.3).

23.7 Diaphragmatic Surgery

Diaphragmatic lesions are observed at high frequency in advanced cases [5].

Therefore, surgical techniques for diaphragmatic lesions are essential for achievement of complete surgery, and one of the techniques that gynecologic oncologists should learn [6]. The diaphragm consists of three-layer structure of the ventral diaphragm (peritoneum), muscle layer, and chest-side diaphragm (pleura).

Removal of diaphragmatic lesions is implemented by two techniques, stripping and full-thickness resection.

For diaphragmatic lesion, it is needed to deal with it on an individual basis depending on the range and depth of the dissemination.

23.7.1 Stripping

Stripping is a method that strips and removes only the ventral diaphragm (peritoneum).

The peritoneum is pulled from a dissection line and stripped from the muscle layer.

One of the essential points of stripping is first to decide the range to be detached and removed. What you should pay attention to at the time is to start the detachment from healthy part slightly apart from the disseminated legion. This is because detachment often does not work well if it is started from a site near the disseminated legion.

When a detachment line is decided, the ventral diaphragm (peritoneal membrane) is incised using an electrosurgical knife. Then, the stump of incision is held using clamps, and the ventral diaphragm (peritoneal membrane) and muscular layers of the diaphragm are detached little by little with applying tension. At that time, it is important to conduct the process with a feeling of "pushing away the muscular layers" rather than intending to "detach them."

After the stripping, no special measures to prevent adhesion are required although the muscular layers are exposed.

The electric ablation may be used to treat the disseminated legions of the diaphragm.

However, such method is restrictive. Striping is more certain for debulking surgery.

Usual disseminated legions are removable by stripping. However, muscle invasion is suspected if the detachment cannot move forward anymore during the stripping. In such cases, it is important to switch the technique to full-thickness resection described below. In this regard, it is thought that the electric ablation is a restrictive technique.

This is because the muscle invasion is not ascertained by the electric ablation.

23.7.2 Full-Thickness Resection

Diaphragmatic lesions in advanced ovarian cancer are often caused by dissemination, but it may also present nodal condition in some cases. Such clinical condition causes infiltration to the diaphragmatic muscle layer as well as the chest-side diaphragm (pleura); therefore, removal by full-thickness resection is required.

Full-thickness resection does not require difficult technique very much.

Muscular layers that cannot be detached are held and stabilized with Kelly clamps, and the muscular layers of the diaphragm are made an incision using an electrosurgical knife to open the chest. Infiltration into the chest-side diaphragm (pleura) is visually confirmed, and then the range of the full-thickness resection is determined.

In the case that visual confirmation is difficult, we observe in the chest cavity using a thoracoscope. Because it is an open chest surgery, we request the Anesthesiology Department to conduct general anesthesia using an intubation tube that enables one-lung ventilation in surgery for advanced ovarian cancer.

Full-thickness resection of the diaphragm is conducted by thoracotomy in cooperation with an anesthesiologist.

23.7.3 Reconstruction of the Diaphragm

Full-thickness resection is implemented through thoracotomy; therefore, reconstruction of the diaphragm is required (Fig. 23.4).

The diaphragm is a well-extensible organ, and usually the chest can be closed using simple suture closure by full-thickness suture. Especially when a large amount of ascites is accumulated, the diaphragm can be adequately sutured even if the diaphragm has a great defect as compared with the hyperextension state.

We conduct simple suture closure by Z interrupted suture of the full thickness using PDS II® 1.0, which is an absorbable suture. However, when the simple suture

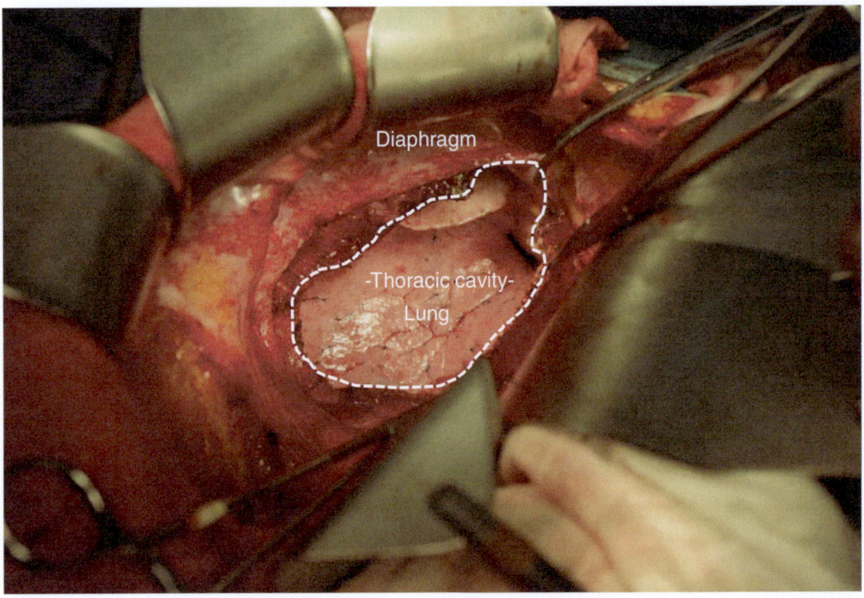

Fig. 23.4 This is the full-thickness resected the diaphragm. The resection range was widespread

closure is impossible due to large defect, we reconstruct the diaphragm using a 1.0 mm thick expanded polytetrafluoroethylene (ePTFE) patch (Gore-Tex soft tissue patch®).

This patch is made of a material excellent in flexibility, extensibility, and durability and is an easy-to-use reconstruction graft in actual surgery. Clinically, it is often used for reconstruction of combined resection of the diaphragm in diffuse pleural mesothelioma and restoration of traumatic hernia of the diaphragm.

It is considered that ePTFE patch has advantages as follows as compared with existing polypropylene mesh: (1) good infiltration of fibroblast from tissues through the patch and excellent biocompatibility; (2) no deterioration, degradation, or elution even in prolonged use; (3) less friction with surrounding tissues due to its flexibility; and (4) less splitting and easy to suture. The patch is sutured with applying tension slightly to the margin of the lost part of the diaphragm by 7–8 mm interval of horizontal mattress suturing using nonabsorbable suture. The key point of reconstruction is to suture a patch, which is cut into a slightly larger size than the absent part, with slightly applying tension to the margin of the absent part of the diaphragm (Fig. 23.5).

The last stitch is held without ligating, and an aspiration tube is inserted from the open chest site for degassing of the thoracic cavity. Ligation is performed, and then the aspiration tube is removed with inflating the lung adequately and keeping that state by requesting it to an anesthesiologist. Pneumothorax condition is improved in this way.

No thoracostomy tube is required.

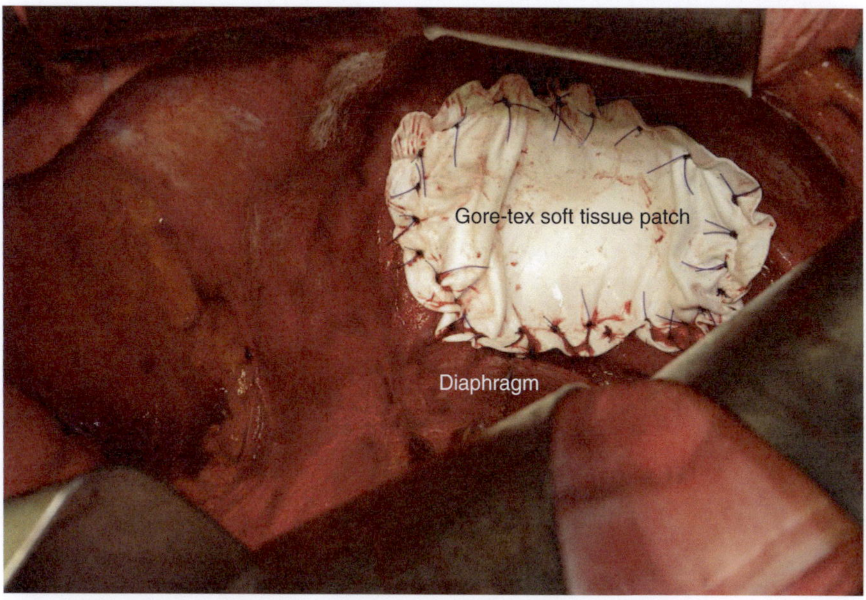

Fig. 23.5 This is the diaphragm reconstructed with Gore-Tex soft tissue patch

A leak test is performed after chest closure to make assurance double sure. The body is laid in Trendelenburg's position with lowering the head. Then, about 500 mL of physiological saline and others is injected into a space under the diaphragm. Enforced ventilation is conducted several times, and air leakage is checked.

23.7.4 Liver Resection

Liver resection includes hepatic segment resection (right lobe resection, extended right lobe resection, left lobe resection, and left lateral segment resection) and partial liver resection, which is nonanatomical resection of a range less than a segment of the Couinaud classification. The latter is usually used in surgery for ovarian cancer.

Surgical treatment is indicated for cases with legions presenting nodular status and invading from the capsule into the parenchyma of the liver.

The procedures of this technique are started with making an incision in a capsule 2–3 cm away from the lesion using an electrosurgical knife.

Cutting into the parenchyma too deep using the electrosurgical knife often causes intense bleeding. Therefore, the incision should be conducted with intending to mark an incision line onto only the capsule. Then, vessels in the liver parenchyma are exposed using an ultrasonic scalpel (CUSA® or SONOTEC®) along the incision line, and congelation and cutting are conducted using a sealing device such as Ligasure® and Harmonic®. These manipulations are alternately repeated, and the tumor is removed eventually.

A sheet-like fibrin preparation is bonded and pressed on the excision site to prevent postoperative bleeding and bile spillage.

It is important to conduct liver resection in a careful manner because hemorrhage control is essential for liver resection (Fig. 23.6).

23.7.5 Splenectomy

For splenic legions, cases that removed the spleen alone are not many, and rather en bloc resection with surrounding organs would be needed in many cases. Therefore,

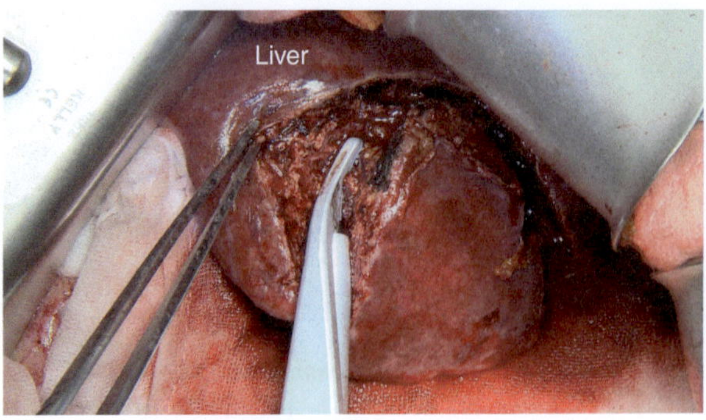

Fig. 23.6 Congelation and cutting are conducted using a sealing device

it is important to check the greater omentum, transverse colon, pancreatic tail, and left diaphragm when a splenic legion is observed. Especially, it is needed to pay attention when the greater omentum has omental cake.

Splenectomy is basically conducted by detaching of the spleen and removing and mobilizing/turning of the spleen from the site. Detachment of the spleen becomes easier when the procedure is started from resection of membranous physiological adhesion site of the splenic flexure of the colon. After that, resection of the splenocolic ligament is implemented, and continuing from the resection line, resection of retroperitoneum and splenophrenic ligament is performed. Then, resection of the gastrosplenic ligament is conducted. Identification of the gastrolienal ligament is easy because the greater omentum is almost completely removed. When the dissection is performed furthermore, short gastric arteries and veins are found near the upper pole. These are ligated and cut.

The spleen locates in a deep part of the left upper quadrant of the abdomen. When adhesions with the retroperitoneum and surrounding organs are removed, the spleen can be completely removed and turned from the site.

A cord-like tissue of the hilum of the spleen is treated with an electrosurgical knife, and the splenic artery and vein are confirmed and then ligated and resected (Fig. 23.7).

In such circumstances, it has been considered that when the splenic arteries and veins are ligated, they should be basically separated and ligated after detaching from the hilum region of the spleen. However, forced detachment causes unwanted bleeding; therefore, it is possible to deal with mass ligation if the course of vessels can be confirmed. When a distance between the hilum of the spleen and pancreatic tail is short, the procedure must be conducted with paying attention not to give excess traction or constrained detachment of the pancreatic tail to avoid damaging the pancreas.

When damage of the pancreatic tail is suspected even if only slightly, a sheet-like fibrin preparation is bonded and pressed on the site.

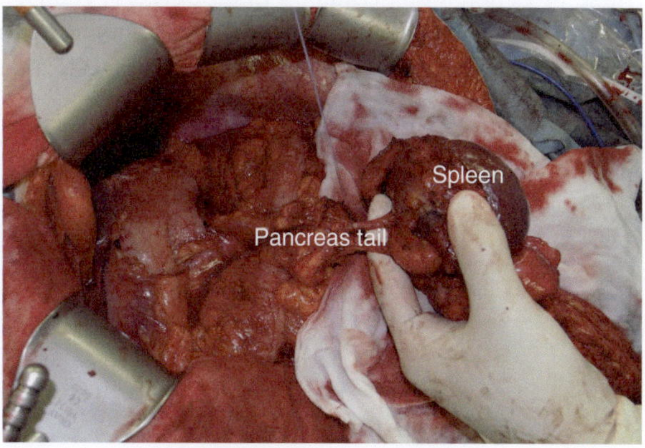

Fig. 23.7 The splenic artery and vein are confirmed and then ligated and resected

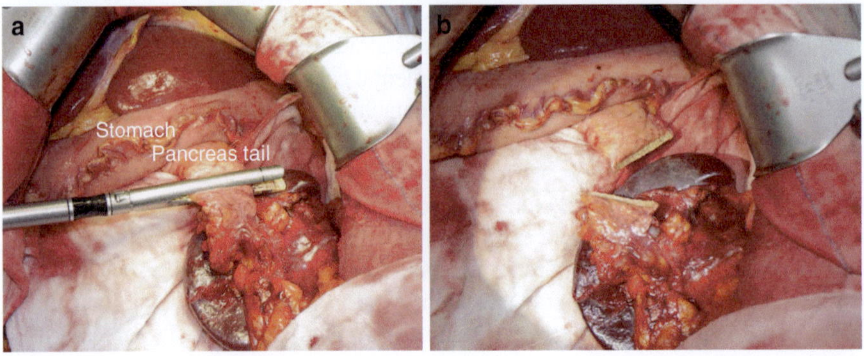

Fig. 23.8 (**a**) The pancreatic tissue is crushed to staple and resected using automatic anastomotic device. (**b**) It is important to thin such like this

23.7.6 Distal Pancreatectomy

When the pancreatic tail is resected in a surgery for ovarian cancer, en bloc resection with the spleen is applied in most of cases.

Opening of the epiploic foramen, which is required for resection of the pancreatic tail, is conducted in advance in many cases because complete removal of the greater omentum is the basic operative procedure of surgery for ovarian cancer.

When en bloc resection of the spleen and pancreatic tail is performed, the surgery is started with detachment and removal and mobilizing/turning of the spleen from the site through the aforementioned procedure. When the spleen is removed and turned from the site, the pancreatic tail is also removed and turned from the site unless there is dorsal development.

The resection line is determined, and the ligation sites of the splenic artery and vein according to the resection line are checked at this step. Surefire prevention of pancreatic leak is the most important in resection of the pancreatic tail.

We conduct the dissection using an automatic anastomotic device with gold cartridge of Echelon 60® (Ethicon Endo-Surgery; Johnson&Johnson). When the pancreatic tissue is crushed to staple and resect in resection of the pancreatic tail using this device, it is essential to conduct this crushing and stapling process slowly and gradually to the fullest (Fig. 23.8).

We conduct preventive measures for all cases by bonding and pressing a sheet-like fibrin preparation on the cutoff stump.

A closed-type information drain is placed under the left diaphragm after the resection of the pancreatic tail.

23.8 Morbidity

23.8.1 After Diaphragmatic Surgery

Pleural effusions are frequently observed. Especially, it is observed after full-thickness resection at a high frequency, but usually no thoracostomy tube is required [7].

In addition, no decrease in the respiratory function is observed after the surgery.

23.8.2 After Liver Resection

Bile spillage usually occurs around 4–5 days after surgery. However, it spontaneously closes within 1–2 weeks if drainage is effective; and it is rare to become a serious condition. If the drainage is poor, drainage under CT guide should be considered.

23.8.3 After Distal Pancreatectomy

Early diagnosis of pancreatic leak is the most important after resection of the pancreatic tail. Observation of properties of drainage from a drain is important. If pancreatic leak occurs, the drainage presents a red wine-like clear color due to hemolyzed red cells. Amylase level in the drainage should be measured on Day 1 after the surgery to observe changes in the level. Usually the value is high on Day 1, and then it gradually decreases. When pancreatic leak is suspected even if only slightly, it is important to abstain from eating first. It is better to remove the drain after observation for several days after restarting oral ingestion.

23.9 Future Prospect

Upper abdominal surgical technique is essential for operative treatment for advanced ovarian cancer.

It is sought that gynecologic cancer specialists make an effort to acquire proficiency in surgical anatomy through human cadaver training, to grasp the surgical techniques and acquire proficiency in surgical procedures through animal lab training, and to master each technique in a convincing way through on the job training in cooperation with digestive system surgery department in the future. It is a shortcut for learning these upper abdominal surgical techniques.

However, this policy is difficult practically and takes time. I think that the centralization of facilities is the best way to save the patient with advanced ovarian cancer at present. The requirement of these facilities is the performance of joint operation with the department of surgery and the making of maximum effort for debulking surgery.

References

1. Hoskins WJ, et al. The effect of diameter of largest residual disease on survival after primary cytoreductive surgery in patients with suboptimal residual epithelial ovarian carcinoma. Am J Obstet Gynecol. 1994;170:974–80.
2. Bristow RE, et al. Survival effect of maximal cytoreductive surgery for advanced ovarian carcinoma during the platinum era: a meta-analysis. J Clin Oncol. 2002;20:1248–59.

3. du Bois A, et al. Role of surgical outcomes as prognostic factor in advanced epithelial ovarian cancer; a combined exploratory analysis of 3 prospectively randomized phase 3 multicenter trials by the Arbeitsgemeinschaft Gynaekologische Onkologie Studiengruppe Ovarialkarzinom (AGO-OVAR) and the Groupe d'Investigateurs Nationaux Pour les Etudes des Cancers de l'Ovaire (GINNECO). Cancer. 2009;115:1234–44.
4. Nick AM, et al. A framework for a personalized surgical approach to ovarian cancer. Nat Rev Clin Oncol. 2015;12:239–45.
5. Cliby W, et al. Diaphragm resection for ovarian cancer; technique and short-term complications. Gynecol Oncol. 2004;94:655–60.
6. Fanfani F, et al. Upper abdominal surgery in advanced and recurrent ovarian cancer; role of diaphragmatic surgery. Gynecol Oncol. 2010;116:497–501.
7. Terauchi F, et al. Incidental events of diaphragmatic surgery in 82 patients with advanced ovarian, primary peritoneal and fallopian tubal cancer. Oncol Let. 2010;1:861–4.

Lymph Node Dissection for Epithelial Ovarian Cancer

24

Kazuhiro Takehara

Abstract

Although peritoneal dissemination is the most common characteristic of ovarian cancer, retroperitoneal lymph node dissemination is also a common route of spread. The highest incidence of nodal metastasis is in the pelvic and para-aortic nodes. Nodal metastases occur in 13–74% of stage III and in 33–88% of stage IV patients. Preoperative evaluation using computed tomography, diffusion-weighted magnetic resonance imaging, and positron emission tomography are not acceptable alternatives to systematic lymphadenectomy regarding sensitivity and specificity for the moment.

Procedures of retroperitoneal lymph node dissection include pelvic lymphadenectomy and para-aortic lymphadenectomy. Each procedure involves development of the retroperitoneal space, recognition of retroperitoneal viscera, and dissection of lymph nodes around vessels. Systematic lymphadenectomy is associated with longer operation times, higher blood loss and transfusion rates, and a longer hospital stay compared with lymph node biopsy or no lymphadenectomy. Common complications of lymphadenectomy are hemorrhage, thromboembolic complications, vessel injury, adhesion, ileus, and injury to the pelvic viscera. Attention is also required for long-term complications, lymph cysts, lymph ascites, and lymphedema.

In patients with advanced epithelial ovarian cancer, maximal cytoreductive surgical efforts for minimizing residual disease contribute to a good prognosis. However, the role of lymphadenectomy as part of maximal debulking surgery is still controversial.

K. Takehara (✉)
Department of Gynecologic Oncology, National Hospital Organization Shikoku Cancer Center, Matsuyama, Ehime, Japan
e-mail: takehara.kazuhiro.ef@mail.hosp.go.jp

M. Mikami (ed.), *Surgery for Gynecologic Cancer*, Comprehensive Gynecology and Obstetrics, https://doi.org/10.1007/978-981-13-1519-0_24

Keywords
Epithelial ovarian cancer · Lymphadenectomy · Surgical procedure

24.1 History

The International Federation of Gynecology and Obstetrics (FIGO) staging was updated in 2013. Cases of ovarian cancer with lymph node metastasis were classified as stage IIIc in FIGO 1988. However, cases with positive retroperitoneal lymph nodes and/or microscopic metastasis beyond the pelvis were classified as stage IIIA [1]. This change highlights the diagnostic and prognostic importance of nodal evaluation, whereas the therapeutic role of lymphadenectomy in ovarian cancer is uncertain.

24.2 Principles and Indications

Peritoneal implantation by exfoliation of cancer cells is the most common feature of ovarian cancer, and retroperitoneal lymph node dissemination is also a common route of spread. Autopsy studies have shown lymph node metastases in up to 80% of patients with ovarian cancer [2, 3]. Para-aortic lymph node metastasis is the most common in ovarian cancer in gynecological malignancies. Therefore, staging surgery with retroperitoneal lymphadenectomy is important for staging, even if in early-stage ovarian cancer. In patients with advanced epithelial ovarian cancer, maximal cytoreductive surgical efforts for minimizing residual disease have been demonstrated in recent studies [4–7]. Cytoreductive surgery should include intraperitoneal and retroperitoneal surgical procedures. However, the role of lymphadenectomy as part of maximal debulking surgery is still controversial. The prognosis of lymph node metastasis is better than that of peritoneal dissemination [8–11].

24.3 Incidence and Pattern of Lymph Node Involvement

Ovarian cancer has three lymphatic pathways for metastasis. The first pathway is to the para-aortic lymph nodes through the infundibulopelvic ligament. The second pathway is to the external iliac nodes, internal iliac nodes, and obturator nodes. The third pathway is to the inguinal lymph node through the round ligament. Various frequencies of lymph node metastasis have been reported because systematic lymphadenectomy is not performed in all cases of advanced ovarian cancer. In patients with apparent stage I/II ovarian cancer, the frequency of lymph node metastasis ranges from 1% to 15% (Table 24.1) [12–16].

Lymph node involvement is more common with advanced ovarian cancer, with nodal metastases being documented in 13–74% of stage III and in 33–88% of stage IV patients [13, 17–20]. The highest incidence of nodal metastasis is in the pelvic

Table 24.1 Frequency of lymph node metastasis in stage I and II epithelial ovarian cancer

				Site of lymph node metastasis		
Author	Stage	*n*	Positive node	Pelvic	Para-aortic	Both
Benedetti-Panici et al. [12]	I	35	5	3	2	0
	II	2	0	0	0	0
Burghardt et al. [13]	I	20	3	2	0	1
	II	7	5	1	1	3
Nomura H, et al. [14]	I*	60	8	1	3	4
	II*	19	2	0	1	1
Ditto et al. [15]	I	84	8	2	8	5
	II	27	7			
Oshita et al. [16]	I*	204	9	2	10	9
	II*	80	14			
Total		538	64 (11.8%)	11 (2.0%)	25 (4.6%)	23 (4.3%)

( ): Rate of lymph node metastasis

and para-aortic nodes, with an occurrence of 53–73% [17, 21, 22]. Isolated metastasis patterns are rare. The incidence of para-aortic node metastasis and pelvic node metastasis is 15–33% and 8–28%, respectively [13, 17, 20, 22–24]. The most common metastatic node in ovarian cancer is the para-aortic node in the area of the inferior mesenteric artery-renal artery, with an incidence of 79% [17, 25].

24.4 Preoperative Evaluation

Although 5 mm or greater enlargement of lymph nodes is often detected with an improvement in computed tomography (CT) image resolution, qualitative diagnosis requires a cautious diagnosis. Diffusion-weighted magnetic resonance imaging (MRI) and positron emission tomography (PET) are useful in assessing qualitative diagnosis of lymph node metastasis. However, diagnosis of lymph node metastasis is frequently difficult in lymph node swelling of 10 mm or less. Final diagnosis is made with findings of postoperative pathology.

A recent systematic review and meta-analysis examined detection of lymph node metastases in patients with ovarian cancer. This study showed that fluorodeoxyglucose-PET/CT or PET showed the highest pooled sensitivity (73%, 95% confidence interval 68–78%) and specificity (97%, 95% confidence interval 96–98%). The corresponding data for CT were 43% (95% confidence interval 36–50%) and 95% (95% confidence interval 93–96%), and those for MRI were 55% (95% confidence interval 44–55%) and 88% (95% confidence interval 85–91%), respectively [26].

24.5 Staging Lymphadenectomy

Staging lymphadenectomy is the gold standard procedure in early invasive ovarian cancer. A total of 23% of women with apparent preoperative stage I ovarian cancer have occult nodal disease [27]. Approximately 30% of patients with early-stage ovarian cancer are upstaged with comprehensive staging surgery [28]. Staging lymphadenectomy affects the indication of adjuvant therapy besides removing lymph node lesions. In early invasive ovarian cancer, some authors have reported that complete surgical staging contributes to a better prognosis [29, 30]. From the point of view of adjuvant therapy, Sankai Gynecology Study Group (SGSG), which is a Japanese local clinical study group, conducted a retrospective study to reveal the survival impact of systematic pelvic and para-aortic lymphadenectomy in patients with pT1 and pT2 epithelial ovarian cancer (EOC) [12]. In this study, the rate of lymph node metastasis in pT2 was 17.5%, which was significantly higher than 4.4% in pT1. The outcome for patients who received adjuvant chemotherapy was significantly improved in patients who had not undergone systematic pelvic and para-aortic lymphadenectomy, but no improvement was observed in patients having undergone lymph node resection. For the above reasons, accurate surgical staging might avoid unnecessary adjuvant chemotherapy in selected early-stage cases.

In previous reports, ipsilateral lymphadenectomy for tumors that appeared to be unilateral was recommended [12]. However, later reports showed that contralateral lymphatic dissemination is often recognized at diagnostic lymphadenectomy. Therefore, even staging procedures of patients with stage I ovarian cancer should include bilateral pelvic and para-aortic lymph node sampling up to the level of the renal veins.

24.6 Systemic Lymphadenectomy

The therapeutic potential of systemic lymphadenectomy for advanced-stage ovarian cancer remains uncertain. A randomized, clinical trial was performed to determine whether systematic aortic and pelvic lymphadenectomy improves progression-free and overall survival compared with resection of bulky nodes only. The authors of this trial concluded that systematic lymphadenectomy improves progression-free, but not overall, survival in women with optimally cytoreductive advanced ovarian carcinoma. In this study, 427 patients with stage IIIB–IV epithelial ovarian cancer and postoperative residual disease less than 1 cm were randomly assigned to systematic pelvic and para-aortic lymph node dissection or resection of bulky nodes only. While systematic lymph node dissection was associated with 7 months' improvement in progression-free survival (22.4 vs. 29.4 months), there was no difference in overall survival (56.3 vs. 62.1 months) [8].

An exploratory analysis of three prospective, randomized trials showed a significant effect of lymphadenectomy on overall survival ($P = 0.0123$) and in patients with small residual tumors up to 1 cm. The effect of lymphadenectomy on overall survival barely reached significance ($P = 0.0497$) [31].

Systematic chemotherapy may not be that effective for retroperitoneal lymph node lesions. A high rate of nodal metastasis has been documented in 26–77% of patients after chemotherapy [32]. Nodal metastatic cancer cells in ovarian cancer are often diploid, and their cell cycle is in the low S phase. Therefore, these cells react poorly to chemotherapy [33].

24.7 Surgical Technique (Fig. 24.1)

24.7.1 Systematic Pelvic Lymphadenectomy Fig. 24.1

24.7.1.1 Development of the Retroperitoneal Cavity

The posterior leaf of the peritoneum is incised from the round ligament to the suspensory ligament of the ovary. To allow adequate exposure to the retroperitoneum, the outside incision of the posterior leaf of the peritoneum is extended. Upon entering the retroperitoneal space, the surgeon should identify the external artery, extend the space along it carefully, and identify the ureter, which crosses over the common iliac artery. The paravesical and pararectal spaces are created.

After separating the gap between the psoas muscle and external iliac artery, the obturator fossa is opened until the obturator nerve is confirmed. The dorsal fat pad of the iliac vein is applied medially and then separated from the wall of the external iliac vein. In this procedure, care should be taken not to damage the obturator vessels and vessels supplying the psoas muscle.

24.7.1.2 Lymph Node Dissection of the External Iliac and External Inguinal Nodes

Dissection is begun with the external iliac nodes. The genitofemoral nerve should be preserved if possible. The node-bearing fat pad is tensioned, and the wall of the

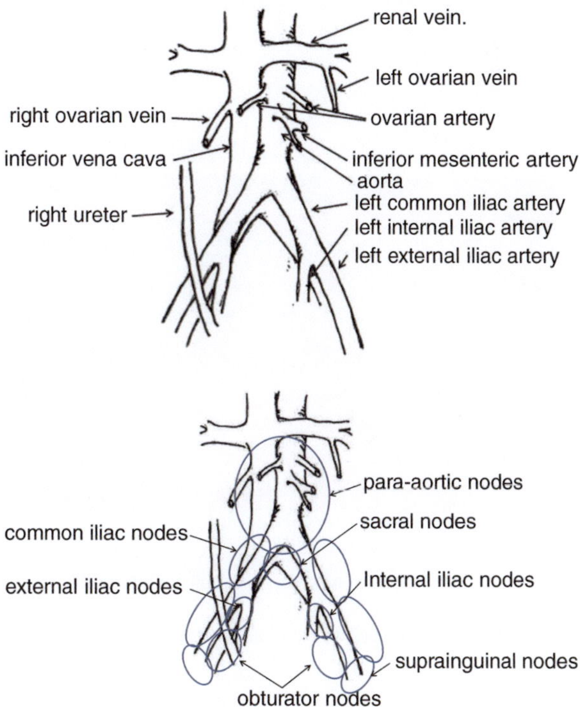

Fig. 24.1 (**a**) Anatomy of the aorta, vena cava, and iliac artery and vein. (**b**) The name of lymph node and anatomical index

external iliac artery is outcropped. After stopping hemorrhage from small vessels, the nodes around the external iliac artery and vein are carefully removed. The dissection is performed from the external iliac vessels down to the level of the deep circumflex iliac vein.

24.7.1.3 Lymph Node Dissection of the Obturator and Internal Iliac Nodes

The obturator fossa is located between the umbilical ligament and the external iliac vessels. Obturator and internal iliac node dissection is performed by displacing the external iliac vessels laterally. The dorsal fat pad of the iliac vein is separated from the external iliac vein and released from the obturator nerve and vessels. The lumbosacral trunk lies next to the lateral internal and external iliac vessels. Therefore, surgeons need to take care to avoid thermal damage by electric devices.

24.7.2 Systematic Para-aortic Lymphadenectomy Fig. 24.2

A midline abdominal incision from beneath the xiphoid process to the pubic symphysis is required for systematic pelvic and para-aortic lymphadenectomy to the level of the renal veins. For a safe operation, a sufficient surgical field and careful visualization of organs are important.

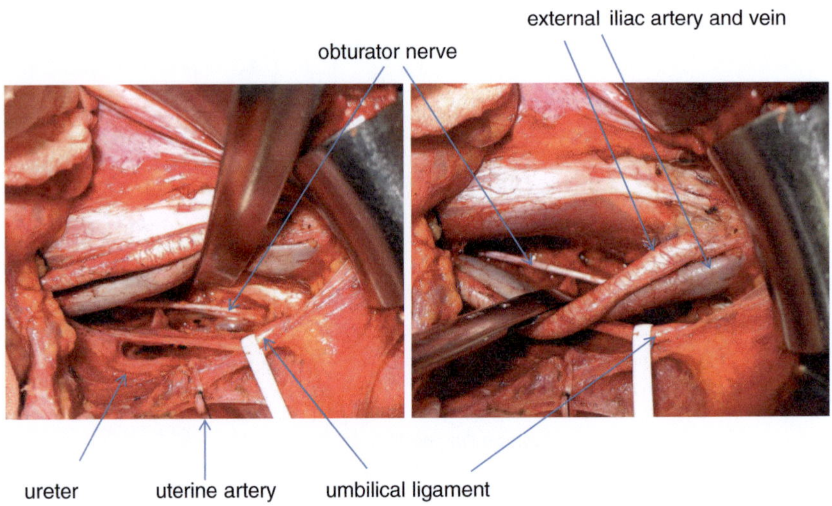

Fig. 24.2 Systematic pelvic lymphadenectomy

24.7.2.1 Development of the Retroperitoneal Space

Some approaches have attempted to develop the retroperitoneal para-aortic space. In the majority of cases, an incision is often made from the infundibulopelvic ligament crossing the vena cava and aorta and ending at the duodenum at the ligament of Treitz. If a larger surgical field is required, the cecum and ascending colon are mobilized from loose underlying connective tissue. The right ureter is identified and retracted laterally. The small bowel is placed in an isolation bag and pulled out of the abdominal cavity.

24.7.2.2 Incision of Connective Tissue Anterior to the Aorta and Treatment of Bilateral Ovarian Vessels

The node-bearing tissue is removed in such a manner as to expose the front wall of the aorta toward the inferior border of the left renal vein. At some point in the procedure, the inferior mesenteric artery is identified. The left ovarian artery is located cephalad to the inferior mesenteric artery, and the left ovarian vein is located lateral to the left renal vein. Therefore, these vessels should be identified and ligated.

24.7.2.3 Dissection of the Right Side of the Inferior Vena Cava

This procedure begins with removal of the fat pad and then exposes the adventitial sheath on the anterior surface of the common iliac artery. Lymph node chains located in the lateral side of the right common iliac vein are dissected from caudal to cephalad. Although only a few vessels, except for the right ovarian vein, are present, perforator veins are sometimes found. Careful attention is required not to tear these veins.

24.7.2.4 Dissection of Nodes Between the Para-aortic and Vena Cava

Some branches of small veins are inside of the inferior vena cava. If bleeding occurs, then the source should be identified, and the bleeding should be stopped without injury surrounding structures. The nodal tissue is gently mobilized and dissected. Special attention needs to be paid not to damage lumbar vessels, which lie in the back of the inferior vena cava and aorta.

24.7.2.5 Dissection of the Left Side of the Para-aortic Nodes

The lymph node chain is removed from the left common iliac vessels, taking care not to damage the lumbar vessels. The node-bearing fat is passed under the inferior mesenteric artery. Lymph node dissection is performed to the level of the inferior border of the renal vein.

24.7.2.6 Removal of the Sacral Nodes

The node-bearing tissue lying between the inside of the bilateral common iliac arteries is carefully dissected from underlying vessels.

24.8 Morbidity

Systematic lymphadenectomy is associated with longer operation times, higher blood loss and transfusion rates, and a longer hospital stay compared with lymph node biopsy or no lymphadenectomy [8, 34]. In retroperitoneal lymphadenectomy, perioperative morbidity and 60-day mortality are higher than those with lymph node biopsy or no lymphadenectomy. Common early postoperative complications of lymphadenectomy are hemorrhage, thromboembolic complications, vessel injury, adhesion, ileus, and injury to the ureter or small and large bowel [35]. Injury to the chyle cistern sometimes leads to chyle leak. The most frequent long-term complications are lymph cysts, lymph ascites, and lymphedema (Fig. 24.3).

24.9 Future Prospects

One of the most important prognostic factors of advanced epithelial ovarian cancer is macroscopic complete resection at initial therapy. From this point of view, systematic lymphadenectomy is considered to improve survival in patients with advanced ovarian cancer who have lymph node metastasis with no visible residual disease [31, 36–38]. However, prospective studies have suggested that systematic lymphadenectomy for epithelial ovarian cancer improves progression-free, but not overall, survival in patients with completely cytoreductive advanced-stage ovarian cancer [8, 34]. The LION trial (AGO OVAR OP3/ENGOT-ov31), which was a prospective, randomized study conducted by AGO, investigated systematic pelvic and

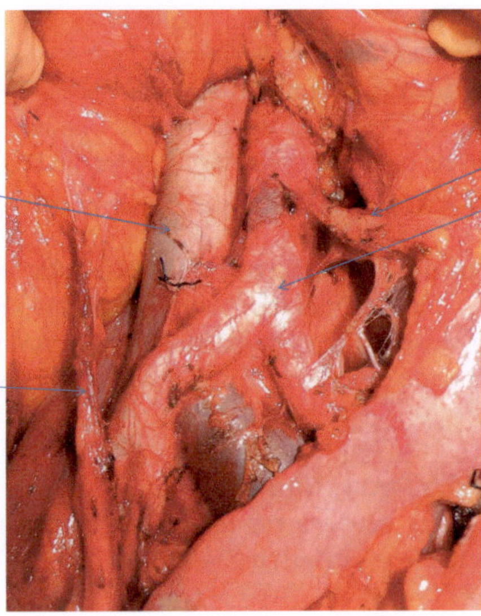

Fig. 24.3 Systematic para-aortic lymphadenectomy

para-aortic lymphadenectomy in patients with advanced ovarian cancer with intra-abdominal complete resection and clinically negative lymph node metastases. These procedures did not improve progression-free (secondary endpoint; lymphadenectomy vs. no lymphadenectomy, 25.5 vs. 25.5 months) or overall survival (primary endpoint; lymphadenectomy vs. no lymphadenectomy, 65.5 vs. 69.2 months), despite the presence (and removal) of subclinical retroperitoneal lymph node metastases in 56% of the patients [39]. Considering this lack of difference in oncological outcome and perioperative morbidity, systematic lymphadenectomy for patients with advanced ovarian cancer and clinical negative lymph node metastasis should not be performed.

Interval debulking surgery followed by neoadjuvant chemotherapy is one of the other therapeutic strategies for advanced ovarian cancer. Whether this method can be applied to patients with neoadjuvant chemotherapy followed by interval debulking surgery needs to be verified. These results could lead to a new clinical staging system.

References

1. Prat J. Oncology FCoG. Staging classification for cancer of the ovary, fallopian tube, and peritoneum. Int J Gynaecol Obstet. 2014;124(1):1–5. https://doi.org/10.1016/j.ijgo.2013.10.001.
2. Bergman F. Carcinoma of the ovary. A clinicopathological study of 86 autopsied cases with special reference to mode of spread. Acta Obstet Gynecol Scand. 1966;45(2):211–31.
3. Abrams HL, Spiro R, Goldstein N. Metastases in carcinoma; analysis of 1000 autopsied cases. Cancer. 1950;3(1):74–85.
4. Bristow RE, Tomacruz RS, Armstrong DK, Trimble EL, Montz FJ. Survival effect of maximal cytoreductive surgery for advanced ovarian carcinoma during the platinum era: a meta-analysis. J Clin Oncol. 2002;20(5):1248–59. https://doi.org/10.1200/JCO.2002.20.5.1248.
5. Aletti GD, Dowdy SC, Gostout BS, Jones MB, Stanhope CR, Wilson TO, et al. Aggressive surgical effort and improved survival in advanced-stage ovarian cancer. Obstet Gynecol. 2006;107(1):77–85. https://doi.org/10.1097/01.AOG.0000192407.04428.bb.
6. Chi DS, Eisenhauer EL, Lang J, Huh J, Haddad L, Abu-Rustum NR, et al. What is the optimal goal of primary cytoreductive surgery for bulky stage IIIC epithelial ovarian carcinoma (EOC)? Gynecol Oncol. 2006;103(2):559–64. https://doi.org/10.1016/j.ygyno.2006.03.051.
7. Kommoss S, Rochon J, Harter P, Heitz F, Grabowski JP, Ewald-Riegler N, et al. Prognostic impact of additional extended surgical procedures in advanced-stage primary ovarian cancer. Ann Surg Oncol. 2010;17(1):279–86. https://doi.org/10.1245/s10434-009-0787-8.
8. Panici PB, Maggioni A, Hacker N, Landoni F, Ackermann S, Campagnutta E, et al. Systematic aortic and pelvic lymphadenectomy versus resection of bulky nodes only in optimally debulked advanced ovarian cancer: a randomized clinical trial. J Natl Cancer Inst. 2005;97(8):560–6. https://doi.org/10.1093/jnci/dji102.
9. Cliby WA, Aletti GD, Wilson TO, Podratz KC. Is it justified to classify patients to Stage IIIC epithelial ovarian cancer based on nodal involvement only? Gynecol Oncol. 2006;103(3):797–801. https://doi.org/10.1016/j.ygyno.2006.08.047.
10. Ferrandina G, Scambia G, Legge F, Petrillo M, Salutari V. Ovarian cancer patients with "node-positive-only" Stage IIIC disease have a more favorable outcome than Stage IIIA/B. Gynecol Oncol. 2007;107(1):154–6. https://doi.org/10.1016/j.ygyno.2007.05.016.
11. Baek SJ, Park JY, Kim DY, Kim JH, Kim YM, Kim YT, et al. Stage IIIC epithelial ovarian cancer classified solely by lymph node metastasis has a more favorable prognosis than other types of stage IIIC epithelial ovarian cancer. J Gynecol Oncol. 2008;19(4):223–8. https://doi.org/10.3802/jgo.2008.19.4.223.

12. Benedetti-Panici P, Greggi S, Maneschi F, Scambia G, Amoroso M, Rabitti C, et al. Anatomical and pathological study of retroperitoneal nodes in epithelial ovarian cancer. Gynecol Oncol. 1993;51(2):150–4. https://doi.org/10.1006/gyno.1993.1263.
13. Burghardt E, Girardi F, Lahousen M, Tamussino K, Stettner H. Patterns of pelvic and paraaortic lymph node involvement in ovarian cancer. Gynecol Oncol. 1991;40(2):103–6.
14. Nomura H, Tsuda H, Susumu N, Fujii T, Banno K, Kataoka F, et al. Lymph node metastasis in grossly apparent stages I and II epithelial ovarian cancer. Int J Gynecol Cancer. 2010;20(3):341–5. https://doi.org/10.1111/IGC.0b013e3181cf6271.
15. Ditto A, Martinelli F, Reato C, Kusamura S, Solima E, Fontanelli R, et al. Systematic para-aortic and pelvic lymphadenectomy in early stage epithelial ovarian cancer: a prospective study. Ann Surg Oncol. 2012;19(12):3849–55. https://doi.org/10.1245/s10434-012-2439-7.
16. Oshita T, Itamochi H, Nishimura R, Numa F, Takehara K, Hiura M, et al. Clinical impact of systematic pelvic and para-aortic lymphadenectomy for pT1 and pT2 ovarian cancer: a retrospective survey by the Sankai Gynecology Study Group. Int J Clin Oncol. 2013;18(6):1107–13. https://doi.org/10.1007/s10147-012-0483-8.
17. Onda T, Yoshikawa H, Yokota H, Yasugi T, Taketani Y. Assessment of metastases to aortic and pelvic lymph nodes in epithelial ovarian carcinoma. A proposal for essential sites for lymph node biopsy. Cancer. 1996;78(4):803–8. https://doi.org/10.1002/(SICI)1097-0142(19960815)78:4<803::AID-CNCR17>3.0.CO;2-Z.
18. Carnino F, Fuda G, Ciccone G, Iskra L, Guercio E, Dadone D, et al. Significance of lymph node sampling in epithelial carcinoma of the ovary. Gynecol Oncol. 1997;65(3):467–72. https://doi.org/10.1006/gyno.1997.4633.
19. Chen SS, Lee L. Incidence of para-aortic and pelvic lymph node metastases in epithelial carcinoma of the ovary. Gynecol Oncol. 1983;16(1):95–100.
20. Morice P, Joulie F, Camatte S, Atallah D, Rouzier R, Pautier P, et al. Lymph node involvement in epithelial ovarian cancer: analysis of 276 pelvic and paraaortic lymphadenectomies and surgical implications. J Am Coll Surg. 2003;197(2):198–205. https://doi.org/10.1016/S1072-7515(03)00234-5.
21. Burghardt E, Pickel H, Lahousen M, Stettner H. Pelvic lymphadenectomy in operative treatment of ovarian cancer. Am J Obstet Gynecol. 1986;155(2):315–9.
22. Wu PC, Qu JY, Lang JH, Huang RL, Tang MY, Lian LJ. Lymph node metastasis of ovarian cancer: a preliminary survey of 74 cases of lymphadenectomy. Am J Obstet Gynecol. 1986;155(5):1103–8.
23. Knapp RC, Friedman EA. Aortic lymph node metastases in early ovarian cancer. Am J Obstet Gynecol. 1974;119(8):1013–7.
24. di Re F, Baiocchi G, Fontanelli R, Grosso G, Cobellis L, Raspagliesi F, et al. Systematic pelvic and paraaortic lymphadenectomy for advanced ovarian cancer: prognostic significance of node metastases. Gynecol Oncol. 1996;62(3):360–5. https://doi.org/10.1006/gyno.1996.0249.
25. Tsumura N, Sakuragi N, Hareyama H, Satoh C, Oikawa M, Yamada H, et al. Distribution pattern and risk factors of pelvic and para-aortic lymph node metastasis in epithelial ovarian carcinoma. Int J Cancer. 1998;79(5):526–30.
26. Yuan Y, Gu ZX, Tao XF, Liu SY. Computer tomography, magnetic resonance imaging, and positron emission tomography or positron emission tomography/computer tomography for detection of metastatic lymph nodes in patients with ovarian cancer: a meta-analysis. Eur J Radiol. 2012;81(5):1002–6. https://doi.org/10.1016/j.ejrad.2011.01.112.
27. Petru E, Lahousen M, Tamussino K, Pickel H, Stranzl H, Stettner H, et al. Lymphadenectomy in stage I ovarian cancer. Am J Obstet Gynecol. 1994;170(2):656–62.
28. Young RC, Decker DG, Wharton JT, Piver MS, Sindelar WF, Edwards BK, et al. Staging laparotomy in early ovarian cancer. JAMA. 1983;250(22):3072–6.
29. Trimbos JB, Vergote I, Bolis G, Vermorken JB, Mangioni C, Madronal C, et al. Impact of adjuvant chemotherapy and surgical staging in early-stage ovarian carcinoma: European Organisation for Research and Treatment of Cancer-Adjuvant ChemoTherapy in Ovarian Neoplasm trial. J Natl Cancer Inst. 2003;95(2):113–25.

30. Chan JK, Munro EG, Cheung MK, Husain A, Teng NN, Berek JS, et al. Association of lymphadenectomy and survival in stage I ovarian cancer patients. Obstet Gynecol. 2007;109(1):12–9. https://doi.org/10.1097/01.AOG.0000249610.95885.ef.
31. du Bois A, Reuss A, Harter P, Pujade-Lauraine E, Ray-Coquard I, Pfisterer J, et al. Potential role of lymphadenectomy in advanced ovarian cancer: a combined exploratory analysis of three prospectively randomized phase III multicenter trials. J Clin Oncol. 2010;28(10):1733–9. https://doi.org/10.1200/JCO.2009.25.3617.
32. Di Re F, Baiocchi G. Value of lymph node assessment in ovarian cancer: Status of the art at the end of the second millennium. Int J Gynecol Cancer. 2000;10(6):435–42.
33. Kimball RE, Schlaerth JB, Kute TE, Schlaerth AC, Santoso J, Ballon SC, et al. Flow cytometric analysis of lymph node metastases in advanced ovarian cancer: clinical and biologic significance. Am J Obstet Gynecol. 1997;176(6):1319–26; discussion 26–7
34. Maggioni A, Benedetti Panici P, Dell'Anna T, Landoni F, Lissoni A, Pellegrino A, et al. Randomised study of systematic lymphadenectomy in patients with epithelial ovarian cancer macroscopically confined to the pelvis. Br J Cancer. 2006;95(6):699–704. https://doi.org/10.1038/sj.bjc.6603323.
35. Trimbos JB. Lymphadenectomy in ovarian cancer: standard of care or unnecessary risk. Curr Opin Oncol. 2011;23(5):507–11. https://doi.org/10.1097/CCO.0b013e32834847e7.
36. Chang SJ, Bristow RE, Ryu HS. Prognostic significance of systematic lymphadenectomy as part of primary debulking surgery in patients with advanced ovarian cancer. Gynecol Oncol. 2012;126(3):381–6. https://doi.org/10.1016/j.ygyno.2012.05.014.
37. Bachmann C, Brucker SY, Kraemer B, Rothmund R, Staebler A, Fend F, et al. The prognostic relevance of node metastases in optimally cytoreduced advanced ovarian cancer. J Cancer Res Clin Oncol. 2015;141(8):1475–80. https://doi.org/10.1007/s00432-015-1945-y.
38. Eoh KJ, Lee JY, Yoon JW, Nam EJ, Kim S, Kim SW, et al. Role of systematic lymphadenectomy as part of primary debulking surgery for optimally cytoreduced advanced ovarian cancer: Reappraisal in the era of radical surgery. Oncotarget. 2017;8(23):37807–16. https://doi.org/10.18632/oncotarget.13696.
39. Harter P, Sehouli J, Lorusso D, Reuss A, Vergote I, Marth C, et al. LION: lymphadenectomy in ovarian neoplasms—A prospective randomized AGO study group led gynecologic cancer intergroup trial. J Clin Oncol. 2017;35(15_suppl):abstr 5500. 2017 ASCO Annual Meeting.

Intestinal Surgery

25

Kazuyoshi Kato and Nobuhiro Takeshima

Abstract

As advanced-stage ovarian cancer frequently involves peritoneal dissemination, the surgical complexity including the intestinal resection is often required to achieve a complete cytoreduction. According to the portion and extent of the tumor involvement, various types of intestinal surgery are applied. This chapter will address the surgical techniques of intestinal resection and anastomosis.

Keywords

Ovarian cancer · Intestinal surgery · Small intestine · Large intestine · Modified posterior pelvic exenteration

25.1 Introduction

The majority of patients with primary ovarian cancer present at an advanced stage and are treated by cytoreductive surgery and platinum-based chemotherapy. The most important predictor of survival in advanced-stage ovarian cancer is residual tumor after primary surgery [1–3]. The ability to achieve a complete cytoreduction to the point of no macroscopic residual disease is a significant factor associated with favorable survival outcomes [4]. As advanced-stage ovarian cancer frequently involves peritoneal dissemination, the surgical complexity including the intestinal resection is often required to increase the extent of cytoreduction.

Heitz et al. reported that among 573 patients with ovarian cancer FIGO IIIB–IVB who had undergone primary debulking surgery, resection of large and/or small intestine was necessary in 434 patients (76%). Consequently, almost 90% of these

K. Kato (✉) · N. Takeshima
Department of Gynecology, Cancer Institute Hospital, Koutou-ku, Tokyo, Japan

M. Mikami (ed.), *Surgery for Gynecologic Cancer*, Comprehensive Gynecology and Obstetrics, https://doi.org/10.1007/978-981-13-1519-0_25

patients underwent a macroscopic complete resection (66.7%) or an optimal (diameter of residual tumor, 1–10 mm) cytoreduction (25.1%) [5].

This chapter will address the surgical techniques of intestinal resection and anastomosis.

25.2 Resection of Small Intestine

In cases of advanced-stage ovarian cancer associated with peritoneal dissemination, small bowel surgery is frequently performed. Gynecologic oncologists should decide the length of small bowel resection according to the portion and extent of the tumor involvement. Bulky disease at the root of the superior mesenteric artery and diffuse disseminated lesions on the mesentery are assessed to be not optimally resectable in primary debulking surgery [5, 6]. For such cases, the use of neoadjuvant chemotherapy has improved the extent of a complete cytoreduction that is possible in interval debulking surgery by reducing the surgical burden [4]. After resection of the small intestine, intestinal anastomosis is performed using a hand-sewn or a stapled technique.

25.2.1 Hand-Sewn Technique

The hand-sewn technique is applicable to an end-to-end anastomosis which is preferable to end-to-side and side-to-side anastomoses, because the end-to-end anastomosis restores the continuity of the small intestine more naturally. However, gynecologic oncologists sometimes select the side-to-side anastomosis due to the presence of sudden intestinal obstruction by a strangulated hernia, tumor dissemination, and so on. There are various hand-sewn techniques such as Albert-Lembert anastomosis, Gambee anastomosis, and layer-to-layer anastomosis.

25.2.2 Stapled Technique

We are presenting the case with a portion of the ileum involved by the recurrent ovarian tumor in the right pelvic wall. When the involved ileum was removed from the tumor, full-thickness resection of the portion of the ileum was needed. Then, the lack of the small intestinal wall was temporarily closed by interrupted 3-0 silk sutures.

Functional end-to-end anastomosis is performed as follows:

1. The proximally and distally transection sites of the small intestine are decided, and the mesentery is divided (Fig. 25.1).
2. Traction sutures are placed near the antimesenteric lines of the proximal and distal segments of the small intestine to allow approximation to each other (Figs. 25.2 and 25.3).

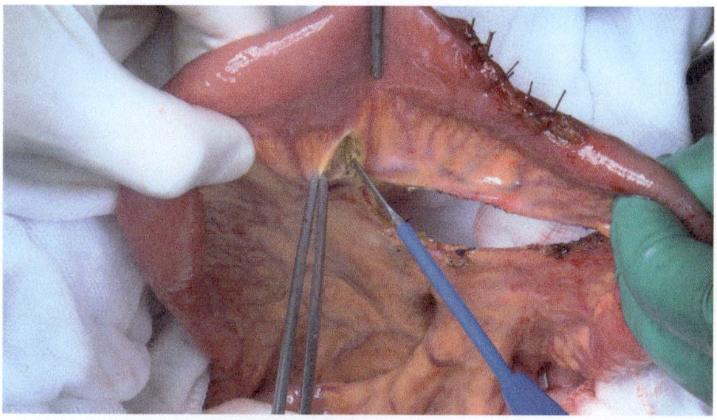

Fig. 25.1 Functional end-to-end anastomosis of the small intestine

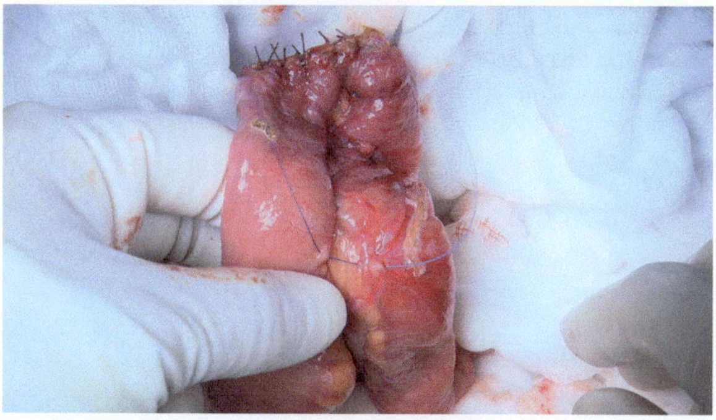

Fig. 25.2 Functional end-to-end anastomosis of the small intestine

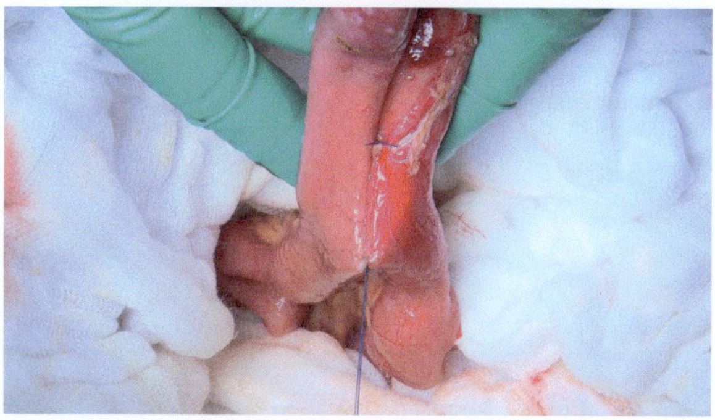

Fig. 25.3 Functional end-to-end anastomosis of the small intestine

3. The linear stapling device is introduced through the holes on the antimesenteric lines of the small intestine (Fig. 25.4).
4. The linear stapler is fired and the common lumen is created (Fig. 25.5).
5. The defect of the segments of the small intestine is clamped and closed using the linear stapling device (Figs. 25.6, 25.7, and 25.8).
6. The enteroenteric continuity can be reestablished (Fig. 25.9).

This method can be applied not only to the enteroenteric but also enterocolonic and colocolonic anastomoses.

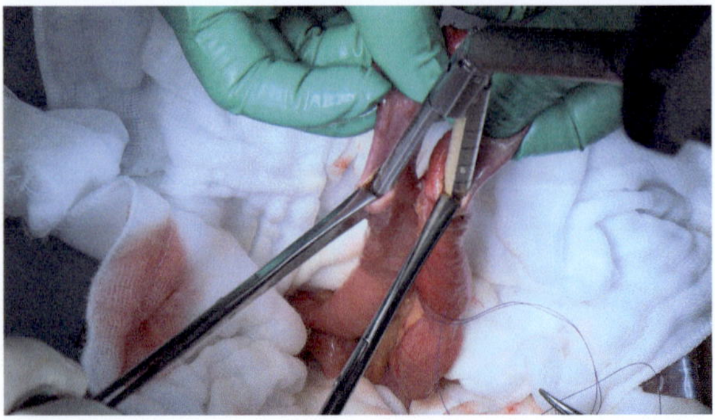

Fig. 25.4 Functional end-to-end anastomosis of the small intestine

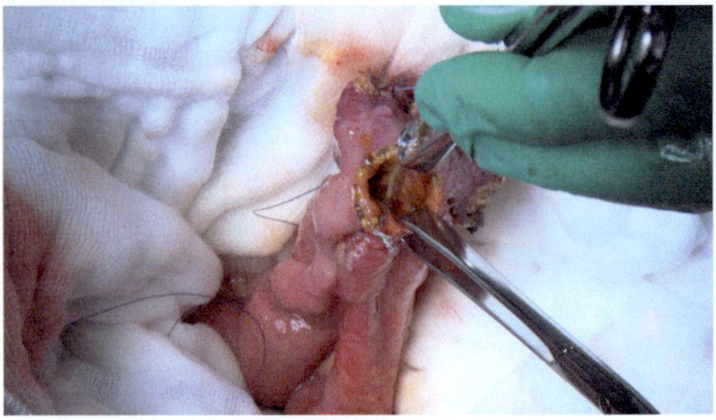

Fig. 25.5 Functional end-to-end anastomosis of the small intestine

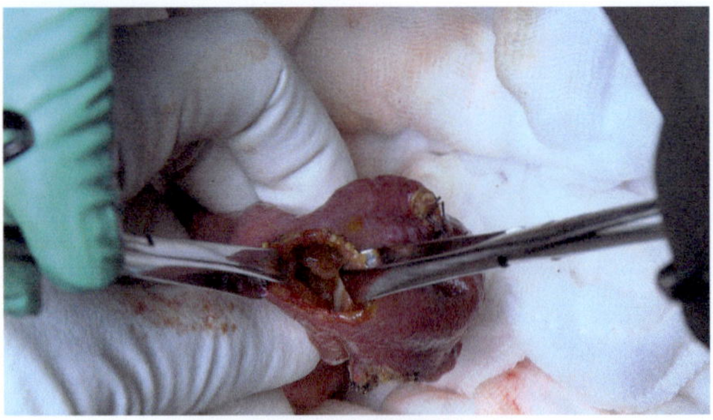

Fig. 25.6 Functional end-to-end anastomosis of the small intestine

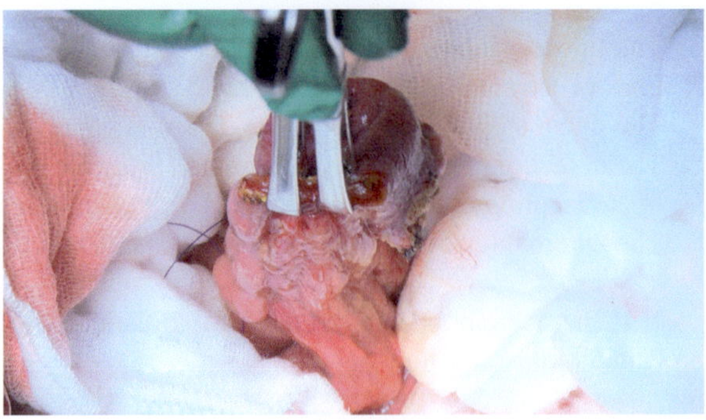

Fig. 25.7 Functional end-to-end anastomosis of the small intestine

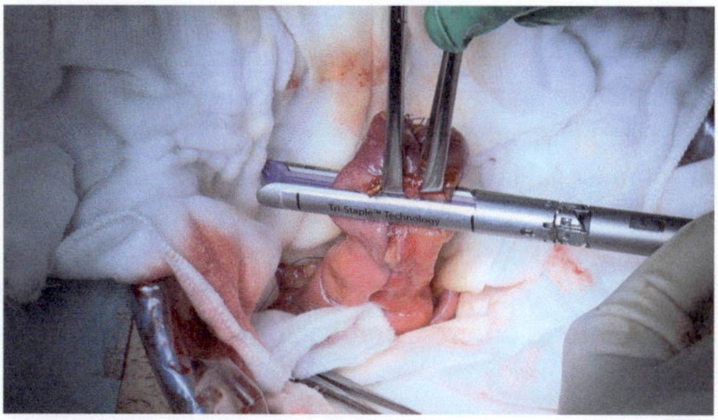

Fig. 25.8 Functional end-to-end anastomosis of the small intestine

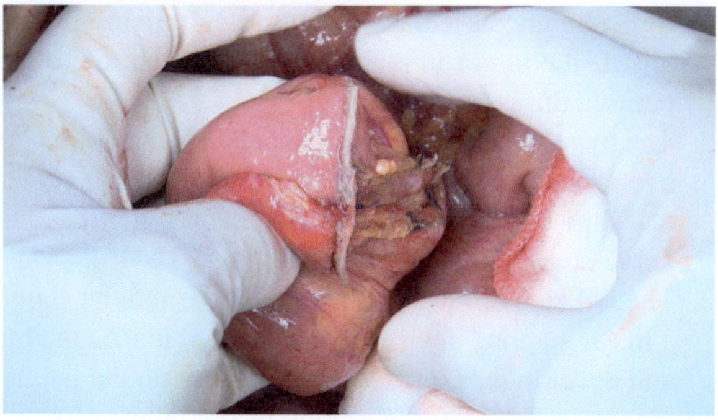

Fig. 25.9 Functional end-to-end anastomosis of the small intestine

25.3 Resection of Large Intestine

During cytoreductive surgery for advanced-stage ovarian cancer, resection of large intestine includes ileocecal resection, right hemicolectomy, transverse colectomy, left hemicolectomy, and sigmoid resection, besides modified posterior pelvic exenteration (anterior resection). Gynecologic oncologists should choose the type of surgical procedure and combine the procedure with each other according to the portion and extent of the tumor involvement. After resection of the large intestine, intestinal anastomosis is performed using a hand-sewn or a stapled technique.

25.3.1 Modified Posterior Pelvic Exenteration

A rectosigmoid resection is the most frequently performed type of bowel surgery because of the anatomic proximity of the rectosigmoid to the female pelvic organs and its frequent involvement in ovarian cancer. Previous investigators have reported that a modified posterior pelvic exenteration, also known as a radical oophorectomy or low anterior en bloc resection, during surgery for ovarian cancer permits a high rate of complete cytoreduction with acceptable morbidity and mortality rates [7–10].

Kato et al. assessed the extents of tumor spreading in the rectosigmoid wall in modified posterior pelvic exenteration specimens from 75 patients with primary ovarian, tubal, and peritoneal cancer [11]. Tumor involvement of the rectosigmoid wall was histopathologically confirmed in 65% of the cases. Invasion to the mucosal or submucosal layer was confirmed in 13%, the muscular layer was in 21%, and the serosal layer was in 31%.

Modified posterior pelvic exenteration was carried out as en bloc resection of the adnexal mass, uterus, pelvic peritoneum, and rectosigmoid. The order of the surgical procedures differs according to the situation. However, we usually perform this surgery as follows:

1. The retroperitoneal space is developed following the ligation and division of the round ligaments and ovarian vessels. Both ureters are identified and moved laterally. If the tumor implants on the anterior side of the pelvis, the anterior pelvic peritoneum is stripped.
2. The hypogastric nerve and the pelvic splanchnic nerves running into the inferior hypogastric plexus are identified in the loose layer hanging down from the ureter, and this layer is preserved in a manner that has been previously described for nerve-sparing radical hysterectomies [12–16].
3. The left side of the colon is mobilized, and the sigmoid colon is transected using a linear stapling device. If primary and metastatic tumors filled the pelvic cavity, and developing a retroperitoneal space on the pelvic sidewall might be impossible, isolation and preservation of the inferior hypogastric plexus are performed following the transection of the sigmoid colon.
4. At the level of the aortic bifurcation, the superior hypogastric plexus is identified. Anterior to the promontory, the superior hypogastric plexus splits into two bundles of hypogastric nerves at the start of the dissection along the parietal pelvic fascia. The dissection is continued laterally and caudally in the avascular plane between the parietal pelvic fascia and the proper rectal fascia. The hypogastric nerves pass inferolaterally along the pelvic sidewall medial to the ureter. The plane of the dissection is then continued to the layer underneath the ureter containing the inferior hypogastric plexus. Consequently, the inferior hypogastric plexus is left to be undamaged on the lateral pelvic wall (Figs. 25.10 and 25.11).
5. After the uterine artery is ligated and divided, the anterior leaf of the vesicouterine ligament is transected, and the ureter is mobilized laterally.
6. If the primary and metastatic tumors in the cul-de-sac invade laterally and posteriorly into the uterosacral ligament and the inferior hypogastric plexus is to be sacrificed, the cardinal ligament and the posterior leaf of the vesicouterine ligament are divided. In the cases with tumor infiltration into the deep retroperitoneal space, the plane of the dissection is placed along the parietal fascia covering the pelvic sidewall and continued to the surfaces of the levator ani and piriformis muscles.
7. The vaginal wall is transected, and the rectum is divided below the peritoneal reflection and inferiorly to a level 1–5 cm below the bottom tip of the tumor

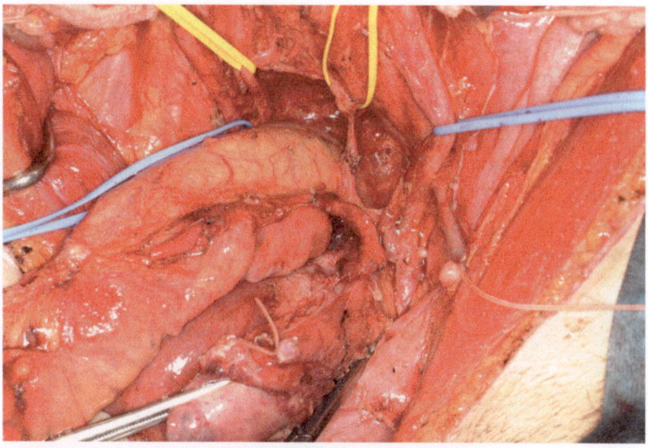

Fig. 25.10 Appearance of the pelvic region during the mobilization of the rectosigmoid. The hypogastric nerves and ureters were isolated and underrun with marker tapes in yellow and blue, respectively

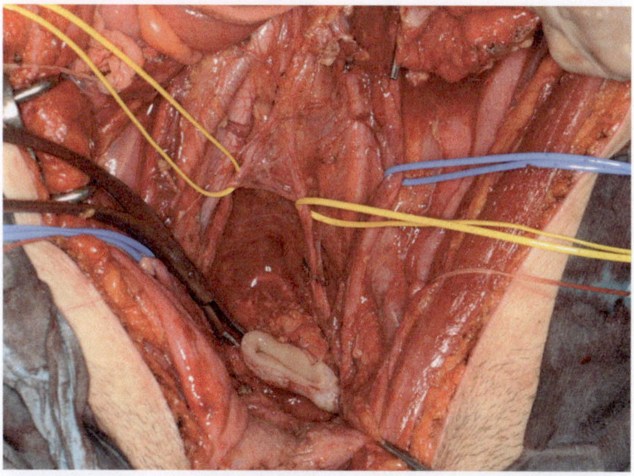

Fig. 25.11 Appearance of the pelvic region following the en bloc resection of the ovarian tumor with the uterus and rectosigmoid. The hypogastric nerves and ureters were isolated and underrun with marker tapes in yellow and blue, respectively

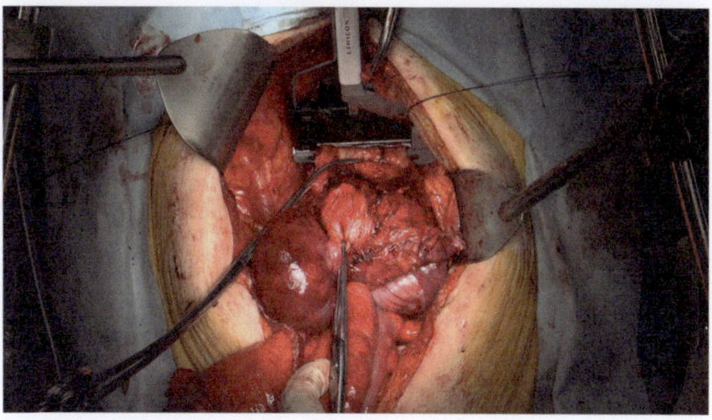

Figs. 25.12 The rectum is transected using the linear stapling device. Then, an en bloc resection of the pelvic tumors together with the uterus and rectosigmoid colon can be performed

(Fig. 25.12). Consequently, an en bloc resection of the pelvic tumors together with the uterus and rectosigmoid colon can be accomplished.

8. Finally, end-to-end or side-to-end colorectal anastomosis is performed using a circular stapling device or a hand-sewn technique (Figs. 25.13, 25.14, and 25.15).

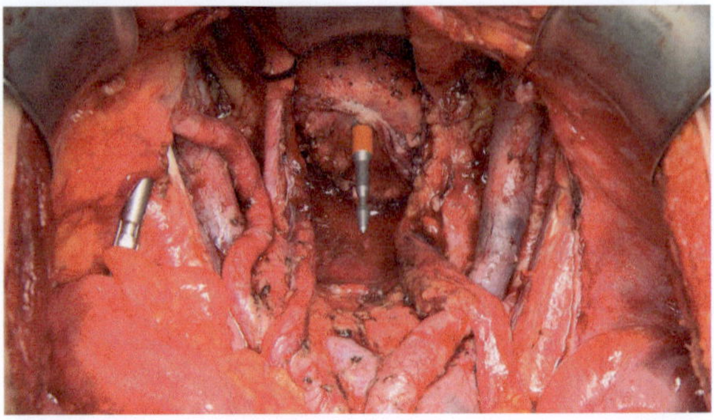

Fig. 25.13 The stapled end-to-end colorectal anastomosis using the double stapling technique. The circular stapling device is transanally inserted, and the rectal stump is penetrated by the central rod

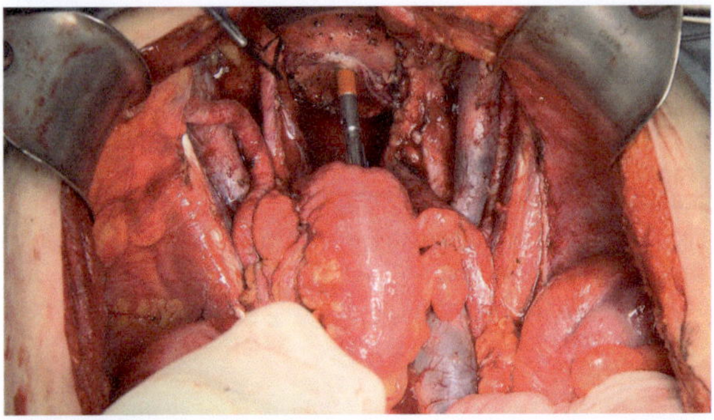

Fig. 25.14 The anvil is inserted into the stump of the left side of the colon, and the anvil shaft is connected to the central rod of the circular stapling device

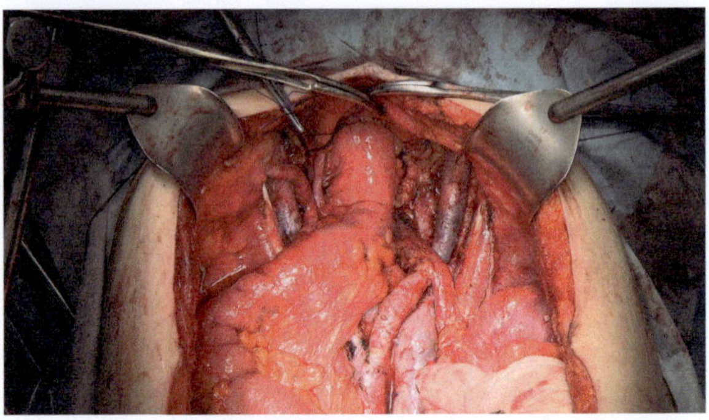

Fig. 25.15 The approximation of the ends of the colon and rectum is completed, and the circular stapling device is fired to create the common lumen

25.3.2 Hand-Sewn Technique

With the advances in medical instrumentation, gynecologic oncologists prefer stapled technique to hand-sewn technique. However, there are cases for which the hand-sewn method is suitable. There are various hand-sewn techniques such as Albert-Lembert anastomosis, Gambee anastomosis, and layer-to-layer anastomosis. In this paragraph, we are focusing a description on procedures during layer-to-layer anastomosis. During the operation of modified posterior pelvic exenteration, the

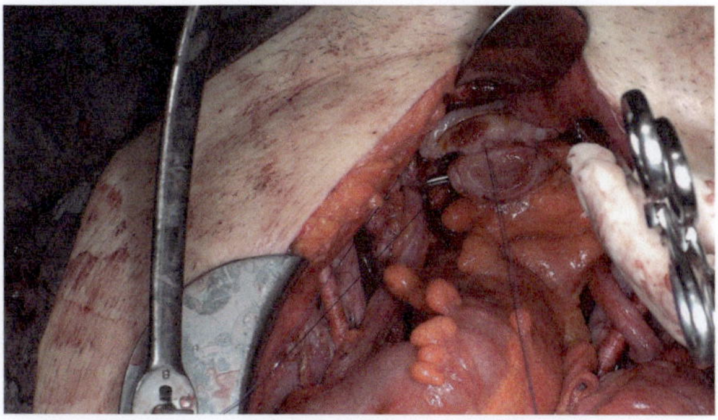

Fig. 25.16 Hand-sewn technique for layer-to-layer colorectal anastomosis

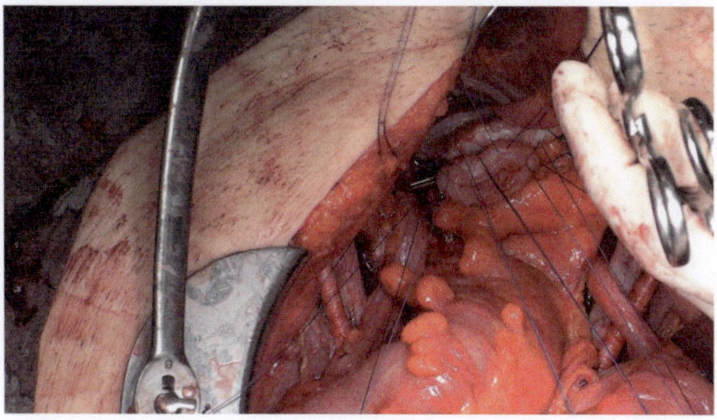

Fig. 25.17 Hand-sewn technique for layer-to-layer colorectal anastomosis

procedures of colorectal anastomosis following the en bloc resection of the ovarian tumor with the uterus and rectosigmoid are presented:

1. To gain approximation to the rectal stump, descending colon is sufficiently mobilized.
2. Interrupted sutures are placed through the posterior seromuscular edges of both the mobilized colon and rectal stump (Figs. 25.16 and 25.17).
3. A double-ended suture is tightened in the lateral edges of the mobilized colon and rectal stump. This continues a running suture through the posterior mucosal and submucosal layers (Figs. 25.18 and 25.19).
4. The anterior mucosa and submucosa are closed by a running suture with the other side of the double-ended suture (Figs. 25.20 and 25.21).
5. The anterior seromuscular layers are closed by interrupted sutures (Fig. 25.22). Then, the colorectal continuity can be reestablished.

25.3.3 Anastomotic Leakage

Previous investigators have reported that intestinal surgery for ovarian cancer permits a high rate of complete cytoreduction with acceptable morbidity and mortality

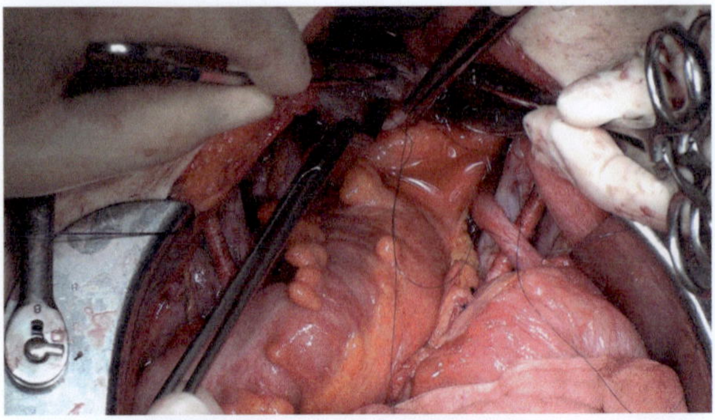

Fig. 25.18 Hand-sewn technique for layer-to-layer colorectal anastomosis

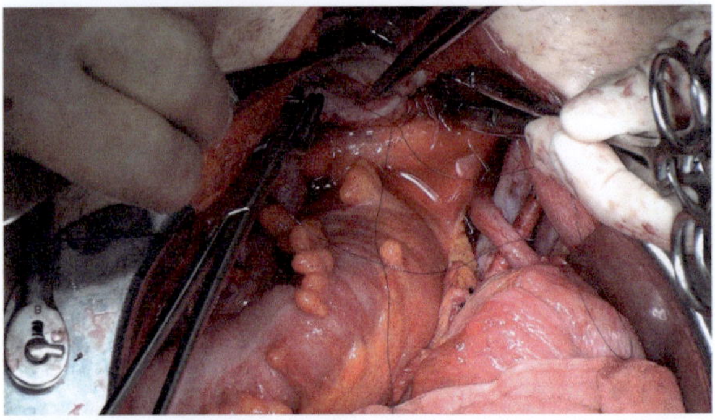

Fig. 25.19 Hand-sewn technique for layer-to-layer colorectal anastomosis

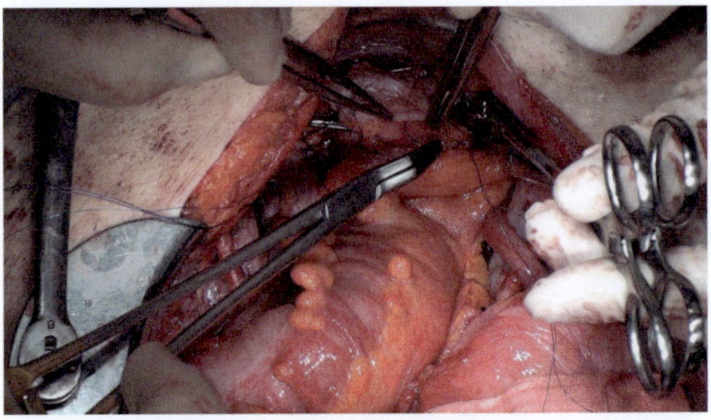

Fig. 25.20 Hand-sewn technique for layer-to-layer colorectal anastomosis

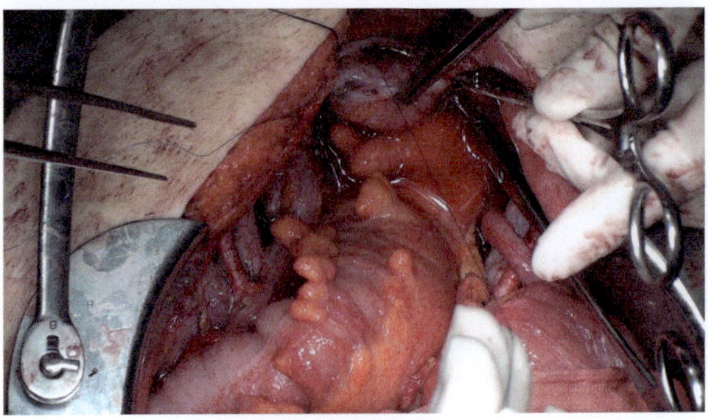

Fig. 25.21 Hand-sewn technique for layer-to-layer colorectal anastomosis

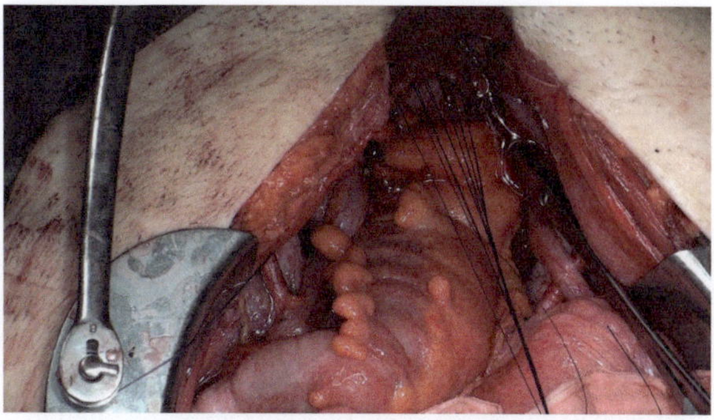

Fig. 25.22 Hand-sewn technique for layer-to-layer colorectal anastomosis

rates [17]. Despite advances in surgical techniques and medical instrumentation, however, anastomotic leakage remains the most serious complication of large bowel resections for ovarian cancer [18]. Especially, the occurrence of anastomotic leakage after modified posterior pelvic exenteration has been relatively higher than that with other various intestinal resections. The incidence of anastomotic leakage has been reported to range between 0.8% and 10% among patients undergoing modified posterior pelvic exenteration for ovarian cancer [9, 18–21].

A diverting colostomy and ileostomy are commonly used in colorectal surgery to reduce anastomotic complications, especially life-threatening ones such as fecal peritonitis or sepsis [22, 23]. In gynecologic literature, some reports have shown that diverting stomas have the potential to decrease the frequency of anastomotic leakage in ovarian cancer patients undergoing rectosigmoid resection. Houvenaeghel et al. analyzed a retrospective data of 305 patients who underwent MPPE during up-front surgery, interval debulking surgery, or secondary debulking surgery from 9 French cancer centers [24]. They reported that 59 patients (20%) received a diverting stoma and the overall anastomotic leakage rate was 8%. In their study, there was no significant difference in the rates of anastomotic leakage according to the presence or the absence of the diverting stoma. Tseng et al. reported that among 331 patients with stage II–IV ovarian cancer who underwent colon resection during up-front surgery, 44 (13%) received a diverting ileostomy [25]. The overall anastomotic leakage rate was 6%. They concluded that patients with a longer operative time and a greater length of rectosigmoid resection more commonly underwent a diverting ileostomy; however, the presence of a diverting ileostomy did not compromise the postoperative outcomes or long-term survival. Kalogera et al. reported that among 77 patients with gynecologic malignancies who underwent rectosigmoid resection, 27 (35%) received a diverting stoma [26]. The rate of anastomotic leakage was 2.6%. They advocated the creation of a diverting stoma if any of the following factors are present: preoperative albumin $\leq$3.0 g/dL; prior pelvic radiation; MPPE plus additional large bowel resection; anastomosis at $\leq$6 cm from the anal verge; non-tension-free anastomosis or signs of bowel ischemia; leakage identified intraoperatively during a proctoscopy or leak test; gross contamination of the pelvis with stool or infection present at time of resection; or a surgeon's intraoperative concerns regarding the integrity of the anastomosis.

25.3.4 Challenges and Future Directions

There have been many reports that elevation of optimal cytoreductive rates in primary surgery resulted in improvement of progression-free and overall survival in advanced-stage ovarian cancer [27, 28]. In order to improve optimal cytoreductive rates, surgical efforts by incorporating extensive upper abdominal surgery into the primary cytoreductive effort are necessary. Surgical procedures included intestinal resection and/or diaphragm peritonectomy resection, splenectomy, distal pancreatectomy, partial liver resection, cholecystectomy, and resection of tumor from the porta hepatis [3]. Also in the Japanese literature, a paradigm shift in surgical approach to advanced-stage ovarian cancer resulted in the elevation of optimal cytoreductive rates and better survival outcomes without causing a significant increase in morbidity and mortality [29]. In their study, the respective median progression-free and overall survival rates increased from 14.6 and 38.1 months before implementing an aggressive surgery protocol in the department of gynecology, respectively, to 25.0 and 68.5 months after implementation, respectively. Of course, such aggressive surgery should not be performed at any institutions. Specialist surgical teams in the department of gynecologic oncology, composed of experts with interests and skills in cytoreductive surgery on multiple organs, should accomplish the operation with surgical complexity [27, 28]. Improvement of the surgical skills and postoperative management of the gynecologic oncologists is necessary to achieve optimal cytoreduction for advanced-stage ovarian cancer. In addition, the passion of the gynecologic oncologists to accomplish the operation with increased surgical complexity is the most important.

References

1. Chang SJ, Bristow RE, Ryu HS. Impact of complete cytoreduction leaving no gross residual disease associated with radical cytoreductive surgical procedures on survival in advanced ovarian cancer. Ann Surg Oncol. 2012;19:4059–67.
2. Du Bois A, Reuss A, Pujade-Lauraine E, Harter P, Ray-Coquard I, Pfisterer J. Role of surgical outcome as prognostic factor in advanced epithelial ovarian cancer: a combined exploratory analysis of 3 prospectively randomized phase 3 multicenter trials: by the Arbeitsgemeinschaft Gynaekologische Onkologie Studiengruppe Ovarialkarzinom (AGO-OVAR) and the Groupe d'Investigateurs Nationaux Pour les Etudes des Cancers de l'Ovaire (GINECO). Cancer. 2009;115:1234–44.
3. Chi DS, Eisenhauer EL, Zivanovic O, Sonoda Y, Abu-Rustum NR, Levine DA, et al. Improved progression-free and overall survival in advanced ovarian cancer as a result of a change in surgical paradigm. Gynecol Oncol. 2009;114:26–31.
4. Chang SJ, Hodeib M, Chang J, Bristow RE. Survival impact of complete cytoreduction to no gross residual disease for advanced-stage ovarian cancer: a meta-analysis. Gynecol Oncol. 2013;130:493–8.
5. Heitz F, Harter P, Alesina PF, Walz MK, Lorenz D, Groeben H, et al. Pattern of and reason for postoperative residual disease in patients with advanced ovarian cancer following upfront radical debulking surgery. Gynecol Oncol. 2016;141:264–70.
6. Fotopoulou C, Richter R, Braicu EI, Schmidt SC, Lichtenegger W, Sehouli J. Can complete tumor resection be predicted in advanced primary epithelial ovarian cancer? A systematic evaluation of 360 consecutive patients. Eur J Surg Oncol. 2010;36:1202–10.

7. Kato K, Tate S, Nishikimi K, Shozu M. Bladder function after modified posterior exenteration for primary gynecological cancer. Gynecol Oncol. 2013;129:229–33.
8. Aletti GD, Podratz KC, Jones MB, Cliby WA. Role of rectosigmoidectomy and stripping of pelvic peritoneum in outcomes of patients with advanced ovarian cancer. J Am Coll Surg. 2006;203:521–6.
9. Bristow RE, del Carmen MG, Kaufman HS, Montz FJ. Radical oophorectomy with primary stapled colorectal anastomosis for resection of locally advanced epithelial ovarian cancer. J Am Coll Surg. 2003;197:565–74.
10. Eisenkop SM, Nalick RH, Teng NN. Modified posterior exenteration for ovarian cancer. Obstet Gynecol. 1991;78:879–85.
11. Kato K, Nishikimi K, Tate S, Kiyokawa T, Shozu M. Histopathologic tumor spreading in primary ovarian cancer with modified posterior exenteration. World J Surg Oncol. 2015;13:230.
12. Raspagliesi F, Ditto A, Fontanelli R, Solima E, Hanozet F, Zanaboni F, et al. Nerve-sparing radical hysterectomy: a surgical technique for preserving the autonomic hypogastric nerve. Gynecol Oncol. 2004;93:307–14.
13. Kato K, Suzuka K, Osaki T, Tanaka N. Unilateral or bilateral nerve-sparing radical hysterectomy: a surgical technique to preserve the pelvic autonomic nerves while increasing radicality. Int J Gynecol Cancer. 2007;17:1172–8.
14. Fujii S, Takakura K, Matsumura N, Higuchi T, Yura S, Mandai M, et al. Anatomic identification and functional outcomes of the nerve sparing Okabayashi radical hysterectomy. Gynecol Oncol. 2007;107:4–13.
15. Sakuragi N, Todo Y, Kudo M, Yamamoto R, Sato T. A systematic nerve-sparing radical hysterectomy technique in invasive cervical cancer for preserving postsurgical bladder function. Int J Gynecol Cancer. 2005;15:389–97.
16. Trimbos JB, Maas CP, Deruiter MC, Peters AA, Kenter GG. A nerve-sparing radical hysterectomy: guidelines and feasibility in Western patients. Int J Gynecol Cancer. 2001;11:180–6.
17. Grimm C, Harter P, Alesina PF, Prader S, Schneider S, Ataseven B, et al. The impact of type and number of bowel resections on anastomotic leakage risk in advanced ovarian cancer surgery. Gynecol Oncol. 2017;146(3):498–503.
18. Richardson DL, Mariani A, Cliby WA. Risk factors for anastomotic leak after recto-sigmoid resection for ovarian cancer. Gynecol Oncol. 2006;103:667–72.
19. Mourton SM, Temple LK, Abu-Rustum NR, Gemignani ML, Sonoda Y, Bochner BH, et al. Morbidity of rectosigmoid resection and primary anastomosis in patients undergoing primary cytoreductive surgery for advanced epithelial ovarian cancer. Gynecol Oncol. 2005;99:608–14.
20. Park JY, Seo SS, Kang S, Lee KB, Lim SY, Choi HS, et al. The benefits of low anterior en bloc resection as part of cytoreductive surgery for advanced primary and recurrent epithelial ovarian cancer patients outweigh morbidity concerns. Gynecol Oncol. 2006;103:977–84.
21. Clayton RD, Obermair A, Hammond IG, Leung YC, McCartney AJ. The Western Australian experience of the use of en bloc resection of ovarian cancer with concomitant rectosigmoid colectomy. Gynecol Oncol. 2002;84:53–7.
22. Matthiessen P, Hallböök O, Rutegård J, Simert G, Sjödahl R. Defunctioning stoma reduces symptomatic anastomotic leakage after low anterior resection of the rectum for cancer: a randomized multicenter trial. Ann Surg. 2007;246:207–14.
23. Tan WS, Tang CL, Shi L, Eu KW. Meta-analysis of defunctioning stomas in low anterior resection for rectal cancer. Br J Surg. 2009;96:462–72.
24. Houvenaeghel G, Gutowski M, Buttarelli M, Cuisenier J, Narducci F, Dalle C, et al. Modified posterior pelvic exenteration for ovarian cancer. Int J Gynecol Cancer. 2009;19:968–73.
25. Tseng JH, Suidan RS, Zivanovic O, Gardner GJ, Sonoda Y, Levine DA, et al. Diverting ileostomy during primary debulking surgery for ovarian cancer: associated factors and postoperative outcomes. Gynecol Oncol. 2016;142:217–24.
26. Kalogera E, Nitschmann CC, Dowdy SC, Cliby WA, Langstraat CL. A prospective algorithm to reduce anastomotic leaks after rectosigmoid resection for gynecologic malignancies. Gynecol Oncol. 2017;144:343–7.

27. Harter P, Muallem ZM, Buhrmann C, Lorenz D, Kaub C, Hils R, et al. Impact of a structured quality management program on surgical outcome in primary advanced ovarian cancer. Gynecol Oncol. 2011;121:615–9.
28. Bristow RE, Chang J, Ziogas A, Randall LM, Anton-Culver HG. High-volume ovarian cancer care: survival impact and disparities in access for advanced-stage disease. Gynecol Oncol. 2014;132:403–10.
29. Tate S, Kato K, Nishikimi K, Matsuoka A, Shozu M. Survival and safety associated with aggressive surgery for stage III/IV epithelial ovarian cancer: a single institution observation study. Gynecol Oncol. 2017;147(1):73–80.

Interval Debulking Surgery

26

Takashi Onda

Abstract

Standard treatment of ovarian cancer consists of debulking surgery and chemotherapy. Primary debulking surgery (PDS) with maximum debulking efforts, followed by chemotherapy, has been the treatment of choice for patients with advanced ovarian cancer. Interval debulking surgery (IDS) is performed in the following two situations: (1) debulking (second challenge) for patients with suboptimal PDS and (2) debulking (first challenge) following neoadjuvant chemotherapy (NAC) in patients for whom PDS is not indicated. The efficacy of IDS after suboptimal PDS is controversial, as shown by three prospective randomized studies. IDS after suboptimal PDS is considered only when primary surgery was not performed by gynecologic oncologists or when the surgery was performed with less extensive efforts. Regarding IDS after NAC, three prospective randomized studies have been conducted. In the first two studies, the survival outcome of patients who underwent NAC treatment (NACT) was non-inferior to those who underwent PDS treatment (PDST). Morbidity in patients who underwent NACT tended to be reduced in one study and significantly reduced in two studies. However, the surgical efforts in these studies investigating NACT compared to PDST have received criticism. A prospective randomized study including only centers with externally proven surgical expertise and audited by experienced surgeons was initiated to compare maximum effort PDS with equally maximum effort NACT–IDS. However, currently, NACT–IDS is becoming widely adopted in advanced ovarian cancer. In contrast, IDS for patients with suboptimal PDS will certainly be decreased as a result of the wide adoption of NACT.

T. Onda (✉)
Kitasato University School of Medicine, Sagamihara, Kanagawa, Japan
e-mail: takashi-tky@umin.ac.jp

M. Mikami (ed.), *Surgery for Gynecologic Cancer*, Comprehensive Gynecology and Obstetrics, https://doi.org/10.1007/978-981-13-1519-0_26

Keywords
Ovarian cancer · Primary debulking surgery · Interval debulking surgery · Neoadjuvant chemotherapy

26.1 Introduction

Standard treatment of ovarian cancer consists of debulking surgery and chemotherapy. Griffiths et al. [1] first reported the correlation between the size of residual tumor after primary debulking surgery (PDS) and the prognosis of patients with advanced ovarian cancer. Thereafter, numerous investigators reported that patients who underwent optimal PDS had better survival compared to those with suboptimal PDS. Optimal surgery was initially defined as surgery with residual tumor less than 1–3 cm in diameter. Suboptimal surgery stands for nonoptimal surgery. PDS with maximum debulking efforts followed by chemotherapy has been the treatment of choice for patients with advanced ovarian cancer. However, optimal PDS is achieved in only 30–60% of patients with advanced ovarian cancer at most institutions. For those who underwent suboptimal PDS, debulking surgery is repeated, as secondary surgery, after two to six cycles of induction chemotherapy. This secondary surgery is termed interval debulking surgery (IDS). On the other hand, patients with very advanced disease—an apparently unresectable tumor or poor performance status (PS) due to the disease itself or medical complications—for whom suboptimal PDS is expected initially receive chemotherapy followed by debulking surgery. This chemotherapy is termed neoadjuvant chemotherapy (NAC), and the first debulking surgery following NAC is also referred to as IDS. These two types of IDS are presented in this chapter.

26.2 IDS Following Suboptimal PDS

26.2.1 Secondary Debulking Surgery for Patients Who Underwent Suboptimal PDS

Initially, secondary debulking surgery for patients who underwent suboptimal PDS was attempted after chemotherapy was completed, e.g., at the timing of second-look operation. However, this secondary surgery performed after the completion of chemotherapy was not linked to a survival advantage, as demonstrated by several studies [2, 3].

Wils et al. [4] compared treatment outcomes of patients who underwent optimal PDS (N = 38) and those of patients with primary non-debulkable disease who underwent secondary debulking surgery after a median of three (range, 2–6) cycles of chemotherapy (N = 18). The difference in histologically confirmed complete remission rates of evaluable patients was not statistically significant between these patient groups (50% vs. 29%, $p = 0.23$). In addition, the 3-year overall survival (OS) rates of these patient groups were similar (60% vs. 50%). Lawton et al. [5] confirmed the feasibility of secondary debulking surgery. Among 36 patients with epithelial ovarian cancer incompletely resected at primary laparotomy, 78% (28/36 patients) underwent secondary debulking surgery following three cycles of chemotherapy. This surgery resulted in 57% (16/28) of patients without macroscopic disease, whereas 18% (5/28 patients) and 14% (4/28 patients) had <1 cm and <2 cm residual disease, respectively. Postsurgical complications were few.

These two studies [4, 5] demonstrated the efficacy of secondary debulking surgery and used the term intervention (debulking) surgery in their reports.

26.2.2 Results of Phase III Studies

Prospective randomized studies have been conducted to further assess the effectiveness of IDS. Thus far, the results of three studies from the UK group, EORTC (European Organization for Research and Treatment of Cancer), and GOG (Gynecologic Oncology Group) have been reported.

26.2.2.1 Study from the United Kingdom

The UK group, including Lawton's institution, conducted the first prospective randomized study of IDS for patients who previously underwent suboptimal PDS. Redman et al. [6] reported the results that are shown in Table 26.1. A total of 79 patients were enrolled in the study. Of those, 37 patients were randomized to IDS, 25 (68%) of whom underwent IDS performed at a median of 13 weeks following PDS. The remaining 42 patients in this study were randomized to chemotherapy alone. The median OS rates for the IDS and chemotherapy alone groups were 15 months (95% confidence interval [CI] 10–20 months) and 12 months (95% CI 8–16 months), respectively. The difference between the groups was not statistically significant (hazard ratio [HR] = 0.71; 95% CI 0.44–1.13). The conclusion of this study was that IDS following suboptimal PDS may not improve survival in patients with advanced ovarian cancer.

26.2.2.2 EORTC Study

The EORTC conducted the first large-scale prospective randomized study of IDS. van der Burg et al. [7] reported the results that are presented in Table 26.1. Of the 319 patients who were enrolled and underwent randomization, 278 were evaluable (140 patients who underwent debulking surgery and 138 patients who did not). They called the surgery just "debulking surgery" in this report. Progression-free survival (PFS) and OS were both significantly longer in patients who underwent IDS compared to those who did not ($p = 0.01$). The difference in median OS was 6 months (26 vs. 20 months, respectively). A 2-year OS was reported in 56% and 46%, respectively. Multivariate analysis showed that IDS was an independent prognostic factor ($p = 0.012$). Overall, after adjustment for all other prognostic factors, IDS reduced the risk of death by 33% (95% CI 10–50%; $p = 0.008$). IDS was not associated with death or severe morbidity. The investigators concluded that IDS

Table 26.1 Prospective randomized studies for the efficacy of IDS in patients with suboptimal PDS

Group	UK group		EORTC		GOG	
Initial stage	IIB–III–IV[a]		IIB–III–IV		III–IV[b]	
Residual tumor by PDS	≥2 cm		≥1 cm		≥1 cm	
PDS performed by gynecologic oncologist	10%		Not indicated		95%	
CTx regimen	CP or PAB		CP		TP	
No. of cycles	≤8 cycles		6 cycles		6 cycles	
Randomization	At enrollment		After 3 cycles		After 3 cycles	
IDS	As soon as possible		After 3 cycles		After 3 cycles	
Arms	IDS(+)	IDS(−)	IDS(+)	IDS(−)	IDS(+)	IDS(−)
No. of Pts evaluated	$N = 37$	$N = 42$	$N = 140$	$N = 138$	$N = 216$	$N = 208$
Median OS	15 M	12 M	26 M	20 M	34 M	34 M
Significance	NS		$p = 0.012$		NS	
Median PFS	NA	NA	18 M	13 M	11 M	11 M
Significance			$p = 0.013$		NS	
IDS performed	68% (25/37)		93% (130/140)		93% (201/216)	
Optimal IDS	51% (19/37)		58% (81/140)		78% (168/216)	

CTx chemotherapy, *CP* cyclophosphamide + cisplatin, *PAB* cisplatin + doxorubicin + bleomycin, *TP* paclitaxel + cisplatin, *EORTC* European Organization for Research and Treatment of Cancer, *GOG* Gynecologic Oncology Group, *IDS* interval debulking surgery, *NS* not significant

[a]Stage IV was restricted to patients with malignant pleural effusion only

[b]Stage IV was restricted to patients with malignant pleural effusion only or resected anterior abdominal wall tumor

significantly prolonged PFS and OS. Based on these findings, IDS following suboptimal PDS and induction chemotherapy was much expected to improve the survival of patients.

26.2.2.3 GOG Study

The GOG conducted a similar large-scale prospective randomized study of IDS. Unexpectedly, Rose et al. [8] contradicted the previous findings reported by the EORTC (Table 26.1). They called the surgery as "interval debulking surgery" or "secondary surgery" in their report. A total of 550 patients were enrolled. Following the completion of three cycles of postoperative chemotherapy, 216 and 208 eligible patients were randomized to receive IDS followed by chemotherapy or chemotherapy alone, respectively. Surgery was declined by or medically contraindicated for 15 patients assigned to the IDS group (7%). The likelihood of PFS in the IDS group, as compared to the chemotherapy alone group, was 1.07 (95% CI 0.87–1.31; $p = 0.54$), and the relative risk of death was 0.99 (95% CI 0.79–1.24; $p = 0.92$). The investigators emphasized the differences regarding the surgical efforts to maximize debulking and the resultant residual tumor size by PDS between their study and EORTC study. PDS was performed by gynecologic oncologist in 95% of patients in the GOG study. Therefore, the investigators concluded that in patients with advanced ovarian carcinoma for whom PDS was considered to be maximal, IDS in combination with postoperative chemotherapy may not improve PFS or OS. In addition, the difference in chemotherapy regimen used was highlighted as a possible cause of the discrepancy observed in the results of these studies. The EORTC study predated the use of paclitaxel for ovarian cancer in Europe; thus the study adopted a combination of cyclophosphamide and cisplatin, which was later replaced by the combination of paclitaxel and cisplatin adopted in the GOG study.

26.2.3 Results of Meta-analyses

Tangjitgamol et al. [9] conducted a systematic review and meta-analysis for IDS following suboptimal PDS and induction chemotherapy. In this systematic review, the three randomized studies discussed earlier in this chapter were selected for analysis. The meta-analysis of these three studies (including a total of 781 patients) for OS found no statistically significant difference between IDS and chemotherapy alone (HR = 0.80, 95% CI 0.61–1.06). Subgroup analysis of two studies (357 patients) in which the primary surgery was not performed by gynecologic oncologists (EORTC study) or was less extensive (UK study) showed a benefit of IDS in OS (HR = 0.68, 95% CI 0.53–0.87). Meta-analysis of two studies (702 patients, EORTC and GOG studies) for PFS found no statistically significant difference between IDS and chemotherapy alone (HR = 0.88, 95% CI 0.57–1.33). The rates of adverse reactions to chemotherapy were similar in both groups (risk ratio = 1.19, 95% CI 0.53–2.66).IDS following NAC.

26.3 Neoadjuvant Chemotherapy

NAC was initially administered as an alternative treatment to PDS in patients with apparently unresectable tumors, poor PS, or medical complications. In addition, some patients received chemotherapy after diagnostic surgery (e.g., exploratory laparotomy). This chemotherapy may also be called NAC in broad sense. Following two to six cycles of NAC and the resulting tumor shrinkage or improvement of PS, IDS (first attempt) was performed. The sequence of treatment initiated with NAC and followed by IDS and postoperative chemotherapy will be referred to as NAC therapy (NACT) hereafter. Similarly, the sequence of treatment initiated with PDS and followed by postoperative chemotherapy will be referred to as PDS therapy (PDST).

26.3.1 Results of Retrospective Analyses

Numerous retrospective studies comparing NACT and PDST have been conducted. These studies compared treatment outcomes and/or complications related to debulking surgery [10–22]. A couple of these studies are presented below.

Jacob et al. [10] conducted a retrospective matched case control study. This may be the first study comparing NACT and PDST. The investigators reviewed their experience with the International Federation of Gynecology and Obstetrics (FIGO) stage III–IV epithelial ovarian cancer in patients referred after initial laparotomy and biopsy only. The planned treatment for the study group ($N = 22$) was two to four cycles of NAC, followed by IDS and six additional cycles of chemotherapy. Two control groups were matched with the study group according to FIGO staging, histologic type, grade (2 or 3), and patient age ±5 years. Treatment for one control group ($N = 18$) was immediate re-exploration and debulking followed by a minimum of six cycles of chemotherapy. All patients received cisplatin-based chemotherapy. Optimal cytoreduction (<2 cm) was achieved in 77% of the study group versus 39% in the control group ($p = 0.02$). The median OS rates were not different (16 vs. 18 months, respectively). Morbidity of the IDS was acceptable. The investigators concluded that patients with bulky residual disease have a uniformly poor prognosis regardless of the timing of further surgery. These results suggest a higher possibility for optimal surgery by IDS and similar outcomes by NACT (study group) and PDST (control group).

Kayikçioğlu et al. [13] compared NACT and PDST. A total of 203 patients among 205 patients with advanced ovarian cancer were divided into the NACT (45 patients) and PDST (158 patients) groups. Two patients were excluded from analysis because they were lost to follow-up. NACT was administered typically in patients with large pleural effusion, multiple metastases at sites that made optimal cytoreductive surgery impossible, presence of large metastatic plaques (e.g., on the diaphragm), or parenchymal liver metastasis. NACT was also administered in patients who were medically unfit for PDS such as those with PS 2 or 3. Patients treated with NACT were older ($p = 0.01$), had worse PS ($p < 0.001$), and more stage IV disease ($p = 0.03$) than patients treated with PDST. Optimal cytoreductive surgery rates (no residual disease) were significantly higher in the NACT group ($p < 0.001$). Multivariate analysis demonstrated that only the residual tumor diameter and appendix involvement affect OS significantly. Five-year and median OS differences between PDST and NACT were not statistically significant. The analysis also demonstrated that patients treated with NACT underwent colon resection ($p = 0.01$, 2% vs. 16%, respectively) and splenectomy ($p = 0.02$, 0% vs. 11%, respectively) less frequently. Based on this analysis, the investigators concluded that NACT in a selected group of patients may not worsen prognosis, permit less aggressive surgery, and improve patient quality of life.

Hou et al. [20] compared survival and perioperative morbidity of patients treated with PDST or NACT. A total of 172 patients (PDST group, 109 patients; NACT group, 63 patients) were retrospectively analyzed. NACT patients, compared to PDST patients, had significantly less intraoperative blood loss (546 vs. 1033 mL, $p < 0.0001$), operating time (211 vs. 276 min, $p < 0.0001$), units of transfusion (1.2 vs. 2.4 U, $p = 0.03$), and shorter hospital stay (5.7 vs. 8.5 days, $p < 0.0001$). Optimal cytoreduction (<1 cm) was achieved in 95% of NACT patients versus 71% of PDST patients ($p < 0.001$). Three patients in the NACT group (5%) versus 27 patients (25%) in the PDST group required aggressive surgery in addition to standard cytoreduction. Within the NACT group, OS was improved in patients who received CP (CBDCA/PTX) compared to CC (CBDCA/CPA) (83 vs. 26 months, $p = 0.008$). Patients with extra-abdominal disease who received CP as NAC had improved PFS and OS compared to those in the PDST group with stage IV disease (15 vs. 9 months, $p = 0.015$, and 31 vs. 20 months, $p = 0.032$, respectively). The investigators concluded that NACT was associated with less perioperative morbidity, less need for further aggressive surgery, and similar survival with PDST. Additionally, in patients with extra-abdominal disease, NACT was associated with improved PFS and OS. Moreover, platinum and taxane were shown to be the therapeutic agents of choice in NAC.

In most studies, NACT was administered to patients who had older age, more advanced disease, or a poorer PS except for a few studies [10, 14, 15]. In these highly biased settings unfavorable to NACT, all studies showed a similar or higher proportion of patients with optimal debulking by NACT compared to PDST, and in most studies NACT yielded outcomes non-inferior to those of PDST. Regarding the invasiveness of debulking surgery, several studies revealed significantly less invasiveness with NACT, including reduced blood loss, lower rate or amount of blood transfusion, lower rate of bowel resection, lower rate of splenectomy, lower rate of surgical morbidities, shorter and less frequent stay in the intensive care unit (ICU), and shorter duration of hospitalization.

26.3.2 Results of Prospective Randomized Phase III Studies

Owing to the favorable outcomes of NACT compared to PDST reported by retrospective studies and other studies, three prospective randomized phase III studies were conducted to confirm the efficacy of NACT. The final results of the EORTC study [23] and CHORUS (*Ch*emotherapy *or* *U*pfront *S*urgery) study [24] by the MRC-CTU (Medical Research Council Clinical Trials Unit) have already been published. The morbidity analysis from the JCOG (Japan Clinical Oncology Group) study [25] was published ahead of the final results.

26.3.2.1 EORTC Study

The EORTC conducted the first prospective randomized study comparing NACT and PDST. The results of this study were reported in 2010 by Vergote et al. [23] They randomly assigned 670 patients with stage IIIC–IV epithelial ovarian carcinoma, fallopian tube carcinoma, or primary peritoneal carcinoma to PDST ($N = 336$) and NACT ($N = 334$). Of those 670 patients, 632 (94.3%) were eligible and initiated PDST ($N = 310$) and NACT ($N = 322$). The largest residual tumor was ≤1 cm in 41.6% after PDS and in 80.6% after IDS. Although a statistical comparison was not performed, postoperative adverse events (AEs) and mortality tended to be more frequent following PDS than IDS (per-protocol [PP] analysis). OS of patients in the PDS and NAC groups was 29 and 30 months, respectively (intention-to-treat [ITT] analysis). The HR for mortality and progressive disease in NACT was 0.98 (90% CI 0.84–1.13; $p = 0.01$ for non-inferiority) and 1.01 (90% CI 0.89–1.15), respectively, as compared to PDST. Multivariate analysis revealed that complete resection of macroscopic disease (PDS or IDS) was the strongest independent variable in predicting OS. The investigators concluded that NACT was non-inferior to PDST for patients with bulky stage IIIC or IV ovarian carcinoma and that complete resection of macroscopic disease remains the objective of cytoreductive surgery whenever surgery is performed.

26.3.2.2 CHORUS Study

The MRC-CTU conducted the second prospective randomized study (CHORUS) comparing NACT and PDST. Kehoe et al. [24] published the results of this study in 2015. Of the 550 eligible patients, 276 were assigned to PDST and 274 to NACT. All patients were included in the ITT analysis. The PP analysis included 504 patients (251 assigned to primary surgery and 253 to primary chemotherapy). The median OS was 22.6 months in the PDS group versus 24.1 months in the NAC group. The HR for death was 0.87 in favor of NAC arm (95% CI 0.72–1.05). Grade 3 or 4 postoperative AEs and deaths within 28 days following surgery were more common in the PDS group than in the NAC group (24% [60/252] vs. 14% [30/209], $p = 0.0007$, and 6% [14/252] vs. <1% [1/209], $p = 0.001$, respectively). The investigators concluded that in patients with stage III or IV ovarian cancer, survival with NACT is non-inferior to that with PDST and NAC prior to surgery is an acceptable standard of care for women with advanced ovarian cancer.

26.3.2.3 JCOG Study

The JCOG conducted the third prospective randomized phase III study comparing PDST and NACT for stage III–IV ovarian, tubal, and peritoneal cancers (JCOG0602). The results for treatment invasiveness were published in 2016 [25]. In this study, patients did not undergo diagnostic laparotomy or laparoscopy prior to treatment. This allowed the investigators to compare the true treatment invasiveness in the two study groups. In the PDS group, IDS was optional for patients who had undergone suboptimal or incomplete PDS, considering the results of the aforementioned EORTC [7] and GOG [8] studies. A total of 301 patients were enrolled and randomized. Of those who were randomized in the PDS group (N = 149), 147 underwent PDS and 49 underwent IDS. In the NACT group (N = 152), 130 underwent IDS. Patients in the NACT group required fewer surgeries (mean 0.86 vs. 1.32, $p < 0.001$) and shorter total operation time (median 273 vs. 341 min, $p < 0.001$) than those in the PDS group. Although they underwent pelvic lymphadenectomy (PLA) and para-aortic lymphadenectomy (PALA) in higher frequency, they required a lower frequency of abdominal organ resection (23.7% vs. 37.6%, $p = 0.012$) or distant metastases resection (3.9% vs. 10.7%, $p = 0.027$). In the NACT–IDS group, loss of blood/ascites was reduced (median 787 vs. 3235 mL, $p < 0.001$), and albumin transfusion and grade 3–4 AEs following surgery were less frequent (26.2% vs. 58.5%, $p < 0.001$; 4.6% vs. 15.0%, $p = 0.005$, respectively). These findings demonstrated that NACT was less invasive than PDST. The final analysis of this study may confirm the non-inferior survival rate of NACT compared to PDST, and NACT may be a possible new standard treatment for advanced ovarian cancer.

26.3.2.4 Summary of Prospective Randomized Phase III Studies

All the studies discussed in this chapter were designed to confirm non-inferiority of NACT compared to PDST, expecting non-inferior survival outcome and lower treatment invasiveness. The EORTC [23] and CHORUS [24] studies successfully demonstrated non-inferior survival of NACT (HR = 0.98 [90% CI 0.84–1.13] and 0.87 [95% CI 0.72–1.05], respectively). Kehoe et al. [24] performed a meta-analysis of the outcome of these two studies. This analysis showed that the HR of NACT for death was 0.93 (95% CI 0.82–1.05, $p = 0.376$) compared to that of PDST. The non-inferiority boundary was 1.18; thus non-inferiority of NACT was demonstrated in this meta-analysis. The final analysis of the JCOG study [25] for survival outcome is anticipated to further confirm the non-inferior survival outcome of NACT.

Regarding treatment invasiveness, the EORTC study showed a trend toward less morbidity by NACT, as shown in Table 26.2. The CHORUS study showed significant less morbidity by NACT, in grade 3–4 postoperative AEs, deaths within 28 days following surgery, and postoperative discharge within 2 weeks. However, the JCOG study revealed several advantages of NACT in morbidity compared to PDST, including number of surgery, duration of total operation time, frequency of abdominal organ or distant metastases resection, blood/ascites loss, frequency of transfusion, etc., as shown in Tables 26.3 and 26.4. Owing to the findings of the JCOG study, the

Table 26.2 Prospective randomized studies for the efficacy of NACT compared to PDST

	EORTC (2010)			CHORUS (2015)		
Arm	PDS arm ($N = 336$)	NAC arm ($N = 334$)	p value for morbidity	PDS arm ($N = 276$)	NAC arm ($N = 274$)	p value for morbidity
Protocol treatment started	92% ($N = 310$)	96% ($N = 322$)		91% ($N = 251$)	92% ($N = 253$)	
Operation time (min)	165 (10–720)	180 (30–560)		120 (12–450)	120 (30–330)	
Surgical outcome (size of residual tumor)						
0 ≲ 1 cm	41.6%	80.7%		41%	73%	
0	19.4%	51.2%		17%	39%	
Perioperative death	2.5%	0.7%	NA	6%	<1%	0.001
Adverse events grade 3–4						
Hemorrhage	7.4%	4.1%	NA	3%	6-7%	NA
Thromboembolism	2.6%	0%	NA	2%	0%	NA
Infection	8.1%	1.7%	NA	6%	3%	NA
Intestinal fistula	1.0%	0.3%	NA	NA	NA	NA
Total postoperative AEs	NA	NA	NA	24%	14%	0.0007
Postoperative discharge within 2 weeks	NA	NA	NA	80%	93%	<0.0001
Survival outcome						
PFS	12 M	12 M		10.7 M	12.0 M	
OS	29 M	30 M		22.6 M	24.1 M	

NA, not available, *NS* not significant

Table 26.3 Surgical procedures in JCOG0602

	Comparison of entire treatment		
	PDS arm ($N = 149$)	NAC arm ($N = 152$)	*p* value
Frequency of surgery (average number per patient)	147 + 49 (1.32)	130 (0.86)	<0.001
Median total operation time (min)	341	273	<0.001
Number of patients who underwent			
PLA	59 (39.6%)	94 (61.8%)	<0.001
PALA	29 (19.5%)	64 (42.1%)	<0.001
Resection of			
Abdominal organ	56 (37.6%)	36 (23.7%)	0.012
Distant metastases	16 (10.7%)	6 (3.9%)	0.027

PLA pelvic lymphadenectomy, *PALA* para-aortic lymphadenectomy

Table 26.4 Blood/ascites loss and transfusion in JCOG0602

	Comparison of main surgery		
	PDS arm PDS ($N = 147$[a])	NAC arm IDS ($N = 130$[a])	*p* value
Median loss (mL) of			
Ascites[b]	2835 ($N = 118$)	0 ($N = 108$)	<0.001
Blood/ascites	3235	787	<0.001
No. of patients who received transfusion			
RCC	75 (51.0%)	70 (53.9%)	0.718
RCC/whole blood	75 (51.0%)	71 (54.6%)	0.630
FFP	39 (26.5%)	25 (19.2%)	0.16
Albumin	86 (58.5%)	34 (26.2%)	<0.001
FFP/PPF/Albumin	106 (72.1%)	55 (42.3%)	<0.001

FFP fresh frozen plasma, *PPF* plasma protein fraction

[a]Patients who did not undergo main surgery were excluded

[b]Patients in whom the amount of ascitic loss was not counted separately from blood loss were excluded from the analyses

lower morbidity associated with NACT compared to PDST was successfully confirmed.

26.3.3 Another Randomized Phase III Study in Restricted Institutions

As mentioned above, the EORTC and CHORUS studies successfully demonstrated a non-inferior survival outcome by NACT. However, these studies have received criticism regarding the surgical effort. Although these were multicenter studies and the target was advanced disease, complete resection of all macroscopic tumor (residual tumor equal to 0) was achieved in as few as 19.4% (61/315) and 16.7% (39/233) of PDS patients in the EORTC and CHORUS studies, respectively. It was pointed out that lower surgical efforts made PDST as similar treatment as NACT after exploratory laparotomy. Thus, the difference in survival outcome between the treatment arms might be decreased. Therefore, the AGO (German Arbeitsgemeinschaft Gynäkologische Onkologie) initiated another prospective randomized phase III study named Trial on Radical Upfront Surgery in Advanced Ovarian Cancer (TRUST, NCT02828618 in clinicaltrials.gov). This study was designed to compare maximum effort PDS performed in centers with proven high surgical quality versus equally maximal effort NACT–IDS. The study includes only centers with externally proven surgical expertise and audited by experienced surgeons. The study was initiated in July 2016, and a total of 686 patients are planned to be enrolled. The final data collection date for the primary outcome measure (OS) is scheduled for April 2023. The results of this study are anticipated with great interest.

26.4 Future Prospect

26.4.1 Adoption of NACT (NAC + IDS)

Meyer et al. [26] reported the results of a multi-institutional observational study on advanced ovarian cancer conducted in six US National Cancer Institute-designated cancer centers. NACT was associated with decreased OS compared to PDST among patients with stage IIIC disease who achieved microscopic or ≤1 cm postoperative residual disease. However, they also stated that the use of NACT increased from 16% (during the period from 2003 to 2010) to 34% (during the period from 2011 to 2012) in stage IIIC disease ($p < 0.001$) and from 41% to 62% in stage IV disease ($p < 0.001$). US cancer centers adopted NACT more frequently following the results of the EORTC study. Meanwhile, Wright et al. [27] published a clinical practice guideline on behalf of the SGO (Society of Gynecologic Oncology) and ASCO (American Society of Clinical Oncology). This guideline stated that (1) patients with high perioperative risks or low likelihood of achieving cytoreduction <1 cm (ideally no visible disease) should receive NACT; (2) NACT is non-inferior to PDST for PFS and OS and is associated with lower peri- and postoperative morbidity and mortality; and (3) primary cytoreductive surgery may offer superior survival in selected patients. The influence of the observational study by Meyer et al. is uncertain. However, based on the additional favorable results observed in the CHORUS and JCOG studies and the recent guideline, NACT is becoming a widely accepted option for the standard treatment of patients with stage IIIC–IV ovarian cancer. Moreover, the final results of the JCOG study are anticipated to confirm the favorable survival outcome of NACT.

26.4.2 Adoption of IDS After Suboptimal PDS

On the other hand, the clinical situation of suboptimal PDS will be certainly decreased as a result of the wide adoption of NACT for advanced ovarian cancer.

Although the efficacy of IDS following suboptimal PDS remains controversial, it is unlikely that further prospective randomized studies will be conducted in this setting. Thus, IDS following suboptimal PDS may be considered only when the primary surgery is not performed by gynecologic oncologists or when the surgery was performed with less extensive efforts.

References

1. Griffiths CT. Surgical resection of tumor bulk in the primary treatment of ovarian carcinoma. Natl Cancer Inst Monogr. 1975;42:101–4.
2. Luesley D, Lawton F, Blackledge G, Hilton C, Kelly K, Rollason T, et al. Failure of second-look laparotomy to influence survival in epithelial ovarian cancer. Lancet. 1988;2(8611):599–603.
3. Vogl SE, Seltzer V, Calanog A, Moukhtar M, Camacho F, Kaplan BH, et al. "Second-effort" surgical resection for bulky ovarian cancer. Cancer. 1984;54(10):2220–5.
4. Wils J, Blijham G, Naus A, Belder C, Boschma F, Bron H, et al. Primary or delayed debulking surgery and chemotherapy consisting of cisplatin, doxorubicin, and cyclophosphamide in stage III–IV epithelial ovarian carcinoma. J Clin Oncol. 1986;4(7):1068–73.
5. Lawton FG, Redman CW, Luesley DM, Chan KK, Blackledge G. Neoadjuvant (cytoreductive) chemotherapy combined with intervention debulking surgery in advanced, unresected epithelial ovarian cancer. Obstet Gynecol. 1989;73(1):61–5.
6. Redman CW, Warwick J, Luesley DM, Varma R, Lawton FG, Blackledge GR. Intervention debulking surgery in advanced epithelial ovarian cancer. Br J Obstet Gynaecol. 1994;101(2):142–6.
7. van der Burg ME, van Lent M, Buyse M, Kobierska A, Colombo N, Favalli G, et al. The effect of debulking surgery after induction chemotherapy on the prognosis in advanced epithelial ovarian cancer. Gynecological Cancer Cooperative Group of the European Organization for Research and Treatment of Cancer. N Engl J Med. 1995;332(10):629–34.
8. Rose PG, Nerenstone S, Brady MF, Clarke-Pearson D, Olt G, Rubin SC, et al. Secondary surgical cytoreduction for advanced ovarian carcinoma. N Engl J Med. 2004;351(24):2489–97. https://doi.org/10.1056/NEJMoa041125.
9. Tangjitgamol S, Manusirivithaya S, Laopaiboon M, Lumbiganon P, Bryant A. Interval debulking surgery for advanced epithelial ovarian cancer (Review). Cochrane Database Syst Rev. 2016;2016(1)
10. Jacob JH, Gershenson DM, Morris M, Copeland LJ, Burke TW, Wharton JT. Neoadjuvant chemotherapy and interval debulking for advanced epithelial ovarian cancer. Gynecol Oncol. 1991;42(2):146–50.
11. Onnis A, Marchetti M, Padovan P, Castellan L. Neoadjuvant chemotherapy in advanced ovarian cancer. Eur J Gynaecol Oncol. 1996;17(5):393–6.
12. Schwartz PE, Rutherford TJ, Chambers JT, Kohorn EI, Thiel RP. Neoadjuvant chemotherapy for advanced ovarian cancer: long-term survival. Gynecol Oncol. 1999;72(1):93–9. https://doi.org/10.1006/gyno.1998.5236.
13. Kayikçioglu F, Köse MF, Boran N, Çalişkan E, Tulunay G. Neoadjuvant chemotherapy or primary surgery in advanced epithelial ovarian carcinoma. Int J Gynecol Cancer. 2001;11(6):466–70.
14. Vrščaj MU, Rakar S. Neoadjuvant chemotherapy for advanced epithelial ovarian carcinoma: a retrospective case-control study. Eur J Gynaecol Oncol. 2002;23(5):405–10.
15. Morice P, Brehier-Ollive D, Rey A, Atallah D, Lhommé C, Pautier P, et al. Results of interval debulking surgery in advanced stage ovarian cancer: an exposed-non-exposed study. Ann Oncol. 2003;14(1):74–7.
16. Loizzi V, Cormio G, Resta L, Rossi CA, Di Gilio AR, Cuccovillo A, et al. Neoadjuvant chemotherapy in advanced ovarian cancer: a case-control study. Int J Gynecol Cancer. 2005;15(2):217–23. https://doi.org/10.1111/j.1525-1438.2005.15206.x.

17. Everett EN, French AE, Stone RL, Pastore LM, Jazaeri AA, Andersen WA, et al. Initial chemotherapy followed by surgical cytoreduction for the treatment of stage III/IV epithelial ovarian cancer. Am J Obstet Gynecol. 2006;195(2):568–74; discussion 74–6. https://doi.org/10.1016/j.ajog.2006.03.075.
18. Inciura A, Simavicius A, Juozaityte E, Kurtinaitis J, Nadisauskiene R, Svedas E, et al. Comparison of adjuvant and neoadjuvant chemotherapy in the management of advanced ovarian cancer: a retrospective study of 574 patients. BMC Cancer. 2006;6:153. https://doi.org/10.1186/1471-2407-6-153.
19. Steed H, Oza AM, Murphy J, Laframboise S, Lockwood G, DEP D, et al. A retrospective analysis of neoadjuvant platinum-based chemotherapy versus up-front surgery in advanced ovarian cancer. Int J Gynecol Cancer. 2006;16(Suppl 1):47–53. https://doi.org/10.1111/j.1525-1438.2006.00472.x.
20. Hou JY, Kelly MG, Yu H, McAlpine JN, Azodi M, Rutherford TJ, et al. Neoadjuvant chemotherapy lessens surgical morbidity in advanced ovarian cancer and leads to improved survival in stage IV disease. Gynecol Oncol. 2007;105(1):211–7. https://doi.org/10.1016/j.ygyno.2006.11.025.
21. Colombo PE, Mourregot A, Fabbro M, Gutowski M, Saint-Aubert B, Quenet F, et al. Aggressive surgical strategies in advanced ovarian cancer: a monocentric study of 203 stage IIIC and IV patients. Eur J Surg Oncol. 2009;35(2):135–43. https://doi.org/10.1016/j.ejso.2008.01.005.
22. Morice P, Dubernard G, Rey A, Atallah D, Pautier P, Pomel C, et al. Results of interval debulking surgery compared with primary debulking surgery in advanced stage ovarian cancer. J Am Coll Surg. 2003;197(6):955–63. https://doi.org/10.1016/j.jamcollsurg.2003.06.004.
23. Vergote I, Tropé CG, Amant F, Kristensen GB, Ehlen T, Johnson N, et al. Neoadjuvant chemotherapy or primary surgery in stage IIIC or IV ovarian cancer. N Engl J Med. 2010;363(10):943–53. https://doi.org/10.1056/NEJMoa0908806.
24. Kehoe S, Hook J, Nankivell M, Jayson GC, Kitchener H, Lopes T, et al. Primary chemotherapy versus primary surgery for newly diagnosed advanced ovarian cancer (CHORUS): an open-label, randomised, controlled, non-inferiority trial. Lancet. 2015;386(9990):249–57. https://doi.org/10.1016/S0140-6736(14)62223-6.
25. Onda T, Satoh T, Saito T, Kasamatsu T, Nakanishi T, Nakamura K, et al. Comparison of treatment invasiveness between upfront debulking surgery versus interval debulking surgery following neoadjuvant chemotherapy for stage III/IV ovarian, tubal, and peritoneal cancers in a phase III randomised trial: Japan Clinical Oncology Group Study JCOG0602. Eur J Cancer. 2016;64:22–31. https://doi.org/10.1016/j.ejca.2016.05.017.
26. Meyer LA, Cronin AM, Sun CC, Bixel K, Bookman MA, Cristea MC, et al. Use and Effectiveness of Neoadjuvant Chemotherapy for Treatment of Ovarian Cancer. J Clin Oncol. 2016; https://doi.org/10.1200/jco.2016.68.1239.
27. Wright AA, Bohlke K, Armstrong DK, Bookman MA, Cliby WA, Coleman RL, et al. Neoadjuvant chemotherapy for newly diagnosed, advanced ovarian cancer: Society of Gynecologic Oncology and American Society of Clinical Oncology Clinical Practice Guideline. Gynecol Oncol. 2016;143(1):3–15. https://doi.org/10.1016/j.ygyno.2016.05.022.

Fertility Preservation

27

Toyomi Satoh

Abstract

The selection criteria for fertility-sparing treatment (FST) in patients with epithelial ovarian cancer (EOC) are (1) stage IA grade 1 (G1) or grade 2 (G2), (2) stage IA clear cell carcinoma (CCC), or (3) stage IC G1 or G2. This indication for patients with stage IC1 remains controversial, and patients with stage IC2 or IC3 CCC, G3, bilateral lesions or stage II, or more advanced tumor are unsuitable for FST. Fertility-sparing surgery (FSS) procedures are similar to standard surgeries, except the uterus and contralateral ovary are preserved. Adjuvant chemotherapy is performed on patients who have received FSS following some guidelines as for patients who have undergone standard surgery. It is essential for the selection of FST that sufficient information on family history is obtained prior to starting treatment. When genetic abnormalities regarding EOC are detected, FST should be selected more carefully. Adhesions in the abdomen after surgery are one factor associated with infertility, so biopsies during FSS should be performed on a minimal basis, even if necessary. JCOG1203 is an ongoing prospective study aimed at confirming the effectiveness of FST in EOC patients with stage IA CCC or stage IC G1/G2 non-CCC.

Keywords

Epithelial ovarian cancer · Fertility-sparing surgery · Selection criteria

T. Satoh (✉)
Faculty of Medicine, Department of Obstetrics and Gynecology, University of Tsukuba, Tsukuba, Ibaraki, Japan
e-mail: toyomi-s@md.tsukuba.ac.jp

M. Mikami (ed.), *Surgery for Gynecologic Cancer*, Comprehensive Gynecology and Obstetrics, https://doi.org/10.1007/978-981-13-1519-0_27

27.1 History

Reports regarding fertility-sparing treatment (FST) for epithelial ovarian cancer (EOC) started to appear in the 1960s and 1970s. Thereafter, until the Gynecologic Cancer Study Group of the Japan Clinical Oncology Group (JCOG) reported a multicenter study of 30 institutions (the JCOG-FST study) in 2010, the only reports analyzed fewer than 60 patients with stage I EOC who received FST. Up to that point, the consensus criteria for FST selection in EOC patients were only stage IA and non-clear cell carcinoma (CCC) grade 1 (G1) or grade 2 (G2) [1].

The JCOG-FST study investigated 211 patients receiving FST for stage I EOC, including 30 patients with CCC and 67 unilateral stage IC patients with G1 or G2 non-CCC. That study confirmed FST as a safe treatment for stage IA patients with CCC (5-year recurrence-free survival rate [5y-RFS]: stage IA, 100%; IC, 66%) and unilateral stage IC patients with non-CCC G1 or G2 (5y-RFS: stage IC1, 92.9%; IC2, 91.7%; IC3, 90.0%), suggesting that FST followed by adjuvant chemotherapy could be feasible for such patients [2]. Several articles regarding FST for EOC that retrospectively analyzed large numbers of patients have since been published [3–6], but no results have been reported to contradict the results of the JCOG-FST study.

However, all evidence for FST of EOC has been obtained from retrospective studies, and evidence levels have thus not been considered particularly high. JCOG has therefore been performing JCOG1203 as a confirmatory prospective study regarding FST for EOC since 2014. The "Future Prospects" chapter provides details of this clinical trial [7].

27.2 Principles and Indications

Fertility-sparing surgery (FSS) procedures include salpingo-oophorectomy of the affected side, infracolic omentectomy or omental biopsy, peritoneal cytology, and pelvic or para-aortic lymph node dissection or biopsy. When metastasis is suspected, biopsy of the contralateral ovary and of various sites in the peritoneum is performed. When the patient is not confirmed to have EOC at the initial surgery, surgery can be limited to FSS without all of the procedures (e.g., salpingo-oophorectomy of the affected side, but excluding lymph node dissection), and after confirming the histological type and grade, restaging laparotomy with complete staging can be conducted [7].

Adjuvant chemotherapy is performed on patients who have received FSS, excluding patients with stage IA and G1 or G2, based on guidelines. The protocol of JCOG1203 specifies the protocol for performing adjuvant chemotherapy, as follows: (1) four cycles of combination therapy with paclitaxel (175 mg/m^2, day 1) and carboplatin (AUC = 6, day 1) are administered every 3 weeks to patients diagnosed with stage IA CCC or with stage IC1 G1/G2 non-CCC and (2) six cycles of the same combination therapy are administered to patients with stage IC2/3 G1/G2 non-CCC [7].

There are consensuses in the indication of FST to patients with stage I EOC based on within recent 10 years retrospective studies as follows: (1) stage IA patients including CCC without G3 and (2) stage IC (unilateral lesion) non-CCC G1 and G2 [2–6, 8]. Consideration of the indication for the patients with stage IB or IC (bilateral disease) is difficult, because very few patients with stage IB or IC with cancer of both ovaries underwent FST and the available data are therefore limited. Indications of FST for patients with stage I G3 and stage IC CCC are slightly confusing. One review article suggested indications for FST such as (1) non-clear cell histology, FIGO stage IA IC, and grade 1–2 EOC or (2) clear cell histology and FIGO stage IA EOC' [9], while another suggested indication such as "FIGO stage I grade 1 and 2, although grade 3 cases could be considered" [10]. The first suggestion was based on the view that FST can be selected only for patients with good prognosis (generally, a 5y-RFS >90%), whereas the second was based on the view that FST can be selected for patients who have the same prognosis as patients undergoing standard surgery, even if the RFS of these patients is not particularly good. FST cannot be recommended for patients with stage IC CCC based on the results of the JCOG-FST study. However, the results of a study clarifying the clinical outcomes of patients with stage IA or more advanced EOC treated with FST found no significant differences in disease-free or overall survival (OS) between patients with stage IC1 and those with stage IA [11]. Another report showed that progression-free survival (PFS) and OS outcomes of patients who underwent radical surgery with stage IA or IC1 CCC were similar (3-year PFS, stage IA and IC, 92.9% and 89.8%, respectively; 3-year OS, stage IA and IC, 93.5% and 96.2%, respectively) [12]. According to the results from those two papers, FST could potentially be performed safely for IC1 CCC patients. Evaluating the situation for patients with stage I G3 is difficult, because most studies from countries other than Japan have counted CCC as G3 disease. However, the number of G3 cases that do not represent CCC can be discerned in some carefully written papers from countries other than Japan [2, 4, 5, 13–17]. When combining the data from those nine papers on stage I G3 patients (excluding CCC patients), the stage I survival rate was an extremely low 68.4% (26/38) (Table 27.1). On the other hand, the 71 chemotherapy patients in the ICON1/ACTION analysis with G3 disease (non-CCC) showed 13 events and a survival rate of 81.7% [18]. This survival rate was far higher than that for patients with G3 disease who underwent FSS (Table 27.1). FST thus cannot be recommended for

Table 27.1 Comparison of survival rates by surgical procedures of patients with stage I non-clear cell carcinoma G3

	Fertility-sparing surgery	Radical surgery
Number (stage)	38 (IA, 8; IC, 7; NR, 23)	71 (NR)
Number of recurrence (stage)	17 (IA, 9; IC, 6; NR, 2)	NR
Recurrence sites	Ovary alone, 0; others, 15; NR, 2	NR
Status of patients with recurrence	NED, 4; AWD, 1; DOD, 12	NED,?; AWD,?; DOD, 13
Survival rate	68.40%	81.70%

NR not reported

Table 27.2 Recommendation for fertility-sparing surgery in young patients with stage I unilateral epithelial ovarian cancer

Stage	Histology/grade		
	Non-clear cell carcinoma G1or G2	Clear cell carcinoma	Non-clear cell carcinoma G3
IA	Offer FSS	Consider FSS + ACT	No FSS
IC	Consider FSS + ACT	No FSS (It may be possible to consider in stage IC1)	No FSS

G1 grade 1, *G2* grade 2, *G3* grade 3, *FSS* fertility-sparing surgery, *CT* adjuvant chemotherapy

patients with stage I G3 disease. Table 27.2 shows recommendations for FSS in young patients with stage I unilateral EOC.

27.3 Preoperative Evaluation

Selection of FST requires sufficient elicitation of the family history before starting treatment. Patients with hereditary breast and ovarian cancer syndrome show a very high risk of recurrence or de novo development of EOC if FST is performed. If necessary, genetic examination should be conducted, and when deleterious BRCA 1 or 2 or other genetic abnormalities associated with EOC are detected, FST should be selected more carefully.

As for EOC arising from endometriosis (such as CCC or endometrioid carcinoma), patients have the possibility of incurring de novo EOC if any endometrial lesions remain after surgery [19]. Imaging examination is important for preoperative detection of contralateral ovarian and extra-ovarian endometriosis.

27.4 Technique Morbidity

Adhesions in the abdomen, particularly in the pelvic cavity, after surgery represent a factor associated with infertility. Biopsies of the contralateral ovary, peritoneum, or any other location should be performed at the minimum number of sites necessary. Extensive lymph node dissection may also cause severe adhesions within the abdominal cavity. In patients with stage I mucinous carcinoma, the rates of lymph node metastasis were reported as 0–4.2% [20–24], and if no enlarged lymph nodes were seen with careful palpation during surgery, omission of the lymph node dissection may be considered.

On the other hand, the long-term prognosis for patients with an isolated ovarian recurrence after FST is much better than for patients with other patterns of

Table 27.3 Oncologic outcomes of stage I patients with isolated ovary recurrence or with extra-ovarian recurrence [1]

Author (year)	*n*	Recurrence *n*	Isolated ovarian recurrence			Extra-ovarian recurrence		
			Status					
			NED	AWD	DOD	NED	AWD	DOD
Fruscio (2013)	237	27	12	1	0	3	0	11
Kajiyama (2010)	60	8	0	1	1	1	0	5
Satoh (2010)	211	18	5	0	0	3	5	5
Park (2008)	59	9	1	0	0	1	3	4
Morice (2005)	33	9	2	0	2	2	2	1
Schilder (2002)	52	5	3	0	0	0	0	2
Zanetta (1997)	56	5	1	0	0	0	1	3
Rate of disease-free survival after salvage therapy			82.1% (23/28)			19.2% (10/52)		

recurrence [1, 25, 26]. A review of seven papers [2, 4, 8, 11, 14, 16, 27] that include clear details of patterns of recurrence and outcomes showed that the disease-free survival rate after salvage therapy was 82.1% (23/28) for patients with recurrence in the opposite ovary alone, compared with 19.2% (10/52) for those with other patterns of recurrence (Table 27.3) [1].

27.5 Future Prospects

JCOG1203 is entitled "A non-randomized confirmatory study regarding selection of fertility-sparing surgery for patients with epithelial ovarian cancer: Japan Clinical Oncology Group Study" [7]. Figure 27.1 shows the shame of JCOG1203. The aim of this study is to confirm the effectiveness of FSS with optimal staging followed by adjuvant chemotherapy in EOC patients with stage IA CCC or stage IC G1/G2 non-CCC. The study is designed as a multi-institutional, non-randomized, confirmatory (phase III) trial. We plan to enroll 250 patients meeting the indications for FSS, and primary analysis is to be conducted for 63 surgical patients with pathologically confirmed stage IA CCH or stage IC unilateral G1/G2 non-CCH. The planned accrual period is 5 years, with the follow-up period set for 10 years after completion of accrual. If the results of JCOG1203 turn out positive, we will be able to perform FST based on high-level evidence for EOC patients who desire to retain the possibility of childbearing.

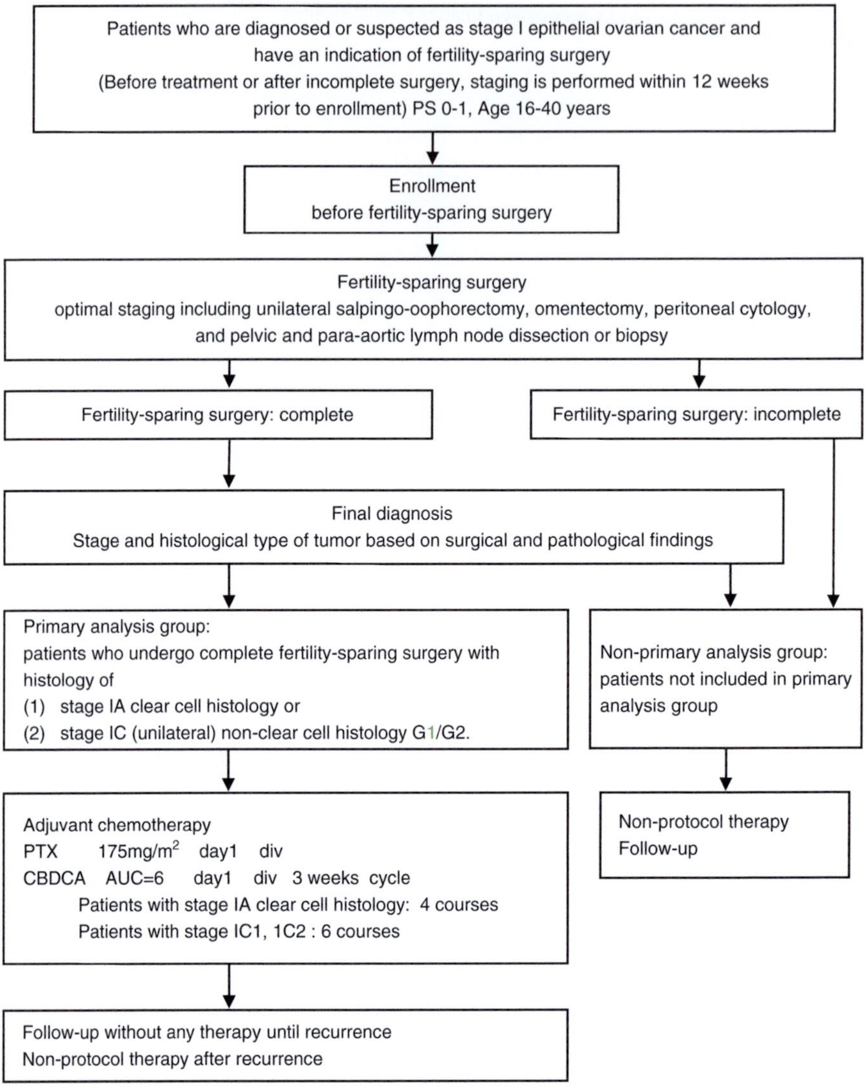

Fig. 27.1 Schema of JCOG1203 study: patient accrual is continued until a total of 63 patients is enrolled to the primary analysis group [6]

References

1. Satoh T, Yoshikawa H. Fertility-sparing surgery for early stage epithelial ovarian cancer. Jpn J Clin Oncol. 2016;46:703–10.
2. Satoh T, Hatae M, Watanabe Y, Yaegashi N, Ishiko O, Kodama S, et al. Outcomes of fertility-sparing surgery for stage I epithelial ovarian cancer: a proposal for patient selection. J Clin Oncol. 2010;28:1727–32.

3. Hu J, Zhu LR, Liang ZQ, Meng YG, Guo HY, Qu PP, et al. Clinical outcomes of fertility-sparing treatments in young patients with epithelial ovarian carcinoma. J Zhejiang Univ Sci B. 2011;12:787–95.
4. Fruscio R, Corso S, Ceppi L, Garavaglia D, Garbi A, Floriani I, et al. Conservative management of early-stage epithelial ovarian cancer: results of a large retrospective series. Ann Oncol. 2013;24:138–44.
5. Kajiyama H, Mizuno M, Shibata K, Yamamoto E, Kawai M, Nagasaka T, et al. Recurrence-predicting prognostic factors for patients with early-stage epithelial ovarian cancer undergoing fertility-sparing surgery: a multi-institutional study. Eur J Obstet Gynecol Reprod Biol. 2014;175:97–102.
6. Melamed A, Rizzo AE, Nitecki R, Gockley AA, Bregar AJ, Schorge JO, et al. All-cause mortality after fertility-sparing surgery for stage I epithelial ovarian cancer. Obstet Gynecol. 2017;130:71–9.
7. Satoh T, Tsuda H, Kanato K, Nakamura K, Shibata T, Takano M, et al. A non-randomized confirmatory study regarding selection of fertility-sparing surgery for patients with epithelial ovarian cancer: Japan Clinical Oncology Group Study (JCOG1203). Jpn J Clin Oncol. 2015;45:595–9.
8. Park JY, Kim DY, Suh DS, Kim JH, Kim YM, Kim YT, et al. Outcomes of fertility-sparing surgery for invasive epithelial ovarian cancer: oncologic safety and reproductive outcomes. Gynecol Oncol. 2008;110:345–53.
9. Nam JH, Park JY. Fertility-sparing surgery for young women with early-stage epithelial ovarian cancer. Gynecol Obstet Investig. 2013;76:14–24.
10. Zapardiel I, Diestro MD, Aletti G. Conservative treatment of early stage ovarian cancer: oncological and fertility outcomes. Eur J Surg Oncol. 2015;140:387–93.
11. Kajiyama H, Shibata K, Suzuki S, Ino K, Nawa A, Kawai M, et al. Fertility-sparing surgery in young women with invasive epithelial ovarian cancer. Eur J Surg Oncol. 2010;36:404–8.
12. Shu CA, Zhou Q, Jotwani AR, Iasonos A, Leitao MM Jr, Konner JA, et al. Ovarian clear cell carcinoma, outcomes by stage: the MSK experience. Gynecol Oncol. 2015;139:236–41.
13. Borgfeldt C, Iosif C, Måsbäck A. Fertility-sparing surgery and outcome in fertile women with ovarian borderline tumors and epithelial invasive ovarian cancer. Eur J Obstet Gynecol Reprod Biol. 2007;134:110–4.
14. Morice P, Leblanc E, Rey A, Baron M, Querleu D, Blanchot J, et al. Conservative treatment in epithelial ovarian cancer: results of a multicentre study of the GCCLCC (Groupe des Chirurgiens de Lutte Contre le Cancer) and SFOG (Societe Francaise d'Oncologie Gynecologique). Hum Reprod. 2005;20:1379–85.
15. Raspagliesi F, Fontanelli R, Paladini D, di Re EM. Conservative surgery in high-risk epithelial ovarian carcinoma. J Am Coll Surg. 1997;185:457–60.
16. Zanetta G, Chiari S, Rota S, Bratina G, Maneo A, Torri V, et al. Conservative surgery for stage I ovarian carcinoma in women of childbearing age. Br J Obstet Gynecol. 1997;104:1030–5.
17. Colombo N, Chiari S, Maggioni A, Bocciolone L, Torri V, Mangioni C. Controversial issues in the management of early epithelial ovarian cancer: conservative surgery and role of adjuvant therapy. Gynecol Oncol. 1994;55:S47–51.
18. Trimbos JB, Parmar M, Vergote I, Guthrie D, Bolis G, Colombo N, et al. International Collaborative Ovarian Neoplasm Trial 1 and Adjuvant ChemoTherapy In Ovarian Neoplasm trial: two parallel randomized phase III trials of adjuvant chemotherapy in patients with early-stage ovarian carcinoma. J Natl Cancer Inst. 2003;95:105–12.
19. Nishida K, Tenjinbayashi Y, Tasaka N, Shikama A, Sakurai M, Nakao S, et al. Possible de novo clear cell carcinoma in the contralateral ovary 9 years after fertility-sparing surgery for Stage IA clear cell ovarian carcinoma. Int Cancer Conf J. 2017;6(2):50–4. https://doi.org/10.1007/s13691-016-0271-9.
20. Cho YH, Kim DY, Kim JH, Kim YM, Kim KR, Kim YT, et al. Is complete surgical staging necessary in patients with stage I mucinous epithelial ovarian cancer. Gynecol Oncol. 2006;103:878–82.

21. Baiocchi G, Raspagliesi F, Grosso G, Fontanelli R, Cobellis L, di Re E, et al. Early ovarian cancer: is there a role for systematic pelvic and para-aoric lymphadenectomy? Int J Gynecol Cancer. 1998;8:103–8.
22. Morice P, Joulie F, Camatte S, Atallah D, Rouzier R, Pautier P, et al. Lymph node involvement in epithelial ovarian cancer: analysis of 276 pelvic and paraaortic lymphadenectomies and surgical implications. J Am Coll Surg. 2003;197:198–205.
23. Suzuki M, Ohwada M, Yamada T, Kohno T, Sekiguchi I, Sato I. Lymph node metastasis in stage I epithelial ovarian cancer. Gynecol Oncol. 2000;79:305–8.
24. Negishi H, Takeda M, Fujimoto T, Todo Y, Ebina Y, Watari H, et al. Lymphatic mapping and sentinel node identification as related to the primary sites of lymph node metastasis in early stage ovarian cancer. Gynecol Oncol. 2004;94:161–6.
25. Marpeau O, Schilder J, Zafrani Y, Uzan C, Gouy S, Lhommé C, et al. Prognosis of patients who relapse after fertility-sparing surgery in epithelial ovarian cancer. Ann Surg Oncol. 2008;15:478–83.
26. Bentivegna E, Fruscio R, Roussin S, Ceppi L, Satoh T, Kajiyama H, et al. Long-term follow-up of patients with an isolated ovarian recurrence after conservative treatment of epithelial ovarian cancer: review of the results of an international multicenter study comprising 545 patients. Fertil Steril. 2015;104:1319–24.
27. Schilder LM, Thompson AM, DePriest PD, Ueland FR, Cibull ML, Kryscio RJ, et al. Outcome of reproductive age women with stage Ia or Ic invasive epithelial ovarian cancer treated with fertility-sparing therapy. Gynecol Oncol. 2002;87:1–7.

28 Surgery for Vulvar Cancer and Vaginal Cancer

Toshiaki Saito

Abstract

Vulvar cancer and vaginal cancer are relatively rare cancer in the field of gynecologic oncology. Nevertheless, several advancements have been achieved in the surgical treatment for these cancers in the past two or three decades, especially in vulvar cancer. Individualization and minimization is the modern trend in the surgical treatment of vulvar cancer. However, the skills and techniques of the surgery for vulvar cancer are derived from the traditional surgery. Especially, the inguinal lymph node dissection is an essential part of the surgery but is not common as a daily practice. It is important for a surgeon to be well acquainted before surgery with the anatomy of the femoral triangle and the skills of the dissection before surgery. Reconstruction surgery is also important to close the wound adequately and safely reducing the postoperative wound breakdown, but is not familiar to most of the gynecologists. In the present chapter, these basic surgical methods in vulvar cancer are mainly described showing examples of the surgery.

Keywords

Radical vulvectomy · Radical local excision · Inguinal lymphadenectomy Vaginectomy · Vulvar reconstruction

28.1 Introduction

Vulvar cancer is a relatively rare cancer in gynecologic malignancies mainly affecting elderly women. The majority of vulvar cancer is squamous cell carcinoma, which accounts for 90% of all vulvar cancer. The curative treatment of vulvar

T. Saito (✉)
Gynecology Service, National Kyushu Cancer Center, Minami-ku, Fukuoka, Japan
e-mail: saito.toshiaki.hf@mail.hosp.go.jp

M. Mikami (ed.), *Surgery for Gynecologic Cancer*, Comprehensive Gynecology and Obstetrics, https://doi.org/10.1007/978-981-13-1519-0_28

cancer requires consideration of both the primary focus of disease in the vulva and the inguinal lymph nodes, which are the regional lymph nodes of the vulva. In current treatment, surgery is the first choice, and the FIGO classification of stages is also based on surgical staging which includes detailed histopathological examinations on lymph node metastasis [1].

Traditionally, "en bloc" radical vulvectomy with bilateral groin node dissection has been the choice of treatment for vulvar cancer since Taussig in the United States and Way in Great Britain introduced this systemic surgical procedure [2, 3]. The rationale of the surgery was based on the analysis of patients with vulvar cancer that the pattern of dissemination of this cancer is predominantly lymphogenic to the inguinofemoral lymph nodes and subsequently to the pelvic lymph nodes. However, many cases accompanied with special site characteristics, very elderly and various medical complications. As a result, the surgery was associated with significant morbidity, including wound dehiscence and infection [4]. In the 1980s it was reported that postoperative complications could be reduced through conservative surgery. Thereafter, surgery of the primary tumor and its lymphatic drainage have drastically changed in the last two decades to the more individualized and conservative procedures with special emphasis on the postoperative QOL of the patients [5, 6]. However, because of the many sites of occurrence and foci of diseases in individuals of vulvar cancer and the low frequency of occurrence, many reports gathered the cases over periods exceeding 20 years. There were no randomized controlled trials of incision methods and no clear evidences of the effect of conservative surgery on vulvar cancer. Therefore, radical vulvectomy is still applied in cases where application of conservative surgery is not clearly indicated, i.e., the tumor is very large, on the side of the pubic bone, the tumors on both left and right sides, multiple foci of disease, or with inguinal lymph node metastasis.

In principle the mainstay therapy for vaginal cancer is radiation therapy. However, surgical therapy is also an option, depending on the location and extent of the focus/foci of disease [7]. In particular, in the case of vaginal cancer occurring in the upper third of the vagina, surgical therapy consisting of hysterectomy extended to the vagina is a good option. If vaginal cancer is accompanied by widespread intraepithelial neoplasia in the vagina, a total vaginectomy may sometimes be selected. Moreover, in carefully selected cases of locally advanced vaginal cancer with no metastasis, pelvic exenteration is sometimes performed.

28.2 Surgery for Vulvar Cancer

28.2.1 Radical Vulvectomy (En Bloc Incision)

Now the standard surgery for the invasive vulvar cancer is the individualized and conservative surgery as it possible. However, the basic techniques for the surgery still lay in the radical vulvectomy with en bloc incision. Therefore, first of all, the skills for radical vulvectomy are shown in detail. The conservative surgery is that some of the procedure of radical vulvectomy is not done and left intact and somewhat easy to do for a surgeon once knowing the procedure of radical vulvectomy.

28.2.1.1 Incision and Inguinofemoral Lymph Node Dissection

The skin incision begins at the right anterior superior spine on the abdominal wall curving down in the inguinal crease. It then crosses in the mons pubis and extends in similar fashion to the left anterior superior spine (Fig. 28.1a). The skin edge of the upper flap was held upward by Allis forceps as the surgeon undermines the skin by beveling through the fat in a plane just above the fascia of abdominal muscles. Additional skin incision is made in upper lines of vulvectomy. Then the lower skin flap was grasped upward to facilitate for the surgeon undermining the skin and dissect through the fat in the same plane in the femoral area. Similar dissection was done on the other side. During the procedure, surgeon must pay attention not to undermine excessively causing the skin very thin without sufficient blood supply (Fig. 28.1b).

The deep layer of fat is then dissected from the underlying fascia which covers the external oblique muscle and rectal muscle. The dissection continues across the midline and on downward to the inguinal ligament. At this point the overlying fat containing lymphatic channels and nodes (superficial inguinal nodes) has been completely mobilized from the underlying fascia but left in continuity with the vulva itself (Fig. 28.1c).

Before dissecting the femoral area, surgeon must identify the position of femoral artery by touching and feeling the pulse and imaging the anatomical structures beneath the fascia lata (Fig. 28.2). The fascia lata is incised along the inguinal ligament in full length with care not to injure the femoral vessels. The surgeon then dissects the femoral area by drawing the mass of fat and nodes medially and downward. At the cribriform fascia of fossa ovalis, the dissection can be continued deeper medial to the femoral vein (sometimes exploring the medial aspect of femoral vein and saphenous vein). Then the femoral sheath is gently incised on its lateral side. The artery immediately comes in view. The sheath surrounding the vessels is opened through its full length from the inguinal ligament downward to the top of the adductor canal where the sartorius muscle laterally and the adductor muscle medially

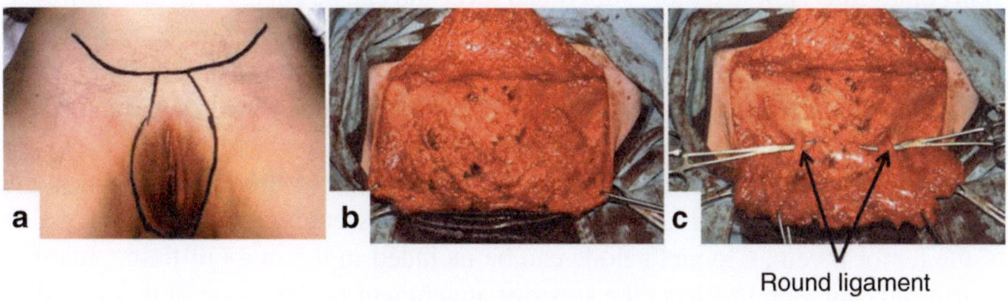

Fig. 28.1 Radical vulvectomy with en bloc incision. (**a**) Incision lines for the groin and vulva. (**b**) Overview of groins and mons pubis after dissection from the overlying skin. (**c**) Overview after dissection of the inguinal fat and lymph nodes showing the bilateral round ligaments

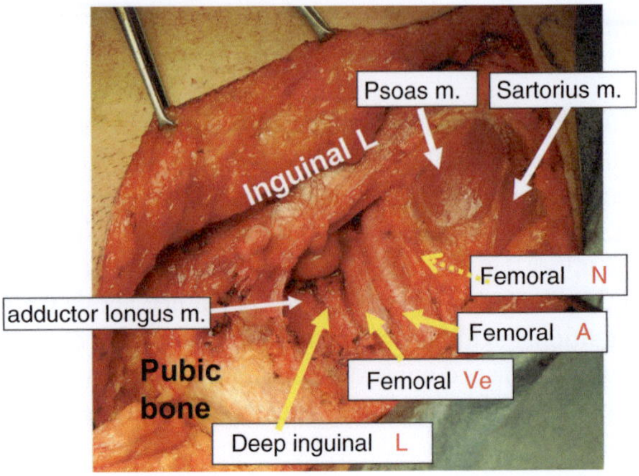

Fig. 28.2 Anatomy of the left femoral triangle beneath the fascia lata. The figure shows the muscles and femoral vessels in the femoral triangle. Note the position and order of each structure; NAVEL: femoral nerve (not explored), femoral artery, femoral vein, and inguinal lymph nodes

come together. A small arterial branch (the superficial external pudendal artery) comes into view on the medial side and is cut and ligated. The femoral artery is exposed up to the inguinal ligament. Care must be taken to identify the superficial circumflex artery which appears on the lateral side of the artery just beneath the inguinal ligament. It will also be cut and ligated. The surgeon continues the separation of the sheath from the artery on the medial side. As the dissection continues, the femoral vein comes into view completely. The sheath is incised and the vein wall exposed. The surgeon dissects the tissue (deep inguinal nodes, femoral nodes) from the femoral vein which lies deep and medial to the artery. The point of entrance of the saphenous vein into the femoral vein may be obscure. The surgeon has exposed probable site of entry of the saphenous vein into the femoral vein. As the dissection progresses, the saphenofemoral junction comes into view. There may be several communicating small veins which empty into the saphenous vein at this location. The surgeon retracts the mass of tissue upward from the femoral sheath and vein. By carrying out this dissection with the sheath, the surgeon can be sure of removing all femoral nodes and lymphatics. Dissection continues as the surgeon cleans off the tissue from the underlying pectineus fascia. As the tissue is freed, the saphenous vein comes into view at a more superficial level and can be cut and ligated. However, saphenous vein can usually be preserved by meticulous dissection along the vein (Fig. 28.3). The surgeon divides the mass of tissue at the lower pole of the dissection. After division, the tissues are secured with a ligature since they contain the main lymphatic channels draining the lower leg.

Just within the femoral canal along the medial side of the femoral vein is the structure designated as Cloquet's node. By gentle dissection along the medial side of the femoral vein, Cloquet's node can be included in the mass of tissue that will be excised. Surgeon transects the superior attachment of the tissue bloc just underneath the inguinal ligament, which connects to the lymphatics in the pelvis. Finally, the mass of tissue including inguinal lymph nodes is now completely freed from the femoral triangle (Fig. 28.2).

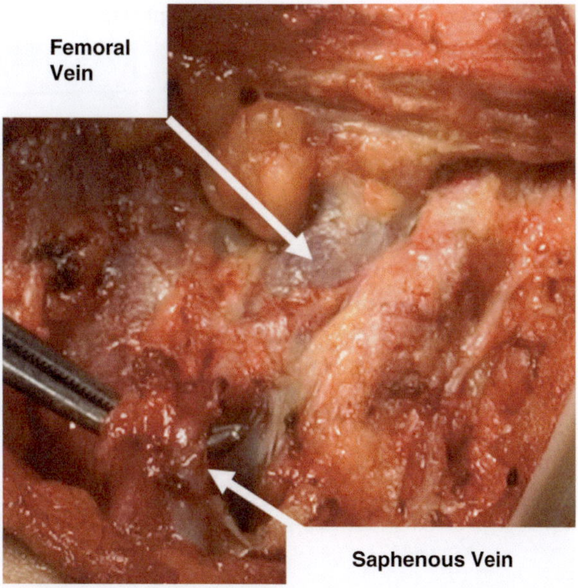

Fig. 28.3 Great saphenous vein joining to the left femoral vein. The saphenous vein is preserved with small branches dissected. Surrounding fat including the lymph nodes is removed

The surgeon dissects the mass free from the underlying surface of the inguinal ligament and mobilizes it toward the midline and the spine of the pubis. As he does so, the round ligament is exposed. The bilateral round ligaments are cut and ligated (Fig. 28.1c).

Before closing the groin wound, sartorius muscle is mobilized to midline to cover the explored femoral vessels. The sartorius muscle is grasped and cut at the attachment to superior anterior spine and moved onto the femoral vessels and tied to the inguinal ligament with mattress sutures (Fig. 28.4). The wound is closed by interrupted subcutaneous absorbable sutures and nylon skin sutures after the placement of suction drainage.

28.2.1.2 Vulvar Phase

The patient is now placed in a lithotomy position to permit the removal of the entire vulva (Fig. 28.5a). The outer incision line is decided to give wide margin to the primary tumor. The inner margin of resection will leave only the urethral and vaginal orifices. The surgeon continues the incision along the lateral wall of the vagina, completely circumscribing the vaginal epithelium. This is the inner incision line. The outer incision lateral to the vulva is deepened to expose the fascia of the underlying muscles. Individual vessels are clamped as they are encountered. The moves are repeated on the opposite side. The entire mass (including the inguinal fat and nodes) is drawn downward as it is dissected from the fascia overlying the symphysis and muscles attaching to the pubic rami. During the procedure, the bilateral round ligaments were stretched, cut, and ligated (Fig. 28.5b). The suspensory ligament of the clitoris must be cut across. By continuing with the dissection in this plane, the

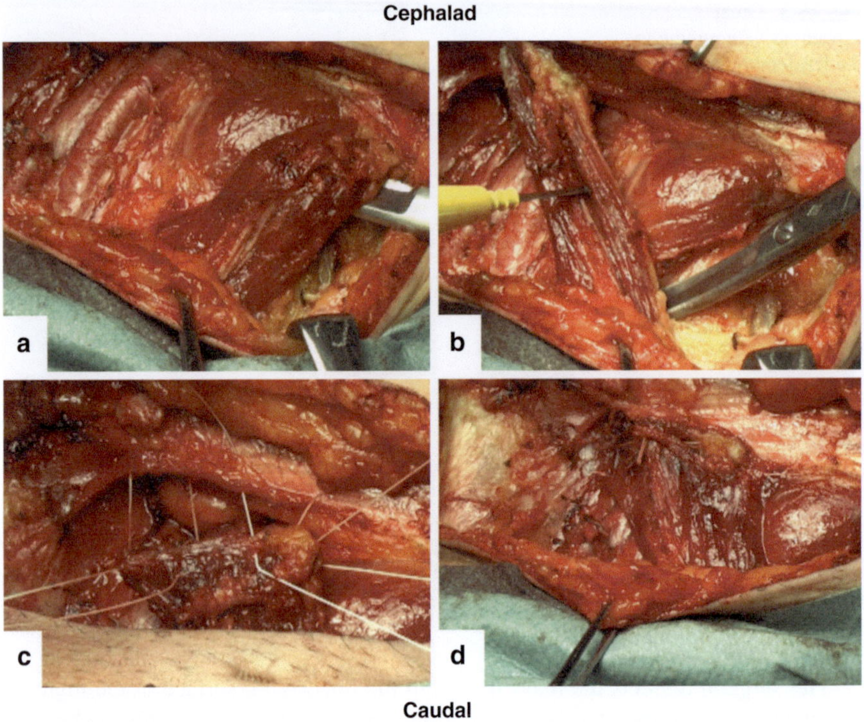

Fig. 28.4 Transposition of sartorius muscle covering the denuded femoral vessels. The figures show the structure of left groin after full lymphadenectomy. (**a**) Sartorius muscle is separated from surrounding tissue. (**b**) Sartorius muscle is divided from anterior superior iliac spine and mobilized for covering the femoral vessels. (**c**) Sartorius muscle is sutured to the inguinal ligament by mattress sutures. (**d**) The femoral vessels are completely covered by sartorius muscle

mass is completely freed from the symphysis, not only on its anterior surface but also underneath the pubic arch. Plexus of vein in this area is also transected and ligated with care of hemorrhage (Fig. 28.5c and d).

The mass of tissue is again drawn to the midline, exposing the branches of internal pudendal vessels appearing below the level of the midpoint of the lateral dissection. The vessels are cut and ligated. The same steps are repeated on the opposite side. The outer aspect of the specimen has now been completely outlined as well as the vaginal aspect on both sides. The perineal incision is now made, and the plane between the perineum/vagina and rectum developed. The surgeon separates the perineum and vaginal wall from the underlying rectum as doing in posterior vaginal repair. Care must be taken not to cut the sphincter ani during the procedure. This dissection is continued well up between the posterior vagina and the rectal wall to permit approximation for the levator muscle at the time of closure. Now the surgeon separates the urethra from the undersurfaces of the specimen. The specimen is now detached from the symphysis and pubic rami except for the small muscle bundle of

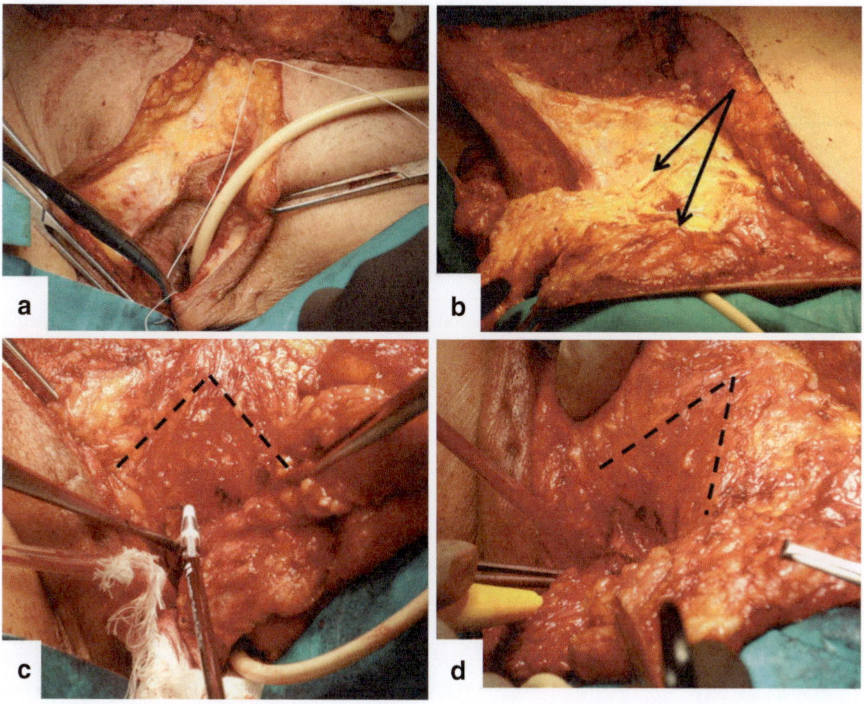

Fig. 28.5 Vulvar phase of radical vulvectomy. (**a**) Outer incision lines of the vulva continued from the groin incision lines. (**b**) Dissection of mass of the inguinal fat over the pubic rami. Note the exposed round ligaments. Arrows indicate the bilateral round ligaments. (**c**) Dissection continued to the tissue under the pubic arch. Dotted lines show the direction of pubic arch. (**d**) Lateral view of the dissection beneath the pubic arch. Dotted lines show the lateral view of the pubic arch

ischiocavernosus which holds it on either side. The bundles are transected and tied in both sides. The tissues overlying the bulbocavernosus muscle are removed downward. Finally the bridge of posterior vaginal wall is divided, and the whole specimen is removed (Fig. 28.6).

Resection of the urethra is sometimes necessary because of invasion of cancer to the lower part of the urethra. The urethra can be resected without disturbing urinary continence when the length of resection is less than 1 cm (Fig. 28.7). The surrounding tissues are separated from lower part of the urethra by meticulous division deeper under the pubic arch. The urethra is cut and removed. The stump of the urethra is everted to the surrounding tissue and sutured to the skin.

28.2.1.3 Closure of the Wound

A series of interrupted sutures is laid into the levator ani muscles in the manner of posterior repair of vaginal wall. The rectum now lies behind the levator muscles, which are approximated in the midline.

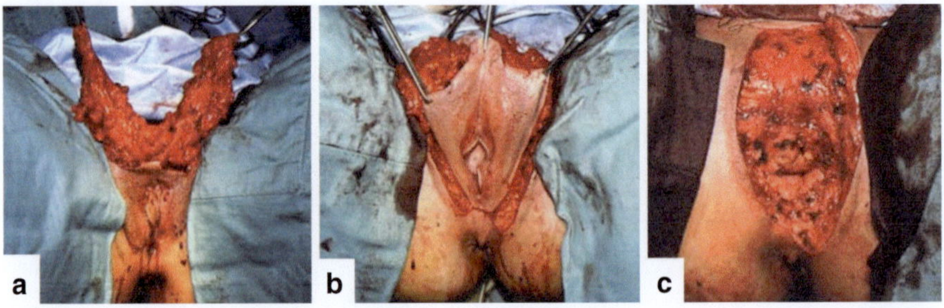

Fig. 28.6 Whole picture of radical vulvectomy. (**a**) Dissected inguinofemoral fat and lymph nodes are continued to subdermal dissection of the vulvar phase. (**b**) Outer incision line of the vulva continued from the groin dissection. (**c**) Removal of entire specimen from vulva after inner incision completed

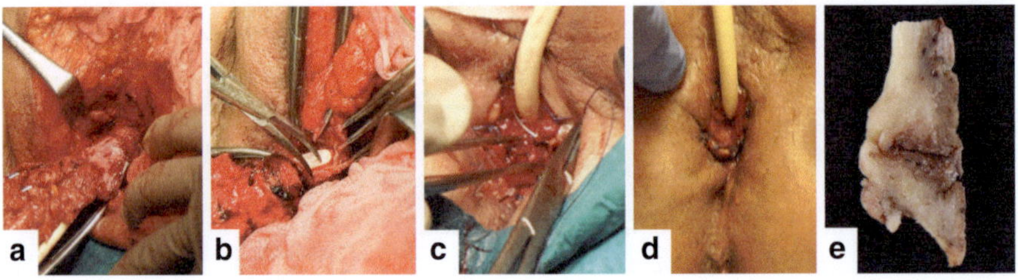

Fig. 28.7 Resection of the urethra invaded by cancer. (**a**) Dissection of surrounding tissue from the urethra under pubic arch. (**b**) Cut and open the upper surface of the urethra revealing the urethral catheter. (**c**) Eversion and suturing the urethral stump to surrounding tissue. (**d**) Reconstructed new meatus urethra. (**e**) Cross section of the fixed urethra resected for 1 cm in length

The drainages for the groin wounds and vulvar wound are essential parts of the wound closure because much dead space created. The insertion of perforated catheter of 3–5 mm diameter with constant suction is necessary for the groin wounds because of long-term postoperative leakage of lymph fluid. The drains are also inserted into the vulvar wounds separately to maintain the suction independently. The edges of the skin in the upper portion of the dissection are brought together with interrupted nylon sutures. The surgeon now approximates the edge of the skin to that of the vaginal wall with interrupted absorbable sutures throughout the circumference. Because of the extensive dissection, the edge will come together with some tension. If they do not fall together easily, one should not hesitate to use reconstructive surgery as mentioned later.

The vaginal wall has been approximated to the skin, and the wound closure is complete. A Foley catheter has been inserted in the bladder. The suction catheters are each fixed to the skin with a suture and connected to small collecting units which maintain constant suction and still permit to the patient to be ambulatory. The wounds are covered by an adequate dressing such as transparent polyurethane film dressing.

28.2.2 Radical Vulvectomy (Separate Incisions)

As an improvement to radical vulvectomy, separate incision (or triple incision) was reported in 1962. In this approach, the excision of vulvar neoplasia is separated from inguinal lymphadenectomy [8]. Later, in the 1980s, a method was developed to leave the suprapubic skin intact as a skin bridge. The prognosis for this procedure was found to be commensurate with historical data in stages I to IV in the old (1988) FIGO classifications, and the frequency of wound complications decreased dramatically [9, 10]. In particular, a comparative matched study was conducted on 32 cases in each localized to the vulva and perineum [11]. Separate incision was shown to be clearly less surgically invasive than en bloc incision. Although skin-bridge recurrence between the vulva and groin was higher for separate incision than for en bloc incision, the survival prognosis after re-excision was good [12, 13]. Also, cases of skin-bridge recurrence between the vulva and groin are less than 1% where no gross lymph node metastasis is present. While recurrence in lymph nodes is lower for en bloc incision, no difference in survival is found. Currently, even when the frequency of recurrence in lymph nodes and of skin-bridge recurrence between the vulva and groin is considered, separate incision is recommended for patients without suspicious lymph node metastasis, due to the lesser degree of impairment caused by treatment [14].

The lines are indicated as the figure (Fig. 28.8). The procedures and skills are identical to those of radical vulvectomy with en bloc incision (Figs. 28.9 and 28.10).

28.2.3 Modified Radical Vulvectomy

Modified radical vulvectomy is defined as any modification of radical vulvectomy en bloc type or separate incision type leaving a part of healthy vulva intact. The

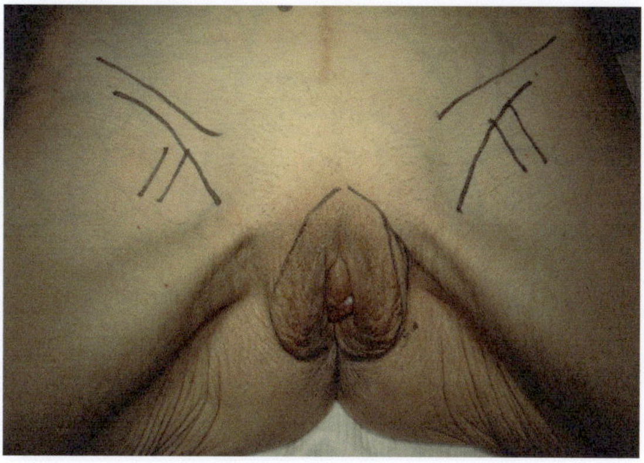

Fig. 28.8 Incision lines of radical vulvectomy with separate incision. Lines indicated the incision lines, inguinal ligaments, and position of femoral arteries

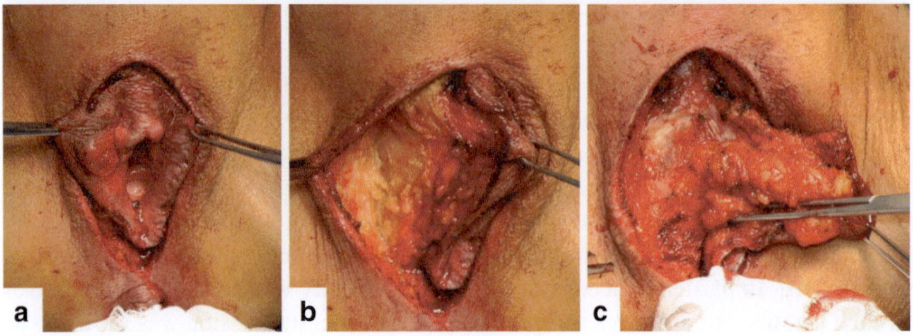

Fig. 28.9 Vulvar phase of radical vulvectomy with separate incision. (**a**) Outer incision line. (**b**) Dissection of subdermal adipose tissue. (**c**) Dissection to the fascia of the bulbocavernosus muscle

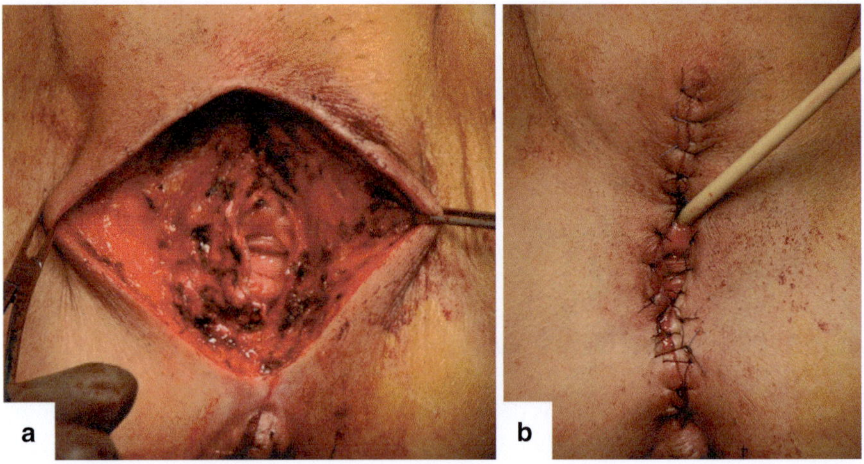

Fig. 28.10 Closure of the vulvar wound of separate incision of radical vulvectomy. (**a**) Vulvar wound after removal of the vulvar specimen with complete hemostasis. (**b**) Primary closure of the vulvar wound without drainage

figure shows an example of radical hemivulvectomy with en bloc incision for the left vulvar lesion and left inguinofemoral lymph node, which extends upward for extraperitoneal resection of gross pelvic lymph node metastasis (Fig. 28.11). The full inguinal lymph node dissection should be done (Fig. 28.2). Full inguinal lymphadenectomy (superficial and deep inguinal) is essential even in these cases, based on the prospective study of GOG074. The study revealed the higher inguinal recurrence rate for superficial lymphadenectomy alone than full inguinal lymphadenectomy [15].

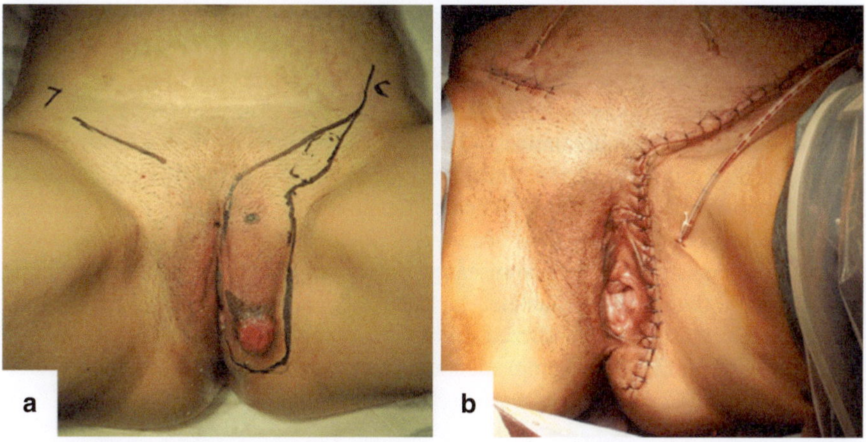

Fig. 28.11 Modified radical vulvectomy for advanced left vulvar cancer with left inguinal and pelvic lymph node metastases. (**a**) Left incision lines indicate the radical hemivulvectomy with en bloc incision for the left vulvar lesion and left inguinofemoral lymphadenectomy, which extends upward for extraperitoneal resection of gross pelvic lymph node metastasis. Right inguinal lymphadenectomy is planned with separate incision. (**b**) Closure of the wounds. Note the placement of suction drainage in each wound

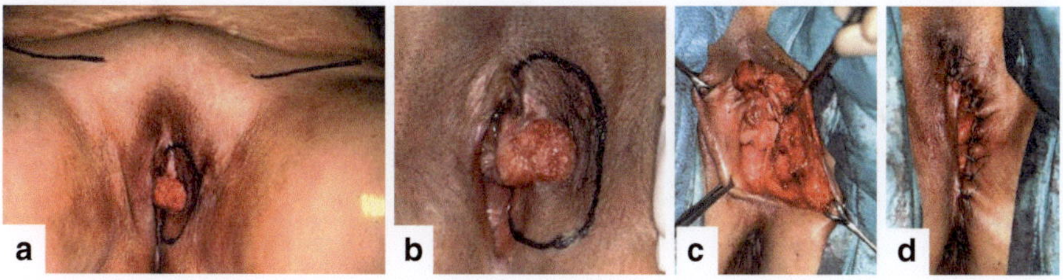

Fig. 28.12 Radical local excision. (**a**) Incision lines of the groin and vulva. The lesion is located lateral but within 1–2 cm from the midline. Bilateral inguinal lymphadenectomy is planned in separate incisions. (**b**) The outline of the excision for vulvar tumor is decided to ensure over 2 cm margins. (**c**) Wound after removal of the vulvar lesion. (**d**) Primary closure of the wound

28.2.4 Radical Local Excision (Fig. 28.12)

Radical local excision can be considered in cases where the lesion is secluded (localized laterally to the vulva), with surrounding skin tissue normal. This surgical technique presents considerably lower frequency of postoperative complications than radical vulvectomy. While the local recurrence rate is reported to be somewhat elevated, no difference is observed in survival prognosis [16–18]. The procedure should be limited to the single-lying tumor which occurs in lateral (defined as 1 cm or more distant from the median line of the vulva).

In this procedure the depth of the excision is similar to that of a radical vulvectomy. The excision margin is closely related to probability of local recurrence. To ensure sufficient excision margin, a gross distance of 2 cm is required [12].

Lymphadenectomy can be limited to the disease side in cases where the tumor is 2 cm in diameter or smaller and is 1–2 cm lateral from the midline structures such as the clitoris, urethra, vagina, perineal body, or anus, and no lymph node metastasis is suspected. While some reports indicate that bilateral lymphadenectomy is necessary if lymph node metastasis has occurred on the diseased side [15], another study reports that metastasis to the non-diseased side is possible only in cases where the tumor is more than 2 cm in diameter, invasion is deeper than 5 mm, and ipsilateral lymph node metastasis is confirmed. In these cases, bilateral lymphadenectomy is essential [19]. Full inguinal lymphadenectomy is also essential as previously mentioned in Sect. 28.2.3.

28.2.5 Reconstructive Surgery for Vulvar Cancer

Radical vulvectomy often requires the sacrifice of large amount of skin and vagina. It may be impossible to cover the defect by merely mobilizing the edges of the remaining skin. In those cases, the surgeon does not hesitate to use the skin or myocutaneous flaps swung across from the region of surrounding area for primary closure. The choice of donor site depends on the site and size of the defect (Fig. 28.13). Although most of the plastic surgery may be accomplished by collaboration with the plastic surgeon, gynecologic oncologist should be prepared for local reconstruction such as Z-plasty and rhomboid flap. Rhomboid flap is an easy procedure for a

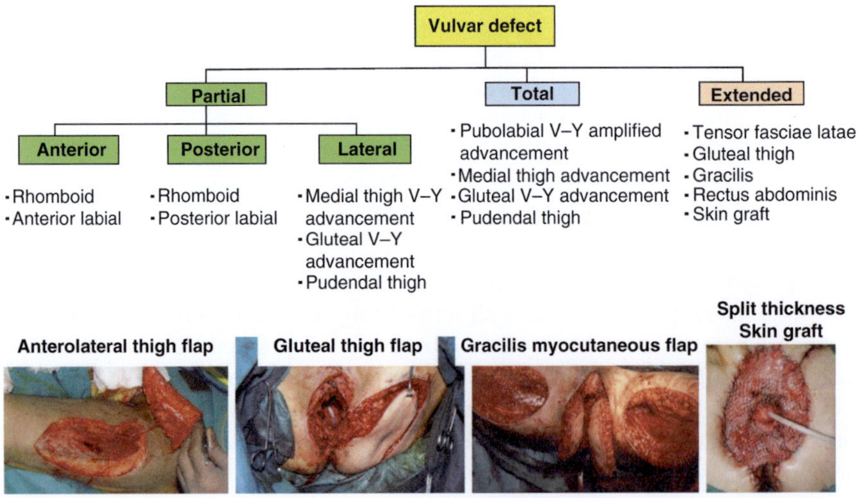

Fig. 28.13 Classification and types of reconstructive surgery applied for vulvar cancer surgery

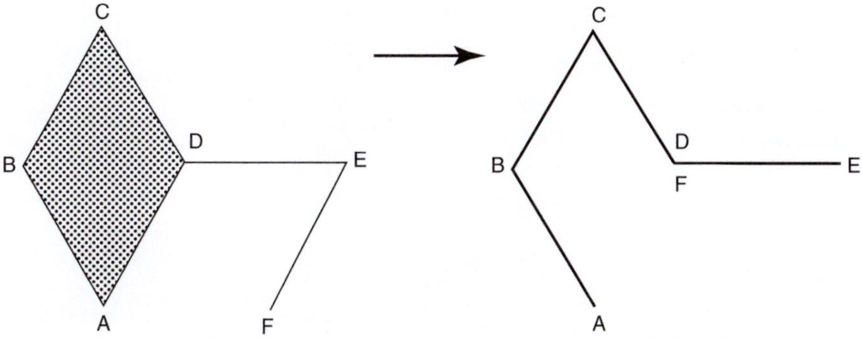

Fig. 28.14 Design of rhomboid flap. Dark area is a defect to be covered. Note the point F being moved to point D and the whole line sutured

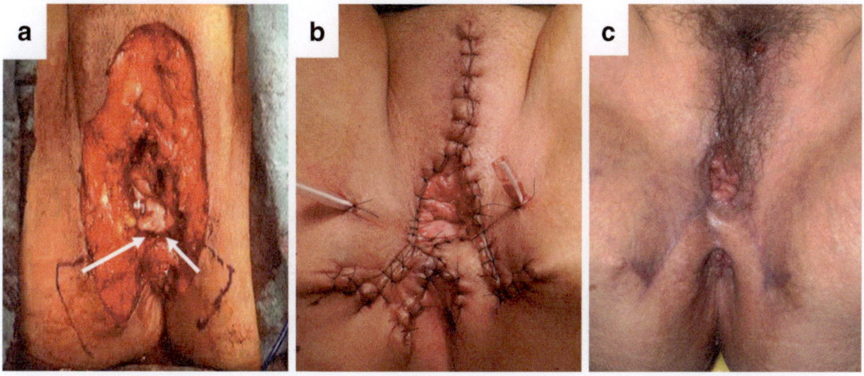

Fig. 28.15 An example of rhomboid flap. (**a**) A vulvectomy wound with a large defect in perineum, which is planned to be covered with bilateral rhomboid flaps. The mark of design is made on the skin. White arrows show the direction of transposition of the flaps. (**b**) Bilateral rhomboid flaps to cover the defect to make new perineum between the vagina and anus. (**c**) Healed wound. Note the good appearance of reconstructed perineum

gynecologist to apply for closure of vulvar defect (Fig. 28.14). It should be planned before surgery what kind of reconstructive procedure is used for primary closure of the defect. Examples of rhomboid flap (Fig. 28.15) and V-Y advancement flap (Fig. 28.16) are shown in the figures.

28.2.6 Postoperative Management and Complications

Most of the patients with vulvar cancer are elderly and frequently associated with medical complications. Postoperative care is of great importance in general management and wound management. Prophylactic antibiotic and suction drainage are the key points for wound healing.

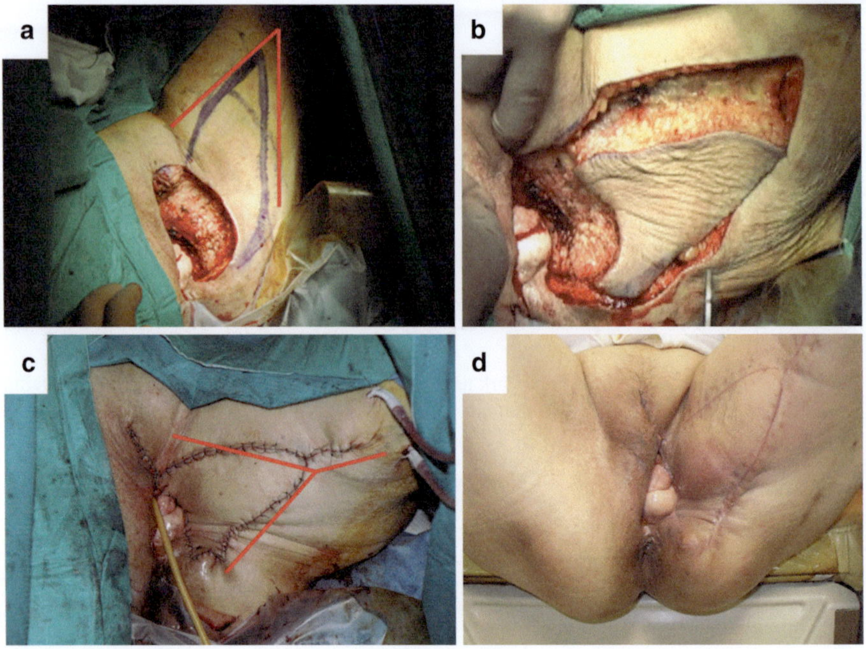

Fig. 28.16 An example of V-Y advancement flap for the irradiated vulvar wound closure. (**a**) A large defect is planned for primary closure using V-shaped flap of adjacent medial thigh. Red line shows the V-shaped flap. (**b**) The skin, subdermal tissue, and fascia of V flap outline are incised to be mobilized toward medial wound. (**c**) Advancement of V-shaped flap and closure by Y-shaped sutures. Red line shows the Y-shaped sutures. (**d**) Appearance of the reconstructed vulva 3 months after surgery

Complications after the radical vulvectomy may result from the procedure itself, from the lymph node dissection, or from the vulvectomy. The most common complications are wound dehiscence and necrosis of the suprapubic or vulvar wound. This complication is attributable to excess undermining of the skin at groin dissection and too much tension at the primary closure of the wound. The second common complication is infection usually accompanied with wound necrosis. Wound dehiscence and infection should be managed by good wound bed preparation. Daily surveillance and debridement of the necrotic tissue is mandatory waiting for healthy granulation elevated from the wound bed. Postoperative hemorrhage and hematoma are also common as in other surgeries. An important delayed complication is due to disturbance of lymph circulation. Lymphocele usually occurs just after removing the suction drainage. Prolonged suction drainage of lymph fluid may reduce the complications. Lymphedema of the lower extremities and pubis is a troublesome complication for a patient reducing her QOL. There's no cure for lymphedema. But it can be managed with early diagnosis and diligent care of the affected limb by using compression garments and compression stockings.

28.3 Surgery of Vaginal Cancer

Fifty-six percent of vaginal cancers have the tumor in the upper one-third of the vagina, and about half of those are located in the posterior wall. If a tumor extends to the middle or lower third of the vagina, it will probably require pelvic exenteration or vulvectomy to remove it completely. Because of the significant reduction in QOL with such an extensive procedure, physicians tend to select radiation therapy. In the case of a stage I or stage II tumor in the upper vagina, a radical or modified radical hysterectomy is often selected, in combination with vaginectomy with sufficient margin, as is the practice with cervical cancer.

In an analysis of 4885 cases of primary vaginal cancer conducted by the US National Cancer Database, the 5-year survival rate was found to be 90% for surgical therapy and 63% for radiation therapy in stage I. In stage II, the figures were 70% and 57%, respectively. These figures indicate a much better trend for surgical therapy than for radiation therapy with probable selection bias [20].

Surgical therapy may consist of vaginectomy preserving a sufficient excision margin, radical hysterectomy and pelvic lymphadenectomy. Curative surgery for a tumor in the lower third of the vagina must be combined with inguinal lymphadenectomy. Postoperatively, if risk factors such as a positive stump or lymph node metastasis are present, radiation therapy is recommended as an adjuvant therapy [21, 22].

When vaginal cancer is discovered after a hysterectomy, surgical therapy may also be considered if the tumor is localized in the vaginal wall. Partial vaginectomy is conducted for CIS. For invasive carcinoma in the upper third of the vagina, a vaginectomy including paracolpium, combined with a pelvic lymphadenectomy, is recommended [21].

Extended surgery such as pelvic exenteration may be considered if the patient has the invasive tumor to the rectum or urinary bladder, a rectovaginal or vesicovaginal fistula, or local recurrent tumors after radiation therapy [21] (Fig. 28.17). According to a report by the US National Cancer Database, the 5-year survival rate in stages III and IV is 47% for surgical therapy alone and 35% for radiation therapy alone. However, the 5-year survival rate rises to 60% when surgical and radiation therapies are combined, indicating a favorable trend when surgery is added [20]. There should be a selection bias not to do surgery for cases with tumors extending to the pelvic wall and to select radiation therapy for highly invasive cases. Consequently surgery may be performed only for the cases with the prognosis tending to be better.

28.4 Future Prospect

Most of vulvar and vaginal cancer is caused by human papilloma virus (HPV) infection. In the future, the incidence of these diseases would be drastically decreased by the widespread of HPV vaccination, hoping surgery to be unnecessary for these

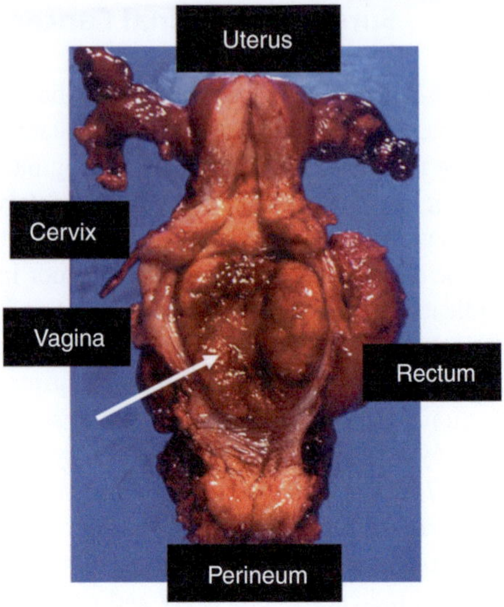

Fig. 28.17 Resected specimen of posterior exenteration for the vaginal cancer. Resected specimen showed a large vaginal tumor occupying the upper and middle of the vagina. White arrow indicates the vaginal tumor

tumors. Until the time comes, efforts should be paid for the development of new strategy for these tumors.

Vulvar cancer surgery drastically changed in the past two decades with individualization and minimization of the surgery. However, there are few prospective studies for the treatment of relatively rare tumor, vulvar cancer and vaginal cancer. Multi-institutional collaborated studies are therefore warranted to establish new surgical treatments.

References

1. Hacker NF. Revised FIGO staging for carcinoma of the vulva. Int J Gynaecol Obstet. 2009;105:105–6.
2. Taussig FJ. Cancer of the vulva: an Analysis of 155 cases. Am J Obstet Gynecol. 1940;40:764–79.
3. Way S. Carcinoma of the vulva. Am J Obstet Gynecol. 1960;79:692–7.
4. Podratz KC, Symmonds RE, Taylor WF, Williams TJ. Carcinoma of the vulva: analysis of treatment and survival. Obstet Gynecol. 1983;61:63–74.
5. Hacker NF, Leuchter RS, Berek JS, Castaldo TW, Lagasse LD. Radical vulvectomy and bilateral inguinal lymphadenectomy through separate groin incisions. Obstet Gynaecol. 1981;58:574–9.
6. Saito T, Kato K. Management of lymph nodes in the treatment of vulvar cancer. Int J Clin Oncol. 2007;12:187–91.
7. Tjalma WA, Monaghan JM, de Barros Lopes A, Naik R, Nordin AJ, Weyler JJ. The role of surgery in invasive squamous carcinoma of the vagina. Gynecol Oncol. 2001;81:360–5.
8. Byron S, Lamb E, Yonemoto R, Kase S. Radical inguinal node dissection in the treatment of cancer. Surg Gynecol Obstet. 1962;114:401–8.
9. Grimshaw RN, Murdoch JB, Monaghan JM. Radical vulvectomy and bilateral inguinal-femoral lymphadenectomy through separate incisions—experience with 100 cases. Int J Gynecol Cancer. 1993;3:18–23.

10. Siller BS, Alvarez RD, Conner WD, McCullough CH, Kilgore LC, Partridge EE, et al. T2/3 vulva cancer: a case-control study of triple incision versus en bloc radical vulvectomy and inguinal lymphadenectomy. Gynecol Oncol. 1995;57:335–9.
11. Helm CW, Hatch K, Austin JM, Partridge EE, Soong SJ, Elder JE, et al. A matched comparison of single and triple incision techniques for the surgical treatment of carcinoma of the vulva. Gynecol Oncol. 1992;46:150–6.
12. De Hullu JA, Hollema H, Lolkema S, Boezen M, Boonstra H, Burger MP, et al. Vulvar carcinoma. The price of less radical surgery. Cancer. 2002;95:2331–8.
13. Burke TW, Stringer CA, Gershenson DM, Edwards CL, Morris M, Wharton JT. Radical wide excision and selective inguinal node dissection for squamous cell carcinoma of the vulva. Gynecol Oncol. 1990;38:328–32.
14. de Hullu JA, van der Avoort IA, Oonk MH, van der Zee AG. Management of vulvar cancers. Eur J Surg Oncol. 2006;32:825–31.
15. Stehman FB, Bundy BN, Dvoretsky PM, Creasman WT. Early stage I carcinoma of the vulva treated with ipsilateral superficial inguinal lymphadenectomy and modified radical hemivulvectomy: a prospective study of the Gynecologic Oncology Group. Obstet Gynecol. 1992;79:490–7.
16. Farias-Eisner R, Cirisano FD, Grouse D, Leuchter RS, Karlan BY, Lagasse LD, et al. Conservative and individualized surgery for early squamous carcinoma of the vulva: the treatment of choice for stage I and II (T1—2 N0—1 M0) disease. Gynecol Oncol. 1994;53:55–8.
17. Burke TW, Levenback C, Coleman RL, Morris M, Silva EG, Gershenson DM. Surgical therapy of T1 and T2 vulvar carcinoma: further experience with radical wide excision and selective inguinal lymphadenectomy. Gynecol Oncol. 1995;57:215–20.
18. Arvas M, Köse F, Gezer A, Demirkiran F, Tulunay G, Kösebay D. Radical versus conservative surgery for vulvar carcinoma. Int J Gynaecol Obstet. 2005;88:127–33.
19. Gonzalez Bosquet J, Magrina JF, Magtibay PM, Gaffey TA, Cha SS, Jones MB, et al. Patterns of inguinal groin metastases in squamous cell carcinoma of the vulva. Gynecol Oncol. 2007;105:742–6.
20. Creasman WT, Phillips JL, Menck HR. The National Cancer Data Base report on cancer of the vagina. Cancer. 1998;83:1033–40.
21. Hacker NF, Eifel PJ, van der Velden J. Cancer of the vagina. Int J Gynaecol Obstet. 2012;119(Suppl 2):S97–9.
22. Tabata T, Takeshima N, Nishida H, Hirai Y, Hasumi K. Treatment failure in vaginal cancer. Gynecol Oncol. 2002;84:309–14.

MIX
Papier aus verantwortungsvollen Quellen
Paper from responsible sources
FSC® C105338

If you have any concerns about our products,
you can contact us on
ProductSafety@springernature.com

In case Publisher is established outside the EU,
the EU authorized representative is:
Springer Nature Customer Service Center GmbH
Europaplatz 3, 69115 Heidelberg, Germany

Printed by Libri Plureos GmbH
in Hamburg, Germany